A Davidson Title

Davidson's
Foundations of
Clinical Practice

Acknowledgements

The following figures are reproduced from Boon et al. 2006 *Davidson's Principles and Practice of Medicine*, 20th edn. Churchill Livingstone, Edinburgh, with permission: Fig. 2.2, Fig. 3.3a, Fig. 3.3b, Fig. 3.4, Fig. 3.5, Fig. 3.6, Fig. 3.7, Fig. 3.8, Fig. 3.9, Fig. 3.10, Fig. 3.11, Fig. 3.12a, Fig. 3.12b, Fig. 3.13, Fig. 7.1, Fig. 10.1, Fig. 10.2 and Fig. 10.3.

Commissioning Editor: Laurence Hunter
Senior Development Editor: Ailsa Laing
Project Manager: Alan Nicholson
Design Direction: Stewart Larking
Illustration Manager: Merlyn Harvey
Illustrator: Graeme Chambers

A Davidson Title

Davidson's Foundations of Clinical Practice

Edited by

Hazel R. Scott MD FRCP
Associate Dean of Postgraduate Medicine,
West of Scotland Deanery, Glasgow;
Director of Medical Education and Consultant
Respiratory Physician,
NHS Lanarkshire, Wishaw, UK

Kevin G. Blyth MD MRCP
Specialist Registrar in Respiratory and General
Medicine, West of Scotland Rotation, UK

Jeremy B. Jones MBChB MRCP
Radiology Registrar,
West Yorkshire Radiology Academy, Leeds, UK

CHURCHILL LIVINGSTONE

ELSEVIER

Edinburgh London New York Oxford Philadelphia St Louis Sydney Toronto 2009

CHURCHILL
LIVINGSTONE
ELSEVIER

ISBN: 978-0-443-06829-4

British Library Cataloguing in Publication Data
A catalogue record for this book is available from the British Library

Library of Congress Cataloging in Publication Data
A catalog record for this book is available from the Library of Congress

Notice
Knowledge and best practice in this field are constantly changing. As new research and experience broaden our knowledge, changes in practice, treatment and drug therapy may become necessary or appropriate. Readers are advised to check the most current information provided (i) on procedures featured or (ii) by the manufacturer of each product to be administered, to verify the recommended dose or formula, the method and duration of administration, and contraindications. It is the responsibility of the practitioner, relying on their own experience and knowledge of the patient, to make diagnoses, to determine dosages and the best treatment for each individual patient, and to take all appropriate safety precautions. To the fullest extent of the law, neither the Publisher nor the Editors assume any liability for any injury and/or damage to persons or property arising out of or related to any use of the material contained in this book.

The Publisher

Printed in China

Preface

It is the first day on the new job and there are many questions...

- What can I remember from University?
- What should I have noted from shadowing or induction?
- What will my Supervisor ask during my assessment?
- And most of all... What am I going to do for the man who has collapsed on the ward?

This book is the answer to questions you may wish you had paid more attention to before. The content is designed as a companion to the initial years of hospital training for doctors in the UK, including, but not limited to, the core elements of the curriculum for Foundation Training.

Patients have co-morbidity and mixed patterns of clinical presentation. In addition, referrals are regularly made between clinical disciplines and the doctors involved need some understanding of the other conditions affecting the patient that they have been called to see.

Therefore, the book brings into one volume key guidance on the presentation and care of patients attending a wide range of disciplines. These appear in the book as they present in real life, according to symptoms. Given the balance of the type of work done by most trainee hospital doctors, the emphasis of the book is on acute, as compared with chronic, symptom presentation and management.

In addition, there is practical step-by-step guidance on a range of core clinical procedures, as well as insight and information not otherwise readily available, on the non-clinical aspects of a clinical career.

The book is written, often by trainees, for trainees. The practical experience of working as a trainee hospital doctor today is blended with senior understanding of conditions and clinical careers.

It is a bag-book, not a pocket-book. This is intentional. You will not wear a white coat with a pocket. You will not want to be seen looking everything up. After the first week, you will need more than scant notes to follow. You will find it useful in the ward office, on-call room, clinic...

With best wishes for your future career.

Hazel R. Scott
2009

Contributors

Helen P. Barclay MRPharmS MSc BSc
Principal Clinical Pharmacist,
Wishaw General Hospital,
Wishaw, UK

Andrew Docherty MBChB PhD FRCP(Glas)
Consultant Cardiologist,
Wishaw General Hospital,
Wishaw, UK

Ian R. Gunn BMSc MBChB FRCPath
Consultant Clinical Biochemist,
Wishaw General Hospital,
Wishaw, UK

Ian Hunter MBChB MRCPCH
Consultant Paediatrician,
Wishaw General Hospital,
Wishaw, UK

Nicholas Kennedy
MD FRCP(Edin) FRCP(Glas) DTM&H
Consultant and Honorary Senior
Lecturer in Infectious Diseases,
Monklands Hospital,
Airdrie, UK

John Paul Leach MD FRCP
Consultant Neurologist,
Institute of Neurological Sciences,
Southern General Hospital,
Glasgow, UK

Graham MacKay
MBChB MRCS MD
Specialist Registrar,
West of Scotland Surgical
Rotation, UK

Alasdair M.J. MacLullich
PhD BSc(Hons) MBChB MRCP(UK)
Professor of Geriatric Medicine,
University of Edinburgh,
Royal Infirmary of Edinburgh,
Edinburgh, UK

K. Donogh Maguire
FRCS(Edin) MRCPI FCEM
Emergency Medicine Consultant,
Monklands Hospital, Airdrie, UK

David M. Matthews (deceased)
BSc(Med Sci) MBChB FRCP(Edin) FRCP(Glas)
Former Consultant Physician,
Monklands Hospital,
Airdrie, UK

Norma C. McAvoy MBChB MRCP
Clinical Lecturer in Hepatology,
Royal Infirmary of Edinburgh,
Edinburgh, UK

Matthew McKernan MBChB MRCOG
Specialist Registrar in Obstetrics
and Gynaecology,
Antrim Area Hospital,
Northern Ireland, UK

Dina McLellan MBChB MRCOG
Consultant Obstetrician
and Gynaecologist,
Wishaw General Hospital,
Wishaw, UK

Elizabeth A. Murphy
BSc MBChB FRCP(Glas)
Consultant Rheumatologist,
Wishaw General Hospital,
Wishaw, UK

John A. Murphy
BSc FRCP(Glas) FRCPath
Consultant Haematologist,
Monklands Hospital,
Airdrie, UK

Gerard L. Picozzi MBChB FRCS
Consultant Ear Nose and
Throat Surgeon,
Wishaw General Hospital,
Wishaw, UK

Susan R. Reid
MBChB FRCP FRCR
Consultant Radiologist,
Wishaw General Hospital,
Wishaw, UK

Roshini Sanders
MBchB DO FRCS FRCOphth
Consultant Ophthalmologist,
Queen Margaret Hospital,
Dunfermline, UK

Freida C.G. Shaffrali
BSc MBBS MSc FRCP(Glas)
Consultant Dermatologist,
Monklands Hospital,
Airdrie, UK

Ilona Shilliday MD MBChB MRCP
Consultant Nephrologist,
Monklands Hospital,
Airdrie, UK

Fiona Sykes BA PGDipCG
Careers Consultant,
Glasgow, UK

Calum J. Thomson BSc RMN RGN
Honorary Lecturer,
Glasgow University School
of Medicine
Clinical Skills Development
Specialist for Medical Education,
Wishaw General Hospital,
Wishaw, UK

Alok Tyagi MBBS MD DNB DM FRCP(Edin)
Consultant Neurologist and
Honorary Senior Lecturer,
Institute of Neurological Sciences,
Southern General Hospital,
Glasgow, UK

Prem Venkatesh MBBS DO FRCSEd(Ophth)
Locum Consultant Ophthalmologist,
Tennent Institute of Ophthalmology,
Gartnavel General Hospital,
Glasgow, UK

Lawrence Walker MD FRCS FRCPS(Glas)Urol
Consultant Urologist, Monklands
Hospital, Airdrie, UK

Contents

SECTION 1

Basic principles of patient care

Initial assessment and emergency management

1

GENERAL HISTORY AND EXAMINATION

History taking and clinical examination form the basis of all clinical assessments. The history enables a short list of differential diagnoses to be generated. Evidence from clinical examination can be used to refine this.

History taking

All clinicians use the same basic history taking template; however, flexibility is essential: be prepared to modify your approach depending on the clinical situation, the patient's concerns or fears and their level of education and understanding.

History of the presenting complaint

This is the most conversational component of the medical history and it is relatively easy to lose focus or drift off into unrelated areas. Therefore, you need to structure the interview in a way that allows you to extract the relevant information, while remaining relaxed and polite. Never lose your temper with a so-called bad historian; good history takers can get the important points of the story from any patient. Use the following routine:

- correctly identify your patient, checking their name, address, date of birth and who referred them
- start with 'open' questions like 'What has happened over the last few days?' or 'When did you last feel well?'
- listen during this first part of the consultation and let the patient talk
- form a differential diagnosis based upon the patient's original description
- during the next part of the history, use 'closed' or direct questions to focus upon the important points and narrow your list of differential diagnoses based on associated features, speed of onset, duration, previous episodes, etc.
- the duration and speed of onset of the patient's symptoms are particularly important, e.g. if a focal neurological defect develops over the course of a few minutes, this could be due to an acute vascular event; if it develops over a number of days there may be infection or demyelination, while a defect that develops over months could suggest an underlying tumour or subdural haemorrhage

- avoid asking more than one question at once, e.g. 'Have you had pain or breathlessness?' should be, 'Have you had any pain?' followed by 'Have you been breathless?'
- throughout the interview, be careful to use language that the patient will understand and avoid medical terminology
- finally, ask if the patient has any worries or concerns: fear and preconceptions often colour the interpretation of symptoms and are always important features of the history.

Systemic enquiry

A few further screening questions are sufficient to identify any areas worthy of additional focus:

- *cardiovascular*: chest pain, palpitations, breathlessness, orthopnoea, oedema
- *respiratory*: breathlessness, cough, sputum, haemoptysis, chest pain
- *GI*: abdominal pain or swelling, bowel habit and bleeding, vomiting, swallowing problems
- *GU*: dysuria, frequency, urgency, haematuria
- *neurological symptoms*: headache, weakness or altered sensation, fits, falls and funny turns, change vision, hearing or speech (see Table 1.1)
- *systemic*: anorexia, weight loss, fever, night sweats, fatigue, sore or stiff joints, itch or rash.

Past medical history

Enquire about the following common illnesses, remembering that patients often employ informal labels (given in parentheses): asthma, COPD (bronchitis, emphysema), ischaemic heart disease (angina), myocardial infarction (heart attack), cardiac failure (fluid on the lung), diabetes mellitus, previous pulmonary TB, previous surgery, previous admissions especially to the intensive care unit (ICU), stroke, epilepsy (fits), hypertension (high blood pressure), hypercholesterolaemia, venous thromboembolism (thrombosis or clots), previous rheumatic fever or significant childhood illnesses.

Drug history

Accurate doses, including the timing of administration, are essential, especially for insulin regimes and patients taking warfarin, along with details of the specific formulation taken, e.g. the type of insulin and the device used; types of inhaler.

Table 1.1 Patterns of speech abnormality in neurological disease

Defect	Description	Cause
Receptive dysphasia	Difficulty in comprehension	Lesion in the dominant cerebellar hemisphere, commonly due to CVA in older patients or trauma in younger patients
Expressive dysphasia	Difficulty in word selection, may be isolated to the naming of objects (nominal) or people	
Dysarthria	Difficulty with the motor execution of speech	Slurred, staccato or scanning speech suggests cerebellar disease, e.g. MS. Slurred speech and a weak voice suggests pseudobulbar palsy (e.g. due to CVA)

If the patient is on a lot of medications, ask if they have an up-to-date repeat prescription with them.

Make specific note of drug allergies. Ask what the patient means by 'allergy': feeling sick or diarrhoea is often mislabelled as such.

In patients with lung disease, check if they are prescribed inhalers and that they know how to use them. Also ask if they are on long-term oxygen therapy (marker of disease severity). Check if the patient is on long-term oral theophylline or phenytoin; if so, you will need to measure a drug level before prescribing any additional IV treatment.

Family history

Enquire about conditions affecting family members, e.g. asthma, ischaemic heart disease, stroke, malignancy, diabetes.

Social history

This is an essential and often overlooked component of the history, especially in older or disabled patients. Accurately document home circumstances, e.g. living alone; independent at home but has social support; residential or nursing home resident. If the patient receives support at home, quantify this in terms of visits per day and the support provided. Ask if the patient has family nearby and if they see them.

Determine the patient's functional capacity and whether they are able to perform the activities of daily living (ADLs), e.g. leaving the house, doing the shopping, housework or cooking. This information allows the setting of realistic discharge goals and is useful when considering treatment escalation or referral to intensive care. Ask about quality of life (QoL). *Remember* that this should be recorded as the patient describes it, not how you judge it; see 'Performance status and quality of life', p. 349.

Ask about recreational drug use. Document cigarette use by current and ex-smokers in pack-years and alcohol consumption in units per week:

- One pack-year equates to a pack of 20 cigarettes per day for a year: someone who has smoked 10-a-day for 50 years has a 25 pack-year history.
- One small glass of wine or one 25 mL measure of spirits is roughly equivalent to 1 unit; 1 pint of ordinary strength lager, beer or cider roughly equates to 2 units; recommended safe limits of alcohol per week for males and females are 21 and 28 units, respectively.

Psychiatric history

Formal psychiatric assessment should be performed in specialist units; however, psychiatric illnesses commonly present to other departments where they should be properly assessed and referred to psychiatry, as appropriate. A detailed history is essential and must include the following (in addition to a standard medical history):

- educational background, religion and occupation, as these may influence interview technique and general approach
- reason and source of referral (self-presentation indicates insight)
- history of the presenting complaint: enquire about the patient's symptoms in their own words, including their effect upon normal function (e.g. work, family, relationships), date of onset, rate of progression and any precipitants identified by the patient
- previous treatments, including drugs, surgery and others, e.g. cognitive behavioural therapy, electro-convulsive therapy
- suicidal ideation.

Personal history should be taken in detail, including:

- childhood problems including parental separation and any history of abuse
- relationships and marital history
- work history, including current level of satisfaction at work and reasons for leaving previous jobs

- illegal activities and any history of violence
- premorbid personality, e.g. anxious, obsessive, solitary
- cognitive assessment should be performed (cognitive dysfunction suggests organic rather than functional pathology)
- abbreviated mental test (AMT) score or the mini-mental state examination (MMSE); see Tables 1.2 and 1.3, respectively
- acute (delirium) and chronic (dementia) cognitive impairment should be distinguished by discussion with family members or social contacts.

Table 1.2 Abbreviated mental test score

Question	Score
What is your age?	1 if correct
What is your date of birth?	1 if complete
What year is it?	1 for exact year
What time of day is it?	1 if correct to nearest hour
What is this place?	1 if correct, e.g. name of hospital or address
Recall a 3-line address (later in consultation)	1 if correctly and completely recalled
Who is the current monarch?	1 if correct
What year was World War I?	1 for either 1914 or 1918
Count backwards from 20 to 1	1 if no mistakes, or corrects without prompting
Can you identify these two people?	1 for both names if known, or both jobs if not

Total score is recorded out of 10; a score <7 suggests cognitive dysfunction.

Table 1.3 Mini-mental state examination

Test	Questions	Maximum score[a]
Time	Day, date, month, season, year	5
Place	County, country, town/city, building, floor	5
Registration	Name 3 objects, e.g. bed, table, book	3
Attention and concentration	Spell 'world' backwards or count out five serial 7s	5
Naming	Show 2 objects	2
Recall	Ask to recall the 3 objects registered earlier	3
Repeating	Repeat 'no ifs, ands or buts': only correct if word perfect	1
3-stage task	Instruct the patient to (1) take this paper in your right hand, (2) fold it in half and (3) drop it on the floor	3
Reading	Write 'close your eyes'; ask the patient to read and obey	1
Writing	Write a sentence: must be complete and grammatically correct	1
Construction	Draw interlocking pentagons	1

[a] Total score recorded out of 30; <23 suggests cognitive impairment.

Recording the history

Many hospitals now provide an admission pack, which includes a history taking proforma for all new admissions. These documents often form part of a unified case record (UCR) or integrated care pathway (ICP). While these tools are useful, there is a danger that they encourage a highly protocolized, 'tick-box' approach to history taking. Take time to work beyond the boxes and fully explore what the patient is trying to tell you.

When recording the history of the presenting complaint, include the main problem and mode of referral. This should be followed by a short paragraph that covers the relevant additional positive or negative points from the history with regard to this presenting problem, e.g. onset, duration, precipitating and relieving factors, previous similar events, as well as relevant admissions or outpatient attendances.

Examination

The guidance given here is necessarily brief. For more detail see *Macleod's Clinical Examination*.

Consider whether you need a chaperone and ensure that the patient's need for privacy is met. Ask for permission to examine them and check if there is any area that is sore to touch. Ensure that the patient is comfortable and in the correct body position for the system you aim to assess:

- *cardiovascular and respiratory*: 45° semi-recumbent
- *abdominal*: lying supine
- *neurological*: semi-recumbent position in bed or sitting in chair, depending on the particular examination performed.

Begin with a general examination, then follow the principles of inspection, palpation, percussion and auscultation as you work through the relevant body systems. Table 1.4 (*overleaf*) highlights important signs to look for during your examination of each body system (the nervous system is addressed separately). Note that when palpating, you should start with the least painful side first and work slowly towards the site of worst pain.

Neurological examination

A flexible approach is essential, especially in patients with receptive dysphasia or cognitive impairment. A working knowledge of basic neuroanatomy is helpful in allowing you to interpret your clinical findings.

A simple neurological examination scheme is summarized below. The order of the tests performed will vary depending on the clinical situation, but should include assessment of cranial nerve function, the motor and sensory components of cerebral function, and cerebellar function.

Inspection

Note any abnormality of resting limb position (contracture or palsy), involuntary movements (seizure activity, tremor and chorea), muscle wasting, fasciculation and gait.

Cranial nerves

Examine cranial nerves II–XII; see Table 1.5. Cranial nerve I (olfactory nerve) is not routinely assessed.

Motor examination

For motor examination, assess tone, power and reflexes, starting proximally and moving distally; compare right with left. Give the patient clear instructions when examining power. It is important to distinguish between upper and lower motor neurone weakness; see Focal neurology, p. 226.

Table 1.4 System examination aid

	Cardiovascular	Respiratory	Abdomen
Hands	Clubbing, temperature of peripheries, pulse rate, rhythm, character		
	Nicotine staining		Palmar erythema Liver flap Leuconychia
	Splinters Capillary refill	Interosseous wasting CO_2 flap	
Face	Conjunctival pallor or suffusion		
	Corneal arcus Xanthelasma Malar flush	Central cyanosis Horner's syndrome	Sclerae (jaundice) Aphthous ulceration Fetor
Neck	Jugular venous pressure		
	Carotid pulsation	Lymphadenopathy	
		Trachea Accessory muscles	Spider naevi
Torso	Scars		
	Thrills and heaves Heart sounds Murmur Radiation Accentuation Radiofemoral delay	Chest expansion Percussion note Breath sounds ± added vocal resonance	Palpation Tenderness or masses Organomegaly/ascites Bowel sounds/bruits Gynaecomastia Caput medusa Inguinal nodes
Additional areas	Pedal oedema		
	Listen at lung bases	Sputum pot	PR exam Genitalia

Table 1.5 Cranial nerves

Cranial nerve	Tests routinely performed
II (Optic)	Acuity, pupillary reflexes (ipsi- and contralateral), visual fields
III (Oculomotor)	Considered together: ocular movements
IV (Trochlear)	
VI (Abducent)	
V (Trigeminal)	Ophthalmic (V_1), maxillary (V_2) and mandibular (V_3) sensory branches; motor function (masseter muscle) rarely tested
VII (Facial)	Five sensory branches (raise eyebrows, close eyes tight, show teeth, puff out cheeks and whistle); taste rarely tested
VIII (Vestibulocochlear)	Rarely tested; hearing deficits best assessed by audiometry
IX (Glossopharyngeal)	Considered together: gag reflex (IX afferent, X efferent); movement of the soft palate (uvula)
X (Vagus)	
XI (Accessory)	Shrug shoulders and resist: rotate head to one side against resistance to test the contralateral sternomastoid muscle
XII (Hypoglossal)	Ask patient to protrude tongue, look for wasting asymmetry and fasciculation

- *tone*: 'normotonia' varies; if hypertonia is genuine, check whether symmetrical or generalized; look for cog-wheeling or associated clonus (hard clinical sign if sustained)
- *power*: grade 0–5, e.g. MRC scale; compare right with left testing individual muscle groups (shoulder, elbow, wrist, fingers, hip, knee and ankle); it is often better to ask the patient to resist you moving their limb than to move it in a certain direction, e.g. when assessing triceps and biceps 'Bend your arms like this and keep them there'
- *reflexes*: strike the tendon, not the muscle; test biceps, triceps, supinator, knee and ankle jerks; an extensor plantar indicates a pyramidal tract lesion; if there is no response, consider using a distraction manoeuvre at the time of striking the tendon, e.g. ask the patient to pull apart inversely clasped hands.

Sensory examination

Sensory examination involves an assessment of pain, light touch, proprioception and vibration sense. Assess pain using a Neurotip® (spinothalamic tract) and light touch using a cotton ball (dorsal columns). Determine whether any abnormality is symmetrical or isolated, whether it corresponds to a particular area on the dermatome map (Fig. 1.1) or is suggestive of a sensory level (spinal cord lesion). Proprioception and vibration sense should be assessed at the distal joints first, moving proximally if an abnormality is detected.

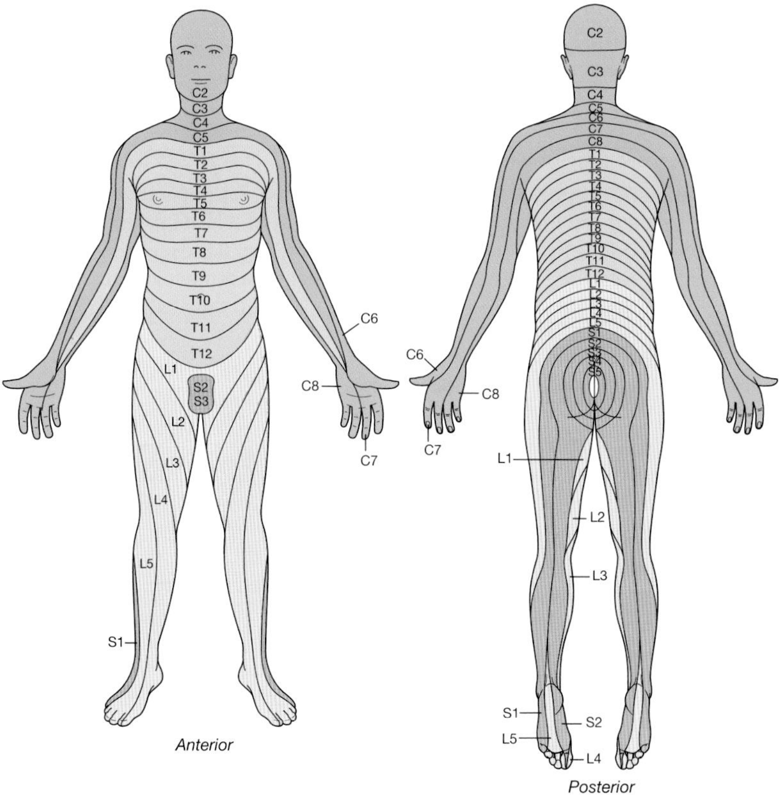

Figure 1.1 Dermatomes.

Cerebellar function

The cerebellum has an important role in the coordination of movement:

- perform the finger–nose test looking for ataxia, past pointing and intention tremor (tremor on approach to the finger); heel–shin test should be performed in lower limb examination
- test rapid alternating movements (dysdiadochokinesis)
- compare right with left
- remember that these tests are unreliable if the limb is weak
- look for nystagmus: horizontal nystagmus suggests cerebellar disease with the fast phase towards the affected side
- assess speech: disjointed and explosive (staccato) speech.

ASSESSMENT OF THE ACUTELY ILL PATIENT

It is vital that the assessment of the acutely ill patient is carried out in a logical and expeditious manner. On arriving at the scene, first check that it is safe to assess and treat the patient on site. This is particularly important in an out-of-hospital environment. Then proceed according to the ABCDE acronym (Airway, Breathing, Circulation, Disability, Exposure).

Airway

Partial airway obstruction may present as stridor, gurgling or wheeze, while a silent chest may indicate complete airway obstruction. Airway compromise is common in acutely ill patients and may be due to:

- CNS depression
- upper airway secretions, blood or vomit
- disruption of upper airway anatomy by trauma
- foreign body
- pharyngeal swelling or laryngospasm.

If the patient's airway appears threatened or unprotected, it is imperative that airway patency be restored and maintained. Inspect the airway; if it is not patent or likely to be compromised in the near future, proceed as outlined in 'Basic life support', p. 12. Remember to protect the cervical spine in any patient with traumatic injuries.

Breathing

While keeping the airway open, look, listen and feel for evidence of spontaneous respiration.

- if the patient is not breathing, put out an arrest call and check whether a cardiac output is present; see 'Circulation' below
- if the patient is breathing, assess the rate and pattern of respiration, and note the extent and symmetry of any chest wall movement; listen to the chest.

High flow oxygen (60–100%) by trauma mask should be given to all critically ill patients pending urgent arterial blood gas results; these results are particularly important in patients with previous type 2 respiratory failure, e.g. COPD. Proximal, upper airway secretions should be removed using a Yanker suction catheter.

Circulation

Impalpable pulse

If the radial pulse is absent, check a more proximal artery, e.g. femoral, carotid; if you still cannot feel a pulse, put out an arrest call and start cardiopulmonary resuscitation (CPR), p. 13.

Palpable pulse

- immediately attach a cardiac monitor, measure the blood pressure, heart rate and rhythm
- look for evidence of poor peripheral perfusion (pallor, cool cyanosed peripheries, a prolonged capillary refill time); prompt treatment of shock is essential; insert at least 2 wide-bore cannulae and start a rapid IV infusion; take routine bloods, including a cross-match and cultures, and follow the guidance given in 'Shock', p. 250
- listen to the heart, perform a 12-lead ECG, identify and treat any arrhythmia; see p. 132
- check for evidence of haemorrhage; if present, this must be controlled following adequate resuscitation; if necessary, contact the relevant on-call surgical team.

Disability

Perform a rapid neurological evaluation of the patient. Quantify the level of consciousness using the Glasgow Coma Scale (GCS); see p. 11. Assess pupillary size, symmetry and responses. Look for any lateralizing neurological signs, or evidence of a spinal cord level.

Look for any reversible causes of neurological abnormality; check the blood glucose and the drug cardex.

Exposure

Expose the relevant parts of the body and examine the patient fully; always preserve the patient's dignity where possible and avoid hypothermia. Take a history, if possible, and ask nursing staff or other witnesses about recent events. Review the case-notes and observation charts: look for trends in pulse, blood pressure, respiratory rate and temperature.

Acute clinical scoring systems

Objective scoring systems are essential tools in identifying patients who are deteriorating clinically, in need of urgent treatment or referral to intensive care. They are also helpful in clinical research, allowing meaningful comparison between patients with varying types of clinical presentation.

Early warning systems

There is a clear correlation between markers of disease severity and subsequent in-hospital mortality. However, the identification of 'sick' patients is a largely subjective process, which is often performed poorly. Early warning systems combine several simple and measurable physiological variables, e.g. respiratory rate, to predict clinical worsening. These systems allow nursing and other staff objectively to assess and monitor ward-level patients, identifying those who need medical review, transfer to HDU/ICU or treatment escalation. The modified early warning score (MEWS) is a commonly used example in UK hospitals; see Table 1.6. Thresholds for action vary between 3 and 5, depending on local policy. Another commonly used example is the patient at risk (PAR) score.

Conscious level

Glasgow Coma Scale

The Glasgow Coma Scale (GCS) is an objective and universally comparable way of quantifying the conscious level of a patient. It can be used as a single point value or monitored over time, and combines scores assigned to three physiological responses: eye opening, verbal responsiveness and motor responsiveness; see Table 1.7.

Table 1.6 The modified early warning score (MEWS)

	Score						
	3	2	1	0	1	2	3
Systolic blood pressure (mmHg)	<70	71–80	81–100	101–199		≥200	
Heart rate		<40	41–50	51–100	101–110	111–129	≥130
Respiratory rate		≤9		8–14	15–20	21–29	≥30
Temperature (°C)		<35		35–38.4		≥38.5	
Urine output (mL/h for 2 h)	≤10	≤30					
AVPU			Confused	Alert	Reacting to voice	Reacting to pain	Unresponsive

Table 1.7 The Glasgow Coma Scale

	Eye opening	Verbal response	Motor response
1	None	None	None
2	To pain	Incomprehensible	Extension to pain
3	To speech	Inappropriate	Flexion to pain
4	Spontaneous	Confused	Withdraws from pain
5		Orientated	Localizes to pain
6			Obeys commands

The GCS was originally used to stratify immediate clinical risk in patients with head injuries. Of those with moderate (9–12) and severe (<9) scores, 63% and 85% respectively remain disabled at 1 year. It is now used in any condition associated with neurological sequelae and has been incorporated into other scoring systems, including APACHE (see below), and standard neurological observations.

AVPU

The AVPU score is an abbreviated scoring system for the assessment of consciousness. It assigns a letter (A, V, P or U) to the patient, depending on whether they are alert, responsive to verbal commands, responsive to pain or unresponsive, respectively. It is commonly used by ambulance crews and forms part of the MEWS; see above. However, it has less of an evidence base than the GCS and is not suitable for longitudinal neurological scoring.

Critical illness

APACHE

The acute physiology and chronic health evaluation (APACHE) scoring system is used to predict in-hospital mortality in patients admitted to ICU. APACHE IV is the most recent version and combines values assigned to acute physiology, age and chronic health. It is extremely accurate, but also complicated to define, and most ICUs use a computer programme for this purpose.

SOFA

The sequential organ failure score (SOFA) is an alternative critical care score that assesses the function of six different organ systems: respiratory, cardiovascular, renal, hepatic, neurological and haematological.

CARDIAC ARREST MANAGEMENT

The UK Resuscitation Council produces regularly updated, evidence-based treatment guidelines for the management of cardiac arrest. Any doctor working in an acute clinical environment should be fully acquainted with them and UK trainees must attend either Basic, Intermediate or Advanced Life Support (BLS, ILS or ALS) training as part of the requirements of their post. If you have not attended such a course, contact your local resuscitation officer who will advise on the appropriate level.

The chain of survival

Survival following cardiac arrest is dependent on four fundamental factors. Arranged chronologically, these are commonly referred to as links in the 'chain of survival':

- early recognition and immediate summoning of help
- early and effective BLS to maintain the perfusion of vital organ systems

- early defibrillation of shockable arrhythmias; see ALS below
- planned, organized and coordinated post-resuscitation care.

Basic life support

On arrival at the scene, first check that the environment is safe for you to assess the patient. If you are the first to discover the patient, check whether they are responsive. If they are, put them into the recovery position and go for help. If they are not, shout for help, but stay with the patient and begin your assessment with ABC.

Airway

Maintenance of adequate tissue oxygenation requires airway patency and the delivery of adequate inspired oxygen to the lungs. Formal intubation of the trachea may not be necessary and is a procedure that requires both skill and practice.

If the patient's airway is occluded and they are not breathing, put out an arrest call. Turn the patient onto their back; clear any obstructing material from the oropharynx by performing a gloved finger sweep. Be cautious in patients with possible head or neck trauma in whom the cervical spine must be protected (see below) and a set of McGill's forceps, rather than a finger sweep, should be used.

Airway manoeuvres

The goal of these manoeuvres is to restore and maintain airway patency. Their effectiveness must be constantly reassessed throughout any resuscitation attempt. The airway should be managed by the most experienced person in the situation at the time.

Head tilt, chin lift

In the absence of suspicion or definite damage to the cervical spine, this is the most effective way in which to open the airway of an unconscious patient. Proceed as follows:

- place the palm/heel of one of your hands on the patient's forehead
- place the fingers of your other hand under their chin (avoid soft tissue)
- gently lift the chin and maintain position by gentle pressure on chin and forehead
- remember that an unconscious patient will always re-occlude their airway if this support is not sustained.

Jaw thrust

Used where cervical spine damage is suspected; see below. Remember that some patients are predisposed to neck trauma at low energy because of osteoporosis or rheumatoid arthritis. Proceed as follows:

- place the middle fingers of both hands under the angle of the mandible
- gently push the mandible forward, opening the mouth with the thumbs.

Airway management in cervical spine injury

If there is a high index of suspicion of cervical spine injury, the head and neck should be immobilized using a semi-rigid collar, lateral head support and taping. Oxygen should be administered via a non-rebreathing facemask or, if necessary, with bag–valve–mask ventilation. If an airway manoeuvre is required, a jaw thrust should be performed, as this will open the airway with minimal chance of cervical spine damage. If this fails to open the airway, you may perform a chin lift without head tilt, with an assistant immobilizing the cervical spine. If basic airway manoeuvres fail to establish airway patency and restore adequate ventilation, intubation may be required; see 'Advanced life support', p. 14.

Airway adjuncts

Oropharyngeal and nasopharyngeal airways can be used with minimal training and practice, and will be available on most 'cardiac arrest' trolleys in the hospital setting and many GP surgeries. These are adjuncts, not alternatives, to standard airway manoeuvres.

Oropharyngeal (Geudel®) airway

This helps to prevent occlusion of the pharynx by the tongue, and maintains patency of the upper airway. Select an airway equivalent in length to the distance from the patient's incisor to the angle of their jaw.

In adults, the airway is inserted upside down until gentle contact with the soft palate is felt. At this point it is rotated into position. In young children, the oropharyngeal airway should be inserted in the orientation that it will sit in the airway; a tongue depressor can be used to hold the tongue out of the way first. An oropharyngeal airway can induce vomiting and aspiration in patients with a preserved gag reflex but a depressed conscious level. In this situation, a nasopharyngeal airway may be safer.

Nasopharyngeal airway

Less rigid than the oropharyngeal airway, the nasopharyngeal airway is less likely to induce vomiting when a gag reflex is present, or the patient is more awake. It is useful in situations where the jaw cannot be opened, or where there are facial injuries. However, nasopharyngeal airways are contraindicated in patients with actual or suspected basal skull fracture or nasal fracture.

Choose an airway equivalent in length to the distance between the patient's incisor and the tragus of the ear. The diameter of the airway should also be similar to that of the patient's little finger. To insert the airway:

- choose the correct size of airway and the largest nostril
- lubricate the outer surface
- attach a safety pin to the flange of the tube to prevent complete entry into the nose
- insert perpendicular to the face along the nasal floor
- stop if there is any resistance
- use a rotating movement back and forth as you insert the tube
- if it does not fit, try the other nostril.

Breathing and circulation

While keeping the airway open, look, listen and feel for breathing and check for a pulse. If there are no signs of life, call for help and ensure that an arrest call has been put out. If you are alone, you will have to leave the patient to do this. Return immediately and commence CPR.

Cardiopulmonary resuscitation

The aim of CPR is to maintain oxygenation and the perfusion of vital tissues until defibrillation is possible or reversible factors can be addressed.

Chest compressions

The blood oxygen content remains high in the first minutes after an arrest, so effective chest compressions to restore perfusion are the most critical component. They should be performed as follows:

- your hands should be placed in the centre of the chest
- compress the chest at a rate of around 100/min and to a depth of around 4–5 cm, in an adult
- between compressions, the chest must be allowed to recoil completely to allow cardiac filling.

Ventilation

Immediate 'rescue breaths' are no longer advised. Instead, 30 compressions should be followed by 2 ventilations and this ratio continued until help, or a defibrillator, arrives. Always use a pocket resuscitation mask if one is available. If mouth-to-mouth ventilation is not possible due, for example, to facial trauma, mouth-to-nose is an effective alternative.

In the hospital environment, the patient should be ventilated with the available bag and mask system entraining high flow oxygen. This is preferential to mouth-to-mouth resuscitation, as the oxygen concentration of a rescuer's expired breath is only 16–17%. When using a bag and mask, one person should perform a jaw thrust/chin lift and maintain a good facial seal while another person squeezes the bag. When performing ventilation:

- deliver each breath over approximately 1 s
- aim to ventilate the chest to what would be an approximately normal volume for the size of the patient
- deliver 2 ventilations after each sequence of 30 chest compressions during CPR with an unprotected (unintubated) airway.

Advanced life support

As soon as the defibrillator arrives, attach the leads or pads, and assess the rhythm (see 'ECG Interpretation', p. 78, and 'Arrhythmias', p. 132). Depending on whether the rhythm is shockable (ventricular tachycardia (VT) or ventricular fibrillation (VF)) or non-shockable (pulseless electrical activity (PEA) or asystole), proceed down the appropriate limb of the ALS algorithm (Fig. 1.2). If the rhythm is shockable, defibrillation must not be delayed.

It is important that the most senior member of the arrest team coordinates the resuscitation attempt. They should direct other team members as indicated below, clinically assess the patient and decide upon the immediate treatment priorities. They should also determine, in consultation with the team, when resuscitation should be discontinued (see 'Decisions regarding resuscitation', p. 399).

Defibrillation in VF or VT

It is essential that you are familiar with the defibrillators used in your hospital (see 'Defibrillation and electrical cardioversion', p. 58). VF and VT should be managed immediately by delivery of a single shock (at 150 J for biphasic defibrillators or 360 J for monophasic machines), followed by immediate resumption of CPR for 2 min (30 compressions: 2 ventilations). Do not reassess the rhythm or feel for a pulse after the first shock. This should be done only after 2 min of CPR, when a further shock can be delivered if indicated. Second and subsequent shocks from a biphasic defibrillator should be delivered at 150–360 J. For all shocks from monophasic defibrillators, 360 J should be used.

If there is doubt as to whether the rhythm is asystole or fine VF, do not attempt defibrillation, but proceed down the non-shockable side of the ALS algorithm.

Intravenous access

IV access should be secured early; this allows fluid resuscitation and the administration of cardiotropic and vasopressor drugs. If at least one large-bore peripheral cannula cannot be sited, a central venous line should be inserted (see 'Procedures', p. 50). In the meantime, 3 mg boluses of adrenaline (epinephrine) should be administered during ALS via the endotracheal (ET) tube (see below), rather than the 1 mg boluses that would have been used IV. In children, intraosseous access should be considered, but this requires appropriate training and competence.

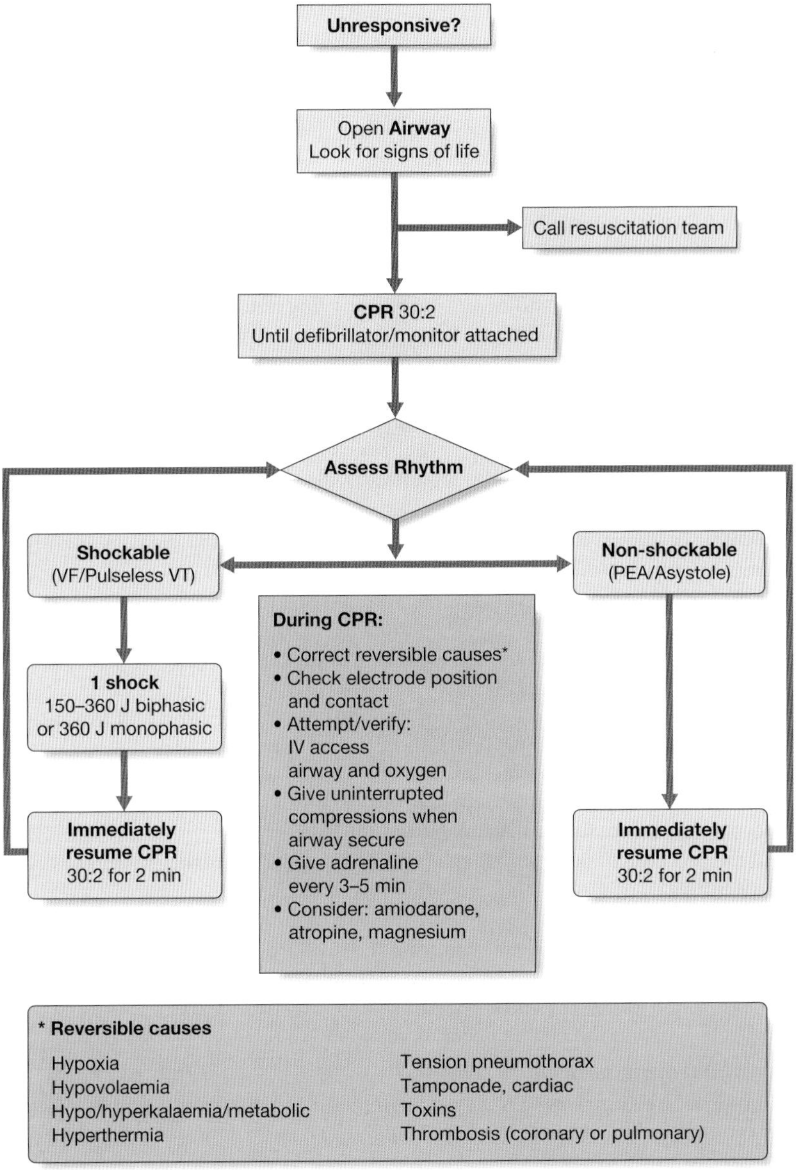

Figure 1.2 Advanced Life Support (ALS) algorithm.

Advanced airway management and endotracheal intubation

Airway patency should be restored and maintained as discussed in 'Basic Life Support', p. 12. In the hospital environment, the patient should initially be ventilated using a bag and mask system connected to high flow oxygen, as above.

Efforts should then be made to intubate the patient as soon as possible (chest compressions should be ongoing and stopped only to allow the ET tube through the cords). This protects the airway and reduces the risk of aspiration. However, failed intubation can lead to profound hypoxaemia and the procedure should be attempted only by someone who is trained and competent to do so. Otherwise, bag and mask ventilation should be continued. Intubation attempts should never delay appropriate defibrillation.

Once the airway has been secured and protected by endotracheal intubation, ventilate the lungs at approximately 10 breaths/min. Note that a laryngeal mask airway (LMA) is not considered a protected airway; see below.

Endotracheal intubation: procedure

- perform checks of breathing and obvious obstruction, as above
- look for signs of possible difficult intubation and seek expert help if necessary, e.g. child, facial trauma, receding jaw, small mouth opening, protruding or diseased teeth, large tongue, previous history of difficult intubation
- obtain a selection of handles and blades (varying size and shape) and a selection of tubes of different sizes
- check the laryngoscope and suction bag are working
- wear gloves and consider the need for eye protection
- select a blade – this should reach between lips and larynx, when held against the face
- pre-oxygenate the patient with high flow oxygen
- position the head: assuming no cervical spine injury suspected, choose a central position with a pillow under the occiput and extend the neck slightly
- remove any dentures and check for loose teeth
- stand behind the head and hold the laryngoscope in your left hand and the ET tube in your right
- insert the laryngoscope over the right side of the tongue using the blade to sweep around the tongue
- put the blade between the epiglottis and the base of tongue and lift (up and away from you, using the whole handle rather than pivoting on the teeth or gums) until you can see the glottis
- slide the ET tube along the right side of the mouth and between the vocal cords; make sure the cuff is beyond the cords
- if the procedure takes more than 30 s, STOP and seek help; bag and mask meantime
- otherwise, inflate the cuff and ventilate with high flow oxygen
- secure the tube by passing a cord from the tube around the patient's neck
- assess for correct position: verify that there is inflation of both sides of the chest; listen for breath sounds on both sides and ensure that there is no gurgling in the stomach on ventilation; obtain CXR.

Laryngeal mask airways

A laryngeal mask airway (LMA) is inserted and inflated blindly into the hypopharynx around the posterior perimeter of the larynx, forming a low-pressure seal around the lumen of the larxynx. Positive pressure ventilation can then take place. Although the LMA is a universally used and effective piece of equipment when used properly, it has some limitations:

- it does not guarantee protection of the airway
- high inflation pressures or over-zealous bagging can lead to inflation of the stomach with an increased risk of aspiration of gastric contents, especially during a cardiorespiratory arrest, when chest compressions are ongoing.

Identification of precipitants

Throughout any resuscitation attempt, precipitating factors must be aggressively sought and corrected. The 4 Hs and 4 Ts (see foot of Fig. 1.2) are particularly relevant in patients presenting with non-shockable arrhythmias, but may also be important in those with VF or VT. It is important that the coordinating member of the cardiac arrest team assesses ABC and performs a rapid clinical survey, using whatever information is available:

- examine the neck veins, chest and abdomen; look specifically for evidence of a tension pneumothorax, tamponade or blood loss (e.g. melaena or blood staining around the mouth)
- check a BM and tympanic membrane temperature
- check FBC, U&E, Ca, Mg, Coag, cross-match, ABG and other clinically relevant tests, e.g. level of digoxin or other potential toxins
- speak to nursing or medical staff who know the patient; enquire about recent events and symptoms, e.g. breathlessness, increasing oxygen requirements.

Management of precipitants

Unless there is a good reason to suspect cardiac failure, and particularly in patients with PEA, start a rapid IV infusion of colloid and respond to the results of the initial blood tests as appropriate. Specific causes should be addressed as directed in the relevant sections of this book. Treatments may include:

- insulin–dextrose infusion (10 units Actrapid in 50 mL 50% dextrose) for hyperkalaemia (see p. 204)
- magnesium sulfate (8 mmol IV over 5 min) for VF/VT associated with hypomagnesaemia or torsades de pointes (see 'Arrhythmias', p. 132)
- sodium bicarbonate (50 mL 8.4% IV), e.g. for profound acidosis, tricyclic overdose
- calcium gluconate for hyperkalaemia (see p. 204), hypocalcaemia (see p. 207), calcium channel blocker overdose
- thrombolytics for suspected MI or PTE, e.g. tenecteplase 500–600 μg/kg IV over 10 s.

2 Use of equipment and procedures

PROCEDURAL COMPETENCE

Competence is a core principle of modern medical education, particularly in relation to clinical procedures. It represents an ability to perform what is required to an expected standard. It is not a measure of excellence and it relates to a specific moment in time, rather than a permanent state.

Competence is not a pre-determined 'end result' imparted by training in any discipline. It is a measure of, or comparison against, a specific standard and therefore, must be assessed to be acquired. For procedural competence to be achieved, an individual will need to demonstrate that prerequisite knowledge about the procedure (anatomy, pathophysiology, method, risks, complications, etc.) has been acquired; that they can perform the procedure correctly and safely; and that they apply appropriate professional attitudes to the patient and other staff. Competence is individual for both the procedure and the doctor. The number of procedures that any one doctor needs to complete to achieve it may differ from that required by their colleagues.

Competence in medical procedures is specific to the environment within which it is acquired. Skills laboratory-acquired 'competence' is not applicable to the clinical setting. It is simply a measure that the doctor performed the practice session satisfactorily, and is ready to progress to supervised learning in the clinical setting. Clinical competency 'at the bedside' must be separately learned and assessed. No doctor should attempt a clinical procedure on a patient, on the basis of skills laboratory-acquired learning, without supervision by somebody who is clinically competent in that procedure.

The process of acquiring competence in any one procedure will usually involve learning theory about it; observing and practising in a 'patient safe' skills laboratory; observing a 'real' procedure; supervision of attempts (by a clinician competent in the procedure); personal reflection, further learning or observation; supervised assessment and either 'sign-off' of achievement of competency, or recommendations regarding specific learning targets before the next assessment (see also 'Assessment', p. 431).

Although competency is 'signed off', it is important to note that this is in regard to performance on one particular day. It does not mean that the doctor involved is safe to do that procedure for ever. Sustaining competence requires regular practice. It may also require periods of further assessment to validate retention of skill.

Doctors must always ask themselves, ahead of any procedure, whether they are competent to undertake it, in that setting. Formal, supervised and validated clinical competency is what is required. Equally, if, despite being 'signed-off', the situation you are facing appears more difficult or risky than one you would usually feel equipped to handle, or some time has passed since you last were assessed or undertook that procedure, or you simply wish to have someone with you, ask for experienced help.

THE STERILE FIELD

Any invasive or surgical procedure must be performed within a sterile field; this minimizes the risk of infection to the patient. This area should include all parts of the patient that will be touched during the procedure, any part of the operator that might touch the procedure site or the sterile equipment being used, and the place used to store any sterile equipment during the procedure. The creation and maintenance of a sterile field is an essential component of aseptic technique.

Preparing the trolley

- wash your hands
- clean the trolley with an antiseptic wipe
- check you have several pairs of the correct size of gloves and the equipment you will need for the procedure
- open the outer cover of the dressing pack and drop the inner pack onto the trolley
- touching only the corners of the pack, pull it open
- open all the other outer packs of things you will need and drop the sterile contents onto the dressing pack
- lastly, open the outer packs of your gloves, gown and towel and drop the inner packs, without touching them, onto the trolley in that order (such that the towel lies at the top).

Handwashing and scrubbing

Before washing or scrubbing in readiness for a procedure, check that you are wearing any other items you require (e.g. hat, plastic or lead apron, mask, visor). (For guidance on surgical scrubbing, see 'Theatre', p. 393.) Simple handwashing should be conducted as follows:

- remove all jewellery and turn on the 'elbow-taps'; if the taps are pushed too far back to reach with your elbows, touch the part where they join the sink, not the 'wings'
- wet your hands, apply soap and rub together for at least 15 s, ensuring you observe the six washing stages: palm to palm; backs of the hands; between the fingers; fingertips; thumbs and wrists; nails (against the palm of the hand)

- rinse off all of the soap from your hands, ideally passing your hands and arms under the water while keeping your fingertips above the level of your elbows
- close the taps using your elbows
- dry your hands with a sterile paper towel (from the gown pack).

Sterile and protective garments

Proper use prevents infective contamination of the patient and doctor and reduces damage to clothes.

Hats, masks and visors

These should be put on ahead of washing/scrubbing. Hats should cover as much of your hair as possible. Make sure the interior of the mask is facing you when you put it on; the metallic strip goes at the top. After fitting the mask, pinch the metal strip to fit closely to the bridge of your nose. Visors/eye-protection should be worn for any procedure that involves potential contact with blood or bodily fluids.

Gowns

Gowns (fabric or paper) should be worn for all sterile procedures. If there is a risk of large amounts of fluid or blood contamination, a waterproof apron should be worn underneath. It is important to unwrap the sterile gown carefully, touching only the inner surface of the gown. Lift it out in such a way as to prevent the front of the gown touching anything else. Push your hands into the sleeves only as far as the elasticated cuffs (see gloves below).

An assistant will help you tie the gown. If you are using a paper gown there will be tapes to close the gown hanging at the front attached to a piece of card. If you are performing a sterile procedure you should not tie these yourself. Instead, once you have your gloves on, you should hold onto one of the tapes and pass the card (attached to the other tape) to someone else to hold. Then you can turn around, which closes the gown, before pulling the tape out of the card (held by your assistant) and knotting the two ties at the front of your gown. Fabric gowns usually have buttons or Velcro® fasteners at the back that your assistant should fasten.

The front of a surgical gown is regarded as sterile from chest level extending down as far as the level of the patient. The sleeves are sterile from 5cm above the elbow to the cuff. The neckline, shoulders, underarms and back of the gown are not thought of as sterile. Once you are gowned and gloved, you should keep your hands 'safe' until the procedure begins, in the rectangle bounded by the mid-sternum, anterior axillary lines and umbilicus.

Gloves

Gloves come in different sizes. If they are too tight they will constrict your fingers; too loose and you will lose dexterity, especially at the fingertips. Standard male size is 7.5 and female is 6.5, but if you do not know your size, try some different ones. Latex gloves are normally provided; however, both patients and staff can be latex-allergic, in which case latex-free gloves should be worn. Gloves should be put on after the gown. Open the inner pack touching only the edges and without touching the gloves themselves. The gloves should be lying with their wrists folded back.

Grasp the inner side of the first glove through the sleeve of your gown and push your hand into it, without folding back the cuff of the glove. Use your now sterile gloved hand to pick up the other glove: this time do not touch the inside of the glove, but slip your gloved hand into the cuff fold of the other. Push your other hand inside the second glove and, with your first gloved hand, flip the second glove cuff over that of your gown. Now use your second gloved hand to flip (from the underside) the cuffed edge of the first glove over the gown sleeve. You must now keep your hands within the sterile field at all times (see p. 19).

Cleaning the skin

Equipment

For injections, cannulation or blood sampling, you will need an antiseptic wipe. For operations, you will need a special sponge-containing instrument, e.g. Rampley's forceps. For procedures, you will need disposable forceps, gauze swabs and a bowl of cleaning solution. This can be an iodine-based preparation such as Betadine®, or a non-iodine preparation if the patient is allergic, e.g. 1% chlorhexidine. You should take care when using non-iodine preparations to ensure the whole area has been cleaned: it will be less easy to see patches that you have missed. Also note that you should not use alcohol-based preparations on the genitalia or mucous membranes.

For ward-based procedures, you might also want to consider placing a disposable absorbent pad under whatever part you are cleaning to protect the bed. Also, tape an open disposable bag onto the trolley handle or nearby, ready to collect your used swabs.

Method

For injections, cannulation or blood sampling

Ensure any obvious dirt is washed off with soap and water. Clean with an antiseptic wipe and allow to dry naturally.

For ward-based procedures

- ensuring sufficient patient privacy, expose the area to be cleaned
- if soiled, wash the area with soap and water; it is no longer thought advisable to shave any area – infection may develop in small cuts or abrasions
- wearing gloves, fold each swab into four and grip with the forceps
- dip the folded swab into the cleaning agent
- start at the centre of the area to be cleaned and, working in a circular motion outwards, clean towards the edge of the area that will be exposed during the procedure; clean about 5 cm beyond the area you intend to frame with drapes; never go back with the same swab towards the centre again
- without touching the swab or bag, drop your forceps into the bag
- take a fresh swab and forceps and repeat the process
- do this again a third time.

For theatre operations

This is much as per the above; however, you will usually have a specific instrument, e.g. Rampley's forceps, to use and you will usually need to cover a larger area. Mark the edge of your 'painting' with one sponge dipped in cleaning agent. Then, with a second, 'fill in' the area, working from the incision site always outwards. Clean any creases/umbilicus last, or with a separate sponge only to that area.

Draping the field

The aim is to cover all of the area that you or your equipment might come into contact with during the procedure. No drape should touch the floor. A variety of drapes are available and your choice should depend on the area you need to work within during the procedure. Standard cloth or disposable paper drapes are deployed around the outside of the work area, working inwards with successive drapes until the edge of the cleaned area is covered entirely by 5 cm of drape. 'Hernia' towels have a central hole that can make it easier to mark off smaller work areas, and steridrapes have a central adhesive-edged hole that is applied to the skin immediately around the area of the procedure. 'Incise' drapes are applied in theatre across the whole operative field and some drapes are impregnated with antiseptic. Towel clips can be used (usually in theatre) to stop the drapes slipping.

Maintenance of the sterile field

It is important to consider the boundaries of the sterile field at all times during the procedure. This allows you minimize contamination and to deal appropriately with any contamination that does occur:

- place only sterile items within the sterile field
- do not allow the sterile parts of you to touch anything that is not sterile or allow any non-sterile part of you, e.g. lower gown or hat, to touch the field (in theatres it is not unusual for your hat to touch the sterile handle of the operating lamps; if it does, the handle will need to be changed)
- take particular care, when items are opened or dispensed onto the trolley or transferred to the patient, only to touch what is sterile and to keep it in the sterile field at all times (note that the edges of any pack holding a sterile item are not sterile)
- ensure other 'non-sterile' personnel do not reach across the sterile field or touch sterile items; likewise do not stretch over a non-sterile area
- avoid unnecessary procedure-related contamination, e.g. bleeding: if a sterile barrier (over operator or patient) has become wet, cut or torn, the area is no longer sterile
- immediately replace any contaminated items
- keep sterile items away from windows or doors.

LOCAL ANAESTHETICS

Local anaesthetic agents are complex drugs which have to be administered with care. You will need to use local anaesthetics when performing basic procedures, e.g. suturing, pleural aspiration. This section provides an introduction to local anaesthetic techniques and practice. It is not a substitute for practice in a skills laboratory environment or supervised clinical experience.

Pharmacology

Local anaesthetic (LA) drugs block conduction of nerve impulses at the level of the axonal membrane with effects on both sensory and motor neurones. Local anaesthetic techniques involve both the administration of the drug and the care of the patient to prevent possible adverse drug effects. Common local anaesthetics are shown in Table 2.1. Most clinically useful LA agents disrupt nerve impulses and act by blocking the cell membrane sodium channel.

Speed of onset of action

The pKa of the drug or 'dissociation constant' is the pH at which a local analgesic drug is 50% ionized and 50% un-ionized. Lipoprotein cell membranes are penetrated by the un-ionized form only and local anaesthetics with a pKa closer to physiological pH tend to have a more rapid time of onset. The pH of the injected solution and the pH at the injection site also alter the balance of ionization and the onset of action. Smaller nerve fibres (pain and autonomic nerve fibres) are blocked earlier than larger ones, such as those for light touch and proprioception.

Duration of action

Systemic re-absorption from the tissue into the bloodstream is important, e.g. in highly vascular or inflamed sites. Also of relevance is the dosage and concentration of the drug, its lipid solubility and protein binding capacity.

Table 2.1 Common local anaesthetics

Drug	Uses	Notes
Lidocaine	Local infiltration and regional	The most commonly used LA; onset in 5–10 min, duration 2–3 h with adrenaline; usually used in 1 or 2% solution max dose: without adrenaline 3–4 mg/kg (approx. 20 mL of 1% solution); with adrenaline 7 mg/kg (approx. 50 mL of 1% solution)
Bupivacaine	Nerve blocks or local infiltration	Long action (3–20 h, depending on area of application and concentration); must not be used for IV regional use
Prilocaine	Local and regional anaesthesia	High doses can cause methaemoglobinaemia; also available as topical cream mixed with lidocaine (Emla®), which is effective after about 1 h
Amethocaine	Topical preparation for venepuncture in children aged over 1 month	Not for use on inflamed, traumatized or highly vascular surfaces
Proxymetacaine	Topical ophthalmic anaesthesia	

Local anaesthetics are usually aminoamides, which are metabolized in the liver, or aminoesters, which are metabolized in the plasma by esterases. Aminoesters are more allergenic than aminoamides because of the metabolite, para-aminobenzoic acid (PABA). Sensitized patients may develop an allergic reaction unrelated to the anaesthetic itself.

Most LAs cause vasodilatation. The addition of a vasoconstrictor such as adrenaline (epinephrine) reduces local blood flow and prolongs its local effect by reducing drug absorption away from the site. Adrenaline must not be used along with local anaesthetics in digits or appendages as it can cause ischaemic necrosis. The total dose of adrenaline must not exceed 200 µg, or a concentration of 1 in 200 000 (5 µg/mL) if more than 50 mL is being used.

Using local anaesthetics

Preparation

Begin by obtaining informed consent. Position the patient for the procedure, prepare the sterile field, and select the appropriate equipment including LA, needles and syringes.

Once you, your field and the equipment are ready, check the drug name and expiry date on the vial of LA held by the assistant. Put a needle with a large bore (green or white) onto your syringe and draw up the drugs required from the vial. The vial is held upside down and you put your needle in at the tip and draw back on the syringe. If it is a fixed glass bottle with a bung rather than a glass tip that can be broken off, first fill your syringe with air, then insert the needle into the bung and inject some air into the bottle: that will allow the same amount of liquid to come back into your syringe without creating a vacuum.

Replace the needle with a small one for skin insertion and check you have any needles required for going deeper. Also check you have any other kit you need ready on the tray, e.g. for the pleural tap or suture.

Administration

Since LA drugs are used to avoid pain, it makes no sense to cause pain in giving the anaesthetic. Use as small a needle as possible, e.g. orange (24 gauge), and warm the vial of solution in your hand before drawing, as fluids closer to body temperature cause less pain when injected.

Consider your route

If you are preparing a track, e.g. for the insertion of a drain, you should be going in a straight line and looking for signs of fluid or air in your syringe. However, if you are trying to numb an area of skin, e.g. for suture, you should approach the area from a variety of angles making small repeated insertion, aspiration and injection moves around it. Nevertheless, try to numb the underlying tissue in several directions from one skin injection point rather than making several skin injections to cover the same area. Likewise if there is already a wound, inserting the needle from the cut edge of the skin, to allow injection of the adjacent subcutaneous tissue, will cause less pain than entering through the intact skin.

Hold the needle and plunger using your other hand as a 'guard'; insert at a shallow angle (20–30°) and advance by no more than 1 cm at a time. As soon as you enter the skin, stop, use your 'guard' hand to brace against the skin and prevent movement forward, and aspirate with the hand holding the plunger. To avoid intravascular injection, look carefully for any sign of blood in the needle. If there is blood, do not inject but remove the needle (the blood in it will make it difficult for you to be sure you have not entered a vessel the next time), replace it and try again in a slightly different point or different direction.

If there is no blood, inject a small amount slowly (slower injections cause less pain), wait a few seconds then start to aspirate again as you advance another 0.5–1 cm. Again, if there is any blood in the needle remove your syringe and needle from the patient, and replace the needle before re-inserting it. Repeat this part of the process until you have covered the area to be numbed.

Bear in mind that local anaesthetic injection into subcutaneous tissue causes it to swell and will make it more difficult to suture: use small amounts spread over an area rather than large volumes in one location. Now allow time for the anaesthetic to work before you proceed with your procedure.

Toxicity

Toxicity relates to the dose of drug given and its uptake from the tissues into the circulation. In addition, pre-existing medical conditions may influence sensitivity to drugs or their delivery. Likewise, accidental intravascular injection may deliver a toxic dose.

Overdose can result in symptoms indicative of CNS and cardiovascular toxicity, often starting with tingling in the lips, ringing in the ears, dizziness, tachycardia, anxiety and excitement, and later leading to sedation, disorientation, restlessness, twitching, convulsions, hypotension, bradycardia, coma and cardiorespiratory arrest.

To avoid toxicity, check the drug and the dose you are using is safe for this procedure and this patient. Always check an up-to-date source of information, e.g. the BNF website, for drug doses, cautions and interactions. Remember to avoid adrenaline for procedures on extremities, e.g. fingers, nose.

Calculate the dose carefully. Remember a 1% solution is 10 mg/mL. Have a trained nurse or another medical colleague check your calculations, drug, strength and use-by date before injecting any drug. Do not use topical anaesthetic creams for broken or inflamed skin as absorption is increased. Do not inject anaesthetic agents into inflamed areas. Before any local anaesthetic is given, especially when large volumes are given or in the case of regional blocks, also insert an indwelling venous cannula and ensure resuscitation equipment is in the vicinity. Observe caution in the presence of heart block, low cardiac output, hepatic insufficiency, porphyria, myasthenia gravis or epilepsy.

Management in suspected toxicity

- stop the procedure
- check the airway is protected and give oxygen
- call a senior colleague if you are concerned about the patient
- check your IV access is still in place
- connect to cardiac, blood pressure and pulse oximetry monitors
- give diazepam if convulsions develop
- give atropine for any bradycardia
- give fluids and raise the end of the bed if hypotensive.

Nerve blocks

Peripheral nerve blocks

A wide variety of nerves are suitable for blockade by local anaesthetic, e.g. median, ulnar, radial, intercostals, maxillary, infraorbital. These require knowledge of anatomy. Lidocaine 1–2% is usually used because of its speed of onset but solutions containing adrenaline should not be used in blocks affecting extremities, e.g. fingers, toes. The most commonly used block in A&E is probably the digital block.

Digital nerve block

- two common digital nerves run along both sides of each finger near the bone and next to the digital arteries, one on the dorsum and one on the palmar aspect; they run closer to the skin than the arteries on both sides
- using a small needle and 1–2% lidocaine, raise a small weal of anaesthetic on the dorsum of the finger just lateral to the bone
- pointing the needle medially, inject 1 mL between the bone and the skin on the dorsal aspect
- advance near the edge of the bone until you can feel the tip of the needle under (but not through) the skin of the palmar/plantar aspect
- aspirate and inject 1 mL in this new position
- withdraw and repeat the procedure on the other side of the joint
- finally, connect the two wheals on the dorsum with 1 mL of solution
- allow about 15 min for the anaesthetic to take effect.

Epidural and spinal blocks

During your initial training, you are unlikely to need to administer these. However, you will need to check with your patient if there are any reasons not to use such an approach when it is being considered. Contraindications include hypotension, abnormal clotting, increased intracranial pressure, fixed cardiac output states, e.g. heart block, aortic stenosis.

You also need to be aware of potential complications, including hypotension, paralysis, hypothermia, shivering, higher rates of obstetric intervention, urinary retention, nausea and itch (if opiates injected). Less common side-effects include nerve palsies, leg pain, spinal headache (if dura punctured), epidural haematoma or infection, drowsiness and respiratory depression – IV injection (convulsions or collapse) and intrathecal injection causing total spinal paralysis.

VENEPUNCTURE AND CANNULATION

Indications

Venepuncture is indicated where blood samples are required. Cannulation is required for the administration of IV fluids, drugs or blood products.

Contraindications

Never take blood from, or attempt to cannulate, a vein where there is paralysis or local sepsis. Do not insert cannulae where there is evidence of lymphoedema or in an arm leading to where axillary lymph node surgery has been performed, e.g. for breast cancer.

Complications

Extravasation

Extravasation or 'tissuing' occurs when the vein wall is breached and the contents of the infusion leak into the surrounding tissues. It is suggested by pain or swelling around the cannula, either during infusion or after injection of a saline flush.

Infection

Cannulae that remain in situ for over 72h are more likely to become infected. Therefore, they should be checked regularly for signs such as pain, swelling and redness and removed after a maximum of 72h. If infection is suspected, the cannula should be removed and a swab of the area sent to the laboratory. Antibiotic therapy is not required unless there are signs of systemic infection.

Procedure

Preparation

Choose the appropriate needles or cannulae (see below). Where you are taking blood, ensure that you have the appropriate vials or Vacutainers®. In addition, you will need a tourniquet, gloves, cotton wool, a dressing, specimen labels and the relevant laboratory request forms. Take a sharps box to the bedside so that you can dispose of your equipment safely and immediately.

Choosing a vein

Before choosing a vein, inspect both hands and arms. Choose a vein that is palpable and refills when depressed. Avoid veins that have been used recently or feel hard and vessels overlying joints as these can be uncomfortable and are more likely to 'tissue'.

In elderly patients and in those who have had chemotherapy, veins are often fragile and tissue easily; consider using a smaller cannula, a tourniquet that is not too tight and a reduced angle of insertion to reduce the risk of exiting the rear of the vessel; a 'butterfly' needle may also help (see below). Where patients are cold or peripherally shut down, veins are more difficult to access; consider encouraging vasodilatation by placing the limb in a basin of warm water.

Choosing needles or cannulae

There are many different sizes of needle and cannula. Green (18 gauge) is the standard needle size, but in elderly patients, children or those who have had chemotherapy, smaller gauges may be necessary. Larger cannulae (grey or white) are used in emergency situations when large volumes of fluids need to be infused. The tubing of 'butterfly' needles allows a much lower angle of vein entry than when a syringe is attached and can be useful where access is poor or veins are fragile.

Method

Phlebotomy

- check the identify of your patient
- in children, consider the application of a local anaesthetic cream, such as Emla®, 30min beforehand
- wash hands and put on gloves
- choose a suitable vein and apply a tourniquet
- encourage venous filling: ask patient to clench and unclench their hand; allow arm to hang at patient's side; tap vein lightly
- anchor vein with free hand applying manual traction of the skin 2–5cm below the proposed insertion site

- with the bevel of the needle upwards, insert the needle into the vein and advance it a further 1–2 mm
- withdraw all necessary blood into the syringe(s) or allow the vacuum to withdraw blood into tube(s) from the vein; ensure that the bottles are filled in the correct order (see 'Artefactual results', p. 70)
- release the tourniquet
- remove the needle and do not re-sheath it; apply pressure with the cotton wool
- label all bottles and forms
- remember to phone the laboratories if you are sending urgent samples.

Cannulation

- identify and position your patient
- wash hands and put on gloves
- choose a suitable vein and apply tourniquet (see above)
- clean the skin over the cannulation site; this is good practice despite limited evidence that it reduces subsequent infection
- anchor vein (as above)
- insert the cannula into the vein at an angle of 25–30°; fragile veins may require a lower angle of insertion
- once you get a flash-back, lower the angle of the cannula to almost skin level
- advance the cannula a few millimetres into the vein, holding it at the wings or protection cap
- withdraw the needle slightly
- hold the flash-back chamber, immobilizing the needle, and advance the cannula forward off the needle into the vein in a single smooth movement
- release the tourniquet
- apply pressure over the vein distal to the cannula tip and remove the needle
- blood samples may be taken at this point if required: be aware that haemolysis is more likely when using small cannulae
- close the cannula with a Luer-Lok injection cap/interlink
- dispose of sharps appropriately
- secure the cannula in position with appropriate dressing
- flush the cannula with saline and check for any signs of extravasation (see p. 26).

BLOOD CULTURES

In any patient with suspected bacteraemia or fungaemia, samples for blood culture should be taken, in addition to appropriate site-specific samples. This allows the prescription of targeted antibiotic therapy and modification of risk factors to prevent future infection. Correct sampling technique is essential as contamination with skin commensals leads to false positive results and may result in unnecessary antibiotic treatment. It involves inoculation into two separate culture bottles, one aerobic and the other anaerobic.

Indications

Features suggestive of possible septicaemia:

- core temperature out of the normal range
- significant focal signs of infection
- abnormal heart rate, blood pressure or respiratory rate
- chills or rigors
- raised or unusually low WBC
- new or worsening confusion: may be the only sign in the elderly or very young.

Contraindications

There are no specific contraindications to taking a sample for blood culture.

Complications

Complications are those related to venepuncture; see p. 26.

Procedure

Timing and number of samples

The collection of multiple sets of blood cultures, ideally from different sites, increases diagnostic sensitivity and is required in cases of suspected endocarditis or pyrexia of unknown origin. However, there is no evidence that sampling during spikes of fever significantly improves sensitivity.

Sampling sites

Blood cultures should be collected from fresh puncture sites rather than existing cannulae or central venous lines. Avoid femoral punctures, since there is a high risk of skin contamination. If multiple cultures are required, sample from at least two different sites, at least 30 min apart, e.g. right antecubital fossa then left antecubital fossa before returning to the right antecubital fossa. If a line infection is suspected, cultures should be sent from both the line and a peripheral site; sampling should be performed from the peripheral site first to minimize contamination risk.

Preparation

Explain the procedure to the patient, and obtain verbal consent. You will need cleaning solution, e.g. 2% chlorhexidine or 70% isopropyl alcohol-impregnated swabs, 2 pairs of examination gloves and a tourniquet. You will also need 3 green needles and a 10 or 20 mL syringe (10 mL is the minimum volume suitable for culture) or a Vacutainer blood culture set.

Method

- put the tourniquet on and identify the target vein
- wash your hands and put on a set of gloves
- clean the skin over the target vein (see p. 21); allow to dry
- remove the plastic caps covering the bottles
- clean the surface of the rubber seals with a fresh cleaning swab; allow them to dry.

Sampling

- remove and discard the first set of gloves, wash your hands again and put on a fresh pair
- being careful not to touch the overlying skin, advance the needle into the target vein
- if a Vacutainer system is being used, load each culture bottle into the Vacutainer shield, onto the covered proximal end of the Vacutainer needle
- if a needle and syringe is being used, withdraw at least 10 mL of blood (ideally 20 mL) into the syringe and inoculate each culture bottle (anaerobic first) with 5–10 mL of blood; there is no need to change the needle between sampling and inoculation
- do not remove the barcode strips on the culture bottles
- record the procedure in the patient's notes, including the date and time
- complete an electronic or paper microbiology request, including patient details, date, time, site sampled and any antibiotic therapy
- arrange for the samples to taken immediately to the microbiology lab; if this is not possible they should be stored in an incubator set at body temperature until analysis.

INJECTIONS AND INFUSIONS

Indications

A variety of drug delivery options are available and their use is dependent on the drug, the reason for delivery, the presence or absence of IV access and the condition of the patient.

Intravenous

There is a rapid onset of action and the entire dose is bioavailable since it does not require absorption and also bypasses first-pass metabolism. A lower dose can often be administered IV rather than orally. Drugs may be administered as a bolus, an infusion or continuously. The route is commonly used for antibiotics, unfractionated heparin, cytotoxic agents and vasoactive drugs.

Intramuscular

Like IV administration, IM drugs avoid first-pass metabolism but absorption using this route is variable and depends on the muscle and blood supply to it. Intramuscular injections are commonly used for administration of analgesics, antiemetics and antibiotics where parenteral administration is required but where there is no intravenous access or where staff are unable to give medication intravenously, e.g. psychiatry or surgical wards. The volume of an IM drug dose should not exceed 5 mL.

Subcutaneous or intradermal

The subcutaneous route is used to deliver 0.5–2 mL of drug. Absorption is slower than for IM injections, but similarly dependent on local blood flow. It is commonly used for insulin therapy or LMWH administration and also for the administration of local anaesthesia.

Intradermal injection (<0.1 mL) is rarely used in hospital medical practice, but indications include vaccination, e.g. BCG, or allergen testing.

Contraindications

Intramuscular (IM), subcutaneous (SC) and intradermal (ID) routes should be used with caution in patients with bleeding diathesis or on warfarin. Care should be also taken only to administer drugs via these routes where tissue deposition of the drug will not cause necrosis.

Complications

In general, complications may result from infection, needle-stick injury and those that relate to the drug injected or the diluent. With doses intended for IM, SC and ID injection, care must be taken not to inject the drug IV. Complications that result from IV injections include extravasation, with resultant tissue necrosis and air-embolus.

Procedure

In all cases, you are responsible for injecting the correct drug into the correct patient and it is good practice to draw up the medication yourself. Always check that the route of administration is appropriate for the drug and dose. Where the drug is being given as an infusion, check that the rate is permissible.

In all cases, explain the procedure to the patient, gain verbal consent and following the injection, ensure that you document that the medication has been given on the cardex.

Preparation

Drawing up medication

- check the name of the medication, the dose and the expiry date
- use a large white needle to draw up drugs (it is quicker)

- dry powder medication: clean the rubber stopper on the top of the medication vial with an alcohol-impregnated wipe and allow it to dry; inject a small amount of (previously checked) diluent into the vial (1.5–2 mL); mix thoroughly by agitating the vial until all the powder has dissolved
- liquid medication: open the ampoule of medication; glass vials have a dot at the point where your thumb should be; take care not to touch the top of the ampoule with your fingers
- carefully insert the needle into the top of the vial/ampoule, taking care not to let the needle scrape the bottom
- invert the ampoule and draw up the liquid into the syringe: if the vial has a rubber bung, you may need to inject some air into the vial to allow fluid to be removed
- once the drug has been drawn up, hold the syringe upright to encourage any air to rise to the top; gentle tap the barrel of the syringe; expel the air until droplets of fluid are seen at the top of the needle
- remove the needle and dispose of it in the sharps bin
- for IM, SC, ID injections, fit a fresh new narrow-gauge needle.

Making up infusions

Infusions require a drug, in powder or liquid form, to be added to a diluent which is then infused at a predetermined rate. Common diluents include 0.9% sodium chloride (normal saline) and 5% dextrose; note that some medications must be used in conjunction with a specific diluent.

- select a bag of the appropriate diluent and volume, e.g. 50, 100, 250 or 500 mL; open it and check the expiry date
- draw up the drug (as above)
- clean the bung on the end of the diluent bag with an alcohol-impregnated wipe and allow it to dry
- hold the diluent bag with the bung at the bottom and insert the needle on the syringe with the drug into it; be careful that you do not pierce the outer skin of the bag
- once the drug has been injected into the bag of diluent, agitate the bag to allow mixing
- write a label which will include patient's name and details, drug name and dose, name and volume of diluent, time of addition and expiry, as well as your signature and that of a witness
- appropriately dispose of any sharps (including vials).

Method

For all injections:

- wash your hands and put on a pair of gloves
- check that the patient is not allergic to the medication and obtain their consent to the injection
- ensuring patient privacy, clean the injection area with an alcohol wipe.

Intravenous injections

In addition to the drug, you will also need 10 mL 0.9% sodium chloride as a flush. Do not use the injection ports attached to giving sets. If a central line is being used, use aseptic technique (see 'Sterile field', p. 19) to clean the injection port before and after injection.

- inject 1–2 mL of flush to ensure cannula patency
- inject the drug at the prescribed rate through the injection port
- inject the remaining flush; if multiple doses of different drugs are being given, a flush should be given between each drug to prevent mixing in the cannula.

Intramuscular injections
Common sites include the outer aspect of the upper arm, outer aspect of the middle third of the thigh and the upper outer quadrant of the buttock:

- stretch the skin with your non-dominant hand
- hold the needle like a dart and warn the patient; insert the needle quickly and smoothly at 90° to the skin, leaving about 1 cm of the needle showing (this will be dependent on the size of the patient)
- with the ulnar border of your hand against the skin, stabilize the syringe
- aspirate to ensure you are not in a vessel; if there is no blood, inject slowly
- once the drug has been injected, withdraw the needle quickly and gently and apply pressure to the area until bleeding stops.

Subcutaneous injection
Common sites for injection include the upper outer aspect of the arms, the anterior aspect of the thighs and the anterior abdominal region:

- pinch the skin using your non-dominant hand
- insert the needle into the subcutaneous tissue; angle of 45° for normal hypodermic needles or 80–90° for ultra-fine needles, e.g. pre-filled insulin syringes
- aspirate to confirm you have not entered a vessel; inject the drug and, on completion, pause briefly to reduce backtracking
- remove the needle and use a tissue to wipe away any blood; do not massage the site.

Intradermal injection
Usually performed on the volar aspect of the forearm or outer aspect of the upper arm:

- pinch the skin using your non-dominant hand
- insert the needle at 10–15°
- inject the drug (usually <0.1 mL), which will raise a small weal
- remove the needle, as above; do not massage the site.

ARTERIAL BLOOD GAS SAMPLING

Indications

Arterial blood gas (ABG) sampling is commonly required in acutely ill patients who may be hypoxic or acidotic. It is also required in the assessment of chronic respiratory disease and necessary for the prescription of long-term oxygen therapy.

Contraindications

Contraindications include those that pertain to venepuncture, in particular localized infection. It is also contraindicated where the pulse is not palpable or in patients with no collateral flow (as indicated by a negative Allen's test, see below).

Complications

Complications include localized bruising, bleeding and, more rarely, infection. There is a small risk of ischaemia, secondary to damage to the artery following puncture (see below).

Procedure

Preparation

Explain the procedure to the patient and gain verbal consent. You will need an ABG syringe, cleaning agent and swab, cotton wool ball, sticking plaster, a pair of gloves, a specimen label and a biochemistry form. This should be filled out including a note of the concentration of inspired oxygen and ventilator settings (IPAP and EPAP), if appropriate.

Collateral blood supply

ABGs are most commonly taken from the radial artery, although they may be obtained from the brachial or femoral artery. If a radial artery puncture is being performed, assess collateral blood supply using Allen's test and document the result in the notes.

Allen's test This assesses the integrity of the collateral ulnar circulation to the hand, and should be performed prior to performing a radial artery puncture or cannulation.

- ask the patient to elevate their hand and make a fist for 20 s
- occlude both the radial and ulnar arteries
- ask the patient to open their hand – it should blanche white
- release compression over the ulnar artery.

If redness/flushing of hand (thenar eminence first) occurs in under 10 s, the ulnar circulation is said to be satisfactory. If the hand fails to flush/return to normal colour, the ulnar circulation may be compromised and a radial artery puncture should not be performed.

Method

- wash hands and put on gloves
- check the expiry date of the syringe, remove syringe guard, fit needle and remove sheath. Note: some ABG syringes are pre-filled with heparin, which should be expelled before the puncture
- place a folded pillow underneath the outstretched wrist such that the arm is supported and the hand can be bent back over the edge; if the patient is drowsy or has difficulty lying still, ask for help to hold the arm
- clean the site with a Medi-Swab™ and allow to dry
- palpate the pulse, placing the index and middle fingers of your non-dominant hand parallel to the vessel; move laterally across the wrist until you are confident of the vessel's maximal impulse; move the fingers back until the fingernails are in line with the vessel and use them as a guide for the insertion point
- insert needle at 45–90°, until blood enters the syringe; in most cases, arterial pressure will be great enough to fill the syringe without additional suction
- draw at least 1 mL of arterial blood
- withdraw the needle and ask your assistant to apply firm pressure with the cotton wool ball directly to the site for at least 5 min and then apply a sticking plaster (if not allergic); where a brachial artery is used, the arm should not be bent at the elbow, but kept straight, raised and pressed
- do not re-sheath the needle: detach it and dispose in the sharps bin
- apply the clear/blue filter to the syringe, hold it upright and expel air; roll gently to mix, label, phone the lab and send the sample
- for interpretation of results, see 'Arterial blood gases', p. 71.

ARTERIAL LINE INSERTION

Indications

Arterial lines allow invasive and continuous monitoring of systolic, diastolic and mean blood pressure (MBP) via a transducer connection. This information is helpful in the management of patients with shock and is particularly useful in tailoring inotropic support to optimize tissue perfusion.

Arterial lines can also be used continuously to monitor or obtain repeated samples for arterial blood gas analysis, e.g. ventilated patients and those with respiratory failure. Patients who require arterial lines should be cared for in an environment where both they and the arterial line can be safely and adequately monitored, e.g. HDU/ITU.

Contraindications

Contraindications to arterial line insertion are the same as for arterial blood sampling (see 'Arterial blood sampling', p. 32). Deranged clotting or a bleeding diathesis will increase the risk of localized bleeding or haematoma.

Complications

Patients are at risk of haematoma, bleeding, infection and damage to the artery.

Procedure

Preparation

Explain the procedure and obtain consent. You will need the following equipment and you should assemble the line, transducer and pressure bag and check that the monitor is working before approaching the patient:

- sterile dressing pack, sterile gloves and gown, protective eyewear
- cleaning solution, e.g. iodine solution or other if the patient has an allergy
- suture pack/equipment
- an arterial line, see below
- transducer cable, pressure bag and appropriate fluids, e.g. 500/1000 mL bag of saline
- local anaesthetic (lidocaine 1–2%)
- 5 mL syringe, 23 or 25 gauge needle
- 2/0 or 3/0 silk suture
- sharps bin, disposal bag.

Arterial lines

There are several different types of arterial line, but they essentially fall into two groups:

- line over wire: the artery is located with a needle, down which a wire is inserted; after removal of the seeker needle, the arterial line is inserted over the guidewire
- line over needle: the arterial line is inserted over a needle, much like a cannula is inserted into a vein; do not use a venous cannula.

Method

- position the patient's hand: dorsiflex at 45–60° and tape in place if necessary; it may be helpful to place a 500 mL bag of fluid under the wrist to optimize position
- wash hands and put on gloves, gown and protective eyewear if required
- clean the site with the cleaning agent
- apply the sterile drape
- check the expiry date of the local anaesthetic and draw up 1–2 mL
- locate the radial artery with your non-dominant hand (see 'Method', p. 32)
- raise a skin bleb of local anaesthetic overlying the radial artery using as small a volume as possible; lidocaine must not be injected into a vessel, so you must always aspirate before injecting (see 'Local anaesthetics', p. 22)
- check the area is numb before proceeding
- insert the arterial cannula with your dominant hand at 40–45°; the technique you use will depend on the arterial line you have, see above
- the pulsation of arterial blood will confirm the correct location of the a-line, at which point you can cap the cannula or close the switch (if present)
- secure the a-line with a silk suture on either side (see 'Suturing', p. 63)
- attach the monitoring line

- calibrate the monitor to zero; if you cannot see an arterial waveform on the monitor, check the arterial line, the transducer, the monitor connections and ensure that the scale on the monitor is appropriate
- dispose of all equipment, including sharps, as per local infection control policy
- record the procedure in the notes with reference to site of insertion, drugs used with doses, initial blood pressure and any complications.

URINARY CATHETERIZATION

Indications

Urinary catheterization may be required as a short-term (<14 days) measure for:

- relief of acute urinary retention
- monitoring of urine output during critical illness
- drainage of urine and/or surgical debris following urological surgery
- urodynamic studies
- intravesical drug instillation.

Long-term (>14 days) catheterization may be necessary in patients with:

- incomplete emptying of the bladder due to neurological disorders or spinal cord damage
- bladder outlet obstruction in whom surgery is not possible
- intractable urinary incontinence.

Contraindications

Contraindications to urinary catheterization or conditions under which discussion with a urologist or more senior colleague are advisable are:

- abdominal or pelvic trauma
- immediately following open prostatectomy
- epididymitis
- haematuria, urethral obstruction, discharge or pus.

Complications

Complications include trauma and infection: most catheters are colonized with bacteria 48 h after insertion.

Procedure

Preparation

Explain the procedure to the patient, obtain consent and ensure privacy. Some hospitals provide a 'catheterization pack', which will include much of the following:

- dressing pack, absorbent pad, sterile bowl
- sterile gloves (2 pairs), disposable plastic apron
- sachet(s) of sterile saline solution (for cleansing)
- sterile local anaesthetic gel
- 2 sterile catheters of suitable type/size
- 10 mL sterile water and syringe, plus an extra syringe if changing catheter (to remove fluid from old balloon)
- drainage bag or valve and urine bag holder if appropriate.

Catheters

Periodic emptying of the bladder by a single catheterization has been shown to be effective and reduces the risk of infection associated with long-term catheterization. This form of catheterization is suitable for patients with chronic retention of urine or incomplete voiding who are sufficiently dexterous, or have a suitably trained carer.

Indwelling urethral catheters can be used when there are no contraindications, such as urethral closure or trauma, and when the patient has no preference for another type of catheter. They are commonly used for short-term catheterization in hospital inpatients. Where long-term catheterization (longer than 14 days) is required, Silastic® catheters should be used.

Catheter diameter The lumen of even the smallest catheter is sufficient to cope with the volume of urine normally produced. Larger catheters are only indicated where a smaller lumen would likely become blocked by debris, blood clots or mucus. To minimize trauma to the urethra, the smallest size possible must be used. In males the recommended standard diameter is size 12–16 F (French or Charrière). However, following transurethral resection of the prostate (TURP), a size 22–24 F catheter may be used to drain blood clots.

Catheter length A male length catheter is typically 45 cm long. A female length is available in most catheter ranges and is 25 cm long. Female length catheters should never be used in men, as the balloon will be inflated in the urethra and may cause urethral rupture.

Catheter balloon Catheter balloons are available in two standard sizes: 10 mL and 30 mL. In most circumstances, the balloon used will be 10 mL. Larger balloons are more likely to cause irritation, induce leakage, damage the bladder neck and cause infection.

Catheter balloons do not inflate uniformly and the total volume required for inflation must be used. Otherwise, the catheter tip may displace to the side, causing pressure on the trigone area, leading to spasm and bypassing.

Lubricant

A lubricant with anaesthetic and disinfectant properties should be used. This will reduce the risk of urethral injury, iatrogenic infection and also produces dilation of the urethral meatus.

Method

Male urinary catheterization

- sit the patient on the absorbent pad, ensuring they are not unduly exposed
- wash hands, put on apron and open the dressing pack
- open the remaining equipment onto the sterile dressing pack
- put on 2 pairs of sterile gloves
- clean the outside of the foreskin and retract
- cleanse urethral meatus and penis, swabbing away from the urethral orifice
- arrange the sterile drape and place so that the penis passes through the hole in the drape
- remove the outer pair of sterile gloves
- using a gauze swab hold the penis gently and laterally behind glans in vertical position
- instill approximately 10 mL anaesthetic gel; warn the patient that slight stinging may be experienced (may be reduced by chilling the gel)
- gently pinch the tip of the penis for at least 1 min before attempting to pass the catheter
- position the sterile bowl to catch urine and tear the top off the protective sleeve around the catheter, leaving the remainder in place to act as a sterile covering
- using a sterile gauze swab hold the penis in an upright position
- the catheter should pass easily and urine should flow within a few seconds; continue to advance to ensure that the balloon is within the bladder
- inflate the balloon with the correct amount of sterile water
- withdraw the catheter gently until slight resistance is felt
- if appropriate, a urine specimen can be collected for bacterial examination at this point
- attach the catheter to a closed drainage system

- it is essential that the foreskin is replaced back over the glans
- dispose of all equipment, as per local infection control policy
- record the following in the patient's records: the reason for catheterization, size of catheter, amount of water in the balloon, gel used, any complications.

Female urinary catheterization

Female catheterization should be performed using a shorter catheter (see above). Method is as per male catheterization with the following variation:

- identify and expose the urethral meatus by separating the labia minora
- cleanse the urethral orifice and surrounding area with cleansing solution (as above): cleansing should be carried out from the superior area in one downward motion)
- it may be necessary to use the index finger of the hand not being used to hold the catheter to 'landmark' the position of the urethra, in relation to the vagina
- once confident that the catheter is in the urethra, advance it approximately 7–9 cm, or until urine flow commences, then advance it a further 2 cm.

Suprapubic catheterization

Indications for suprapubic catheterization include urinary retention, chronic urethral infection, urethral stricture or trauma. It should not be attempted where there is an empty or indefinable bladder. Other contraindications include bladder malignancy and lower abdominal scarring.

Prepare and consent as above, except that cleaning should be of an area from symphysis pubis to umbilicus. Localization of the bladder is the most important part of this procedure. The use of a bladder scanner can help to determine the volume of the urinary bladder and bedside ultrasonography may be used to assist localization. If the bladder is not palpable and ultrasound is not available, the procedure should not be attempted.

Equipment is the same as for a transurethral approach, with the addition of local anaesthetic, 5 mL syringe and green needle, a suprapubic insertion kit with peel-away introducer sheath and a urinary catheter 1 Ch smaller than the introducer kit:

- palpate the symphysis pubis
- determine the entry site: 2 cm above the symphysis over a palpable bladder, or at a suitable site identified using ultrasound
- raise of bleb of local anaesthetic under the skin (see 'Local anaesthetics', p. 22) and then anaesthetize deeper subcutaneous tissues
- check that the skin is numb
- into the previously located bladder (see above), insert the introducer needle attached to a syringe
- if appropriate, a urine specimen can be collected for bacterial examination at this point
- remove the syringe and insert the guidewire through the needle
- make a small incision at the point of insertion and remove the needle
- thread the introducer over the wire and into the bladder
- remove the wire and then introduce the catheter through the introducer; a large volume of urine may escape through the introducer sheath unless the catheter is inserted efficiently
- inflate the balloon with the correct amount of sterile water
- remove the peel-away sheath introducer
- withdraw the catheter gently until slight resistance is felt
- secure the catheter to the abdominal wall with a sterile dressing
- connect the catheter to a closed drainage system and document the procedure in the notes.
- dispose of all equipment, including sharps, as per local infection control policy

LUMBAR PUNCTURE

The spinal cord lies within the spinal column, from the foramen magnum to the level of the L1–2 vertebrae. To avoid damage to the spinal cord, lumbar puncture must be performed below this level, into the CSF lying in the subarachnoid space between the arachnoid and pia mater.

Indications

- *diagnostic*: suspected meningitis or encephalopathies, subarachnoid haemorrhage, MS, Guillain–Barré syndrome
- *therapeutic*: spinal anaesthesia, intrathecal drug administration (e.g. steroids, antibiotics, chemotherapy), benign intracranial hypertension.

Contraindications

- *absolute*: infected skin over the needle entry site; raised intracranial pressure suggested by reduced GCS, focal neurological findings, papilloedema or abnormal brain imaging
- *relative*: intraspinal mass, coagulopathy, platelets <50, immunocompromised state, agitated or drowsy, severe degenerative spinal joint disease.

Complications

- headache (in up to 40%, may last for up to 8 days), backache
- CSF leakage, haemorrhage, bruising or infection at the puncture site
- coning: tonsillar or transtentorial herniation, suggested by severe headache, vomiting, focal neurology, papilloedema
- nerve root irritation, herniation and transection.

Procedure

Preparation

Explain the procedure and gain consent, ideally written. Ask the patient to adopt a curled position, lying on their side, as close to edge of the bed as possible with their knees raised to their chest and clasped by their hands (ask a second staff member to help support them). Expose the lumbar region and identify the posterior iliac crests; palpate the L4 spinous process lying on virtual line between them and mark it.

Equipment

- sterile gloves (2 pairs) and gown
- cleansing agent, local anaesthetic and sterile dressing pack with drapes
- 5 mL syringe and selection of ordinary needles
- lumbar puncture needles
- manometer and three-way tap (if pressure measurement required)
- glucose tube and 4 sterile universal containers, pre-numbered 1–4
- sterile occlusive dressing.

Method

- wash and dry hands, put on gown, 2 pairs of gloves and, with the help of an assistant, prepare the trolley and lay out the equipment in a sterile field
- connect the manometer to the three-way tap
- cleanse the skin: start at intended site of injection and work outwards in a circular motion, never returning to the centre with a used swab
- remove and discard the top set of gloves
- place sterile drapes around the exposed area

- raise a weal of local anaesthetic under the skin and infiltrate the subcutaneous tissue in relation to the L3–L4 interspace (see 'Local anaesthetic', p. 22); the needle should be held parallel to the floor and directed towards the umbilicus
- allow time for the anaesthetic to take effect
- slowly and firmly insert thc LP needle (as small as possible, e.g. 22 G) along the same tract as the local anaesthetic needle; you may feel a 'give' as you enter the subarachnoid space
- if you are unsure that you have entered the subarachnoid space, withdraw the stylet to check for a CSF flash-back
- if resistance is felt, e.g. due to contact with bone, the needle should be withdrawn and repositioned
- if a pressure measurement is required, attach the manometer before samples are taken (normal value: 5–20 cmH_2O)
- collect 10 drops of CSF into each into each of the pre-numbered containers in sequence (the container for the xanthochromia specimen should be filled last; see CSF, p. 74)
- once all specimens have been collected, remove the needle, apply pressure to the puncture site and then cover with an appropriate dressing
- dispose of all equipment, including sharps, as per local infection control policy
- instruct the patient to lie flat in bed for 4–6 h
- record the event in the notes and, if relevant, the pressure and samples taken.

PLEURAL ASPIRATION

Indications

Used for diagnostic sampling or therapeutic drainage of pleural effusions (see p. 150) and for the treatment of pneumothoraces (see 'Breathlessness', p. 148). Where a patient has abnormal clotting, consider the relative risks and benefits before proceeding.

Contraindications

There are no absolute contraindications, although care should be taken if the patient is anticoagulated or coagulopathic. Ideally, correct this first and proceed when the INR is <1.5.

Complications

Complications include pneumothorax and bleeding. Profound vagal responses may also occur and are particularly common in young men.

Procedure

Preparation

Review a recent chest radiograph to ensure correct location of the pathology. In the case of pleural fluid, clinical corroboration of the lung/fluid margin is necessary. Where this is not apparent on percussion and auscultation, a pleural ultrasound should be used to locate the fluid for safe aspiration, e.g. to avoid needle insertion below the diaphragm. Aseptic conditions are necessary (see 'Sterile field', p. 19). You will need an assistant to work with you and to reassure and monitor the patient.

Patient

Obtain written consent where possible, and document in the notes. Position the patient appropriately:

- for large clinically identifiable collections, sit the patient at the side of the bed with their arms crossed in front of them over a chair back or bedside table; use a pillow between the chair or table and patient for comfort
- in patients who are less fit, sit them forward in bed, leaning over pillows and supported by a nurse

- where ultrasound has been used to identify the aspiration site, you will need to adapt the position to reflect this.

Equipment

The equipment required to perform these procedures will depend on whether a diagnostic or therapeutic procedure is being performed. When performing a diagnostic aspiration 20–50 mL of pleural fluid should be withdrawn and sent to appropriate laboratories (see 'Pleural fluid', p. 76).

- sterile dressing pack, gloves and apron or gown
- lidocaine 1 or 2%
- 5–10 mL, 20 mL and 50 mL syringes
- cleaning solution, e.g. iodine solution or other if the patient has an allergy
- assortment of hypodermic needles
- occlusive dressing.

If you are performing a therapeutic aspiration, you will also need:

- size 14–16 gauge cannula
- 3-way tap
- tubing (e.g. drip set with bag cut off) and container to collect fluid (only if effusion present).

Method

Regardless of whether this is a therapeutic or diagnostic procedure, the following steps should be followed:

- choose site: for fluid, as determined by ultrasound or clinically within the region of the posterior axillary line and 1–2 intercostal spaces below the upper edge of the effusion; for air, 2nd intercostal space, midclavicular line or within the triangle of safety (see 'Chest drain insertion', p. 40)
- put on gloves and apron or gown
- clean the skin (see Fig. 2.1, p. 41)
- choose an approach above the rib to avoid the neurovascular bundle that lies beneath
- infiltrate down to the parietal pleura with local anaesthetic (see 'Local anaesthetic', p. 22); the presence of pleural fluid or air in the syringe confirms that you are within the pleural space
- check the area is numb before proceeding
- replace the needle with a 14 or 16 F cannula in the same way as you would cannulate a vein; take care to cover the cannula portal when removing the needle to prevent air being drawn in.

Diagnostic fluid aspirate

- connect your 20 or 50 mL syringe to the cannula
- fill your containers with the aspirate
- remove the cannula and cover the site with an occlusive dressing
- dispose of all equipment, including sharps, as per local infection control policy
- label the containers
- fill out appropriate forms, e.g. biochemistry, bacteriology and cytology (see 'Pleural fluid', p. 76)
- repeat the CXR to confirm no pneumothorax has developed
- document the procedure.

Therapeutic aspiration

- follow the instructions under 'Method' above
- connect the 3-way tap
- connect the 50 mL syringe to one side of the 3-way tap and the tubing to the other
- alternately aspirate fluid or air from the chest and expel it into the container or atmosphere

- if diagnostic samples are also required, collect these directly from the tubing into the tubes now
- note the number of aspirations to calculate the volume removed
- continue until resistance is felt or until 1.5–2 L of fluid or air have been removed (it is unwise to take more than this at one aspiration) (see 'Chest drain insertion', below)
- remove the cannula and cover the site with an occlusive dressing
- dispose of all equipment, including sharps, as per local infection control policy
- repeat the CXR to confirm lung re-expansion
- measure pulse and blood pressure
- document the procedure.

CHEST DRAIN INSERTION AND MANAGEMENT

The investigation and management of pleural disease is covered in 'Breathlessness', p. 139. The drainage of air or other material from the pleural space is desirable in patients with a variety of pleural diseases. This is usually achieved by inserting a chest drain, as repeated pleural aspiration is time-consuming, unpleasant for the patient, more likely to lead to complications and, in many cases, less effective.

Indications

- tension pneumothorax, following needle decompression
- primary spontaneous pneumothorax: after failed aspiration or where the pneumothorax is large and poorly tolerated
- secondary spontaneous pneumothorax: chest drain usually first-line; aspiration can be attempted first if minimal symptoms and patient <50 years old and pneumothorax small
- traumatic pneumothorax or haemothorax
- empyema: as indicated by pus on aspiration or pleural fluid pH <7.2 or positive pleural culture
- malignant effusions: for relief of symptoms; also to facilitate ward pleurodesis in patients not fit enough for VATS procedure.

Contraindications

- lung adherent to chest wall, e.g. previous pleurodesis
- bleeding tendency (relative): if possible correct and aim for INR <1.5; routine checking of Coag and Plt not required unless risk factors are present.

Complications

- pain: this is common, see below
- vaso-vagal reaction on entry into the pleural space: more common in young men; lie the patient flat
- malposition: may require withdrawal; never advance a drain that is sticking out
- organ damage, e.g. liver, spleen, lung, heart, great vessels, stomach
- re-expansion pulmonary oedema: especially young patients who present late with a large pneumothorax and in rapidly drained effusions; less likely if the amount drained suddenly is limited to 1 L; may be associated with haemodynamic compromise, treat as pulmonary oedema, see p. 146
- haemorrhage into the drain: malignant effusions can be very bloody; large volume, high pressure drainage suggests intercostal vessel or organ damage; clamp drain, image urgently and liaise with a cardiothoracic surgeon
- surgical emphysema: more likely in patients with a pneumothorax; check whether there is an air leak around the drain or whether the drain has become displaced such that the side-holes lie subcutaneously

- intrapulmonary placement: suggested by bleeding and a large continuous air leak; occurs in 3% of trauma patients
- infection: empyema rate is 1%, higher in traumatic pneumothorax
- late displacement: drains should rarely (if ever) fall out if secured properly.

Procedure

Preparation

Patient

Before you start, examine the patient, review the CXR and any other imaging; check the side that the drain is required. Explain the procedure and its risks to the patient; obtain consent (ideally written) and IV access.

The patient should be positioned sitting in bed at 30°. Rotate the affected side slightly upwards and ask the patient to hold their arm behind their head. This opens the intercostal spaces slightly.

If possible, a chest drain should be placed laterally in the triangle of safety (Fig. 2.1). This may not be possible in localized posterior pleural fluid collections, but minimizes the chance of damaging intercostal vessels. These structures run in the middle of the intercostal space posteromedially and only tuck underneath the ribs as they move anterolaterally. A laterally situated drain is also more comfortable for the patient, as they can sleep on their back.

Equipment

Chest drain There are two principal types of chest drain. The traditional, Argyle, drain is a relatively stiff chest drain mounted on a sharp metal trocar. Placement of this type of drain requires blunt dissection through the subcutaneous and intercostal tissues down to the pleura. A defect is then made in the parietal pleura and

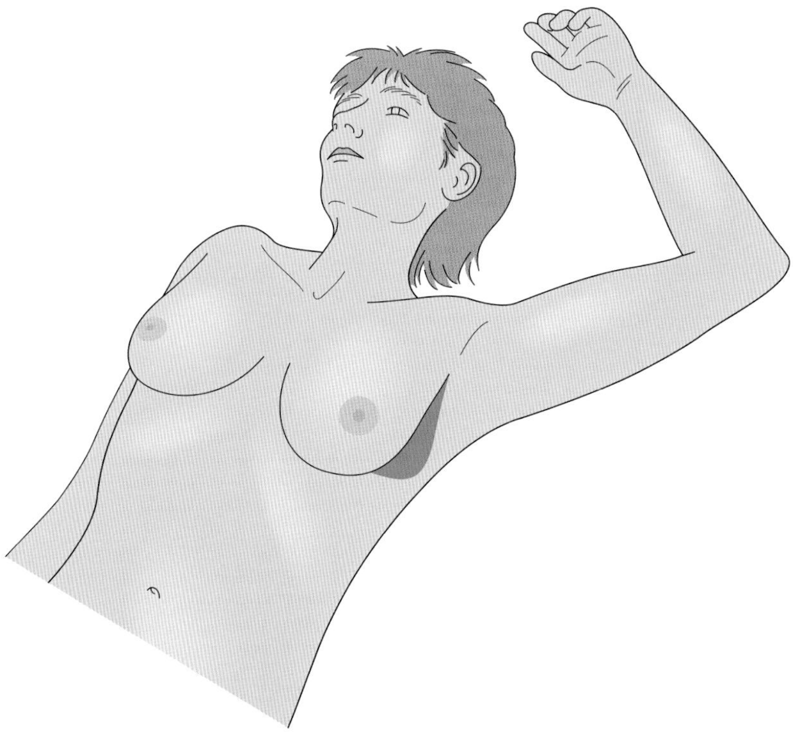

Figure 2.1 Triangle of safety for chest drain insertion. The marked area is bounded anteriorly by the lateral border of pectoralis major, posteriorly by the anterior border of latissimus dorsi and inferiorly by the 6th rib.

the drain inserted after removing (i.e. not using) the trocar. This technique can be dangerous and has been largely superseded by the more modern Seldinger-type drain. These are inserted over a guidewire and are safer and less unpleasant for the patient. A 'dial-up' system of dilators can facilitate placement of large-bore chest tubes using this technique.

Small drains (12–16 F) are more comfortable for the patient and are as effective as large bore tubes in the majority of circumstances. Larger drains (28–32 F) are indicated in the following situations:

- pneumothorax with a large, persistent air leak indicating a broncho-pleural fistula
- surgical emphysema despite a functioning small bore tube
- empyema: the turbidity of the fluid leads to an increased chance of tube blockage
- haemothorax: due to the likelihood that blood clot will block the tube.

Trolley

You will need the following:

- a selection of needles and a 10 mL Luer-Lok syringe
- 10 mL 2% lidocaine, pre-medication if appropriate, e.g. 1–2 mg midazolam IV and opiate analgesia, e.g. 2.5–5 mg morphine IV
- chest drain pack, e.g. Cook® or Portex®, including tubing which is often wrapped separately, and either a 3-way tap, if this fits your drainage set, or a set of chest drain clamps
- underwater seal drainage bottle and sterile water
- sterile dressing pack and cleaning solution, e.g. Betadine®
- sterile drape, gown and hand-towel and sterile gloves
- 2 stitches, scissors, pack of swabs and adhesive, e.g. Hypafix® or a specific chest drain fixing dressing (not available in some units).

Method

- wash your hands while your assistant opens and places on the trolley the sterile dressing pack, needles, syringe, drapes and the gown and hand-towel
- dry your hands and put on the gown and gloves
- open your sterile dressing pack and ask your assistant to pour out some cleaning solution and open the vials of lidocaine
- clean the skin over the insertion site
- anaesthetize the skin and subcutaneous tissues down to the pleura (see 'Local anaesthetics', p. 22); entry into pleural space is indicated by the withdrawal of air bubbles or pleural fluid into your syringe
- while your local anaesthetic takes effect, open the chest drain set and tubing and ask your assistant to fill the drainage bottle with water up to the appropriate level
- check the skin overlying the insertion site is numb
- pass your introducer needle into the pleural space with the bevel pointing upwards to direct the guidewire to the apex of the lung (pneumothorax) or downwards to direct it to the base (pleural fluid); as before entry into the pleural space is indicated by the withdrawal of air bubbles or pleural fluid into your syringe
- once you are confident the tip of your needle is in the pleural space, twist off and remove your syringe and load your guidewire onto the back the introducer needle
- pass the guidewire into the pleural space: do not do so unless you are confident you are in the pleural space
- use the scalpel blade in the chest drain set to make a small stab incision at either side of your needle/wire assembly; only cut the skin, do not try to cut muscle; keep the face of the blade pointing away from needle/wire
- keeping the wire in place, remove the introducer needle

- feed your introducer(s) over the wire into the pleural space using a twisting steady pressure and then remove them using the opposite action; large-bore drains use a series of 'dial-up' dilators which progressively increase in diameter and should be used sequentially; control any leakage of fluid/air at the insertion site using a swab and if necessary increase the size of your skin defect as the diameter of the dilators increase
- once the last introducer, which is usually 2 F wider in diameter than the drain, has been removed, feed your drain over the guidewire and into pleural space; estimate how far to insert your drain by comparing to the size of patient's chest; ensure you insert the drain far enough so that all of the side holes lie in the pleural cavity
- remove the central stiffening rod from the centre of the chest drain bore: holding it in the first three fingers of your hand, and clamping the wire against your palm with your little finger, you can remove the wire at the same time
- connect the drain to the tubing, which should be attached to the underwater seal and placed below the insertion site; use a 3-way tap between the drain and tubing if possible, this facilitates easy flushing and pleurodesis if required
- if a large volume (>1 L) of pleural fluid drains immediately, consider clamping the drain or closing the 3-way tap to avoid re-expansion pulmonary oedema; this can also ease severe pleuritic pain which can accompany rapid re-expansion of the lung
- pleural fluid or condensation in the tubing, in pneumothorax and pleural effusions respectively, confirms correct placement in the pleural space
- insert a loose stitch to the left of the drain site (a tight stitch will cause skin necrosis and fall out) and leave both ends of equal length; wrap one, then the other end of the stitch around the drain and tie securely where they meet; repeat this to the right of the drain
- dress the drain securely using a specific chest drain fixing; alternatively use a strong adhesive dressing, e.g. Hypafix®: run a strip from the chest up each of the four sides of the drain and then connecting strips across where these meet the chest
- tape the connection between the drain and the tubing
- create a securing loop: attach the middle of a further piece of Hypafix® to the tubing near the drain connection; fold and oppose about 5 cm of the tape leaving two free ends to attach to the skin
- dispose of all equipment, including sharps, as per local infection control policy
- request a CXR to document position of the drain
- document the procedure in the notes.

Drain management

Patients with chest drains should be managed on a specialist ward if possible. The drainage bottle must always be kept below the insertion site. Chest drain observations should be recorded including pain, RR, SaO_2, HR, BP, volume of fluid in the bottle and whether the drain is swinging and/or bubbling.

A swinging drain indicates the drain is in the pleural space and functioning. A drain that is not swinging is kinked, blocked, clamped or out. If the drain still looks in the right place, consider flushing the tube with 30 mL of sterile saline and remove any drain that is still not functioning.

A persistently bubbling drain (when the patient breathes or coughs) indicates that there is a communication between the lung and the water in the drainage bottle. This is most commonly due to a bronchopleural fistula (i.e. a tear in the visceral pleura), but may also reflect an air-leak in the drainage system. Therefore, check the connections in the system and the skin wound. Do not ever remove a bubbling drain.

Clamping chest drains

Generally speaking, you should not clamp chest drains. In particular, never clamp a bubbling drain, as this may precipitate a tension pneumothorax. Occasionally, drains are clamped to control the rate of pleural fluid drainage and avoid re-expansion pulmonary oedema. On specialist units, drains are occasionally clamped temporarily, and under close supervision, as a 'trial before removal' in patients with pneumothorax in whom drain re-insertion would be extremely difficult. However, this should not be performed routinely and without senior consultation.

Drain removal

Following a pneumothorax, the drain should be removed once the lung has completely re-expanded, the drain has stopped bubbling (indicating closure of the precipitating pleural tear) and at least 24h has elapsed since it was inserted. For pleural effusions of any type, the drain should be removed once the pleural cavity is dry or when pleural fluid drainage falls below 150mL/day, assuming the drain is not bubbling. Any chest drain that is not functioning should be removed.

There is no clear consensus on how to remove a chest drain. Whether the drain is removed at maximum inspiration or expiration probably does not matter. Have some swabs, a fresh stitch and dressing ready. Wearing gloves and an apron, use a stitch-cutter to remove the stitches. Advise the patient to hold their breath and extract the tube smoothly. Seal the hole, using the stitch if necessary; this is often not the case with small-bore tubes. Apply an occlusive dressing and request a CXR to document lung position. Record the event in the case-notes.

NASOGASTRIC TUBE INSERTION

Indications

Nasogastric (NG) or Ryle's tubes are passed without guidance into the stomach via the nasopharynx and oesophagus. They are most commonly used to deliver short-term nutritional support and oral medications to patients who are unable to swallow. If the ability to swallow does not return within 6 weeks, placement of a percutaneous feeding tube should be considered. NG tubes can also be used to decompress and empty the stomach in patients with bowel obstruction or gastroparesis.

Fine-bore tubes (<9 F) are better tolerated and are less commonly associated with complications (see below). However, if large volumes of drainage are expected, e.g. in small bowel obstruction, a larger-bore tube should be used.

Contraindications

A NG tube should not be passed in patients with:

- known gastric stasis or severe gastro-oesophageal reflux
- oesophageal stricture
- basal skull fractures, facial or nasal trauma.

Complications

Complications include incorrect placement (e.g. in a proximal airway), reflux, aspiration and local irritation (e.g. rhinitis, pharyngitis, oesophageal erosions).

Procedure

Preparation

Before you start, explain the procedure to the patient and gain their consent. Check your trolley: you will need a NG tube (usually fine bore, see above), lubricant anaesthetic jelly, e.g. Instillagel®, and tape to secure the tube at the nose.

Position the patient in bed, sitting at 45° with their neck in a neutral position. Examine the nose and verify that the nostrils are patent. Estimate how much of the tube you will have to pass; this is done by measuring the tube from the bridge of the nose to the earlobe and then down to a point halfway between the xiphisternum and umbilicus. Mark the required length with a marker or note the measurement on the side of the tube corresponding to the point identified.

Method

- lubricate the distal 3–4 cm of the tube
- insert the tube gently into the most widely patent nostril
- advance the tube smoothly and ask the patient to swallow when they feel a sensation at the back of their throat; if they have difficulty or the tube coils in the mouth give them a glass of water to sip at the same time
- if resistance is felt, try twisting the tube as you advance, but do not force it
- if the patient coughs or becomes distressed, stop and withdraw
- advance the tube to the marked distance and secure it with tape at the nose
- check tube position before use; this can be done by either performing a CXR or testing the pH of aspirated material using Litmus paper (pH <4 indicates gastric contents, but higher values may be found in patients on acid suppressing drugs).

PEG TUBE RE-INSERTION

Indications

PEG tubes may be dislodged intentionally or accidentally. Where this does occur, the tract can close relatively quickly and it is therefore important that a urinary catheter is inserted into the tract until a PEG tube can be re-inserted.

Contraindications

There are no specific contraindications.

Complications

Complications relate to trauma associated with attempted replacement, or infection of the site.

Procedure

Preparation

Before you start, explain the procedure to the patient and gain consent. You will need:

- a sterile dressing pack and sterile gloves
- cleaning solution, e.g. iodine solution (or other if the patient has an allergy)
- PEG tube (same size as original)
- sterile water (for balloon inflation), 5 mL syringe and lubricant gel
- disposal bag.

Once you have prepared your trolley, position the patient lying on their back with the PEG site exposed.

Method

- if a catheter has been inserted to maintain tract patency, remove it
- wash hands and put on gloves
- clean the site with swabs and the cleaning agent
- check that the balloon on the PEG tube inflates correctly and deflate it again
- draw the correct volume of water into the syringe for balloon inflation later

- lubricate the end of the PEG tube and insert into tract, applying pressure and gently rotating; if the PEG tube will not advance, try a small-diameter tube
- insert the tube completely and inflate the balloon (with the specified volume of water); draw back gently until resistance is felt
- secure in place (usually with the device attached to the PEG tube)
- dispose of all equipment as per infection control policy
- record the procedure in the notes.

ASCITIC TAP AND DRAIN INSERTION

Indications

A diagnostic ascitic tap (also known as abdominal paracentesis) should be performed in patients with ascites of unknown aetiology. This allows measurement of the protein, albumin and cellular content of ascitic fluid. It is particularly important in patients with decompensated chronic liver disease, in whom spontaneous bacterial peritonitis and malignancy must be actively excluded.

Removal of larger volumes of ascitic fluid may also be desirable for symptomatic relief in patients with tense ascites unresponsive to medical therapy (around 5% of patients). Repeated small volume paracentesis is time consuming and increases the risk of ascitic leakage and infection. Therefore, it should be avoided and a large volume paracentesis (LVP) performed instead.

Contraindications

LVP should be avoided, if possible, in patients who are hypovolaemic or have low blood pressure. Contraindications for LVP and ascitic tap include:

- infection of the overlying skin
- severe uncorrected coagulopathy
- known intra-abdominal adhesions
- distended bowel (e.g. obstruction) or bladder
- pregnancy.

Complications

Ascitic tap or LVP may result in trauma to vascular or intra-abdominal structures, introduction of infection or a persistent fluid leak from the aspiration/insertion site.

The risk of infection following LVP can be minimized by removal of the drain within 6 h of insertion. Other complications of LVP include hypernatraemia and circulatory disturbance which may result in hepatorenal syndrome. This risk can be minimized by appropriate fluid replacement, including administration of albumin (see below).

Procedure

Preparation

Explain the procedure to the patient and gain consent, ideally written. Confirm that ascites is present by eliciting shifting dullness. If the bladder is palpable consider urinary catheterization, see, p. 34. Identify an appropriate site for diagnostic aspiration or drain insertion (see below). Ensure that the patient has an intravenous cannula in situ and position them on their back with pillows under the opposite side to rotate them slightly towards you.

Site

Identify a point 2 cm lateral to the intersection of a line running transversely across the abdomen from the umbilicus and another running longitudinally from the mid-inguinal point. Avoid any previous surgical scars and ensure there is underlying dullness to percussion. If you are unsure about the presence or absence of fluid, consider requesting ultrasonography to guide positioning.

Diagnostic ascitic tap

Equipment

- sterile dressing pack and sterile gloves
- cleaning solution
- 20 mL or 50 mL syringe with an appropriate needle; see below
- sterile specimen containers
- containers for any additional fluid that may be removed
- sterile dressing
- sharps bin, disposal bag.

Needle choice This will depend on the volume of fluid to be removed and the thickness of the abdominal wall. In obese patients, a longer needle will be required; use a white needle, a large-bore cannula or a metal LP needle.

Method

- wash hands and put on sterile gloves
- cleanse the area of insertion and position the drape, (see 'Sterile field', p. 21)
- local anaesthetic is often not necessary, but should be offered: if required raise a skin bleb and then anaesthetize skin and subcutaneous tissue; wait for the local anaesthetic to take effect (see also 'Local anaesthetics', p. 22)
- using your non-dominant hand, stretch and displace the insertion site to one side; this 'z-track' reduces leakage of ascitic fluid after withdrawal of the needle
- with your dominant hand slowly and smoothly insert the needle and syringe aspirating intermittently; insert the needle by no more than 5 mm between aspirations
- on aspiration of ascitic fluid, stop advancing the needle and aspirate an appropriate volume of fluid; remove the needle
- transfer the fluid to sterile containers and label them
- dispose of all materials according to local protocol; fill out the laboratory form and send the samples
- record the procedure in the patient's notes.

Large volume paracentesis

Equipment

- sterile dressing pack and sterile gloves
- cleaning solution
- local anaesthetic, e.g. 1% or 2% lidocaine
- 5 mL and 10 mL syringes with a variety of needles (a long needle will be needed if the patient is obese; see above)
- Banano®, or other suitable drainage catheter
- catheter bag and appropriate tubing
- sterile dressing
- salt-poor albumin for IV administration; see below
- sharps bin, disposal bag.

Albumin To avoid infection, fluid should be drained rapidly. However, LVP can result in huge fluid shifts, leading to a fall in right atrial pressure and systemic vascular resistance, particularly during the first 3 h. This can be dangerous in patients with chronic liver disease, who may already be intravascular deplete as a result of diuretic therapy. This risk can be reduced by intravascular volume expansion with salt-poor albumin solution.

Albumin is a blood product and, therefore, you will need to order it through the haematology lab. This should be done before starting the procedure and you may have to discuss its use with the on-call haematology consultant (see 'Blood Products', p. 122).

Guidance on the amount of albumin replacement necessary varies. Usually, following the first 3 L of ascitic fluid drainage, 1 vial of albumin is administered for every subsequent 3 L of fluid drained. However, check your local protocol and ensure you have all the patient's details available when making the phone call to haematology.

Method

- unpack the Banano® catheter; some packs have an plastic sheath over the catheter that keeps it straight if the needle is not in situ; this should be removed
- check that the drainage tubing attaches to the catheter appropriately
- follow the instructions given for ascitic tap above
- assemble the Banano® catheter and hold it at the insertion site, at 90° to the skin
- insert the catheter with your dominant hand; hold the catheter with your non-dominant hand close to where it enters the skin; this allows you to control the rate of insertion
- you will feel a 'give' as the needle enters the peritoneal cavity and ascitic fluid will start to flow
- holding the needle with one hand, advance the catheter over the needle (much akin to inserting a cannula) until the catheter is fully inserted
- remove the needle and connect the drainage bag
- apply a sterile dressing
- dispose of all materials according to local protocol; if samples have been taken, fill out the laboratory form and send the samples
- record the procedure in the patient's notes and ensure they have adequate analgesia prescribed
- the drain should be removed as soon as possible, ideally within 6 h of insertion.

JOINT ASPIRATION AND INJECTION

Indications

Joint aspiration should be performed where septic arthritis, haemarthrosis or crystal arthropathy is suspected. This allows inspection of the synovial fluid (for pus and blood) and laboratory analysis for inflammatory cells, microorganisms and crystals. Joint aspiration may also provide symptomatic relief in patients with large effusions due to degenerative joint disease.

Corticosteroid injection is an effective means of controlling pain and reducing inflammation in single joints affected by osteoarthritis, rheumatoid arthritis and other inflammatory arthropathies.

Contraindications

- infection overlying the joint
- severe uncorrected bleeding disorders
- joint injection with corticosteroid is absolutely contraindicated if there is any possibility of septic arthritis; this must be actively excluded.

Complications

- introduction of infection (risk <1 in 10 000 if strict asepsis is maintained)
- synovial trauma and bleeding
- injury to tendon or nerves, due to incorrect needle placement
- local reaction to injected corticosteroid, e.g. atrophy of overlying skin, post-injection symptom flare (due to synovitis), joint destruction
- systemic affects of corticosteroid injection, e.g. tendon weakening/rupture, muscle wasting, facial flushing or deterioration in diabetic control (more common if multiple joints are injected frequently with high doses of steroids).

Procedure

Most peripheral joints can be aspirated simply and safely on the ward, or in A&E. However, less accessible joints, such as the hip or spine, may require image-guided or surgical aspiration in theatre. Prosthetic joints should only be aspirated in theatre, because of the consequences of introducing infection.

Preparation

Explain the procedure to the patient and gain consent, ideally written. Prepare your trolley; you will need a sterile dressing pack, cleaning solution, e.g. Betadine® or 1% chlorhexidine, a pair of sterile gloves, 5–10 mL of 1% or 2% lidocaine, a selection of needles and two 10 mL syringes (three if you plan to inject steroids into the joint).

Before you wash your hands and put on sterile gloves it is essential that you examine the joint, identify the relevant bony landmarks, see below, and mark your needle insertion point.

Injection points and patient positioning

Knee joint

- lie the patient on a bed or examination couch with their leg straight
- identify the superior lateral border of the patella; mark the skin 1 cm caudal and 1 cm lateral to this point
- the angle of insertion will be at 45° caudally and 45° below the patella.

Shoulder: glenohumeral joint (anterior approach)

- sit the patient with the arm resting at their side and the shoulder externally rotated
- palpate the head of the humerus, coracoid process and acromion
- the insertion point is medial to the head of the humerus and 1 cm lateral to the coracoid process; during insertion the needed should be directed posteriorly and slightly superiorly and laterally.

Method

- once you have examined the joint and marked the insertion point, wash your hands and put on the sterile gloves
- wash the skin overlying the insertion site with cleaning solution (see 'Cleaning the skin', p. 21)
- draw 5–10 mL of lidocaine into a 10 mL syringe
- infiltrate the skin and subcutaneous tissues with local anaesthetic
- change to a fresh syringe and needle; after verifying that the overlying skin is numb, insert the needle into the joint space, aspirating as you advance.

Diagnostic aspirate

- once synovial fluid enters the syringe, stop advancing and collect 10–20 mL
- fill the sterile sample containers, dress the wound and dispose of your equipment safely
- send samples for analysis to microbiology (Gram-stain and culture), biochemistry (protein, glucose, crystal microscopy) and cytology (white cell count, including differential)
- record the procedure in the patient's notes; document the colour and viscosity of the fluid aspirated.

Joint injections

- if there is an effusion, entry into the joint space will be verified by aspiration of fluid; if there is no effusion, accurate placement of the needle in the joint space may be more difficult
- keeping the needle in place, remove the aspirating syringe and replace it with the syringe containing corticosteroid; inject this slowly into the joint space
- remove the needle and syringe, dress the wound and dispose of your equipment safely.

Post-procedure

Physical activity should be limited for 24 h because increased circulation may cause medication 'wash out' and increased activity increases the risk of complications. In the setting of septic arthritis, complete drainage of infected synovial fluid is essential and may require repeated aspiration.

CENTRAL LINE INSERTION

Indications

Central venous line insertion allows measurement of central venous pressure (CVP) and access to the central veins for administration of cardiotropic and vasopressor drugs and irritant, hypertonic solutions (e.g. TPN). A broadly similar insertion technique can be used to site a haemodialysis line or an introducer sheath for transvenous pacing or pulmonary artery catheterization.

Measurement of CVP is often desirable in critically ill or shocked patients. CVP is commonly used as a surrogate of left heart filling pressures. As such, it can guide intravenous fluid resuscitation and balance the risks of hypotension due to under-filling against those of pulmonary oedema due to fluid overload. CVP measurements are also useful in identifying patients with distributive forms of shock, who tend to be hypotensive despite a normal or high CVP; see 'Shock', p. 250.

CVP measurements may not accurately reflect intravascular volume in patients with pulmonary hypertension (most commonly due to severe lung disease and mitral valve disease) or impaired RV function, e.g. following RV infarction.

Contraindications

Superior vena cava obstruction, or infection over the proposed insertion site, are absolute contraindications. Relative contraindications include abnormal coagulation (which should be corrected if possible beforehand), recent cannulation of the target vein and carotid disease.

Complications

Advice on the management of insertion-related early complications is given below. These include arterial puncture, cardiac arrhythmias, perforation or tamponade, pneumothorax and air embolism. Complications that occur later include venous thrombosis, infection, chylothorax (due to thoracic duct injury) and haemothorax (due to vascular or lung injury).

Procedure

Preparation

Patient

Consent, ideally written, should be obtained beforehand, although this may not be possible in critically ill patients. For internal jugular (IJ) and subclavian (SC) lines, the patient should lie supine, with their head at the top of the bed, which should be tilted head down (this reduces the chance of an air embolus). However, the amount of time the patient will be able to spend in this position may be minimal if they are breathless. If an IJ line is being inserted, the patient should be advised that a drape will cover at least part of their face, but reassured that a member of staff will be nearby if they feel claustrophobic or distressed. If a femoral line is being inserted, the patient should lie flat, with the leg on the side to be cannulated abducted by around 30°.

Ultrasound guidance

Two-dimensional ultrasound scanning (US) has been shown to reduce failure rates and the incidence of complications during internal jugular line placement. As a result, NICE guidelines have recommended that all internal jugular lines should be placed using US guidance where a suitable device is available, e.g. Site-Rite®.

This assumes appropriate training and competency and should not delay line placement in an emergency.

Site of insertion, surface anatomy and approach

Cannulation of the internal jugular vein or subclavian vein allows placement of the line tip in the superior vena cava and measurement of central venous pressure. This is not possible using a femoral line, which should only be sited for intravenous access.

The choice between an IJ and a SC line depends on a number of factors including the operator (choose the site that you have most experience with), any lines that are already in situ (or have been recently removed) and anatomical factors (see below). IJ lines are often considered to be the safest of the alternatives as US guidance is feasible and pneumothorax is less likely. In addition, in contrast to the subclavian artery, the carotid artery is directly compressible, if it is punctured accidentally during IJ vein cannulation.

Internal jugular vein The IJV runs in the carotid sheath just posterolateral to the carotid artery. It lies medial to the body of the sternocleidomastoid (SCM) muscle in the upper part of the neck, passes between the two heads of sternocleidomastoid in the middle third of the neck and then joins with the subclavian vein, under the sternal end of the clavicle.

Locate the IJ vein at the level of the thyroid cartilage around the division of the two heads of sternocleidomastoid. When using ultrasound, the IJ vein can be identified by the following characteristics:

- it is usually bigger than the carotid artery
- it will be compressible
- it will increase in size if the patient performs a Valsalva manoeuvre.

If you are using surface anatomy alone to locate the IJ vein, palpate the carotid artery at the level of the thyroid cartilage at two points. The IJ vein should run just lateral to a line joining these points. Insert the needle at a 45° angle to the skin, aspirating as you go.

Subclavian vein The subclavian vein is a continuation of the axillary vein. It lies below and parallel to the clavicle. The subclavian artery is superior and posterior to the vein and is separated from it by the anterior scalene muscle.

US guidance is not generally helpful when inserting a SC line. Instead, after turning the head to the opposite side and adopting a head-down position as above, the vein can be located by inserting a needle 1 cm below the junction of the middle and medial thirds of the clavicle. While aspirating, keep the needle horizontal and direct it medially, under the inferior border of the clavicle, towards the suprasternal notch. It is safest to hit the clavicle with your needle initially; this will allow you to find and slip under its inferior border. As you move medially, the vein should be found after about 4–5 cm.

Femoral vein The femoral vein runs alongside the femoral artery in the thigh and drains into the external iliac vein at the level of the inguinal ligament. It lies medial to the femoral artery in the femoral triangle. While US may be used to locate vessels, there is little evidence to suggest it improves either cannulation rates or complications.

Feel for the femoral pulse in the groin at the mid-inguinal point (midway between the symphysis pubis and anterior superior iliac spine). The femoral vein can be found 1 cm medial and 1 cm caudal to the artery at this point. Insert your needle at a 20–30° angle to skin, pointing in a cephalic direction. Aspirate continually until you enter the vein.

Equipment

You will need the following:

- US machine, e.g. Site-Rite®, if available, including sterile sheath, rubber bands and sterile contact gel

- central line pack including the line, a dilator, guidewire, introducer needle and syringe
- sterile dressing pack, sterile gloves and gown, protective eyewear
- hernia towel, if available
- cleaning solution, e.g. Betadine® or 1% chlorhexidine
- 5–10 mL of 1% or 2% lidocaine and a selection of needles and syringes
- scalpel and 2 sutures
- sterile dressing
- sharps bin and disposal bag.

Method

Before you scrub up or put on the sterile gown and gloves, you should position the patient appropriately and identify the surface landmarks you will use to locate the vein (as above). If an US machine is available you should identify the target vein at this point and ensure that it is patent before proceeding. It is not necessary to sterilize the skin or US machine at this point.

The following description is for the insertion of a central line using the Seldinger technique:

- position the patient and identify the relevant surface landmarks as above
- if you have used US to identify the target vein, wash off any excess contact gel from the patient's skin and the probe before you proceed
- ask your assistant to open the equipment; take each item and place the sterile contents of each, including the central line kit, onto your trolley (see 'Sterile field', p. 19)
- put on protective eyewear, if required, wash your hands and put on the sterile gown and gloves
- remove (and keep) the caps from each lumen of the line, open the clips on each lumen and flush each one with sterile saline; then lock them and replace each cap
- if you are using an US machine, instruct your assistant to apply sterile contact gel to the surface of the probe; this ensures an air-free interface between skin and probe
- open the sterile sheath and gather it such that your assistant can carefully lower the transducer by its cable onto the inner surface of the end of the sheath; you should then carefully extend the cover over the US cable taking care not to touch it with your gloved hands; secure the sheath by wrapping the sterile rubber bands round the transducer and place the, now sterile, assembly on your trolley
- clean the skin over the target vein (see 'Cleaning the skin', p. 21) and apply a hernia towel, or at least 2 sterile drapes to cover the surrounding area
- draw up 5–10 mL of 1% or 2% lidocaine (see also 'Local anaesthetics', p. 22)
- identify the target vein, using US or the surface landmarks given above
- infiltrate the skin and overlying tissues with local anaesthetic, taking care to aspirate before each injection; if you enter the target vein with the LA needle, withdraw the needle and be careful not to inject any anaesthetic
- put down the LA needle and, after verifying that the overlying skin is numb, insert the introducer needle attached to a 5 or 10 mL Luer-Lok syringe
- advance the needle, aspirating as you go (see 'Surface anatomy and approach' above)
- if you are using US guidance the needle should be placed in the guide channel on the transducer and the vein should be kept in the centre of the screen
- venous puncture is confirmed by easy aspiration of dark red blood into the syringe chamber; you may see the vein deform on US as the needle punctures it

- carefully remove the syringe from the introducer needle without altering its position and attach the guidewire assembly (in some systems you may be able to thread the guidewire directly through a channel in the centre of the syringe without having to remove it)
- slowly and smoothly advance the guidewire to around 10–15 cm; if resistance is felt, remove the wire and reattach the syringe to verify that you are still in the vein; do not push blindly; atrial ectopics suggest you are in too far, so withdraw a little
- take the scalpel and slide it down each side of the guidewire (still covered by the introducer needle for extra protection), making small stab incisions to accommodate the dilator and line
- holding the wire, slide the introducer needle back off the guidewire and control any local bleeding with a swab
- thread the dilator onto the guidewire
- while holding the proximal end of the guidewire with your non-dominant hand, advance the dilator using a twisting motion through the skin and subcutaneous tissues; you do not need to advance it all the way down the vein
- remove the dilator with your dominant hand, ensuring that the wire is held at all times with your other hand; expect some local bleeding and control this with a swab
- thread the central line over the guidewire, holding onto the wire near the skin as you do so; once the line reaches the skin, stop advancing the line and start withdrawing the guidewire
- as the wire passes up the line it will enter one of the central lumens; remove the cap, open the clip occluding this lumen and withdraw the wire; only when you can hold onto the end of the guidewire with your non-dominant hand should you advance the line over the wire through the skin
- insert the central line to around 15 cm
- gently withdraw the guidewire and close the clip of the relevant lumen
- check that blood can be aspirated freely from all lumens and flush them with saline
- stitch the line in place using a suture on either side
- cover with a sterile dressing
- dispose of all sharps carefully and document the procedure in the notes
- before the line is used organize a CXR to verify the position of the line tip: it should sit at the junction between the superior vena cava and right atrium.

Management of complications during insertion

- arterial puncture: suggested by bright red, or highly pressurized, blood in the introducer syringe or lines; this may be less obvious in patients who are hypoxic or hypotensive; if in doubt, check an ABG on blood from the line; if confirmed remove the needle/line and apply direct, firm pressure (not possible from subclavian approach)
- pneumothorax: suggested by acute breathlessness and aspiration of air into the introducer needle; treat as per outlined in 'Pneumothorax', p. 149.
- air embolus: may occur if the needle or cannula is left open to the air; more common in hypotensive patients, but preventable by ensuring the patient is positioned head down
- the wire will not come out through the introducer needle: remove the needle with the wire in it; this reduces the risk of the end of the wire being severed by the needle tip
- arrhythmias: usually occur if the line has been inserted too far (into the right atrium); the average distance to the right atrium is 15 cm; withdraw the line a little

- persistent bleeding: apply firm and direct pressure to the site; bleeding should stop unless there is a coagulopathy; persistent and severe bleeding may require exploration by the surgical team if there has been an arterial or venous tear.

TEMPORARY CARDIAC PACING

Temporary cardiac pacing is used when heart block and other bradyarrhythmias compromise cardiac output. These rhythms may arise as a consequence of acute myocardial infarction, metabolic upset or drug overdose, and guidance on their identification and management is provided in 'Rhythm disorders', p. 80, and 'Arrhythmias', p. 132, respectively. Temporary pacing delivers a pulsed electrical stimulus to the heart by either a transcutaneous or transvenous route.

Modes of temporary pacing

Transcutaneous cardiac pacing

Transcutaneous, or external, cardiac pacing delivers electrical energy to the heart via gel pads attached to the patient's chest. These should be placed at the upper right sternal edge and over the cardiac apex. Most modern biphasic defibrillators have a mode specifically designed for this purpose. However, the electrical energy delivered induces painful contraction in the intercostal and pectoral muscles and the patient will require sedation and analgesia if they are fully conscious. Therefore, it should be used only in an emergency, and continued only until transvenous pacing can be arranged.

Transvenous cardiac pacing

Transvenous pacing can be used temporarily to restore a regular rhythm at a satisfactory rate. It is usually well tolerated by the patient and should be considered the definitive emergency treatment for dangerous bradyarrhythmias. However, if restoration of a functional native rhythm appears unlikely, arrangements should be made as soon as possible for the insertion of permanent pacemaker system. This reduces the risk of complications, particularly infection or lead displacement (see below), that increase the longer a temporary pacing line (TPL) is in situ.

Transvenous pacing requires considerable training and experience (see 'Procedural competence', p. 18); this means that the vast majority of TPLs are placed by cardiology trainees or consultants. Nevertheless, an understanding of the indications, contraindications, complications and practical use of TPLs is essential for any trainee in medicine, intensive care or accident and emergency. If you think your patient needs to be paced, contact cardiology or your consultant immediately and discuss the case.

Types of transvenous pacing

There are two types of transvenous pacing: atrial and ventricular. The vast majority of TPLs are guided into the right ventricle by fluoroscopy via an introducer sheath placed in either the right internal jugular, subclavian or femoral vein. The pacing electrode is connected to an external pacing box which can be used to control the rate and voltage output of the electrical pulse. On the ECG, this arrangement produces a left bundle branch block pattern, preceded by a pacing spike (Fig. 2.2).

Atrial pacing has the advantage of maintaining atrioventricular synchrony which can improve cardiac output by up to 20%. This may be of critical importance in patients with severely impaired cardiac function or patients with extensive RV infarction, diseases that result in stiff, non-compliant ventricles, e.g. HOCM, amyloidosis and patients with recurrent atrial tachyarrhythmias.

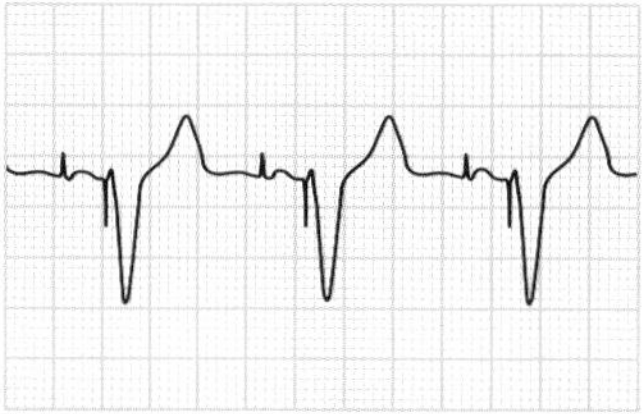

Figure 2.2 Paced rhythm (temporary pacing line (TPL) in the right ventricle).

Pacemaker modes

The international generic pacemaker code is used to define the operational mode of any pacemaker system (Table 2.2). Almost all TPLs function in 'demand' mode; this equates to a VVI mode, meaning the chamber paced is the ventricle (V), the chamber sensed is the ventricle (V) and pulse generation will be inhibited (I) if a spontaneous QRS complex is sensed.

Indications

Following acute myocardial infarction

- asystole
- symptomatic 2nd- or 3rd-degree (complete) heart block
- trifascicular block
- following anterior MI: complete or Mobitz type II 2nd-degree heart block, even if asymptomatic
- symptomatic sinus bradycardia unresponsive to medical therapy (see 'Bradyarrhythmias', p. 138)
- over drive pacing for refractory VT unresponsive to medical therapy (see 'VT', p. 137).

Indications unrelated to myocardial infarction

These assume medical therapies have failed (see 'Arrhythmias', p. 132) and include:

- symptomatic sinus or junctional bradycardia
- symptomatic 2nd- or 3rd-degree (complete) heart block
- sinus arrest
- torsades de pointes
- refractory ventricular tachycardia
- drug overdose, e.g. β-blockers, digoxin, rate-limiting calcium antagonists
- to facilitate a permanent pacemaker change in a pacemaker-dependent individual
- prophylactic pacing should be considered before general anaesthesia in patients with symptomatic sinoatrial disease, 2nd-degree heart block or complete heart block.

Table 2.2 The international generic pacemaker code

Chamber paced	Chamber sensed	Response to sensing spontaneous electrical activity
0 = none	0 = none	0 = none
A = atrium	A = atrium	T = triggered
V = ventricle	V = ventricle	I = inhibited
D = dual	D = dual	D = dual (atrium triggered, ventricle inhibited)

Contraindications

A TPL should not be inserted if the patient is hypothermic. Hypothermia results in increased myocardial irritability and a significant risk of ventricular fibrillation on contact between the pacing wire and heart muscle. Other contraindications are relative as the patient is likely to be critically ill. These include digoxin and other drug toxicity, which also increase myocardial irritability, and prolonged asystole, in which there is little chance of success.

Complications

- those related to central line insertion, including pneumothorax and vascular injury (see 'Central line insertion', p. 50)
- ventricular ectopics and non-sustained ventricular tachycardia: ectopics are common as the wire crosses the tricuspid valve and do not require treatment; persistent ectopics or runs of VT may indicate that the wire is stretched across the tricuspid valve; try increasing the amount of slack in the wire; persistent VT suggests pacing of the RV outflow tract and mandates repositioning
- failure to pace or sense: this is particularly likely in patients with extensive (particularly inferior) myocardial infarction or those who have used class Ia anti-arrhythmic drugs, e.g. procainamide, quinidine. If the position of the wire looks satisfactory it is reasonable to accept a higher than normal pacing threshold in these patients (<1.5 V)
- sudden loss of capture: this may indicate an increase in the threshold of the system (commonly doubles in the first 24 h due to local myocardial oedema) or lead displacement; try increasing the output on the pacing box, if this fails attach the external, transcutaneous pacing leads, roll the patient onto their left side (this can move the wire back into the myocardium) and arrange repositioning of the wire
- infection or septicaemia, most commonly with *S. aureus*
- pericarditis
- myocardial perforation ± tamponade: presents with pericarditic chest pain, a pericardial rub, falling BP with or without signs of cardiac tamponade, enlarging cardiac shadow on CXR and diaphragmatic pacing at low voltage; urgent echo and pericardial aspiration required (if tamponade); reposition the wire
- diaphragmatic pacing: may be asymptomatic or present with painful twitching and breathlessness; may complicate normally placed wires if a high voltage is required; if develops at a low voltage suggests myocardial perforation.

Procedure

Preparation

After discussion with cardiology and agreement that a TPL is indicated, transfer the patient to the pacing suite or coronary care unit. There are few other areas in most hospitals that will have the necessary fluoroscopy equipment, facilities for monitoring and resuscitation, and nursing experience. You may need a radiographer to operate the fluoroscopy system in your unit; if so contact them as soon as possible.

Explain the procedure and its risks to the patient if they are conscious and obtain consent (ideally written) and peripheral IV access. If sedation for transcutaneous pacing is necessary before insertion of a TPL, you should explain and consent the patient for transvenous pacing while they are still conscious, if possible. Check that there is a functioning defibrillator, ECG monitor and pacing box available. Ensure that your assistant has experience in connecting and operating the pacing box.

Insertion site

It is easiest to direct the pacing wire into the right ventricle from a right internal jugular vein approach. However, it is more comfortable for the patient if a right subclavian vein approach is used. A right femoral vein approach may be used but requires the operator to loop the wire in the right atrium to direct it into the right ventricle. Femoral vein cannulation is also associated with a greater risk of local infection and DVT. The left internal jugular vein approach is best avoided because of a series of tight bends that the wire would have to negotiate. If possible, also avoid the left subclavian vein, which is the preferred site for permanent pacemaker system access.

Equipment

Most coronary care units will keep a trolley prepared for emergency pacing; this should include the following:

- a selection of needles and a 10 mL Luer-Lok syringe
- 10 mL 2% lidocaine and pre-medication if appropriate, e.g. 1–2 mg midazolam IV
- a lead apron for everyone in the room
- pacing wire: most pacing wires are 5 or 6 F and come in a pack containing an introducer kit; if those available to you do not, you will need a separate introducer kit, see below; for ventricular pacing use a ventricular wire, these have an 'open-J' at the tip; atrial wires have a tight 'closed-J' that facilitates easy placement in the atrial appendage, but are difficult to site in the ventricle
- 6 or 7 F introducer kit: this should contain a sheath, introducer needle, guidewire and syringe; if you are using a separate introducer kit ensure that is at least one size larger than the pacing wire
- sterile water or heparinized saline to flush the introducer
- sterile dressing pack and cleaning solution, e.g. Betadine
- 2 sterile drapes, a gown and hand-towel set and sterile gloves
- 2 stitches, scissors, pack of swabs and a clear adhesive dressing.

Method

- put on a lead apron
- wash your hands while your assistant opens and places on the trolley the sterile dressing pack, needles, syringe, drapes, gown and hand-towel
- dry your hands and put on the gown and gloves
- open your sterile dressing pack and ask your assistant to pour out some cleaning solution and open the vials of lidocaine
- clean the skin over the insertion site
- anaesthetize the skin and subcutaneous tissues; see 'Local anaesthetics', p. 22
- open the pacing and/or introducer kit and flush the side arm on the introducer with heparinized saline
- cannulate a central vein and advance the guidewire as described in 'Central line insertion', p. 50
- make a small nick in the skin with the scalpel blade in the pacing/introducer kit and advance the introducer/sheath into the vein, along the guidewire
- remove the guidewire and introducer, and confirm the sheath is in the vein by aspirating blood from the side arm; flush the side arm again with heparinized saline
- advance the pacing wire through the introducer sheath (not the side arm) via the expandable sterile cover that accompanies it: do not unfurl and attach the rest of sterile cover to the proximal wire yet; this makes the wire more difficult to manipulate
- pass the wire into the right atrium (RA) and identify it on screening
- for ventricular wires, advance the tip of the wire across the tricuspid valve into the right ventricle (RV)
- watch the monitor for ventricular ectopics or VT as you cross the tricuspid valve and enter the RV; see complications above

- once through the valve, advance and then site your wire so that it points inferiorly at the most lateral point of the RV
- if your wire does not cross the tricuspid valve easily you will need to make a loop in the right atrium; from an internal jugular or subclavian approach, twist the wire through 180° so that the tip points at the lateral wall of the RA, make a complete loop in the RA and advance the wire into the RV; from a femoral approach, after rotating the wire tip to point at the lateral wall of the RA, advance the wire and make an incomplete J loop, then flip the wire through 180°, across the valve and advance into the RV
- once in a satisfactory position, leave some slack in the wire so that it is not stretched across the tricuspid valve; the final fluoroscopic appearance should resemble the outline of a foot, with the heel in the RA, the arch across the tricuspid valve and the toe in the RV
- ask your assistant for help with the next stages so you can stay sterile: they should connect the wire to the pacing box; for most systems there are two leads – the black lead is connected to the black terminal and the red lead to the red terminal – and turn the box on at 3 V
- check for 'capture': a paced broad complex rhythm
- ask your assistant to check the threshold (the lowest voltage that will initiate electrical activity), by slowly turning down the voltage; a value of <1.0 V is ideal but <1.5 V may be acceptable in some circumstances; see complications above
- check for positional stability: have the box set at a rate higher than the patient's own heart rate; ask them to sniff or cough; if capture is lost, reposition
- the box should then be set to 'demand pacing'; the voltage output should be at least twice the threshold, e.g. 3 V, the rate set as desired for the clinical situation, e.g. 70–80 b.p.m. for most bradyarrhythmias
- use the expandable sterile cover to enclose the length of the pacing wire distal to the introducer
- stitch the sheath and wire to the patient's skin; coil up the rest of the covered wire and stick it down using the clear adhesive dressing
- dispose of all equipment, including sharps, as per local infection control policy
- organize a CXR to confirm the position of the wire and exclude a pneumothorax.

DEFIBRILLATION AND ELECTRICAL CARDIOVERSION

Defibrillation refers specifically to the emergency electrical treatment of VF and pulseless VT. The shock delivered depolarizes a critical mass of ventricular myocardium, terminating the arrhythmia and allowing restoration of normal conduction through the sinoatrial and atrioventricular nodes.

Electrical cardioversion involves a more controlled and synchronized delivery of electrical energy at a specific time in the cardiac cycle. It is indicated for the urgent treatment of atrial or ventricular tachyarrhythmias associated with haemodynamic compromise and is also used electively in patients with persistent atrial tachyarrhythmias.

Indications

- *emergency*: e.g. decompensated tachyarrhythmias, see 'Arrhythmias', p. 132
- *elective*: e.g. conversion of stable AF or flutter of greater than 48 h duration.

Contraindications

In the emergency situation, contraindications are relative. In elective situations, it is unwise to attempt cardioversion in patients with dysrhythmias secondary to enhanced automaticity, e.g. digoxin toxicity. In this setting, it is unlikely to be successful and is associated with a significant risk of VT/VF.

Complications

- rhythm deterioration into VT or VF
- embolic: the return of sinus rhythm and atrial contraction may dislodge thrombi that have formed in the atria; adequate anticoagulation is required before the procedure; see below
- discomfort: delivery of a high energy electric shock is painful and the patient requires adequate analgesia and sedation
- burns: if paddles (rather than adhesive defibrillation pads) are used, gel pads must be applied to the chest first
- complications relating to the sedation, e.g. aspiration.

Procedure

Preparation

Connect the patient to appropriate monitoring equipment in a clinical area that is safe, ideally CCU. Obtain IV access, check the defibrillator, as above, and ensure that airway management and resuscitation equipment is nearby.

Emergency procedures

In an emergency, written consent may not be possible but you should explain the procedure and its risks to the patient, if possible. Anticoagulation should be considered; see 'Anticoagulation', p. 134. Fast page the anaesthetist, who will manage the patient's airway and sedate them, unless they are unconscious.

Elective procedures

The patient should be anticoagulated, usually with warfarin, for at least 3 weeks prior to cardioversion. Anaesthetic assistance should be arranged before admission. Explain the procedure to the patient and gain written consent. Ensure that they have fasted, check their INR and electrolytes. If they are on digoxin, a level should be checked: if they are digitoxic, cardioversion should be delayed.

Equipment: types of defibrillator

At the earliest opportunity you should familiarize yourself with the defibrillators used in your hospital. There are several different models. The principal differences between the types of system used relate to the mode of energy delivery and the interface with the patient.

Monophasic versus biphasic In traditional monophasic systems, the current travels in one direction (from positive to negative). However, in biphasic systems, there is rapid alteration of the direction of electrical current. A shock delivered by a biphasic system is more likely to terminate an arrhythmia. Hence, lower energy shocks can be delivered, reducing the incidence of skin burns or myocardial damage.

Pads versus paddles Paddles have largely been superseded by the use of adhesive gel pads which have the following advantages:

- improved safety: there are no trailing cables or live metal plates
- improved contact: the pads stick to the chest wall; defibrillation is more likely to be successful
- better ECG monitoring: improved continuity of the ECG trace since they do not need to be removed between defibrillation attempts
- transcutaneous pacing is possible depending on the machine being used.

Safe practice

The operator of the defibrillator is responsible for the safe delivery of the electrical energy to the patient. They must warn other members of staff to stand clear as they charge the machine and should perform a visual check before defibrillation to ensure that everyone has done so. Once the defibrillator has been charged, a second warning should be given, followed by a further visual check. At the same time they must ensure that any oxygen tubing has been removed from the patient.

Method

Additional guidance on emergency defibrillation can be found on p. 14.

- attach the three leads from the defibrillator in addition to other external monitoring equipment
- attach the adhesive electrode pads to the patient's chest: place one electrode to the right of the upper sternum and one over the apex in the midaxillary line; if the patient has an implanted pacemaker or chest drain, place the electrodes away from this
- turn the machine on and select the appropriate energy (Table 2.3).
- ensure that a clear trace is visible: lead II often provides the best trace
- switch on 'sync' mode: this synchronizes any delivered shock with the patient's own rhythm and reduces the risk of 'R on T', which can precipitate VT or VF
- once the sync mode is active, a mark should appear on each QRS complex: if a mark does not appear, increase the gain on the defibrillator
- allow the anaesthetist to administer the necessary sedation
- once the anaesthetist is happy that the patient is adequately sedated, charge the defibrillator and ensure that everybody is clear of the bed, patient and leads
- deliver a shock by pressing and holding the 'shock' button; you may need to keep it depressed for up to a second as the defibrillator waits for a safe point in the cardiac cycle to deliver the shock, see 'sync' mode above; the length of the delay will depend on the patient's heart rate
- if a further shock is required, check that 'sync' is still on: some machines default back to 'off' after a shock is delivered; if the initial shock fails to terminate the rhythm, try a further two shocks before increasing the energy
- after sinus rhythm is restored, check and maintain the patient's airway and monitor their vital signs until they regain consciousness; perform a 12-lead ECG.

Cardioversion problems

If sinus rhythm is not restored after two shocks, consider increasing the energy. If you have not been successful after three shocks give an IV bolus of amiodarone and consider changing electrode position. The gel pads should be moved to the anterior–posterior position: anterior pad lying at the lower left sternal border and the posterior below the left scapula.

In VT synchronization may be difficult. If the defibrillator will not allow you to deliver a synchronized shock and the patient is clinically unstable, deliver unsynchronized shocks instead.

Recovery

Emergency procedures

Following emergency cardioversion, further treatment will depend on the clinical situation. Reversible precipitants should be sought and treated appropriately. Consider also an infusion of amiodarone as a means of maintaining sinus rhythm; see 'Chemical cardioversion', p. 135.

Elective procedures

Electively cardioverted patients usually require 2–3 h observation prior to discharge. They should be reviewed in clinic in 4–6 weeks to check that sinus

Table 2.3 Initial energy settings for cardioversion

	Monophasic (J)	Biphasic (J)
Broad complex tachyarrhythmias Atrial fibrillation	200	120–150
Narrow complex tachyarrhythmias Atrial flutter	100	70–120

rhythm has been maintained and should continue on anticoagulation until then. They should not drive or operate machinery for at least 24 h following their sedation.

WOUND CLOSURE AND DRESSINGS

Wound healing

Successful wound healing is dependent on a number of factors. The most fundamental of these is effective and prompt closure of the original tissue defect. This promotes repair and healing; however, the strength of the damaged tissues never fully returns to normal. The rate of recovery in tissue strength has been estimated at 5% after 1 week, 25% after 1 month and 80% after 1 year. Factors that are likely to impair wound healing should be actively sought and addressed; these include:

- skin-related factors, e.g. tissue ischaemia, infection or necrosis; foreign material in the wound; excessive mobility, tension or swelling around the wound; recent radiotherapy
- general factors, e.g. increasing age; malignancy, cachexia and nutritional deficiencies; immunosuppression and steroid therapy; diabetes mellitus, smoking or hypoxia.

First-intention healing

This occurs after a clean incision, or when the edges of a wound have been closely and directly opposed. There are three recognized phases:

- *inflammatory*: cells migrate across the surface of the wound, histamine and prostaglandins are released promoting tissue permeability and vasodilatation; the wound is only weakly opposed at this point and very dependent upon the support of closure devices, such as sutures
- *proliferative*: neovascularization occurs within the healing tissues and granulation tissue forms; there is also epithelialization, early scar formation and some contraction of the wound, which is associated with an increased risk of dehiscence about 7–10 days after injury
- *remodelling or maturation*: connective tissue re-organization and further contraction of the wound.

Second-intention healing

This occurs where the edges of the wound are ragged and unopposed. As a result the wound defect fills with clot which matures into a scab. Beneath this, waves of epithelization advance towards the centre of the wound edges until it can be lifted off the surface of the healed tissue. The process is slower than for first-intention healing and more likely to result in scar formation.

Abnormal scar formation

In a small number of cases, keloid or hypertrophic scars can develop. The former extends beyond the boundary of the original wound and is more common in black or darkly pigmented skin. Treatment can include the use of silicone gel sheets to flatten and fade the scar, or steroid-containing tapes or injection into the scar.

Wound closure

Materials

A variety of materials can be used to achieve wound closure including sutures, staples, tapes and glue.

Sutures

See 'Suturing', p. 63.

Staples

Staples may be used for wound closure in theatre or A&E, often over wounds under high tension, e.g. trunk or scalp. They offer the advantage of speed for wound closure. They should not be used in delicate areas or over bony prominences or highly mobile areas. The resultant wound is also more prone to cross-hatch scarring. However, this can be reduced by correct placement of the staples at 45° or 60° angles. The usual staple size is 4–6 mm wide and 3.5–4 mm high. Larger staples are used in thicker skin. Removal is with a designated staple extractor.

Tapes

These are effective at opposing the wound, provided it is dry and superficial. Steri-Strip® skin closures are commonly used. They can also be used to support other sutures or to facilitate their earlier removal.

Glue

Cyanoacrylates, e.g. octylcyanoacrylate (Dermabond®; Ethicon®) are often used for simple lacerations in children, for facial wounds and for rapid closure of wounds under casts. They should be avoided in wounds over highly mobile areas.

Wound dressings

The type of wound dressing used should reflect the age of the wound and the relevant phase of healing; see above. It is also important to consider how dry or deep the wound is. A wound dressing serves a number of functions.

Protection, moisture and temperature control

Any dressing helps to isolate the wound from further physical contact and reduce disturbance of the epithelial re-growth. Some can also help to retain moisture, which makes scab formation less likely and allows more rapid epithelialization. Dressings also reduce heat loss from a wound, which improves tissue oxygen availability by shifting the oxygen–haemoglobin dissociation curve to the right.

Barrier to microorganisms

Air-borne bacteria can infect a wound and a dry dressing helps to prevent this, e.g. simple gauze dressings. However, if it becomes affected by 'strike-through', the passage of blood or exudate from a wound to the outside of a dressing, a channel is created permitting bacterial travel back to the wound. In such a situation, the dressing's protective function has been lost and it should be changed. Polymeric films, e.g. Opsite®, Tegaderm®, are transparent adhesive dressings that provide protection while allowing simultaneous monitoring of the underlying wound and are often used for sutured areas.

Debridement

Debridement, especially of necrotic slough-forming wounds such as chronic ulcers, can be achieved with the help of a dressing by various means:

- mechanical: the traditional method of applying a wet saline dressing to soften the wound surface that adheres as it dies and debrides when removed
- chemical or enzymatic: such as streptokinase-containing dressings, e.g. Varidase®; the duration of application is limited by their effect on healthy surrounding tissue and they should not be used on granulating or epithelizing wounds; a secondary dressing may be necessary
- autolytic, e.g. hydrocolloids, hydrogels (see below) or films creating a moist environment.

Absorption of exudate, blood and odour

Wound exudate is helpful to the normal healing process. However, wounds producing excessive amounts of exudate can be troublesome and may also be at increased risk of infection. Infected exudate or slough, especially by anaerobic organisms such as *Pseudomonas*, causes odour. Deep wounds will collect exudate or blood and need to be packed. Various dressing types provide absorbancy to assist in the management of such wounds:

- simple dressings (e.g. gauzes with low adherent coverings such as Melolin®, or tulles such as Jelonet®) quickly become saturated and require frequent

changing; by themselves they do not provide a moist environment; can be used during epithelization, for the final process of healing or as secondary dressings
- hydrophilic bead-based dressings, e.g. Debrisan® or Iodosorb®, are best used for moderate to heavy exudate producing necrotic, infected or sloughy wounds (provided these are not very deep, are not granulating and do not contain narrow sinuses); a secondary dressing is needed
- Lyofoam®, a polyurethane foam sheet is hydrophilic and used for shallow granulating wounds with low to moderate exudate, e.g. sacral sores
- Silastic® foam can be used to pack deeper granulating cavity wounds with low to moderate exudate production, provided there is no sinus or track within which pieces of the foam can remain and cause problems later
- hydrogels, e.g. Geliperm®, IntraSite®, absorb low to moderate amounts of exudate and, being semipermeable, also allow gas exchange; can be used to pack necrotic deep granulating or epithelizing wounds, even those with sinuses; Geliperm® should not be used if there is a *Pseudomonas* infection
- hydrocolloids, e.g. Granuflex®, Comfeel®, can be used for shallow wounds with light or moderate exudate production; the hydrocolloid layer liquefies into a gel as it absorbs exudate and produces a distinctive odour
- fibrous polymers, e.g. Kaltostat®, Sorbsan®, are absorptive alginate-based dressings and can be used for deep, heavily exuding or bleeding wounds; they should not be used where there are low amounts of exudate where they can adhere; a secondary dressing may be needed.

Reduction of pain

Dressings can limit pain by reducing physical contact and moisture loss. Some also provide a gel-derived cushion comfort or wound support. However, dressings that adhere to a wound can cause considerable discomfort when removed and analgesia may be required. Low-adherence dressings are needed in the case of wounds with little or no exudate, e.g. Melolin®. Pain is also a symptom of infection and, where the wound is infected, an iodine-based low-adherence dressing such as Inadine® could be used.

Wound support

Support of a closed wound, e.g. by sutures or tapes, is useful in the initial stage of healing to reduce opening. Dressings that adhere to the surrounding tissue may also reduce skin stretch and offer some support to the wound. Other dressings, e.g. Blue Line Webbing, can be used to compress the wound and reduce oedema. Care must be taken when using compression bandaging to ensure vascular supply is adequate. The dressing should be removed at night and re-applied in the morning.

SUTURING

Terminology

- bite: the amount of tissue taken either side of the wound edge when placing a suture
- percutaneous/skin closure: sutures (non-absorbable) tied on the surface of the skin
- dermal closure: suture (absorbable) and knot in the subcutaneous tissue or dermis
- continuous/running closure: a suture running the entire length of the wound where knots are only tied at either end; entry and exit have a tendency to scar
- interrupted closure: single sutures tied separately that together close the wound; cross-hatched scarring can occur from the tension created
- subcuticular stitch: suture running under the skin with bites from the subcutaneous layer; best choice for wounds on sternum or trunk to reduce scarring.

Procedure

Preparation

Wounds should be clean and a sterile approach adopted during the procedure (see 'Sterile field', p. 19). They should be dry (haemostasis should be meticulous) and foreign bodies or devitalized material should be removed. Local anaesthetic ± analgesia should be considered; see 'Local anaesthetics', p. 22. Patients should be aware of the risks of subsequent scarring.

Equipment

Absorbable sutures are often used for dermal or subcuticular closure. Surgical gut, formed from the intestine of sheep or cows, was the first absorbable suture material used, and is still used. It is available in three forms: fast-absorbing (used for facial wounds), plain and chromic (both used for mucosal surfaces or vessel ligatures). These preparations vary in the length of time that they will maintain their initial tensile strength (5–7, 7–10 and 10–21 days, respectively).

Synthetic absorbable sutures are also available, e.g. polyglycolic acid (Dexon®), polyglactin (Vicryl®), polydioxanone (PDS®), polytrimethylene carbonate (Maxon®), poliglecaprone (Monocryl®). Tensile strength, ease of handling and rate of hydrolysis varies. Some are relatively stiff and require extra throws during knot tying, but tensile strength is generally greater than for gut and they can be used effectively when dermal support is needed in deeper wounds.

Non-absorbable sutures are predominantly used for percutaneous closure (see below) and include silk, nylon, polyester, polypropylene and polybutester. Silk or polyester is best used for suturing of mucosal or other delicate areas, as nylon can cut through them. However, polyester is expensive and silk sutures are more prone to cellular invasion and pain on removal. Nylon also has poorer handling and knot security properties. Polypropylene and polybutester, e.g. Novafil®, slip easily through tissue and are often used in running subcuticular sutures. Despite their synthetic nature, they both retain elasticity and can accommodate for wound oedema.

Method

General points

- as fine a suture as possible should be used
- layers should be matched across the wound from deepest upwards
- the 'dead space' of any deep wound should be closed where possible using absorbable sutures or a drain led from the area prior to closing more superficial layers
- the bite is dependent on the area, e.g. face 1–2 mm; abdomen 5 mm
- the wound edge should be held with toothed forceps; needle entry and exit should be as close to perpendicular as possible
- where interrupted sutures are used, avoid any gaping between sutures but do not use excessive numbers
- wound edges should be everted: scars contract with time and a slightly raised wound edge will flatten to a more acceptable appearance than the linear pit created by a suture line that is inverted or opposed
- tension across the wound should be avoided: edges should just touch and any planned incisions should follow or parallel natural crease lines.

Techniques for wound-edge eversion

In addition to ensuring a vertical needle incision into the skin as above, vertical and horizontal mattress sutures can help promote wound-edge eversion. An interrupted suture technique, they use a combination of large deeper bites with smaller epidermal bites. In the vertical mattress suture a 1.5 cm dermal bite is taken away from the wound edge A, and a corresponding bite from the opposite edge B. Then the needle reverses taking a small 1–2 mm bite from the epidermal/dermal junction of wound edge B and the same from wound edge A.

Suture removal

If non-absorbable sutures or strips have been used, standard removal times would be:

- face and neck: 4 days
- scalp: 7 days
- abdomen and chest: 7–10 days
- limbs: 7 days
- feet: 10–14 days.

ECG RECORDING

Indications

An electrocardiogram (ECG) can contribute to the diagnosis of many conditions. However, it may be normal despite the presence of conditions such as MI and ACS, paroxysmal arrhythmias, ventricular hypertrophy, electrolyte disturbances, pericarditis, or drug toxicity. The sensitivity varies and is rarely 100% and there are several recognized normal variants within different populations. Therefore, an ECG should be viewed in the context of an assessment that includes the age, sex of the patient, the history, any findings on clinical examination, current medications and recent laboratory results. Common indications for ECG recording include:

- chest pain or suspected cardiac disease
- arrhythmias: remember that a normal ECG does not exclude pathology if the patient complains of intermittent symptoms; consider a subsequent 24-h recording
- following recovery from cardiac arrest
- collapse or drug overdose
- preoperatively or for health screening, e.g. in pilots
- confusion in the elderly.

For guidance on the interpretation of the ECG, see p. 78.

Procedure

Preparation

Explain the procedure to patient, enquire about skin allergies and obtain consent. Position the patient sitting at a 45° angle. If required, shave the skin and ensure it is clean and dry prior to placing electrodes.

Equipment

Check the ECG machine has paper and enough electrodes (if the electrodes are non-disposable, you will also need electrode gel). Switch the machine on and check that it does a self-test analysis. Ensure the Filter is switched 'on'; if not set by default. You may also need a razor or scissors and tissue.

Method

- apply electrodes to the appropriate anatomical sites: outer aspect of each forearm (RA, LA), medial aspect of each lower leg (LL, RL), chest leads (V1–V6)
- connect leads to electrodes as per colour or numbers
- advise the patient to relax, to let their arms lie loose and to breath gently
- if prompted to do so, enter relevant patient information
- when ready, push the 'auto' button to start recording
- observe the recording as the paper emerges: check that lead placement was correct, that the recording is free from artefact (such as a wandering baseline), paper speed was 25 mm/s and normal standardization was used (1 mV, 10 mm)
- turn off the machine and disconnect the leads from electrodes

- carefully peel off the electrodes and wipe off any gel from the patient's skin with gauze or tissue; dispose of the electrodes in the clinical waste bin
- ensure the ECG is labelled with all patient details, the time and date, and is signed
- mark on the ECG any symptoms the patient was experiencing at the time, e.g. pain or palpitation.

OXYGEN DELIVERY

Indications

The principal indications for oxygen therapy include respiratory failure, shock and significant carbon monoxide poisoning.

Contraindications

There are no specific contraindications to oxygen therapy. Uncontrolled oxygen therapy should be avoided in patients who demonstrate unfavourable ventilatory responses. This is most common in patients with chronic type 2 respiratory failure in whom hypoxic drive may be the principal stimulus to ventilation (see 'Breathlessness', p. 144). Oxygen therapy should be avoided during laser bronchoscopy because of a risk of ignition.

Complications

- ventilatory depression may occur in patients reliant on hypoxic drive; see above
- inhalation of high oxygen concentrations (FiO_2 >0.6) has been associated with absorption atelectasis, oxygen toxicity and depression of ciliary function; however, these problems are rarely clinically evident
- neovascularization, retrolental fibroplasia and blindness may develop in neonates treated with high oxygen concentrations.

Delivery systems

Various types of oxygen delivery system are available; these can be broadly grouped into controlled and uncontrolled types.

Controlled oxygen therapy

Venturi mask

This is a fixed performance system, meaning that a prescribed inspired oxygen fraction (FiO_2) can be delivered to the patient regardless of their breathing pattern. Such a system is particularly useful in patients who rely on hypoxic drive to maintain ventilation and who may respond poorly to high oxygen concentrations, e.g. chronic type II respiratory failure. The Venturi® system can deliver a FiO_2 between 0.24 and 0.6 depending on the mask and oxygen flow rate. When using this type of mask the patient does not re-breathe their own expired carbon dioxide.

Uncontrolled oxygen therapy

Non-re-breathing mask

Also known as a 'trauma mask', this system is commonly used in emergency situations to administer high doses of oxygen (FiO_2 >0.6). High oxygen flow rates (>10L/min) are required and the reservoir bag must be fully inflated before the mask is put on the patient. The maximum FiO_2 that can be delivered using this system is around 0.85, at an oxygen flow rate of 15L/min. A non-re-breathing mask incorporates a one-way valve to ensure that the patient does not re-breathe their own expired carbon dioxide.

Hudson mask

This system is often used in postoperative recovery areas for short-term oxygen therapy in patients with uncomplicated medical problems. It is a variable performance system, i.e. the amount of oxygen delivered will depend on the patient's breathing pattern. Expired carbon dioxide will be re-breathed and the system is not suitable for use in acutely ill patients or those with chronic respiratory failure.

Nasal cannulae

These are often used in patients who are unable to tolerate a mask and do not have to be removed to allow talking, eating and drinking. Their principal disadvantage is that only low inspired oxygen fractions can be delivered. Flow rates above 4 L/min produce little additional rise in FiO_2 >0.3 and may damage the nasal mucosa. As for the Hudson mask, nasal cannulae are a variable performance system. In particular, the amount of oxygen delivered will vary depending on a patient's ratio of mouth to nasal breathing. The patient does not re-breathe their expired carbon dioxide.

Choice and adjustment of oxygen flow rate

Patients with acute hypoxaemia should be commenced on high oxygen concentrations, unless there is a reason to suspect chronic CO_2 retention and a reliance on hypoxic drive. In such patients, e.g. those with COPD, a lower inspired oxygen concentration should be delivered using a Venturi mask.

All patients with respiratory failure requiring oxygen therapy should have urgent arterial blood gasses checked. Where possible, an initial sample should be taken 'on air' and used to guide their initial oxygen dose. This should aim to maintain a normal PaO_2 in patients without previous lung disease, or a PaO_2 that is normal for the patient in those with chronic respiratory impairment. This can be estimated from previous ABGs; in many patients a PaO_2 of 6–8 kPa is adequate; for more information on oxygen prescription in COPD, see p. 144.

Oxygen is a drug and like any other it should be prescribed and monitored closely. In doing so, staff should be aware of the limitations of simple oxygen saturations. If there is any evidence of clinical deterioration or a drop in oxygen saturation, a sample for ABG should be taken. Equally, in patients who may develop worsening of type 2 respiratory failure, the ABG should be checked about 1 h after initiating oxygen therapy.

NEBULIZERS

Indications

Nebulizers can be used to deliver a variety of drug therapies to the airways, including bronchodilators, steroids and antibiotics. The indications for nebulized treatment depend upon the drug that is being administered.

Bronchodilators, e.g. salbutamol and ipratropium, are the most commonly prescribed nebulized treatments. They are useful in patients with acute bronchospasm who are too unwell to use inhaled treatment and also for long-term symptom relief in patients with severe COPD on otherwise optimal therapy.

Steroids, e.g. budesonide, are occasionally used in patients with steroid-responsive airways disease who are unable to use inhaled therapy. Nebulized antibiotics, e.g. gentamicin, are a useful therapeutic option in patients with bronchiectasis, CF and recurring lower respiratory tract infection. Occasionally other drugs, such as morphine, are given by the nebulized route.

The decision to supply a long-term nebulizer is normally made in consultation with a chest physician.

Contraindications

Long-term nebulized bronchodilators should not be prescribed for patients with COPD unless they produce a clear improvement in lung function, symptoms or exercise capacity.

Complications

- salbutamol may result in tremor, nausea, hypokalaemia or arrhythmias
- ipratropium delivered by a mask can precipitate glaucoma
- steroids may result in oral thrush.

Procedure

Equipment

There are various different nebulizer systems in clinical use and it is important to familiarize yourself with the equipment used locally. All will consist of an air compressor, a drug reservoir, an interface device (mask or mouthpiece) and the necessary tubing. A mask interface is commonly used in the acute setting, but both options should be available to patients on longer term treatment. A mouthpiece is preferable when delivering ipratropium because of the risk of precipitating glaucoma with a mask delivery.

Air or oxygen?

A minimum gas flow rate through the drug reservoir (of around 6 L/min) is necessary to generate the aerosolized drug vapour that the patient inspires. The nebulizer unit itself is a simple air compressor that delivers the necessary flow rate of room air. However, oxygen can also be used, by connecting the tubing from the reservoir to a piped oxygen supply set at 6 L/min. This should be avoided in patients who require controlled oxygen therapy (e.g. those with chronic type 2 respiratory failure) who should, instead, have 1–2 L/min of oxygen delivered by nasal cannulae and the nebulizer driven by air.

Method

- pour the medication into the reservoir and screw this into the base of the mask or mouthpiece
- attach the tubing from the reservoir into the nebulizer or wall oxygen (set at 6 L/min)
- switch on the nebulizer or oxygen
- the patient should breathe as normally as possible; over-breathing will adversely affect lung deposition of the drug (the patient will tend to breathe less deeply); therefore anxious or very breathless patients may benefit from some reassurance and guidance in the early stages of treatment
- continue until all of the drug solution has gone; if this takes >10 min, the machine should be serviced
- the reservoir should be rinsed out with water after each dose
- all nebulizers should be part of an annual service programme.

PEAK FLOW AND SPIROMETRY

Peak flow

The peak expiratory flow rate (PEFR) is a measure of the maximum air flow during a forced expiration. See 'Spirometry', p. 89, for indications and further information.

Procedure

Attach a disposable mouthpiece to the peak flow meter and check that the pointer is at zero. Some patients find it difficult to perform a peak flow manoeuvre and your instructions will be key to their success. Show them how to hold the meter so that their fingers do not impede the movement of the pointer. Ask the patient to sit on the edge of the bed or stand and instruct them to:

- exhale fully first
- take the deepest breath possible, then close their lips tightly around the mouthpiece
- 'blow out as hard and fast as you can … as if you were blowing out a candle'.

Take note of the PEFR (L/min), return the pointer to zero and repeat the measurement three times. Record the best reading and dispose of the mouthpiece.

Spirometry

For indications and interpretation, see 'Spirometry', p. 89. Forced expiration causes large increases in abdominal, thoracic, intracranial and ocular pressure. National guidance advises avoiding spirometry in those who have had abdominal, thoracic or ocular surgery, a myocardial infarction or CVA within the past 6 weeks. Spirometry should be performed by an appropriately trained technician and the following is not a substitute for practical training.

Procedure

Attach the disposable mouthpiece to the spirometer and ensure that you have a trolley or chair in case the patient feels faint. Use a machine that has been regularly and properly calibrated.

Method

- the patient should exhale fully and then take as large a breath as possible before putting the mouthpiece to their lips (nose clips should be used to prevent air leakage)
- the technician should ensure there is an adequate seal around the mouthpiece
- the patient should exhale again as hard and fast as possible; they will need encouragement to keep blowing until they cannot exhale any more.

A practice run may be necessary before a proper reading. The exhaled volume at 1 s (FEV1) and the total exhaled volume (FVC) are recorded. An average of the patient's three most consistent results should then be compared with the age and height adjusted values.

3 Interpreting tests

LABORATORY TESTS

Using the laboratory

Laboratory tests should only be requested for specific reasons such as:

- diagnosis of disease in a patient with suggestive clinical features
- screening for disease in an asymptomatic or at risk population
- monitoring of changes in a patient's condition
- assessing prognosis.

Communication with the laboratory

Check any local policies that relate to routine, urgent and emergency sampling. Remember that most laboratories are busy in the early morning and early afternoon when routine samples arrive from the wards and GP surgeries, respectively. If you are sending an urgent or emergency sample it is essential to warn the lab beforehand, otherwise your urgent sample could end up at the bottom of the routine pile.

Refer to local protocols regarding the use of pneumatic tube systems for the delivery of samples. Never send samples that have been difficult to obtain by this method, e.g. CSF.

Artefactual results

Effect of the sample container

Contamination of the yellow-topped electrolyte Vacutainer with EDTA can occur if sampling with the EDTA-containing, purple-topped Vacutainer is performed first. This leads to falsely elevated potassium and low calcium.

Effects of poor sampling technique

Some results may be significantly altered by poor technique in collecting or handling a specimen:

- haemolysis may occur due to use of narrow-gauge needles, excessive shaking of the specimen and rapid transit in an air-tube system; several tests results are affected, e.g. potassium, LDH

- clotting of EDTA specimens due to inadequate mixing affects the FBC result
- incorrectly taking a specimen near to a site of an intravenous infusion (may occur downstream or upstream)
- not cleaning the skin thoroughly before taking samples for blood culture may result in contamination
- incorrect labelling of the sample.

Effects of acute illness

The acute phase response can make the interpretation of blood tests difficult in acutely ill patients. Its function is to promote the clearance of infection and tissue healing. Liver synthetic function is directed away from albumin synthesis towards the production of more useful proteins, e.g. immunoglobulin and serum binding proteins. This enhances immune function and reduces the free concentration of elements such as iron and zinc, which are essential for bacterial metabolism. The acute phase response may last for several weeks and results in:

- low serum albumin, iron and zinc
- high serum ferritin, copper and CRP
- altered thyroid function tests.

Effects on reference ranges

Threshold values that suggest 'disease' must always be interpreted with an understanding of the false positive and false negative rates of the test and other factors that may affect its result. Examples of these include:

- age and gender, e.g. serum creatinine and alkaline phosphatase
- time of day, e.g. cortisol
- monthly cycle, e.g. LH, FSH
- posture, e.g. aldosterone, urine albumin
- food, e.g. glucose, creatinine.

Venous blood tests

Information about specific blood tests can be found in the chapters relating to the conditions that cause their derangement:

- electrolytes, see p. 202
- renal function, see p. 209
- liver function, see p. 178
- glucose, see p. 187
- thyroid function, see p. 197
- full blood count, see p. 276
- coagulation.

Arterial blood gases

Arterial blood gases (ABG) are used to assess circulating blood oxygen levels, the adequacy of ventilation and the presence or absence of any acid–base imbalance.

ABG analysers can measure, or calculate, a number of important values. The most clinically useful of these are the hydrogen ion concentration, the arterial partial pressures of oxygen (PaO_2) and carbon dioxide ($PaCO_2$), the bicarbonate concentration and base excess. An understanding of these individual values is essential for the interpretation of ABG results.

Individual values

Hydrogen ion concentration

Most analysers will quote both hydrogen ion concentration ($[H^+]$) and pH (this is the negative logarithm of the hydrogen ion concentration). These indicate whether the patient is acidaemic (H^+ >45 nmol/L or pH <7.35) or alkalaemic (H^+ <36 nmol/L or pH >7.45) as a consequence of both the primary disease state and any respiratory or renal compensation that has taken place.

$PaCO_2$

Carbon dioxide is extremely water soluble and diffuses rapidly from the bloodstream into the alveolar spaces. Therefore, for a constant metabolic rate, the level of $PaCO_2$ will be determined entirely by alveolar ventilation.

The normal range for $PaCO_2$ is 4.6–6 kPa. Hypoventilation will result in a rise in this value (hypercapnia), while hyperventilation will result in a fall (hypocapnia). Since CO_2 forms carbonic acid when it is dissolved in water, hypercapnia leads to acidosis and hypocapnia to alkalosis. Such primary defects are respiratory in origin and, therefore, these patterns are referred to as respiratory acidosis and respiratory alkalosis, respectively.

PaO_2

Oxygen is less water soluble than carbon dioxide, so it diffuses less readily from the alveoli into the bloodstream. This means that a number of factors must be in place for adequate oxygenation: a large alveolar surface area; adequate, effective and well-matched ventilation and perfusion within the lung; sufficient oxygen in the inspired air. The interpretation of a PaO_2 value must take these different factors into account; see below.

The normal range for PaO_2 is 10.5–13.5 kPa. A PaO_2 <8 kPa defines the presence of respiratory failure, which can be further classified as type 1 or type 2.

Type 1 respiratory failure

This is isolated hypoxaemia with a normal or low $PaCO_2$. A low PaO_2 value can be caused by numerous conditions, but only five main physiological mechanisms:

- ventilation/perfusion (V/Q) mismatch: this is the reason for hypoxia related to most common conditions, e.g. pneumonia, heart failure, the early stages of acute asthma
- impaired diffusion: due to loss or thickening of the gas exchange surfaces of the lung, e.g. emphysema and pulmonary fibrosis, respectively
- shunting: may be intra-cardiac or extra-cardiac
- a low inspired oxygen fraction, e.g. at altitude
- alveolar hypoventilation: $PaCO_2$ is usually high, in which case type 2 respiratory failure is present.

Type 2 respiratory failure

This is hypoxaemia associated with a high $PaCO_2$. Hypercapnia always indicates alveolar hypoventilation, which may be due to:

- reduced respiratory drive due to impaired brainstem function, the sedative effects of drugs or a metabolic alkalosis
- respiratory pump failure due to respiratory muscle weakness, obesity, chest wall abnormalities or airways disease (often a combination is present).

Type 2 respiratory failure is rarely due to hypoventilation alone, the exceptions being respiratory muscle weakness or over-sedation of a patient with normal lungs. Instead, in most patients with this pattern, a component of their hypoxaemia is due to V/Q mismatch or other physiological abnormalities associated with their acute illness; see above.

Bicarbonate and base excess

The kidneys regulate acid–base balance by secretion of hydrogen ions and resorption and production of bicarbonate ions. The bicarbonate on an ABG sample is usually calculated from the measured pH and $PaCO_2$ and the normal range is 21–28 mmol/L.

Failure to produce bicarbonate in the kidney, or the buffering of excessive body acids produced elsewhere (e.g. lactate in sepsis or renal failure, β-hydroxybutyrate in DKA) will lead to a low bicarbonate level, known as a metabolic acidosis.

Excessive loss of hydrogen ions (e.g. from the gut due to vomiting, or the kidney due to hypokalaemia) will result in a high bicarbonate level, known as a metabolic alkalosis.

The base excess is an alternative, and probably better, measure of the metabolic component of any acid–base disturbance. It can be thought of as the amount of acid that you would have to add to a blood sample to return it to a normal pH of 7.4. Thus, a negative base excess indicates a metabolic acidosis, while a positive base excess indicates a metabolic alkalosis. The normal range of base excess is −3 to +3 mEq/L, depending on the analyser.

Compensation

'Compensation' is the homeostatic mechanism that seeks to restore normal blood pH. In a respiratory acidosis, the kidneys will reabsorb or generate additional bicarbonate ions to buffer excess carbon dioxide in the bloodstream. However, this is a slow process and complete renal compensation may take days. Respiratory compensation is much quicker, e.g. the metabolic acidosis associated with DKA will immediately stimulate increased (Kussmaul's) ventilation, by activation of central and peripheral chemoreceptors, resulting in hypocapnia.

In order to recognize compensation, look for a change in the buffering system (respiratory or renal) that was not involved with the primary problem. Guidance on how to do this is given below.

Interpretation scheme

It helps to approach things from the perspectives of acid–base physiology and respiratory physiology separately. The following scheme uses a hydrogen ion concentration ([H^+]), rather than pH, and bicarbonate, rather than base excess.

Acid–base physiology

Look at the [H^+]

Determine whether the patient is acidaemic (>45 nmol/L) or alkalaemic (<36 nmol/L).

Look at the $PaCO_2$

- if it is abnormal and has shifted in the same direction as the [H^+], then the primary problem is respiratory in origin, either respiratory acidosis ($PaCO_2$ ↑, [H^+] ↑) or respiratory alkalosis ($PaCO_2$ ↓, [H^+] ↓)
- if it is abnormal, but has shifted in the opposite direction to the [H^+], then the primary problem is metabolic, the change in $PaCO_2$ being compensatory.

Look at the bicarbonate

- if it is abnormal and has shifted in the opposite direction to the [H^+], then the primary problem is metabolic in origin, either metabolic acidosis (bicarbonate ↓, [H^+] ↑), or metabolic alkalosis (bicarbonate ↑, [H^+] ↓)
- if it is abnormal, but it has shifted in the same direction to the [H^+], then the primary problem is respiratory, the change in bicarbonate being compensatory.

Respiratory physiology

Look at the $PaCO_2$

Determine whether alveolar ventilation is adequate; hypoventilation is indicated by a high $PaCO_2$, hyperventilation by a low $PaCO_2$.

Look at the PaO_2

Determine whether the patient has respiratory failure (PaO_2 <8 kPa) and if it is type 1 or type 2. The causes of these are given above.

Examine the acid–base balance

As above, assess whether there is evidence for a primary respiratory or metabolic problem and whether there is any evidence of renal compensation to suggest chronicity.

CSF

Normal CSF is clear, colourless and sterile. A number of conditions result in altered appearance and/or composition of CSF and laboratory analysis of the fluid can be diagnostic (Table 3.1) Specific points related to the analyses performed in each clinical situation are discussed below.

Suspected subarachnoid haemorrhage

Bleeding into the subarachnoid space leads to yellow discoloration of the CSF, known as xanthochromia. However, this is an inexact and subjective term and objective analysis of the CSF is mandatory. Laboratories will usually look for two compounds:

Oxyhaemoglobin (OxyHb)

This is released from erythrocytes within an hour or two of bleeding into the subarachnoid space. It is sensitive but not specific, as OxyHb does not discriminate between a genuine subarachnoid bleed and a traumatic tap.

Bilirubin

Bilirubin is produced by in vivo metabolism of OxyHb. It is a more specific marker of SAH than OxyHb; however, it may not appear in the CSF for 12 h after the event. Therefore, if SAH is suspected an LP should not be performed before this time. False positive results may occur if previous failed LP attempts have introduced blood into the CSF causing in vivo formation of bilirubin.

Suspected meningitis or brain abscess

A CT should be performed before CSF sampling in patients with focal neurological signs, suspected abscess, or an abnormal GCS. Where there is no immediate indication for CT, CSF sampling should be undertaken as early as possible, ideally before antibiotic administration. However, in either case, ensure antibiotics are given promptly. Typical CSF results are shown in Table 3.1.

When sending the sample to the lab, indicate any antibiotics that have been administered, on the form. An additional sample should be sent for AAFB staining and culture if tuberculous meningitis is suspected.

Multiple sclerosis

Multiple sclerosis is a condition associated with local production of immunoglobulins in the central nervous system. This may be reflected by the presence of oligoclonal protein bands in the CSF. Where appropriate, send an additional sample for this to biochemistry, accompanied by a blood sample for serum protein analysis.

Urine

Ward analysis

Urinalysis on the ward involves the use of a dipstick test-strip and comparison of the results with a colour chart. The amount of time the urine is in contact with the strip and the time it is read can affect the result and the instructions on the bottle should be read. The dipstick measures several things:

- glucose: present in, but not diagnostic of, diabetes
- protein: only partly quantitative but is highly sensitive and a negative test virtually excludes proteinuria (except for light-chains); detects albumin and can indicate infection or renal dysfunction; persistently high levels should be quantified with a 24 h collection analysis (see below); note, a dipstick test cannot detect microalbuminuria
- blood: intact red cells and free haemoglobin may be found in infection and a range of primary or secondary renal conditions; note myoglobinuria (e.g. in rhabdomyolysis) leads to a false positive result

Table 3.1 CSF features

Features/ conditions	Normal	SAH	Bacterial meningitis	Viral meningitis	TB meningitis	MS	Malignancy
Pressure	50–180 mmH_2O	Increased	Normal or increased	Normal	Normal or increased	Normal	Can be raised
Colour	Clear	Blood-stained or xanthochromic	Cloudy	Clear	Cloudy	Clear	Clear
Red cell count	0–4/mm^3	Raised	Normal	Normal	Normal	Normal	Normal
White cell count	0–4/mm^3	Normal or slightly raised	1000–5000 polymorphs	10–2000 lymphocytes	10–5000 lymphocytes	0–50 lymphocytes	0–100 lymphocytes
Glucose	>60% blood level; 2.5–4.0 mmol/L	Normal	Decreased	Normal	Decreased	Normal	Decreased
Protein	<0.45 g/L	Increased	Increased, can be over 1 g/L	Normal/ increased	Increased, can be over 1 g/L	Normal or increased; oligoclonal bands may be present	Normal or increased
Microbiology	Sterile	Sterile	Organisms on Gram-stain and/or culture	Sterile	AAFB may be seen or TB culture +ve	Sterile	Sterile

- leucocytes: white cells suggestive of infection or trauma to kidneys or urinary tract
- ketones: present in fasting states and in diabetic ketoacidosis
- nitrites: sensitive test for infection; produced by Gram-negative bacteria
- pH: normally 4.5–8 and affected by changes in systemic acid–base balance
- specific gravity: indicative of urine concentration and reflects states of body fluid overload or depletion; normal 1.005–1.020.

Laboratory analysis

Microscopy

- more than 10 white blood cells/mm^3 is abnormal and suggests infection or trauma
- more than 2 red blood cells/mm^3 is abnormal (see 'Haematuria', p. 185)
- protein or cell casts may be present; hyaline casts are proteinaceous but insignificant; red cell casts are found in acute or chronic glomerular disease; granular casts are found in acute tubular necrosis or nephritis
- bacteria may indicate infection above the relevant laboratory threshold, particularly if associated with white cells and nitrites; check local protocols.

Culture

Urine specimens for culture should be collected into a container with boric acid as a preservative. Patients should be advised on techniques to avoid contamination with perineal commensal organisms, such as collecting a midstream urine specimen. Early morning urine specimens for AAFB should only be collected if renal TB is suspected; they are not useful in pulmonary or nodal disease.

Biochemistry

Table 3.2 summarizes the more common biochemical tests performed on urine. 'Spot' urines for biochemical investigation should be collected into plain (white top) 'universal' containers. The concentration of urine in spot samples is variable and better standardization of the test can be achieved by collecting an early morning specimen. The laboratory will usually report any results relative to the urine creatinine, e.g. albumin:creatinine ratio (ACR), protein:creatinine ratio (PCR).

Alternatively, a urine specimen can be collected over a 24 h period. To allow this, your local laboratory will issue a container with the appropriate preservative, e.g. urine metadrenalines collection requires a low sample pH, so hydrochloric acid will be added to the bottle as a preservative. In such cases, it is important to inform the patient that there is supposed to be something in the bottle and that they should not allow it to touch their skin.

Pleural fluid

The colour and viscosity of the pleural fluid should be noted and documented in the case sheet. Normal pleural fluid is straw-coloured and non-viscous. Important abnormal appearances include:

- blood or blood-stained fluid suggests malignancy, PTE or a haemothorax (defined by a pleural fluid haematocrit >50% of blood haematocrit)
- pus or turbid fluid suggests empyema
- milky fluid suggests chylothorax or empyema.

Pleural fluid should be sent for the following routine investigations.

Biochemistry

Protein and LDH

In patients with a normal serum protein level, an exudate is defined by a pleural protein level >30 g/L and a transudate by a level <30 g/L. In borderline cases

Table 3.2 Chemical analysis of urine in adults

Test	Spot or 24 h	Normal value	Notes
Sodium concentration	Spot 24 h	20–40 mmol/L 100–200 mmol	Low in pre-renal ARF; high in ATN and obstructive uropathy
Osmolality	Spot	500–800 mmol/kg	A serum sample is also required for comparison; used in the diagnosis of SIADH (p. 204), diabetes insipidus (p. 204) and pre-renal failure versus ATN (p. 209)
Calcium	24 h	1.2–12 mmol depending on diet	Increased in hypercalcaemia (p. 206) and also in hypercalcuria with normal serum calcium in stone-formers
Protein	24 h	≤0.3 g/L	Excess suggests renal protein loss, e.g. nephropathy
Metadrenaline	24 h	0.3–1.7 μmol	Increased in phaeochromocytoma (p. 201); specific diet, e.g. avoiding vanilla, required during testing
Urate (uric acid)	24 h	1.2–3.0 mmol	Measure while on a low purine diet; excess causes gout, renal stones and urate nephropathy
Copper	24 h	≤0.6 μmol	High in Wilson's disease and usually accompanied by low serum ceruloplasmin

For creatinine clearance, see p. 115. For urine toxicology, see p. 238.

(25–35 g/L) or when the serum protein level is abnormal, Light's criteria should be used to identify exudates, defined by:

- a pleural protein:serum protein ratio >0.5 or
- a pleural LDH:serum LDH ratio >0.6 or
- a pleural LDH over two-thirds of the upper limit of normal serum LDH.

Glucose

Pleural glucose is low in pleural infection, rheumatoid pleurisy and malignancy (where it indicates that pleurodesis is less likely to be successful).

pH

A pH should be requested on all non-turbid samples; analysis of turbid samples is unnecessary and may damage the blood gas analyser. Heparinize the sample in a blood gas syringe and alert the laboratory that the sample is pleural fluid. A pleural pH <7.2 suggests pleural infection and is a powerful indication for intercostal drainage.

Others

Analyses that may be useful when specific aetiologies are suspected include amylase (pancreatitis, oesophageal rupture), haematocrit (haemothorax), rheumatoid factor (rheumatoid effusions), triglycerides and cholesterol (chylothorax and pseudochylothorax, respectively).

Cytology

May identify malignant cell populations and provides a differential cell count:

- neutrophils: any acute effusion, e.g. parapneumonic, PTE
- lymphocytes: TB, especially if >80% of the total population; malignancy, including lymphoma
- mesothelial cells: often seen in transudates, but not a helpful aetiological discriminator.

Microbiology

Pleural fluid should be sent in blood culture bottles for Gram and auramine staining and culture, including for TB. Positive results with coagulase negative staphylococcus and mixed organisms may indicate contamination.

Synovial fluid

Normal synovial fluid is clear, colourless to pale yellow and contains very few cells. Features on analysis suggestive of disease are:

- pus or increased total cell (particularly neutrophil) count: found in inflammation and infection
- white colour: suggests urate crystals or cholesterol
- crystals on light microscopy: urate crystals are needle-shaped and have negative birefringence; calcium pyrophosphate crystals are rhomboid with positive birefringence; note, local anaesthetic used in the procedure may appear as negatively birefringent crystals
- uniform blood staining: florid synovitis or trauma
- organisms on Gram-stain or culture.

Ascitic fluid

Normal ascitic fluid is clear. Cloudy fluid suggests infection; blood is in keeping with malignancy; bile suggests a bilious communication and milky fluid, lymphatic obstruction. Features on analysis suggestive of disease are:

- protein: ascites with a protein concentration below 25 g/L is usually due to cirrhosis, whereas a protein concentration above this (or serum: ascites albumin ratio below 1.5) can be found in infection, malignancy and hepatic venous obstruction
- amylase: a high amylase level (>1000 U/L) is found in pancreatic ascites
- glucose: a low level suggests malignancy or TB
- white cells: a leucocyte count above 250/mm^3 suggests infection, e.g. spontaneous bacterial peritonitis (see p. 163)
- cytology: may reveal a malignant cell population.

ECG INTERPRETATION

An electrocardiogram (ECG) is a graphic representation of the electrical activity of the heart and does not necessarily indicate myocardial contractility. ECG machines record the electrical activation of cardiac muscle cells which results in the depolarization of cell membranes. The difference in polarity between the activated cell membrane and adjacent cells results in electrical currents that can be detected by electrodes attached to the patient's skin.

This section reviews the features that define a normal ECG trace, provides examples of common ECG abnormalities and proposes a structured approach to ECG interpretation. Guidance on performing an ECG can be found in 'Procedures', p. 65. Details on the management of arrhythmias and cardiac ischaemia can be found in 'Arrhythmias', p. 132, and 'Chest pain', p. 125, respectively.

ECG analysis

Modern ECG machines produce '12-lead' ECG recordings using 10 electrodes. This apparent discrepancy reflects the fact that the word 'lead', in this context, refers to a virtual line along which electrical signals travel, rather than a physical electrical connection.

A typical ECG trace of a normal single heart beat is shown in Figure 3.1. Einthoven assigned the letters P, Q, R, S and T to the individual deflections of the ECG trace in 1901. Each waveform corresponds to a step in the propagation of electrical signals through the heart. The voltage baseline of the trace is known as the isoelectric line.

The ECG is a key diagnostic tool in the investigation of many cardiac, pulmonary and metabolic conditions. The order in which you look at the individual features on the trace is less important than making a complete and comprehensive assessment. However, the scheme of 'rate, rhythm, axis, waves and intervals' is commonly used because the rate and rhythm can help to direct further assessment.

Rate and rhythm

Rate

To determine the heart rate, divide 300 by the R-R interval, counted in the number of large boxes. The normal heart rate is 60–100 b.p.m. In tachycardia, the heart rate is >100 b.p.m.; in bradycardia it is <60 b.p.m.

The ECG trace should be regular and every P wave should be followed by a QRS wave after a constant time interval. However, normal variations are common, including:

- sinus arrhythmia: phasic alteration of the heart rate with respiration
- sinus bradycardia: may be normal in athletic individuals, but can be due to pathological processes or drugs; see below
- sinus tachycardia: usually due to an increased sympathetic drive associated with exercise, emotion, pregnancy, but also associated with pain or general systemic upset.

Rhythm

Look at the rhythm strip or, if none is available, lead I, II or V1 where P waves should be clearly visible. Determine:

- *whether the rhythm is regular*: mark the peaks of consecutive R waves on a piece of paper placed on top of your trace; the interval should remain constant when you move the piece of paper onto another section of the ECG

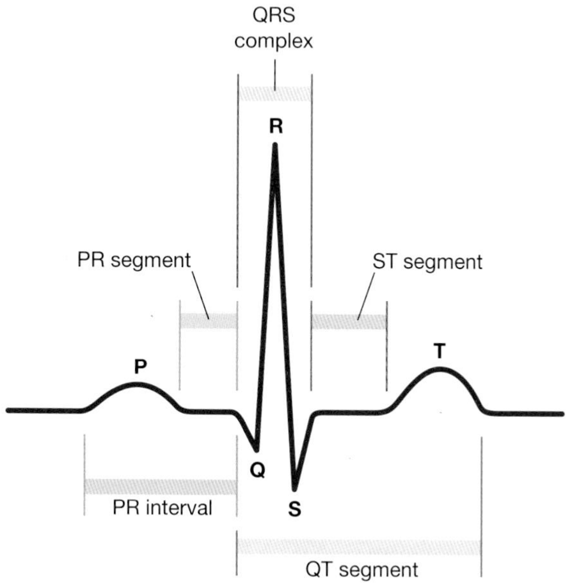

Figure 3.1 The PQRST complex.

- *whether the rhythm is sinus*: for sinus rhythm to be present the P wave must be visible and positive in leads II and aVF and negative in aVR
- *the rate*: calculate this based on the R-R interval as suggested above; for irregular rhythms calculate an average value or range.

Rhythm disorders

An arrhythmia describes a rhythm other than sinus rhythm and should be categorized according to the following:

- rate: tachyarrhythmias (>100 b.p.m.) and bradyarrhythmias (<60 b.p.m.)
- regularity
- likely origin: narrow or broad complex.

These distinctions are largely self-explanatory and the first two have been covered earlier in this section. The differentiation between broad and narrow complex arrhythmias is an important one. Narrow complex rhythms originate above the AV node and are therefore conducted down the normal route through the ventricles. Broad complex arrhythmias are defined by a QRS duration >0.12 s (three small boxes) and originate either within the ventricles, or above the AV node with aberrant conduction down a pre-existing bundle branch block. They are important to identify as true ventricular arrhythmias are often poorly tolerated and more dangerous. A description of the common types of arrhythmia is found in 'Identification of arrhythmias', below.

Axis

Leads I, II, III, aVR, aVR and aVL can be used to determine the electrical axis of the heart in the frontal plane. This reflects the overall direction of the depolarization wavefront as it travels through the heart.

The electrical axis is determined by a hexaxial reference system (Fig. 3.2). To use this system, identify which lead of the six above has the most equiphasic QRS complex (where the positive and negative deflections of the QRS complex appear roughly equivalent). Select the lead that runs perpendicular to this lead on the hexaxial reference diagram. The electrical axis is then determined by looking at the polarity of the QRS complex in this perpendicular lead on the ECG trace. If the QRS deflection in the perpendicular lead is positive, the electrical axis is positive. For example, if the most equiphasic lead is I, the perpendicular lead will be aVF; if the QRS deflection on the ECG is positive in aVF, the electrical axis will be +90°.

- normal axis: −30° to +90°
- left axis deviation: −30° to −90° may indicate left anterior fascicular block or Q waves from a previous inferior MI
- right axis deviation: +90° to +180° may indicate right ventricular strain, Q waves from a high lateral MI or left posterior fascicular block.

Left or right axis deviation in association with right bundle branch block indicates bifascicular block (trifascicular block if also associated with 1st-degree heart block).

Waves and intervals

P wave

This is initiated by firing of the SA node, which itself cannot be detected by the ECG trace. The P wave represents organized depolarization of the atria, right then left. A normal P wave, indicative of sinus rhythm, must be positive in leads II and aVF and negative in aVR. This deflection should be smooth and up to 2.5 mm tall and 0.12 mm wide (three small boxes). P-wave abnormalities include:

- *P mitrale*: left atrial enlargement in mitral valve disease may result in an enlarged, notched P wave
- *P pulmonale*: increased right heart pressures and right atrial enlargement in chronic hypoxic lung disease
- *P wave inversion*: retrograde activation through the AV node may result in an inverted P wave in a lead in which it should be positive, e.g. lead II.

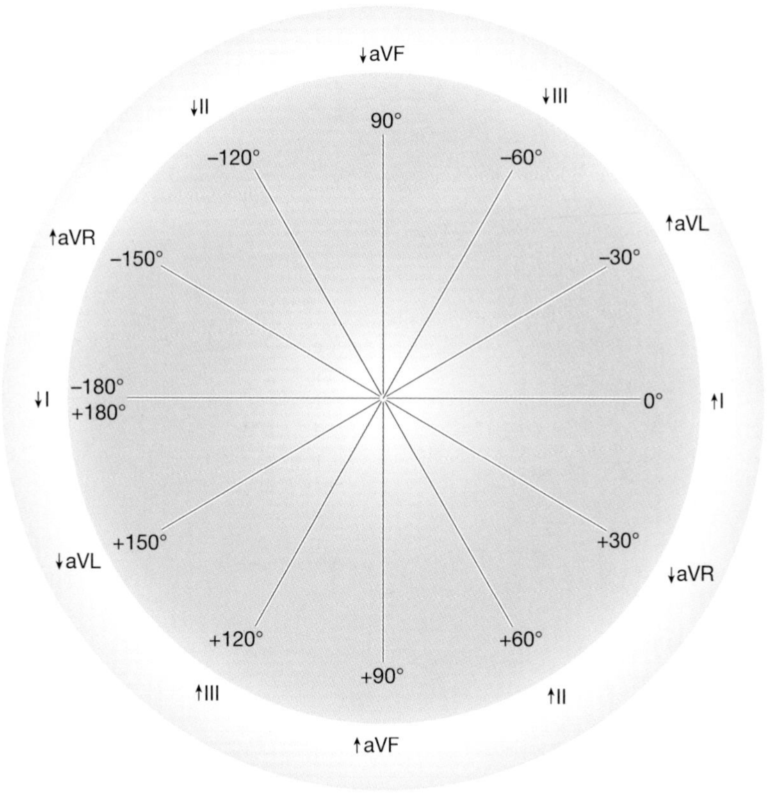

Figure 3.2 The hexaxial reference system.

PR interval

This is the interval from the beginning of the P wave to the beginning of the QRS complex. PR is used rather than PQ because, on a normal trace, most leads will not record a Q wave (see below). The PR interval should be between 0.12 and 0.2 s (3–5 small boxes). However, the PR interval will shorten physiologically in response to high heart rates. Abnormalities of the PR interval include:

- a prolonged, or variable, PR interval may occur in AV node disease which results in varying degrees of heart block; see below
- a shortened PR interval may occur in pre-excitation syndromes which result in early activation of the ventricles, e.g. Wolff–Parkinson–White syndrome, or where this is an ectopic atrial pacemaker, situated closer to the AV node than the SA node.

QRS wave

This represents depolarization of the ventricles. Normal conduction through the high-speed electrical conducting tissues (bundle of His, bundle branches and Purkinje fibres) creates a narrow QRS wave; normal duration 0.06–0.1 s (maximum duration of three small boxes). Note that not all leads will record a Q wave and, if present, these may be physiological or pathological. Physiological Q waves are seen in I, aVL, V5 and V6 and represent septal depolarization, hence the name 'septal Q waves'. Common abnormalities of the QRS complex include LVH, poor R-wave progression and bundle branch block.

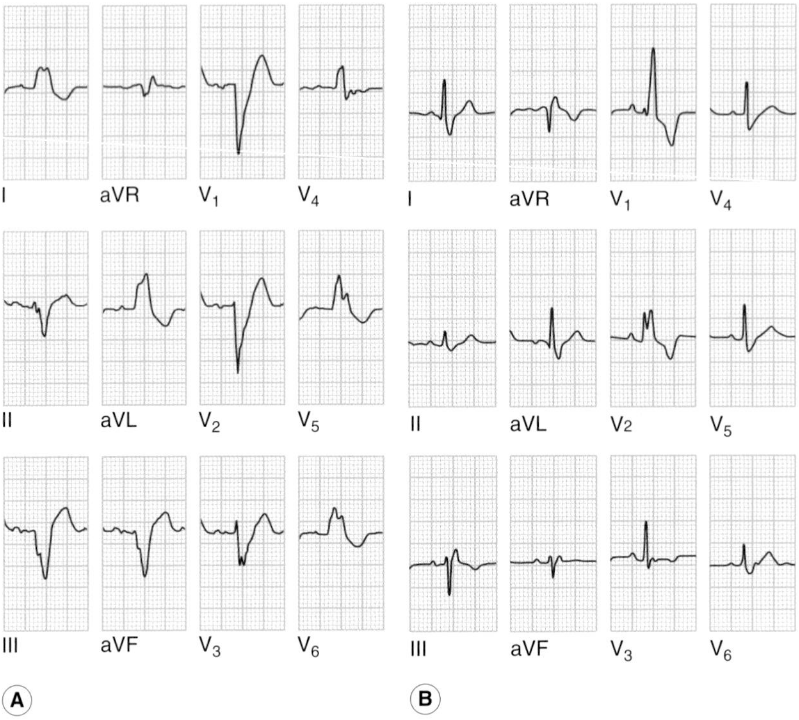

Figure 3.3 (a) Left bundle branch block (LBBB). (b) Right bundle branch block (RBBB).

Left ventricular hypertrophy (LVH)

The increased muscle bulk creates an increased voltage when it depolarizes. Voltage criteria for LVH include a combined amplitude of the S wave in V1 and the R wave in V5 >35 mm or an R wave amplitude >12 mm in aVL.

Poor R wave progression

The QRS complex should be negative in V1, positive in V6 and there should be a smooth increase in R wave amplitude between leads V1 and V4. Poor R wave progression is a non-specific finding, but suggests underlying cardiac disease.

Bundle branch block

Interruption to right or left bundles of the bundle of His delays conduction, broadens the QRS complex (>0.12 s defines complete bundle branch block) and produces characteristic ECG patterns; see Figure 3.3a for left (LBBB) and Figure 3.3b for right bundle branch block (RBBB). RBBB may be a normal variant, but LBBB indicates significant underlying cardiac disease.

ST segment

This connects the QRS complex to the T wave; the origin of the ST segment is known as the J point. The ST segment often has a slightly upward concavity, but should be isoelectric and in-line with the preceding PR and subsequent TP segments. ST segment deviation is an important indicator of myocardial ischaemia and infarction.

Depression may indicate myocardial ischaemia. However, this may be rate-related in the setting of tachyarrhythmias or a reflection of excessive muscle bulk in LVH ('strain' pattern). Widespread, up-sloping, 'reverse-tick' ST depression is a typical consequence of digoxin use.

ST elevation may indicate myocardial infarction, especially if territorial and associated with reciprocal ST depression in other areas. Knowledge of the relationship between coronary artery perfusion territories and the standard ECG leads is essential when interpreting ECGs in patients with chest pain:

- anteroseptal leads, V1–V4: left coronary artery system (Fig. 3.4)
- lateral leads, I, aVL, V5–6: left coronary artery system
- inferior leads, II, III, aVF: right coronary artery (Fig. 3.5)
- high lateral leads, I, aVL: circumflex artery.

Other causes of ST segment elevation include pericarditis (where the elevation is smoother, concave upwards and widespread across the leads) and ventricular aneurysm (where it persists indefinitely) and 'high-take-off'. An artificial and insignificant upsloping elevation is seen during rapid heart rates.

T wave

This represents ventricular repolarization or 'recovery'. The T wave may be up to 5 mm in height in the limb leads (10 mm in chest leads). T waves are usually positive in all leads other than aVR, III and V1. The interval from the beginning of the QRS wave to the peak of the T wave is termed the 'absolute refractory period'. The last half of the T wave is termed the 'relative refractory period' or vulnerable period; ectopic beats occurring during this time can lead to dangerous arrhythmias.

T wave inversion may occur in cardiac ischaemia (see 'Chest pain', p. 125) and changes in morphology may occur with electrolyte disturbances, e.g. 'tented T waves' in hyperkalaemia (see 'Electrolytes', p. 204).

QT interval

This is the time taken between depolarization and repolarization. The normal QT interval is around 0.4 s; however, this is inversely proportional to heart rate. To correct for the heart rate use the following: corrected QT interval (QTc) = $QT/\sqrt{\text{R-R interval}}$, where the R-R interval is the time interval, in seconds, between R waves.

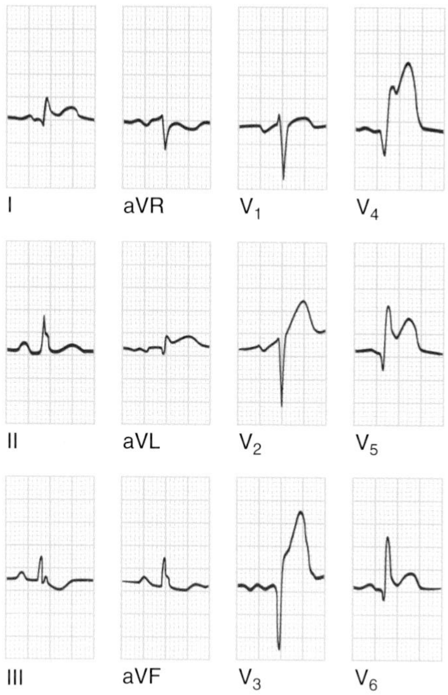

Figure 3.4 Anterior myocardial infarction (MI).

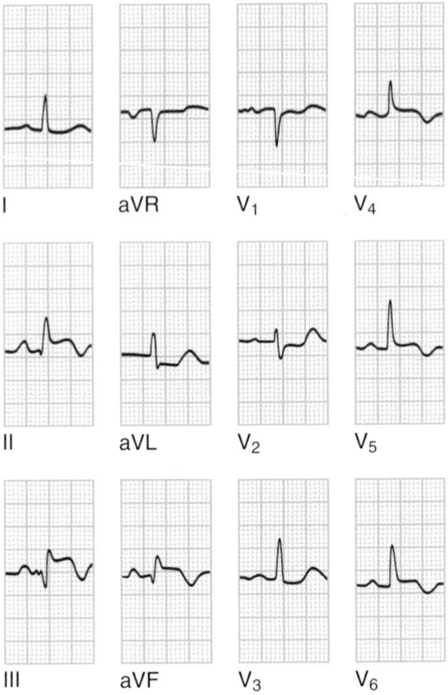

Figure 3.5 Inferior myocardial infarction (MI).

Pathological lengthening occurs in hypokalaemia, hypocalcaemia, hypomagnesaemia, a side-effect of drugs, e.g. erythromycin, clarithromycin, haloperidol, and in congenital long QT syndrome. This results in delayed ventricular repolarization and an increased risk of ventricular arrhythmias, particularly torsades de pointes. QT shortening (<0.3 s) occurs in congenital short QT syndrome which can result in VF and sudden death.

R-R interval

This is the time interval between sequential R waves and is used to determine the heart rate from the ECG trace. R-R variability is also used as a measure of arrhythmogenic potential in a variety of conditions.

U wave

Visible in 50–75% of normal ECGs, this represents depolarization of the papillary muscles and Purkinje fibres. Prominent U waves are seen in patients with hypokalaemia, hypercalcaemia, digoxin toxicity and thyrotoxicosis.

Identification of arrhythmias

Narrow complex tachyarrhythmias

The alternative name for these is supraventricular tachyarrhythmias (SVT), as any arrhythmia originating above the bifurcation of the bundle of His will be narrow complex, unless there is concomitant bundle branch block. However, the term SVT is usually reserved for the regular narrow complex tachycardia caused by an AVNRT or AVRT; see below.

When faced with a narrow complex tachyarrhythmia, the important early distinction to make is between regular and irregular rhythms.

Irregular narrow complex tachyarrhythmias

Irregular rhythms will be either atrial fibrillation or atrial flutter with variable block.

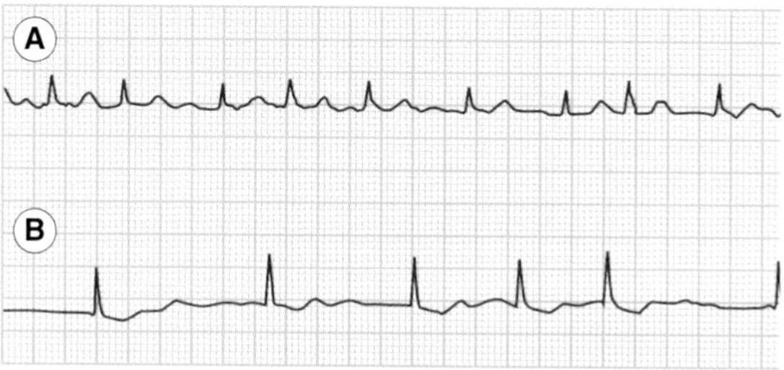

Figure 3.6 Atrial fibrillation with a fast (A) and slow (B) ventricular response.

Atrial fibrillation

P waves will be absent and the ventricular rate will depend on the proportion of atrial beats conducted to the ventricles (Fig. 3.6). There may be ST segment or T wave changes due to underlying cardiac disease, heart rate or digoxin therapy.

Atrial flutter with variable block

See 'Atrial flutter', below.

Regular narrow complex tachyarrhythmias

Sinus tachycardia

This reflects excessive sympathetic drive and may be a physiological response. It may accompany any pathological condition associated with an increased sympathetic drive, e.g. thyrotoxicosis, phaeochromocytoma, pain or distress. The rate is rarely above 150 b.p.m.

Atrial tachycardia

This is due to an ectopic atrial pacemaker and, therefore, P wave morphology will be abnormal. The rate is usually 150–250 b.p.m. and AV block may be present. In multifocal atrial tachycardia, several pacemakers exist and P wave morphology will be variable and, therefore, ventricular rate may be more irregular.

AV nodal re-entrant tachycardia (AVNRT)

Where an accessory pathway exists within the AV node itself, this can result in a re-entrant rhythm. This accounts for the majority of the commonly seen SVTs and results in a narrow complex tachycardia where P waves may be inverted and occur after the QRS or be hidden within it.

AV re-entrant tachycardia (AVRT)

Caused by an abnormal band of rapidly conducting tissue (accessory pathway) connecting the atria and ventricles. Examples where the accessory pathway has been identified include Lown–Ganong–Levine syndrome (the James bundle) and Wolff–Parkinson–White syndrome (the bundle of Kent). In the latter pre-excitation of the ventricles results in a 'slurred' δ-wave before the QRS.

Atrial flutter with fixed AV block

Flutter waves in the atria circulate at about 300 b.p.m. and are visible on the ECG trace as a 'saw-tooth' baseline. The AV node is unable to conduct all impulses and, therefore, limits the ventricular rate with a block that may be fixed or variable. The ventricular response rate will be around 75, 100 or 150/min if there is 4, 3 or 2:1 block, respectively. If the extent of AV block is variable, the ventricular rate will be irregular. Commonly, 2:1 AV block occurs; therefore, atrial flutter should always be suspected with a regular tachyarrhythmia of around 150 b.p.m. (Fig. 3.7).

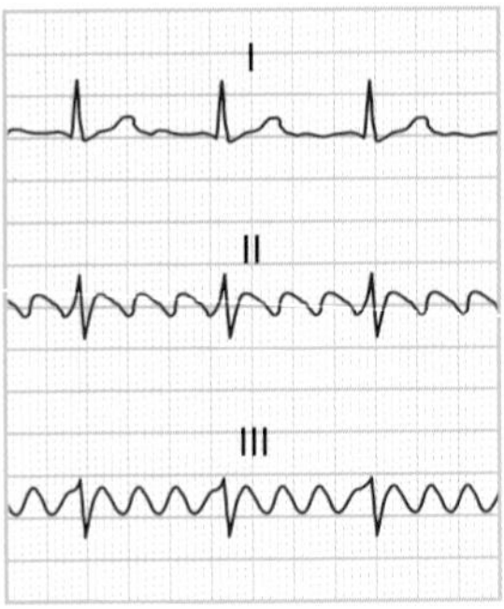

Figure 3.7 Atrial flutter, as shown for leads I, II and III.

Broad complex tachyarrhythmias

Defined by a QRS duration >0.12 s (3 small boxes), as described above. Examine the rhythm strip and determine if the trace is regular or irregular.

Regular broad complex tachyarrhythmias

These will either be ventricular tachycardia (VT) or SVT with aberrant conduction, discussed above. VT is defined as a regular broad complex tachycardia, over 120 b.p.m., and may be self terminating or 'unsustained' (defined by a duration <30 s) or persistent and 'sustained' (Fig. 3.8). It may be difficult to differentiate VT from an SVT with aberrant conduction, but ECG features that favour VT include:

- QRS complex >140 ms (3.5 small squares)
- a recent ECG showing normal conduction
- marked left axis deviation (negative complex in lead II)
- AV dissociation
- fusion or capture beats: in VT the SA node will be firing independently; occasionally an atrial beat will be conducted to the ventricles resulting in a normal looking (narrow) QRS complex
- QRS concordance (same pattern across all leads): if the QRS is predominantly positive this strongly suggests VT.

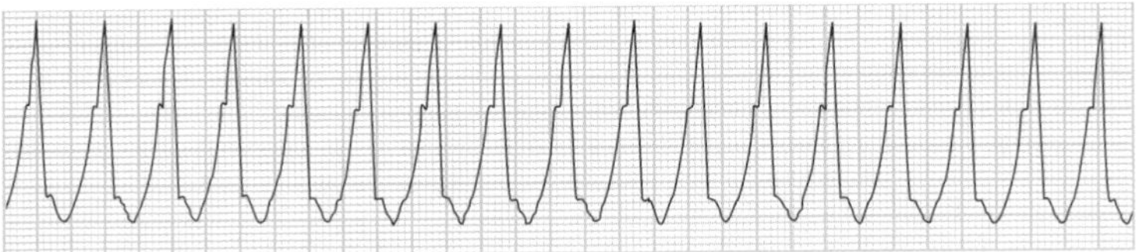

Figure 3.8 Ventricular tachycardia (VT).

Irregular broad complex tachyarrhythmias

These are likely to be AF or multifocal atrial tachycardia with bundle branch block or polymorphic VT. VF would also produce an irregular broad complex rhythm.

Polymorphic VT

This is a complication of delayed ventricular repolarization, identifiable by a prolonged QT interval (Fig. 3.9). Commonly known as torsades de pointes (translated

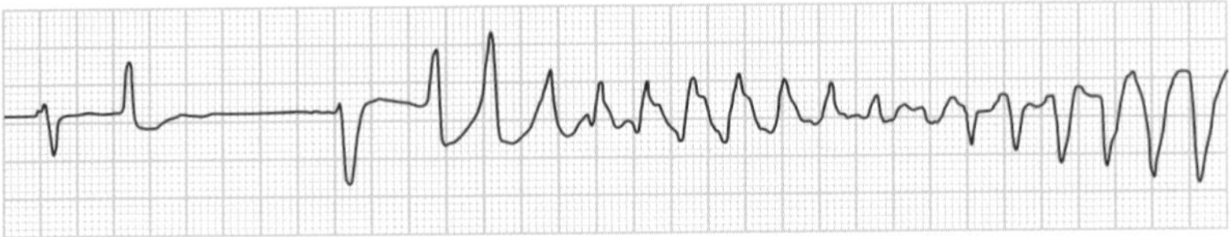

Figure 3.9 Polymorphic ventricular tachycardia (VT) following an R or T ectopic.

as twisting of the points) and characterized by variation in QRS amplitude resulting in a trace that appears to twist around the isoelectric baseline. Usually non-sustained, but can degenerate into VF.

VF

There is a chaotic irregular rhythm with indiscernible PQRS morphology (Fig. 3.10). It is incompatible with a cardiac output and rarely seen on a 12-lead ECG.

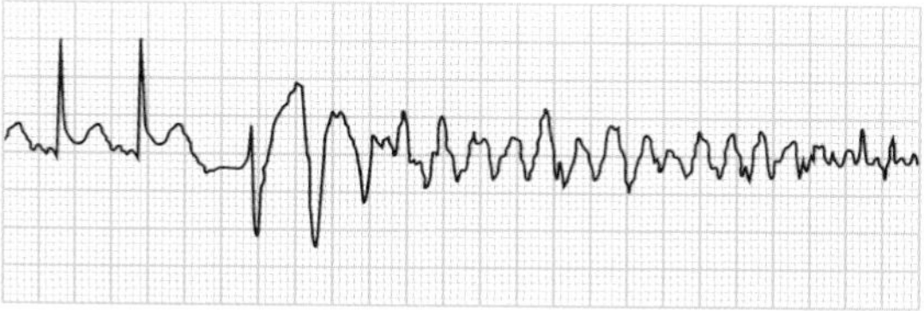

Figure 3.10 Ventricular fibrillation.

Bradyarrhythmias

Defined by a heart rate <60 b.p.m. Sinus bradycardia may be physiological in athletes or in response to drugs, e.g. β-blockers, diltiazem, verapamil. However, it may reflect AV or heart block as a result of disease. In profound bradycardia escape rhythms may develop.

Escape bradyarrhythmias

This is a regular collection of junctional or ventricular escape beats (see below), which fire at the usual rate for that part of the heart (40–60 for junctional; 20–40 for ventricular). They occur when the SA or AV node persistently fails to generate or conduct a beat and a new intrinsic cardiac 'pacemaker' must take over. The resulting rhythms are called junctional bradycardia and idioventricular rhythm, respectively. The former has narrow, normal size beats and may have P waves that are inverted; the latter has larger, broader beats and P waves are usually absent. In accelerated idioventricular rhythm, the rate is between 41 and 100/min.

Heart block

This can cause a mixture of regular and irregular bradyarrhythmias depending on the level of AV block. Delay in conduction through the AV node may increase the PR interval and, in some cases, conduction through the node may not occur, leading to a failure of ventricular depolarization.

First degree

There is an increase in the time taken for AV conduction. PR interval is increased (>0.2 s, three small boxes) which may occur physiologically or as a result of medication (Fig. 3.11).

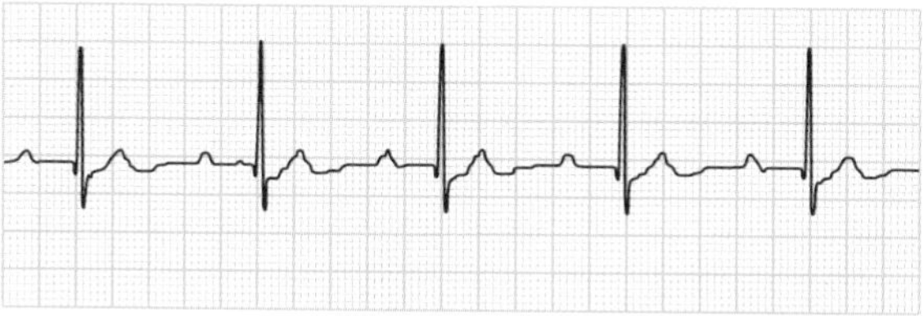

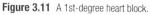

Figure 3.11 A 1st-degree heart block.

Second degree

Some, but not all, P waves are conducted through the AV node resulting in 'dropped' beats. There are two forms:

- *Mobitz type I (Wenckebach)*: there is progressive prolongation of the PR interval until a P wave occurs without an accompanying QRS complex

(Fig. 3.12A); usually repeated; may be physiological in fit young adults but can result from any condition that causes AV conduction delay, including ischaemia

- *Mobitz type II*: the PR interval is constant, but not all P waves are followed by QRS complexes (Fig. 3.12B); usually caused by disease within the conducting system and carries a high risk of progression to asystole; may appear random (variable block) or there may be a regular relationship between the P waves and conducted QRS complexes, e.g. 2:1 block, where every second P wave is followed by a QRS

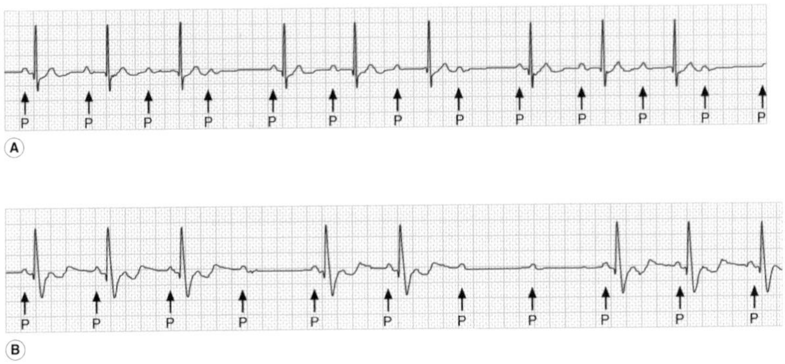

Figure 3.12 A 2nd-degree heart block. (a) Mobitz type I. (b) Mobitz type II.

Third degree

There is complete dissociation of P waves and QRS complexes: atrial and ventricular depolarization occur independently from separate pacemakers (Fig. 3.13). The site of the ventricular pacemaker will determine the ventricular rate and QRS duration. The lower the ventricular rate, the higher the risk of symptoms and degeneration to asystole.

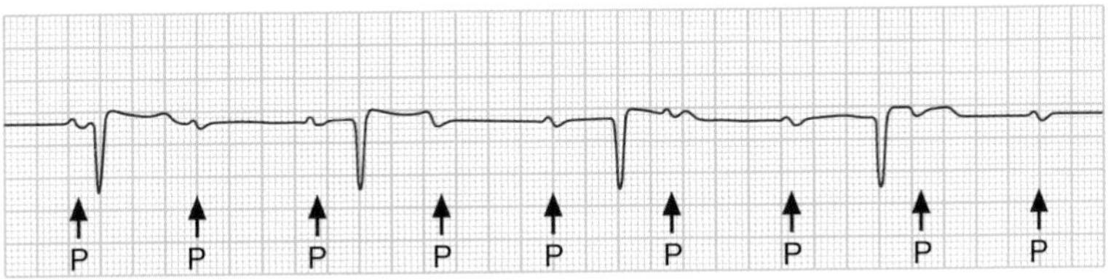

Figure 3.13 A 3rd-degree heart block.

Transient beat to beat arrhythmias

If the rhythm appears irregular, examine the relationship between P and QRS waves. If this appears normal, look for 'extra' ectopic beats that might explain the irregularity. Ectopic beats are due to premature excitation and occur before the next expected beat. In general they are benign:

- supraventricular ectopics: narrow QRS complex; may be atrial (P waves present) or junctional (P waves absent or inverted) in origin
- ventricular ectopics: broad QRS complex; can occur singly or in groups; two together are called a 'couplet'; three or more appearing sequentially are called a 'salvo'; when every normal beat is followed by a ventricular ectopic, bigeminy is said to be present (the term trigeminy is used if this occurs after every two normal beats).

PEAK FLOW AND SPIROMETRY

Peak flow

Peak flow, or peak expiratory flow rate (PEFR), is the most commonly used test of lung function. PEFR (L/min) is reached within the first fraction of a second during a maximum forced expiratory manoeuvre and reflects the calibre of the large, proximal airways.

Although cheap and apparently simple to perform, peak flow is very dependent upon patient effort. For this reason, normal ranges or 'predicted' peak flows are notoriously unreliable and it is difficult to draw definitive conclusions regarding airway calibre from isolated measurements. Serial PEFR measurements are much more useful, but even then should be interpreted relative to a patient's 'best' rather than a predicted value read from a chart. Under these circumstances, PEFR can be useful as a measure of airway calibre, and therefore of control in both acute and chronic asthma. All asthmatics should be encouraged to know their best PEFR.

In the acute asthmatic inpatient, PEFR can be used to assess severity and monitor treatment (see 'Asthma', p. 141). In chronic asthma, PEFR variability (a variation of >20% on at least 3 days in a given week) can be used as an aid in diagnosis and as part of an asthma self-management plan.

Spirometry

Spirometry plots depict change in lung volume against time during a forced expiratory manoeuvre, describing airflow and basic lung volume. Three measurements can be derived from a spirometry curve:

- FEV_1: forced expiratory volume exhaled within the first second
- FVC: forced vital capacity; this is total volume of air that can be exhaled; the FVC (the point at which the trace flattens) is reached in normal subjects within 3–4 s
- FEV_1/FVC ratio: this is self-explanatory; in healthy lungs, 70–80% of the FVC can be exhaled within the first second of the manoeuvre and the normal FEV_1/FVC ratio is 0.7–0.8.

These values, also known as the dynamic lung volumes, can be used to distinguish between two broad groups of lung disease that affect airflow and lung volumes differently: obstructive and restrictive lung disorders. Figure 3.14 overleaf, shows the typical spirograms obtained in normal patients and those with obstructive and restrictive lung disease.

Obstructive lung disease

In obstructive lung disease, expiratory airflow is reduced due to a reduction in airway calibre, most commonly due to COPD or asthma. The FEV_1 is reduced because airway narrowing results in a slower expiratory manoeuvre. FVC is usually normal (although it will take longer to reach) and, therefore, the FEV_1/FVC ratio is reduced.

Reversibility in obstructive lung disease

Obstructed airways that can respond to bronchodilator stimuli are said to display 'reversibility', which is characteristic of asthma. Reversibility is measured by repeating spirometry after a nebulized bronchodilator (e.g. 2.5 mg salbutamol) or a course of inhaled or oral steroids. 'Significant' reversibility can be defined as a 15% increase in FEV_1 (and/or FVC), or an absolute increase of ≥ 200 mL if the FEV_1 is <1 L.

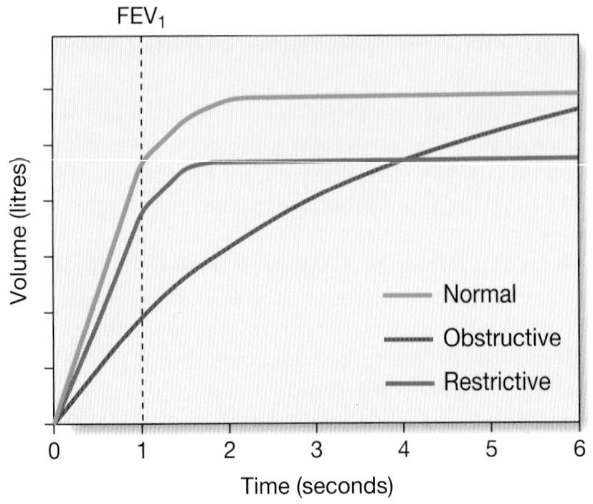

Figure 3.14 Typical spirograms.

Restrictive lung disease

In restrictive lung disorders, the primary defect is within the interstitium of the lung (e.g. pulmonary fibrosis), or the chest wall (e.g. kyphoscoliosis), not the airways. The volume of air that can be drawn into the lungs is reduced, either due to lung stiffening and reduced lung volumes, or because of reduced mechanical efficiency of the chest wall. Therefore, the physiological hallmark of restrictive lung disease is a reduction in FVC.

The rate at which air is exhaled is either normal (because the airways are normal), or increased (due to increased elastic recoil of stiffened lungs). Therefore, although FEV_1 is usually reduced to a similar extent to FVC, it can be normal or even elevated in restrictive disease. As a result, the FEV_1/FVC ratio is either preserved or increased.

RADIOLOGICAL TESTS

Legal and safe requests

As a junior doctor, you will be responsible for the vast majority of imaging requests for patients under your care. Therefore, it is important that you are aware of the legal responsibilities of requesting such examinations as detailed in the DH 'Ionising Radiation (Medical Exposure) Regulations 2000'.

Take care to:

- request the correct examination for the correct patient
- provide as much relevant patient information as possible, as this will influence the choice of investigation and the interpretation of the images
- avoid making duplicate requests for the same test.

Consent

Radiological tests expose the patient to radiation, intervention or examination. They should be regarded as procedures, not just investigations. It is important that informed consent is obtained (see 'Capacity, consent and competence', p. 404). In addition, requests for high radiation-dose, complex examinations such as CT scans should be made in consultation with a senior member of the medical team. Table 3.3 provides a list of radiation dose equivalents for some common investigations.

Table 3.3 Radiation dose equivalents

Procedure	Typical dose (mSv)	CXR equivalent
Chest (PA) X-ray	0.02	1
Lumbar spine X-ray	1.3	65
Abdominal X-ray	1.0	50
IVU	2.5	125
Barium enema	7	350
CT head	2.3	115
CT chest	8	400
CT abdomen OR pelvis	10	500
Bone scan (technetium-99m)	4	200

Intravenous contrast

Intravenous access

If intravenous access is required for a procedure, a cannula should be inserted before the patient leaves the ward.

Renal impairment

Iodine-based IV contrast agents used in CT, urography and angiography are potentially nephrotoxic, especially in patients with pre-existing renal impairment in whom you should:

- warn radiology staff of the renal impairment, prior to the investigation
- postpone, where possible, the examination until renal function is restored
- consider alternative investigation strategies
- adequately hydrate the patient with IV fluid where appropriate.

The IV contrast agent used for MRI (gadolinium) should also be avoided in patients with significant renal failure. In addition, patients taking metformin are at a greater risk of renal impairment and the department should be notified.

Contrast reaction

Iodine-based contrast agents may also rarely induce an allergic reaction. Asthmatics and those who have had a previous contrast reaction are at an increased risk and the department should be notified.

Magnetic resonance imaging

MRI does not involve ionizing radiation; however, some patients find lying in the scanner claustrophobic and the noise unpleasant. The magnetic field is permanently switched on and, therefore, access to the MRI suite is restricted. Most examinations last for 20–30 min. Consider the following:

- you must always inform the unit that a patient has a pacemaker: MRI may not be safe in some cases, although, most modern devices are MRI compatible
- MRI staff should be informed of any metallic implants or foreign bodies to allow an assessment of MRI compatibility, e.g. intracranial clips or coils, joint replacements
- patients with known or suspected intraocular metallic foreign bodies will require plain X-ray; if confirmed, the examination will be cancelled since movement of these objects in the magnetic field may cause severe disability or even death.

Pregnancy

If possible, examinations involving ionizing radiation or MRI should be deferred until after delivery. Where this is not possible they should be arranged by senior staff and the patient must be made fully aware of the risks.

Using specific radiological tests

Plain X-rays

The most commonly requested plain films are of the chest and abdomen; see pp. 94 and 101 for detailed guidance on these. Back and neck pain are extremely common symptoms in the general population. However, plain radiography of cervical, thoracic and lumbar spine is not routinely indicated, unless there has been trauma, or there is a suspicion of neoplasm or osteomyelitis. MRI of the spine is used even less frequently, but should be performed in patients with persistent pain if associated with long tract signs or clinical suspicions of cord involvement or disc herniation.

Except following trauma, plain imaging of joints is rarely required. Indications include investigation of degenerative and/or erosive arthropathies and episodes of suspected joint infection. CT, MRI and isotope bone scanning have a role in the further investigation of some patients, as directed by relevant clinical specialists.

Barium examinations

In addition to plain radiography, contrast agents may be given to highlight structures that are not normally visible. In the GI tract, intraluminal masses, obstructive or constrictive lesions can be identified with the use of water-soluble contrast:

- barium swallow: contrast is swallowed while X-rays are taken of the upper GI tract in 'real time'; this allows the radiologist to assess the effectiveness of the swallow and identify any obstructing lesions
- barium follow-through: contrast is swallowed and images are taken after a suitable interval, allowing the barium time to enter the small bowel
- barium enema: contrast is injected per rectum; the patient is then moved into different positions on a mobile unit to encourage the flow of contrast throughout the large bowel; air is then instilled per rectum to create contrast; some patients report colicky abdominal discomfort and trapped wind.

Preparation

Appropriate consent should be gained from patients before they have these procedures carried out and you should ensure that they are fit enough. Bowel preparation is usually requested to optimize barium enema views. Where there is a risk of perforation, other agents such as Gastrografin® are used in place of barium.

Ultrasound

Ultrasound scanning is non-invasive, generally simple to perform, requires minimal patient preparation and does not involve ionizing radiation. Mostly used for investigation of intra-abdominal or pelvic organs and pathology, ultrasound is particularly useful in assessing the gallbladder and biliary tree. It is also ideal for assessing fluid collections in the abdomen and pleural spaces and can be used as a guide to aid drainage. Young female patients presenting with pelvic pain should be investigated using ultrasound, as this gives much better detail of the ovaries and cystic or solid adnexal masses than other investigations, such as CT. However, the image quality and diagnostic yield of ultrasound are limited in some clinical situations:

- excessive fat, either in obesity or due to fatty deposition in tissues
- gas within bowel loops, e.g. obscuring aorta or pancreas
- free intraperitoneal gas or subcutaneous emphysema
- densely calcified or osseous structures.

Preparation

Patients attending for ultrasound scanning of upper abdomen will usually be asked to fast for up to 6h. This helps to reduce small bowel gas and prevents contraction of the gallbladder, aiding assessment of calculi and inflammation of the gallbladder wall.

Patients attending for ultrasound scanning of the pelvic organs will be asked to have a full bladder. This aids imaging by lifting the gassy small bowel loops up out of the lower pelvis and uses the fluid-filled bladder as an 'acoustic window' through to the pelvic organs. This characteristic, plus the lack of ionizing radiation, makes this one of the best ways to assess the female pelvic organs and also the developing fetus.

CT scanning

CT scanning uses ionizing radiation to build up a cross-sectional image of the scanned area. Increasing image resolution and reconstruction potential has greatly widened its range of applications. However, it is associated with a significant radiation dose to the patient and alternative lower dose methods of investigation should always be considered. Your radiology department may offer advice about preparation for patients undergoing CT scanning, but see also that under 'Intravenous contrast' above.

Trauma

CT scanning is especially useful in the early assessment of patients following trauma or head injury and, once the patient is sufficiently stable, aids rapid assessment of internal injuries and the planning of any surgical intervention.

Oncology

CT scanning is used in oncology for the initial staging of solid tumours, demonstrating metastases to distant sites such as the lungs and liver and detecting nodal involvement. It is also used following chemotherapy or radiotherapy regimes to assess treatment impact and detect tumour recurrence.

Neurology

CT is invaluable in the assessment of patients with head trauma or those with a neurological deficit. Likewise, its ability to detect intracranial haemorrhage, in the acute phase of a suspected cerebral infarction, is important when considering antiplatelet therapy or thrombolysis. It may also reveal previously unsuspected pathology, such as an arteriovenous malformation or intracranial neoplasm.

In those patients in whom there is a clinical suspicion of abscess or space-occupying intracranial lesion, IV contrast will usually be given.

Thoracic conditions

In addition to the staging and follow-up of bronchial carcinoma, CT is used to assess the mediastinal structures, such as the thoracic aorta for aneurysm formation or dissection. In addition, CT pulmonary angiography is a first-line investigation for suspected pulmonary embolism (see p. 152); high resolution CT scanning of the lungs is used to assess fibrosis or bronchiectasis, and cardiac imaging, using multi-slice CT, is increasingly developing.

Abdominal imaging

In more complex cases of abdominal pain, e.g. abscesses following diverticulitis, CT scanning may be helpful. In addition, in those with peritonism, small amounts of free intraperitoneal gas not seen on an erect CXR may be detected on CT. Retroperitoneal pathology may also be better established with CT than by ultrasound. Where a ruptured aortic aneurysm is suspected, CT scanning should be the first-line investigation. A non-contrast CT of the abdomen may also be used to identify renal stones.

MRI

MRI is able to generate cross-sectional images in any plane using a large magnetic field and non-ionizing radiofrequency signals. MRI utilizes the signal returned from water protons within the tissue of interest to generate images. Therefore, tissues that have a low water content, e.g. bone, may be better imaged using CT. Contrast agents such as gadolinium can be given IV but should be avoided in patients with renal failure.

Neurological

Brain MRI has a greater diagnostic yield than CT and allows improved visualization of white matter, the brainstem, pituitary and posterior fossa. MR angiography can also be performed and the images reconstructed to visualize the cerebral circulation. MRI is the investigation of choice where spinal cord damage is suspected. It can also detect subtle changes that result from infection or tumour.

Fibromuscular

MRI obtains detailed images of joints, intra-articular structures, ligaments and muscles.

Hepatobiliary

MRCP (magnetic resonance colangio-pancreatography) provides non-invasive assessment of the biliary tree and pancreatic duct. It also gives detailed images of the liver, pancreas and other abdominal organs.

Gastrointestinal

Detailed images of the small bowel can be acquired using MR enteroclysis. Several litres of water-based contrast are injected by a NG tube into the patient's small bowel. It can also help in the diagnosis of small bowel Crohn's disease.

Cardiac

This provides exceptionally detailed structural images of the heart. It is used in the assessment of congenital heart disease, heart failure, valvular and ischaemic heart disease.

CHEST X-RAYS

When interpreting chest X-rays, it is useful to adopt a systematic approach.

Initial assessment

Film quality

Projection

The standard interpretation of a chest film is based on a postero–anterior (PA) view, where the X-ray beam is directed from behind the patient. The patient stands with their chest against the plate and their arms held forwards to remove the scapulae from the field of view. However, if the patient is too unwell to go to the X-ray department, an antero–posterior (AP) view can be taken with the patient sitting or lying with the X-ray plate behind them.

Since the PA view is regarded as the 'norm', only the AP view is usually marked to show its type. The quality of a proper departmental PA view is usually better than the more portable AP view. Where possible, a PA view should be obtained.

Penetration

You should be able to see the lower vertebral bodies through the heart shadow, but only just. If you can see them clearly, the film is probably over-penetrated; if you cannot see them, it is probably under-penetrated. Either will impair your capacity to assess the lungs properly.

Rotation
The medial ends of the clavicles should be the same distance apart from the spinous processes.

Inspiration
A correctly inspired film shows the anterior end of the 6th vertebra and the posterior end of the 10th vertebra just above the diaphragm. Any more and the patient is hyperinflated. If you cannot see these ribs above the diaphragm the X-ray has not been taken during a full inspiration. This may make the heart look artificially larger, or cause the false appearance of shadowing at the lung bases.

The 'quick scan'
Before examining the detail of any one area, it is helpful to have an overview of the whole film.

Trachea
This should be central, but deviate to the right near the aortic knuckle.

Mediastinum
Check the general shape: it should have a narrow 'bottle-neck' shape at the top and broaden gently like a wine bottle. Check for indistinct edges which indicate loss of the air–tissue interface with normal lung (known as the 'silhouette' sign; see 'Position', p. 97).

Hila
The left hilum should be slightly higher than the right; they should be concave and a similar shape and density to each other.

Heart
Check the shape is normal and look for cardiomegaly (i.e. maximum diameter > half the thoracic diameter on a PA view); as for the mediastinum, check for a distinct edge on both sides.

Diaphragm
The right should be slightly higher than the left and the edges smooth, slightly domed and distinct. The highest point of each dome should be in the middle of the right hemithorax, but slightly to the left of the midline on the left. A triangle of clear lung should be visible at each costophrenic angle.

Lung fields
These should look similar, both from side-to-side and top-to-bottom. Compare each side with the other in thirds or 'zones': upper, middle, lower. Identify any obvious difference. Look for:

- any discrete opacities or an area of more general opacification/shadowing and which 'zone' it is in, e.g. right upper zone, bilateral lower zone shadowing
- differences in the shape of the upper third as framed by the ribs: check whether they are similarly inflated or whether one side is slightly less full, with its ribs slightly flatter than the other side; if so there may be reduced lung volume on that side
- the position of the horizontal fissure: if visible, this should go from the right hilum to the 6th rib in the axillary line; if it is higher, there may be volume loss in the upper lobe.

Bones
Run your eye over the edges of each rib looking for interruption of the smooth outline and/or missing bits from the edge, e.g. tumours, fractures. Likewise, look out for any dark 'holes', e.g. lytic lesions. Check over the other bones for any other 'black' bits or indistinct edges. Look at the overall density and for evidence of osteoporosis (difficult on a chest film).

Soft tissues

Look for evidence of obesity or cachexia, and for differences in soft tissue from one side to the other.

Normal film

If there is nothing obvious, double check for:

- shadowing or absent lung markings in the lung apices (Pancoast carcinoma or apical pneumothorax respectively)
- absent breast shadow(s) in females (mastectomy)
- free air under the diaphragm (perforation)
- air along either edge of the mediastinum (pneumomediastinum)
- shadows behind the heart, e.g. an air/fluid level (hernia) or an additional straight line (left lower lobe collapse)
- dextrocardia.

Detailed CXR examination

The hila

It will take some time viewing lots of normal films to be confident about whether hila are a normal size or not. However, it is quite straightforward to spot unilateral enlargement or gross bilateral enlargement. Generally speaking, the hila should be the same size and density and both should be concave in shape. If in doubt, it is always useful to review previous chest films for any sign of change. Remember to check that the film is not rotated as this can make one hilum look bigger. Genuine hilar abnormalities should be described as one of the following:

Unilateral enlargement

- lymphadenopathy (often well defined or lobulated)
- tumour (may be speculated and extend out into the lung tissue)
- pulmonary artery aneurysm (rare).

Bilateral enlargement

- lymphadenopathy as a result of malignancy (e.g. lymphoma), sarcoidosis, TB, silicosis (eggshell calcification)
- prominence of the proximal pulmonary arteries in pulmonary hypertension.

Aetiology

If the hila appear abnormal look for clues elsewhere on the CXR to the underlying pathology:

- tumours or lymphoma may also cause mediastinal lymphadenopathy: look for broadening of the mediastinum along the side of the trachea (paratracheal nodes)
- other signs of lung tumour: intrapulmonary mass, lobar collapse, effusions
- other signs of cardiac disease, e.g. cardiomegaly
- other evidence of sarcoidosis, e.g. nodular pulmonary infiltrates.

The heart

It is important to comment on heart size when reporting CXRs. Cardiomegaly is defined as a cardiac shadow more than half the total diameter of the chest. If the heart is enlarged consider whether it is global or localized to one area, or quadrant.

Global enlargement

This suggests either:

- LV dysfunction, often ischaemic or hypertensive heart disease; look for other signs of heart failure and ischaemic heart disease, including pulmonary oedema, pleural effusions, upper lobe venous diversion and median thoracotomy clips from a previous CABG
- pericardial effusion: look for a globular 'filled-sac' shape.

Localized enlargement of one quadrant

- *Top left:* may reflect LA enlargement, look for evidence of pulmonary venous engorgement and interstitial fluid; consider mitral valve disease
- *Top right:* may reflect a dilated right pulmonary artery or an engorged superior vena cava
- *Bottom right:* consider RA enlargement; may be due to an ASD or pulmonary hypertension
- *Bottom left:* may reflect LV enlargement (if apex depressed; may be due to ischaemia or cardiomyopathy), RV enlargement (if apex elevated; may be due to chronic pulmonary hypertension or pulmonary stenosis) or ventricular aneurysm.

Something 'in' or 'behind' the heart

Classical densities seen in this area include:

- a triangular opacity with a straight edge: left lower lobe collapse
- a ring or disc-like shadow: prosthetic valve replacement
- wires attached to a box near the shoulder; a pacemaker, remember that one wire indicates a single chamber device, two indicates a dual chamber system.

White areas in the lung fields

Lumps

Consider the size, number, outline, position and density of any white lumps visible on the CXR:

Small lumps

- single: a small single lump is a pulmonary nodule
- multiple: multiple very small lumps raise the possibility of miliary TB; slightly larger ones are seen in patients who have had chickenpox pneumonia or who have pulmonary metastases or fibrotic nodules.

Larger lumps

- smooth edges: benign tumours (e.g. hamartoma); inflammatory lesions (e.g. Wegener's granuloma, rheumatoid nodule); 'coin' renal metastases or an aspergilloma (which can have a fluid level)
- irregular edges: suggestive of tumour, infarct or pneumonic masses; check for cavitation since necrosis or infection can occur in any lump, and especially in tuberculous masses, tumours and infarcts.

Areas of opacification

Consider the density, extent and position of any more confluent areas of opacification, and whether there is associated volume loss.

Density

Dense opacification suggests collapse or fluid, e.g. pleural effusion (Fig. 3.15), fluid-filled post-pneumonectomy space. Hazier shadowing indicates that there may still be pockets of air within the tissue, due, for example, to consolidation, pulmonary oedema or fibrosis.

Extent

Conditions that are due to systemic processes, e.g. drug toxicity, vasculitis, sarcoidosis, or those that affect both lungs equally, e.g. pulmonary oedema, are more likely to result in bilateral and symmetrical changes (Fig. 3.16). More localized problems, such as pneumonia or bronchial carcinoma, rarely have symmetrical appearances.

Look at the appearance of the top of any suspected pleural effusion. An up-sloping meniscus should be visible at the lateral aspect of the collection.

Position

Areas of opacification on the chest film can be localized to a specific lobe by use of the 'silhouette sign'. On a normal CXR there is clear, well defined contrast between the air-filled lungs and the structures that surround them (mediastinum, heart, hemidiaphragms and chest wall). Opacification of an area of lung directly

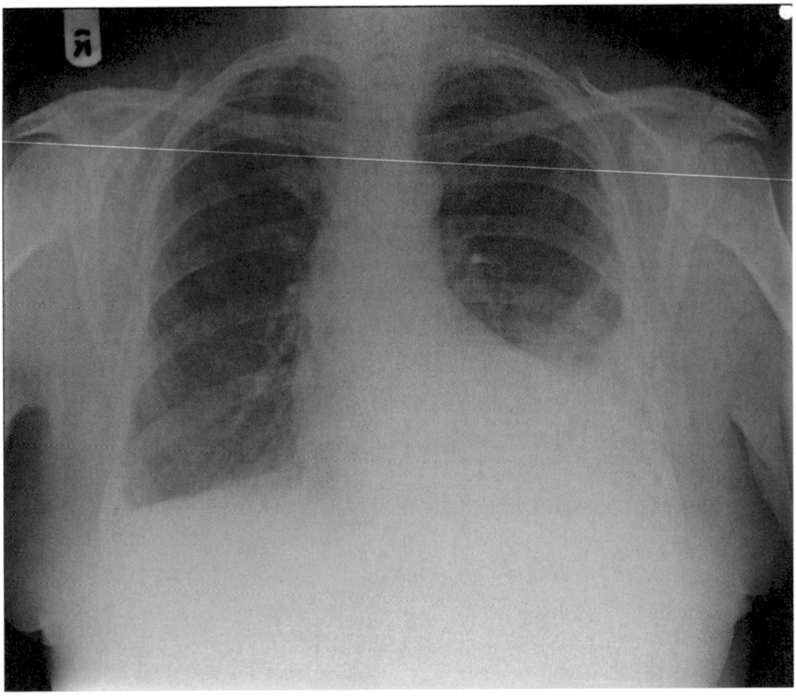

Figure 3.15 Left pleural effusion with adjacent consolidation.

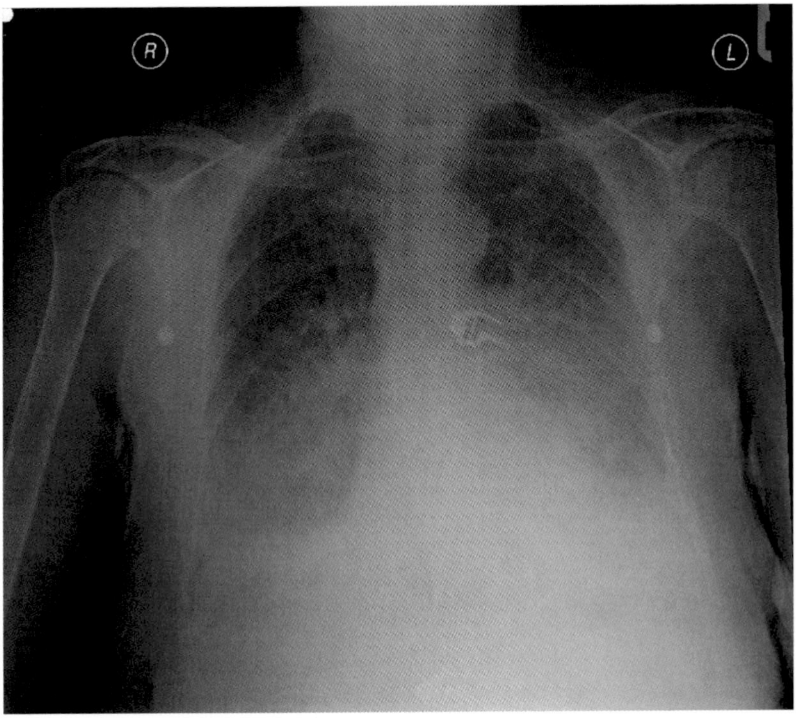

Figure 3.16 Pulmonary oedema.

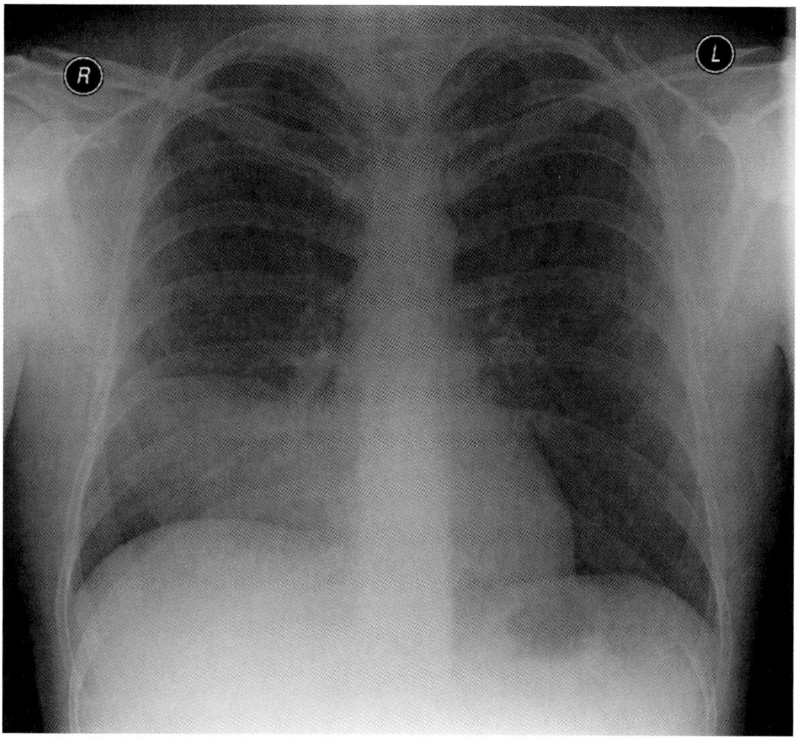

Figure 3.17 Right middle lobe consolidation.

adjacent to one of these results in loss of this sharp air–tissue interface. Thus, loss of clarity at the:

- right heart border = right middle lobe pathology (Fig. 3.17)
- left heart border = lingular pathology
- right hemidiaphragm = right lower lobe pathology
- left hemidiaphragm = left lower lobe pathology
- right side of the upper mediastinum = right upper lobe pathology
- left side of the upper mediastinum = left upper lobe pathology.

Volume loss

Volume loss, indicated by mediastinal shift, a raised hemidiaphragm, or displacement of adjacent fissures, suggests associated lung collapse. This may be due to a proximal obstructing lesion, diaphragmatic palsy or previous surgery, e.g. lobectomy. Occasionally, massive pleural effusions, especially those associated with little or no underlying lung collapse, may result in mediastinal shift away from the affected side.

Black areas in the lung fields

Black lung fields can occur when the film is over-penetrated. However, a black appearance within the lung fields may reflect lung pathology, including:

- emphysema: usually bilateral reflecting air trapping and reduced density of lung parenchyma
- pneumothorax: usually unilateral (Fig. 3.18); look for a lung edge and the absence of lung markings beyond it; in a tension pneumothorax, the mediastinum may be shifted away from the side involved
- pulmonary embolism: due to reduced blood flow to the affected lung segment (pulmonary oligaemia).

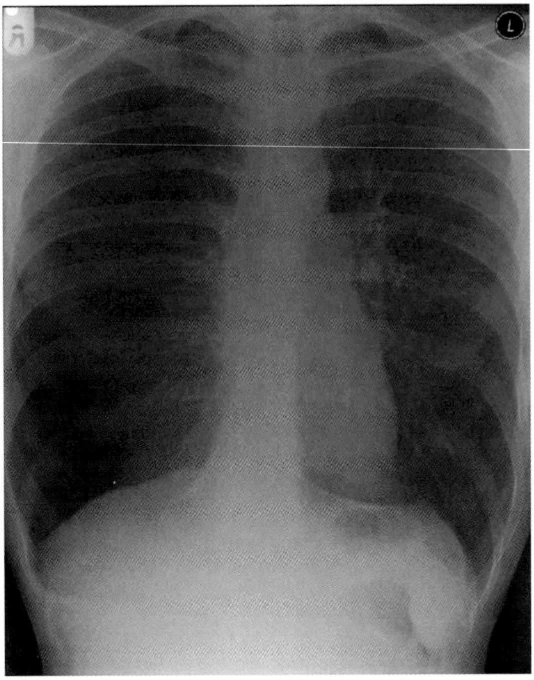

Figure 3.18 Right-sided pneumothorax.

PACS display systems may have a limited screen resolution on the smaller viewing platforms provided in ward areas. This makes it very difficult to see small pneumothoraces. If there is a clinical suspicion or reason for a pneumothorax, you should check a film's appearance with a radiologist (who will have access to higher definition reporting screens) before discharging the patient.

The ribs

The ribs should look uniformly white throughout the chest. Each rib should have a distinct and smooth top and bottom edge along its length. Metastases are often indicated by the absence of a section of rib. Such dark holes can be lost against the blackness of the lungs unless the edge is followed carefully.

Fractures

Fractures are a common finding. Old fractures are indicated by surrounding radio-opaque callous; several may lie in a row as a result of significant blunt trauma. There may be numerous fractures in several areas across the chest from repeated minor injury. Both patterns are common in heavy drinkers and are usually the result of falls.

New fractures are less easy to spot, but if you follow the edge of the ribs you will see these as a break or step in the rib edge. If you see fractures consider that the following associated features may be present:

- a flail segment: where two or more ribs are involved in two or more places (see p. 255)
- a pneumothorax ± surgical emphysema or haemothorax (see p. 148)
- an underlying lung mass or metastases
- damage to the liver, spleen or kidney (lower rib fractures)
- other trauma: upper rib fractures are rare and indicate that a large amount of force has been encountered.

The soft tissues

There should be a 'frame' of soft tissue that is equal on both sides. A very scanty layer of soft tissue may imply cachexia from severe illness or tumour. A lump on one side but not on the other may be due to a soft tissue mass or, alternatively, removal of a breast.

'Bubbles' of blackness in the soft tissue and a haziness lying over the lung fields could be due to surgical emphysema. Check if there has been a history of trauma, oesophageal injury or intervention or chest surgery/drain insertion.

The lateral view

You are unlikely to be asked to comment on a lateral view. There are relatively few reasons for choosing to do one and most clinicians would wait for the formal radiology report before taking a decision using one.

ABDOMINAL X-RAYS

The plain abdominal radiograph (AXR) allows assessment of bowel gas patterns and internal organs by identifying their interface with the surrounding, lower density, intra-abdominal fat planes.

Bowel gas patterns on AXR

Normal gas patterns

Normal small and large bowel contain a variable amount of gas. When assessing the pattern created by this, it is important to establish whether the gas is in the large bowel or the small bowel. The latter is generally in the central abdomen and pelvis, and has valvulae conniventes: mucosal folds running the full circumference of the small bowel producing fine, regular indentations. Large bowel loops can usually be found around the periphery of the abdominal cavity and have haustrations: smooth muscle bands which are further apart than the valvulae and cross only a third of the circumference of the bowel.

Abnormal gas patterns

Obstruction

Small bowel loops are less distensible than large bowel, and they should not normally have a diameter of >3.5 cm. The caecum and ascending colon have the greatest capacity to distend, with an upper limit of normal of 7 cm, while the diameter of the transverse colon is normally <5 cm.

The site of obstruction may be suggested by a change in calibre: from dilated to collapsed or normal. Although a plain film may provide the diagnosis of bowel obstruction, it rarely indicates the cause. However, associated features may provide some clues.

In small bowel obstruction central dilated loops of small bowel occur with air–fluid levels and an absence of colonic gas (Fig. 3.19). In the small bowel, the valvulae conniventes completely cross the lumen of the bowel as compared to the haustral folds of the large bowel which do not. In large bowel obstruction, bowel gas is seen proximal to the level of obstruction, but no gas is seen in the rectum. If there is dilated small bowel with air in the biliary tree, consider gallstone ileus.

Caecal volvulus

The caecum twists around on its short axis causing obstruction and resulting in a distended, gas-filled caecum lying in an unusual position, usually the left upper quadrant. The large bowel distal to this will be collapsed down and relatively gasless.

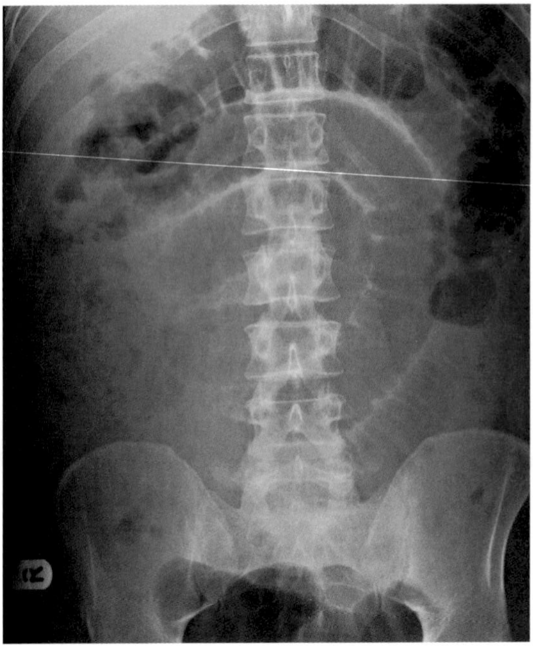

Figure 3.19 Small bowel obstruction.

Sigmoid volvulus

This usually occurs in patients with a large volume sigmoid and elongated sigmoid mesentery. There is much more gaseous distension in a sigmoid volvulus than in a caecal volvulus and an almost vertical line passing through the gas-filled sigmoid gives the typical 'coffee-bean' configuration in mid-abdomen (Fig. 3.20).

Inflammatory bowel disease

Mild inflammatory change, although symptomatic, may not produce any changes on the abdominal film. In small bowel inflammation, thickened, flattened valvulae conniventes (picket fence appearance) may be seen in the affected segment. More often, dilated small bowel proximal to a stricture may be the only finding.

Severe inflammation of the large bowel causes loss of the normal haustral pattern, with bowel wall oedema and a lack of faecal residue within the colon. The colon appears featureless and gassy with characteristic 'thumb-printing'. In some cases, the colon dilates resulting in an entity called 'toxic megacolon' which is at risk of perforation. A sign of imminent perforation is gas within the bowel wall.

Bowel ischaemia

The bowel gas pattern may be normal in cases of small or large bowel ischaemia. Even detailed contrast-enhanced CT scanning may fail to show any abnormality in the bowel and a series of normal radiological investigations should not preclude laparotomy if there is reasonable clinical suspicion of bowel ischaemia.

Gas not within the bowel on AXR

If gas is identified within the abdomen, but cannot be localized to the bowel loops, the appearance and position may give an indication of the underlying cause.

Free intraperitoneal gas will not be seen on a supine abdominal radiograph unless there is a very large amount. Hence, an erect chest X-ray is the examination of choice in suspected perforation of a hollow viscus. Gross pneumoperitoneum

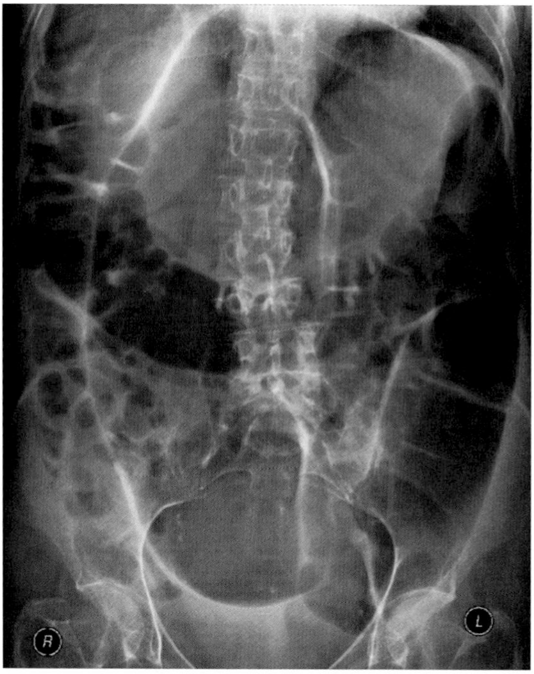

Figure 3.20 Sigmoid volvulus.

may be detected when both the outer and inner wall of the bowel loops can be visualized. This feature is known as 'Riggler's sign'.

Intra-abdominal abscesses can occur anywhere within the abdomen and a fairly rounded, circumscribed gas bubble, separate from the bowel, may be seen, if there is a significant gas component within an abscess.

Gas in abdominal organs

Gas in the biliary tree is visible as a branching pattern over the liver shadow in the right upper quadrant. This is occasionally seen in elderly patients, but is more commonly seen after biliary intervention such as sphincterotomy. If accompanied by features of small bowel obstruction, gallstone ileus should be considered.

A well circumscribed bubble of gas in the right upper quadrant over the liver can be seen in cases of emphysematous cholecystitis, a condition that is more likely to occur in diabetic patients and should be treated as a surgical emergency.

Gas may be seen in the urinary bladder if there is a fistulous connection to the bowel. A bubble of gas is commonly seen following instrumentation, including catheterization.

Soft tissues on AXR

The outline of the intra-abdominal organs and other soft tissues will not always be visible. Fat is of lower density than soft tissue. Therefore, its lesser ability to attenuate the X-ray beam makes fat appear relatively darker on X-ray images. As a result, the fat surrounding the intra-abdominal organs will often outline them, aiding assessment of their position and size.

Enlarged organs or masses may also be apparent through their displacement of bowel loops: an enlarged liver will push the hepatic flexure of colon medially and toward the pelvis, producing a large, gasless, homogeneous area in the right upper quadrant.

If an abnormal soft tissue mass is perceived on AXR, it is useful to consider which structures would normally be expected to lie in that area. An enlarged liver, spleen and kidneys or a distended bladder can often be diagnosed by the typical shape and position of the mass 'shadow' that they create.

Other masses such as matted loops of bowel in Crohn's disease, tumours or enlarged lymph nodes may be visible on plain AXR but will require further imaging to help establish the diagnosis. Ultrasound scanning is a very useful tool for the investigation of suspected intra-abdominal masses, whether they are picked up on clinical examination or AXR, and will usually be the next investigation of choice. CT scanning may be required ultimately.

Calcification on AXR

Calcification detected on AXR may help to guide further investigation. However, it is important to be able to identify areas of incidental or benign calcification which do not require further investigation or consideration.

Often, speckled areas of calcification can be seen scattered across the upper abdomen. Costal cartilage calcification is a normal and variable process. Once the relationship to the ribs and costal cartilage is appreciated, these can be dismissed.

Nodes and vessels

Mesenteric lymph nodes may calcify, but are not of any clinical concern. The appearance is generally very typical, with a dense focus of rounded or 'popcorn' calcification. Vascular calcification is linear (in the vessel wall) and follows the normal course of the arterial branches. The common vessels to calcify are the aorta, iliac arteries and the splenic artery.

Calcified venules low in the pelvis are called phleboliths and are typically small and round with a central area of lucency. Sometimes, it can be impossible to differentiate on AXR between a phlebolith and a small distal ureteric calculus in a patient presenting with renal colic.

Gallstones

Most gallstones are cholesterol stones and are not radio-opaque. Where calcification does occur, they generally produce the typical appearance of a group of multi-faceted stones, each with a calcified rim in the right upper quadrant. The wall of the gallbladder itself may calcify resulting in a smooth, ovoid ring over the liver. Ultrasound scanning is the investigation of choice for suspected biliary pathology, as this can also demonstrate inflammatory thickening of the gallbladder wall, or biliary dilatation if the common duct is obstructed.

Urinary tract

When the indication for abdominal imaging is suspected renal colic, the image focuses on the urinary tract and is called a KUB (kidneys ureters bladder).

Most urinary calculi are radio-opaque and visible on plain film. However, if renal colic is suspected from the clinical presentation, absence of a visible calculus on KUB cannot exclude the diagnosis and further imaging (usually a CT KUB) will be required.

Urinary calculi range from large, amorphous 'staghorn' calculi filling the pelvicaliceal system to tiny foci of calcification. Calculi may also form in the bladder. When looking at a film from a patient with suspected renal colic, it is useful to locate the renal outlines if possible and find any calcified densities projected over this area. Check the line of the ureters on either side of the lumbar spine down into the pelvis, and look for calcified areas. Prostatic calcification is normal in elderly male patients and can be seen as multiple small foci of calcification at the base of the bladder.

Gynaecological organs

In female patients, calcification may be seen in the ovaries and in uterine fibroids. Calcified fibroids have a fairly typical dense, conglomerate appearance and lie low in the pelvis.

Ovarian calcification may be seen in patients with dermoid cysts. These cysts arise from primitive elements and may contain any combination of soft tissue, teeth, hair and fat. Any teeth will be calcified and are clearly visible.

Upper abdominal organs

The pancreas may become calcified in chronic pancreatitis. This typically produces fine, stippled calcification, projected over the body of the 12th thoracic vertebra extending across to the left of midline. The other upper abdominal organs may occasionally contain small foci of calcification in cysts, or following previous trauma or infection. Small rounded calcified foci here can generally be considered to be incidental.

Drugs and prescribing

4

GENERAL PRESCRIBING

Patients trust that they will be prescribed the correct medicine, at the correct dose, to be taken at the correct time and by the correct route.

Choosing treatment

The potential benefit of any medication must be weighed against the risk of side-effects or other problems associated with its use. This requires a knowledge and understanding of the results of clinical trials (see 'Statistics', p. 445) and commitment to the practice of evidence-based medicine.

Assuming they are competent, the patient should be included in this decision-making. A well informed patient is likely to be more compliant and tolerant of side-effects. For every new medication, consider the following:

- allergy: check this with every patient before you start a new medication
- potential duplication of similar medicines, e.g. adding diclofenac to ibuprofen
- opposing effects, e.g. prescribing a β-blocker for an asthmatic patient taking salbutamol
- interactions, e.g. clarithromycin in a patient on theophylline
- relative contraindications: these need to be weighed against the necessity for the treatment
- absolute contraindications: these prohibit treatment altogether, e.g. warfarin in pregnancy
- the best route of administration, e.g. a patient with a cerebral infarct could have aspirin per rectum if they cannot swallow safely
- specific dose adjustments: these may be required when certain medications are used in patients with renal or hepatic impairment and also during pregnancy and lactation; see the appropriate appendices in the BNF and 'Drug use in special circumstances', p. 119.

Legible and clear prescribing

Although people joke about doctors' writing, drug administration errors are a serious issue. If a nurse or pharmacist gives a patient the wrong medication or dose because they cannot read the prescription, the prescriber will be liable for any harm that results. All doctors have a responsibility to prescribe medications correctly and legibly:

- use generic names: only specify a brand if you need to, e.g. modified release preparations, such as Tildiem LA® or Isotard®
- use English only: do not use Latin or other abbreviations, except perhaps for PRN
- use appropriate units: write 500 micrograms rather than 0.5 mg
- write 'micrograms' in full: handwritten 'mg' and 'µg' can look very similar.

Using a cardex

Drug cardex (prescription chart) design may vary from hospital to hospital, but the principles for using them remain the same. The patient details section must be completed in full, including the relevant unique patient identifier and documentation of allergy status. All medicine cardexes will have sections for once-only prescribing, regular IV and oral medications and PRN (as required) prescribing. It is important to:

- use the correct section of the document when prescribing
- clearly complete each box and sign and date each new addition or removal
- if the medication is not given every day, document this
- sign and date when stopping medications
- rewrite the line if a dose or frequency changes: do not alter the first prescription
- ensure all medications used are prescribed on the cardex, including those written on other infusion charts, e.g. insulin prescription
- use your local formulary: choose medication that is easily available.

Discharge prescriptions

These can be in paper or electronic form:

- use unambiguous identification, e.g. a unique identifier such as the 'NHS number' or 'Community Health Index (CHI)', rather than a hospital-specific number
- list all medications, even if they do not need to be dispensed: when medications are not listed, GPs may assume that they have been discontinued
- correctly document the drug name, dose, preparation and frequency
- detail how long each treatment should continue for, e.g. an antibiotic course
- provide enough description of the medication format, e.g. the type of inhaler the patient needs; a minimum dose interval in 'as required' prescriptions
- warfarin prescriptions: give a date for the next INR check
- note that controlled drugs need to be prescribed in a specific way by law; see the BNF.

COMMON PRESCRIBING

Acute pain

Analgesia will be required by many patients for simple complaints such as headache, backache or minor wound pain. However, you should always assess the patient before prescribing analgesia, especially at the request of others. Check whether the patient's symptoms are new, when and how they developed and whether they indicate a significant change in their condition.

Mild pain

Simple analgesia alone is often sufficient, e.g. paracetamol 1 g orally 4-hourly (max. 4 g/24 h) assuming there is no significant hepatic impairment. It may be necessary to provide additional types of analgesia to target specific types of pain.

Inflammatory and musculoskeletal pain

Consider prescribing a NSAID, e.g. ibuprofen (400 mg PO 8-hourly; max. 1.2 g/24 h). However, such preparations should not be used in patients with a history of GI bleeding, asthma or renal disease. In the elderly or those who will need a prolonged course, consider the use of a proton pump inhibitor, e.g. omeprazole (20 mg daily).

Back pain and other spastic muscle pains can be alleviated by a muscle relaxant, e.g. diazepam (2 mg 8-hourly). Avoid this in patients with respiratory muscle disorders or severe COPD causing respiratory failure.

Colicky pain

Colicky pain may be better managed with an antispasmodic, e.g. oral, IM or IV hyoscine butylbromide (20 mg 6-hourly; a parenteral dose can be repeated after 30 min). This is especially the case if pain is due to constipation, which opiate analgesia will exacerbate. Note that these drugs are contraindicated in glaucoma, myasthenia, paralytic ileus, prostatic enlargement, pyloric stenosis and porphyria; also avoid in Down's syndrome, the elderly or pregnant/breast-feeding women, in children and those with ulcerative colitis, pyrexia or cardiac disease.

Moderately severe pain

Patients with more intense pain, e.g. postoperative, may need a stronger analgesia, such as a 'weak opioid', e.g. dihydrocodeine (30 mg PO 6-hourly; max. 120 mg/24 h) or tramadol (50 mg PO 4-hourly; max. 400 mg/24 h). This should be given in combination with paracetamol, unless otherwise contraindicated. Numerous combination preparations exist, e.g. co-codamol 30/500 (2 tablets 4-hourly; max. 8 tablets/24 h).

Weak opioid preparations may cause nausea, constipation or respiratory depression. Therefore, in addition to the usual cautions in patients with renal or hepatic disease, the elderly or pregnant women, these preparations should be used cautiously in patients with head injury, COPD or disorders of respiratory muscle function. Laxatives may be required (see 'Constipation', p. 173).

Severe pain

Patients with an acute organ injury (e.g. MI, renal colic), postoperative pain, labour or trauma will have acute severe pain, and will usually require strong opiate analgesia. They are often unable to eat, vomiting and require prompt relief of symptoms. Therefore, parenteral analgesia should be used and combined, if necessary, with an appropriate antiemetic (see 'Vomiting', p. 172) and laxative. See 'Prescribing in palliative care', p. 376, for patients with chronic severe pain and for notes on opiate side-effects and cautions.

Patient-controlled analgesia

PCA is commonly used for the control of postoperative pain, in which setting it offers potential advantages over 'on request' dosing. A syringe driver is configured to deliver small, usually top-up, doses of analgesia on demand by the patient. The device is controlled by a hand-held trigger and can be set to a maximum dose frequency, above which no further doses will be delivered. PCAs should only be set up and altered by those with specific training and the necessary competencies.

Morphine

Morphine may be given via various routes. Intravenous dosing bypasses first-pass metabolism and the onset of action is more rapid. Therefore, doses are usually two-thirds of those required by IM or SC routes, e.g. 10 mg IV equates to 15 mg IM. Suggested dosing:

- elderly: initial dose of 5 mg with adjustment according to clinical condition
- adults: 10 mg adjusted to response and repeated every 4–6 h
- children (12–18 years): 2.5–10 mg
- children (2–12 years): 200 µg/kg
- infants (1–24 months): 100–200 µg/kg.

Pethidine

Pethidine has a shorter duration of action than morphine, is less potent, but is also less likely to cause constipation. It is useful in severe colicky abdominal pain, e.g. biliary colic, renal colic, and is often preferred for the management of obstetric pain. Common regimes include:

- postoperative pain: 25–100 mg, repeated 2-hourly
- obstetrics: 50–100 mg SC, repeated after 1–3 h, up to a maximum of 400 mg/24 h
- other acute pain: 50–150 mg PO, 4-hourly; 25–100 mg SC/IM, 4-hourly; 25–50 mg slow IV bolus 4-hourly.

Reversal of opiate analgesia

This may be necessary if respiratory depression or a disproportionate fall in conscious level results from administration. Naloxone (0.4–2 mg IV) can be given at intervals of 2–3 min up to a maximum of 10 mg. Use this with caution in patients with cardiac instability and opiate dependency, since an acute withdrawal reaction can be precipitated in the latter group.

Anticoagulation

Anticoagulation prescribing is best done by a doctor who knows the patient. If you are called to initiate or modify an existing prescription, you should review recent coagulation results and ensure that there has been no change in the patient's condition, any injury or evidence of bleeding. Note especially any history of intracranial haemorrhage, haemophilia or other bleeding disorder, severe hypertension, peptic ulcer or significant renal or hepatic disease, each of which would contraindicate or complicate the use of any anticoagulation. Consider potential interactions with concomitant medications that increase the risk of GI bleeding, e.g. NSAIDs. Only prescribe the drug if there is written documentation in the case-sheet that this is required, or you have checked with a senior.

Heparin

Before prescribing heparin consider the following:

- contraindications: recent major trauma or surgery, especially to the eye; severe liver disease; thrombocytopenia
- cautions: renal impairment; pregnancy; hypersensitivity to low molecular weight heparins (LMWH); spinal or epidural anaesthesia
- platelets and potassium, see 'Side-effects', below
- which formulation of heparin should be used, i.e. LMWH versus unfractionated (intravenous) heparin (UFH).

Side-effects of all heparins

In addition to bleeding, heparin may cause thrombocytopenia and hyperkalaemia, as well as local and systemic drug reactions such as skin necrosis and urticaria.

Thrombocytopenia is an immune-mediated phenomenon beginning 5–10 days after the onset of treatment. Platelet counts should be measured before treatment and every 4 days thereafter. Treatment should be discontinued if the platelet count drops by 50%, especially if this is associated with evidence of bleeding, bruising or petechiae. LMWH should be avoided and alternative anticoagulants commenced, e.g. lepirudin and danaparoid.

Hyperkalaemia results from heparin inhibition of aldosterone and patients with renal failure, diabetes, acidosis or those on potassium sparing drugs are more susceptible. Potassium should be measured at the initiation of heparin treatment and monitored regularly if treatment continues for more than 7 days.

LMWH

Most hospitals will have specific local guidelines or prescription charts that reflect the drugs in use locally. Common examples are given below, but the doses stated assume normal renal and hepatic function and the absence of any contraindication.

- preoperative prophylaxis (moderate risk): enoxaparin SC 20 mg 2 h pre-surgery; 20 mg/24 h for 7 days
- preoperative prophylaxis (high risk): enoxaparin SC 40 mg 12 h pre-surgery; 40 mg/24 h for 7 days
- general DVT prophylaxis: enoxaparin SC 40 mg 24-hourly until ambulant (max. 14 days)
- acute coronary syndrome: enoxaparin SC 1 mg/kg twice daily
- DVT/PTE treatment: tinzaparin 175 units/kg SC daily until established on oral anticoagulants.

Unfractionated heparin

Indications

Unfractionated heparin (UFH) has a short half-life, fast onset of action and can be reversed with protamine. However, it requires regular monitoring of the patient's APTT and has a limited number of indications in current clinical practice. These include anticoagulation of patients presenting with new onset atrial fibrillation (see 'Management of AF', p. 134) and following administration of fibrin-specific thrombolytics. UFH is used instead of warfarin perioperatively where discontinuing anticoagulation completely would lead to an unacceptably high risk of thrombotic complications, e.g. those with mechanical heart valves. The patient's warfarin can be discontinued a few days before surgery and replaced with IV heparin. This can then be stopped 6 h before surgery and restarted a few hours afterwards.

Prescription and monitoring

Intravenous heparin comes in preparations of 1000 IU/mL (20 000 IU in 20 mL). Many hospitals have specific protocols for its use and you should adhere to these. Where these are not provided, and assuming normal renal and hepatic function and no other contraindications, give a bolus of 80 IU/kg (usually rounded to 5000 units) over 5 min, followed by an infusion of 18 IU per kg per h (usually 1000 IU/h, but note: in adults under 50 kg or children the loading dose should be reduced to 50 IU/kg, followed by an infusion of 15–25 IU per kg per h).

Measure the APTT after 6 h and thereafter every 10 h. Adjust the dose as determined by the APTT, ideally according to a local protocol. Aim for an APTT of 1.5–2.5. If the APTT is >7, stop the infusion and check again 3 h later. If it is between 2.6 and 7, stop the infusion for 30–60 min and, for every increment of 1.0 above 2.5, reduce the infusion rate by 100 IU/h.

Intravenous heparin can be reversed with protamine sulphate (10 mg/mL): 1 mg will tend to reverse 90 IU of heparin. Do not exceed a total dose of 50 mg protamine. Note protamine may not fully reverse LMWH and, if given quickly, can cause hypotension.

Warfarin

Before prescribing warfarin consider the following:

- contraindications: pregnancy; peptic ulcer; bacterial endocarditis
- cautions: recent surgery; hepatic disease; breast-feeding
- interactions: a variety of drugs can affect warfarin metabolism, e.g. amiodarone, simvastatin, carbamazepine, rifampicin.

Initiating warfarin

Warfarin causes a paradoxical increase in thrombotic tendency initially; therefore, its introduction is normally 'covered' with heparin for a few days.

Local initiation protocols should be consulted, but a commonly used regime is 10 mg given at 1800 h daily, for 2 days (5 mg in the elderly, underweight, those with heart or liver failure or with other reasons for increased warfarin sensitivity). After 2 days, check INR at 0900 daily and adjust dose as per local protocol. The recommended INR range depends on the reason for anticoagulation:

- 2.0–3.0: first DVT/PTE (6 months); AF; dilated cardiomyopathy; rheumatic heart disease; mural thrombus post-MI
- 2.5–3.5 in mechanical aortic valves
- 3.0–4.0 and lifelong in recurrent DVT/PTE while adequately warfarinized (INR >2.0), or mechanical mitral valve.

Reversal

Any decision to reverse warfarin anticoagulation should be taken with caution and not simply undertaken because of a high INR. It makes re-anticoagulation very difficult and can be dangerous in patients with mechanical valves. In patients who are well and not actively bleeding, consider simply stopping the warfarin and admitting for observation.

If reversal is deemed necessary, vitamin K (5–10 mg PO or 0.5–2 mg IV) can be given, although it will take 6–12 h to become effective. If the patient is bleeding and immediate reversal is required, use fresh frozen plasma (see 'Blood products', p. 122) after discussion with haematology.

Night sedation

Hospital is a noisy environment and sleep disturbance is common. This impairs recovery and, although night sedation may be helpful, it does not offer the same quality of rest as natural sleep. Be aware that:

- patients may experience 'hangover' side-effects the next day
- some patients, especially the elderly, may develop confusion or psychosis
- sedation may worsen respiratory failure and should be avoided in those with respiratory failure or any condition that may cause this, e.g. COPD, myasthenia
- sedation should not be used in pregnant or breast-feeding patients or those with significant hepatic or renal disease
- a new prescription of sedation should only be used for a short period
- prescriptions started in hospital should not normally be continued on discharge.

Commonly used night sedation options include:

- lorazepam 1–4 mg at night
- lormetazepam 0.5–1.5 mg at night (0.5 mg in the elderly)
- nitrazepam 5–10 mg at night (2.5–5 mg in the elderly)
- zopiclone 7.5 mg at night (3.75 mg in the elderly).

Oxygen

Oxygen therapy should be thought of as a drug, with indications, contraindications and side-effects. Oxygen should be prescribed for patients, in whom it is indicated, using the cardex. This prescription should be at an appropriate dose (FiO_2) and the treatment should be appropriately monitored (see 'Oxygen delivery', p. 66).

COMMON INTERACTIONS

A drug interaction occurs when the effect of one drug is altered by another drug, herbal medicine or food substance. These interactions can be either pharmacokinetic or pharmacodynamic and vary in their expression between individuals. Several routes of metabolism and elimination may be involved in the removal of a specific medication and the amount of a given drug that is cleared is dependent upon a variety of physiological factors.

Types of interaction

Pharmacokinetic interactions

Absorption

The rate of absorption or the total amount of drug absorbed is altered, e.g. antacids can reduce the absorption of quinolone antibiotics and reduce their effects.

Distribution

Where drugs are highly protein bound, they may be displaced from their protein binding site by other drugs resulting in an increased concentration of the unbound and active molecule; in practice this is rarely significant.

Metabolism

The cytochrome P450 group of isoenzymes can be either inhibited or induced during the metabolism of drugs in the liver:

- inhibition: two medications compete for the same route of metabolism; either one or both of the medications may be affected and there is a resulting rise in plasma concentration, e.g. erythromycin inhibits the metabolism of theophylline, resulting in a higher than expected plasma concentration of theophylline
- induction: the liver responds to the presence of certain drugs by increasing the production of metabolizing enzymes, altering the metabolism of other medications, e.g. rifampicin accelerates warfarin metabolism, reducing the anticoagulant effect.

Elimination

Active tubular secretion in the kidney can be influenced by the presence of other drugs that compete for the same elimination pathway, e.g. aspirin reduces the excretion of methotrexate, increasing the risk of methotrexate toxicity.

Pharmacodynamic interactions

These interactions occur between drugs that have similar pharmacological effects, or side-effects, and are due to direct competition at a receptor site, or action on the same physiological system. They may be classified as:

- synergistic, e.g. potassium sparing diuretics and potassium supplements both increase serum potassium
- antagonistic, e.g. ACE inhibitors and NSAIDs which both impair autoregulation of glomerular blood flow in the kidney but by opposing mechanisms; ACE inhibitors inhibit angiotensin-mediated vasoconstriction of the efferent glomerular arterioles while NSAIDs inhibit prostaglandin-mediated vasodilatation of the afferent arterioles
- drug uptake, e.g. tricyclic antidepressants prevent reuptake of noradrenaline (norepinephrine) into peripheral adrenergic neurones, increasing the response in a patient given noradrenaline.

Interactions in clinical practice

Clinically significant interactions are those that cause an increase or decrease in the efficacy of the medication, or an increase in side-effects. They are more likely to occur when using drugs with a narrow therapeutic range. Interactions can also occur with herbal medicines such as St John's wort (phenytoin), foodstuffs such as grapefruit (simvastatin) and tobacco smoking (theophylline).

Table 4.1 Examples of drug interactions

Interacting drugs		Clinical effect
Amiodarone	Antipsychotics	Increased risk of ventricular arrhythmias
	Digoxin	Digoxin concentration increased: reduce dose
	Phenytoin	Phenytoin plasma concentration increased
Imidazole antifungals, e.g. ketoconazole	Phenytoin	Ketoconazole plasma concentration reduced
	Simvastatin	Increased risk of myopathy because clearance of simvastatin is reduced
	Mirtazapine	Plasma concentration of mirtazapine increased
Digoxin	Itraconazole	Reduced digoxin clearance: consider dose reduction
	Verapamil	Reduced digoxin clearance: consider dose reduction
Macrolides, e.g. clarithromycin and erythromycin	Carbamazepine	Increased plasma concentration of carbamazepine
	Simvastatin	Increased risk of myopathy due to increased simvastatin concentration: avoid combination
	Warfarin	Increased anticoagulant effect
Quinolones, e.g. ciprofloxacin	Theophylline	Theophylline metabolism inhibited by ciprofloxacin: consider dose reduction
	Tricyclics	Prescription with moxifloxacin increases the risk of ventricular arrhythmias (both prolong QT)
	Warfarin	Increased anticoagulant effect with ciprofloxacin
Statins	Fibrates	Increased risk of myopathy when co-administered
	Verapamil	Increased risk of myopathy: reduce dose
Theophylline	Phenytoin	Theophylline plasma concentration reduced
	Rifampicin	Theophylline metabolism is increased leading to a lower plasma concentration
Warfarin	Amiodarone	Increased anticoagulant effect
	Fluconazole	Increased anticoagulant effect

Where interactions are expected or develop, medications may have to be discontinued or, if the clinical situation warrants use of both medications, increased monitoring will be required. A list of some common interactions can be found in Table 4.1.

PRESCRIBING ERRORS

Most errors are the result of not knowing enough about the drugs that are being prescribed or the patient who is to receive them. Always consider concomitant therapy to avoid accidental drug duplication or errors resulting from drug interaction. Never prescribe medication at the request of someone else, without knowledge of the patient.

Common errors

- ACE inhibitors: care needs to be taken when prescribing with other agents that also increase potassium levels like potassium sparing diuretics and potassium supplements
- contraindications, cautions and dose reductions: co-morbid disease can influence how the medicine will affect the patient; if you do not know the drug restrictions in detail, check the BNF or product information first
- drug duplication: combination preparations can lead to double prescription, e.g. paracetamol and co-codamol
- gentamicin: two common dosing regimes exist, a standard dose may be given twice daily or a larger dose every 24–48 h (see 'Dose calculation', p. 115)
- insulin: stipulate the specific form of insulin and the correct 'mix' where appropriate (e.g. Human Mixtard® 30) and never abbreviate 'units' to 'u' since it can be misinterpreted as a zero, increasing the dose 10-fold; fatalities have occurred with prescribing errors involving insulin
- inhalers: care must be taken to specify correctly the inhaled medication (e.g. Serevent® versus Seretide®) and the administration device (e.g. Seretide® Accuhaler® versus Seretide® Evohaler®)
- infusions: incorrectly prescribing the rate at which an infusion should be given can have serious results so it is mandatory that another doctor or registered nurse double-checks your calculations and prescription
- modified-release (MR) preparations: the pharmacokinetics of the MR preparation will differ from those of the standard preparation of the same drug, so specific knowledge of each preparation is required; check with ward pharmacists if you are unsure
- warfarin: loading and maintenance doses of warfarin can be affected by a variety of factors including age, liver function and interactions with other medications.

DRUG REACTIONS

A drug reaction is defined as an unwanted or harmful reaction experienced following the administration of a drug or combination of drugs. It can be an expected side-effect, or it may be one that has not been recognized before. Reactions can range from mild to serious; for the management of anaphylaxis (see 'Anaphylaxis', p. 253).

It is important to consider reporting all reactions, serious or otherwise, to the Medicines and Healthcare products Regulatory Agency (MHRA). New medicines will only have been trialled in relatively small numbers of patients and their full side-effect profile may not become apparent until the wider population has used them. The reaction you have seen could be an important part of the information needed to shape that. Information on reactions relating to older medicines is also still important to collect as the prevalence of a reaction may change how often that medicine is used.

The 'Yellow Card Scheme' is the main system reporting scheme in the UK. Proof of association between the drug and the reaction is not required. Where you have a reasonable suspicion that the drug, or combination of drugs, was involved, you should consider making a report using an MRHA yellow card or online. You can find a yellow card in each BNF and also on the MHRA or Yellow Card Scheme websites. All reactions to any new medicines (with a black triangle symbol against them in the BNF) should be reported. For other medicines, serious reactions should be reported, i.e. fatal, life-threatening, disabling, incapacitating, resulting in or prolonging hospitalization, congenital abnormalities and any others you consider as significant. Any reaction in the elderly, in children or in pregnant patients is also worth reporting.

DOSE CALCULATION

For a variety of drugs, you will be required to calculate a starting dose ± an infusion concentration and rate. When determining these parameters, it is often necessary to calculate ideal body weight (IBW) and creatinine clearance (CrCl) (Box 4.1).

Box 4.1 Useful calculations

Ideal body weight

2.5 kg for every inch over 5 feet + 50 kg in males or 45.5 kg in females.

Creatinine clearance

$$\frac{140 - \text{age (years)} \times \text{IBW (kg)} \times K}{\text{serum creatinine } (\mu\text{mol/L})}$$

where K = 1.23 in males or 1.04 in females.

Aminoglycosides

Most hospitals will have specific protocols for the dose calculation and monitoring of these drugs. However, if such protocols are not provided the following guides may be used.

Gentamicin

Initial dose

This depends on IBW and CrCl (Table 4.2). Put the dose in 100 mL 0.9% saline and administer it over 1 h. Subsequent dosing depends on serum drug levels and renal function, but is based on a 24 or 48 h interval between doses as specified in the table.

Table 4.2 Gentamicin dosing

CrCl	Ideal body weight (kg)				
	40–49	50–59	60–69	70–79	≥80
<21	2.5 mg/kg (max. 180 mg)				
21–30	120	140	160	240[a]	260[a]
31–40	160	180	200	280[a]	280[a]
41–50	200	220	240	260	280
51–60	220	240	260	280	320
61–70	240	260	300	340	380
71–80	260	280	320	360	400
81–90	280	300	340	380	440
>90	280	340	400	440	500

[a]This dose is to last 48 h not 24 h.

Monitoring and subsequent dosing

In patients with a creatinine clearance <60 mL/min, discuss before initiating treatment with pharmacy. In patients with a creatinine clearance >60 mL/min, measure the level and U&E between 6 and 14 h after the first dose. Include the time the sample was taken and the previous dose administered on the request form. Use the graph in Figure 4.1 to plot the measured concentration against the time the sample was taken. If the measurement is below the line, continue the current dose and dose interval. If it is above the line, withhold the next dose, re-check within 12–24 h and seek advice from the pharmacy.

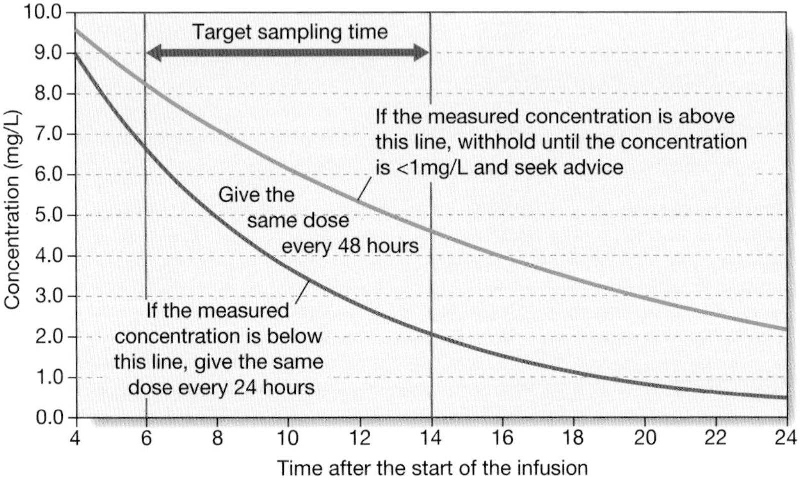

Figure 4.1 Gentamicin dosing graph.

Vancomycin

Initial dose

Calculate ideal body weight and creatinine clearance as above, and then calculate the initial dose according to Table 4.3. Reconstitute vancomycin with water (10 mL for 500 mg vial; 20 mL for 1 g vial) and add to a bag of 0.9% sodium chloride or 5% dextrose (100 mL for 500 mg; 250 mL for higher doses). Vancomycin should be infused SLOWLY and can cause anaphylaxis if give faster than 10 mg/min. Give over an infusion time of 10 min/100 mg total dose.

Table 4.3 Calculation of initial dose of vancomycin

CrCl	Ideal body weight ≤60 kg	Ideal body weight >60 kg
<20	1000 mg; sample after 24 h	
20–29	1000 mg every 48 h	
30–49	750 mg every 24 h	1000 mg every 24 h
50–59	1000 mg every 24 h	
60–69	500 mg every 12 h	
70–79	750 mg every 12 h	
80–100	750 mg every 12 h	1000 mg every 12 h
>100	1250 mg every 12 h	

Monitoring and subsequent dosing

Monitor U&E daily and check the trough concentration just before the fourth dose (within 48 h) or sooner if the renal function is worsening or unstable. The target trough concentration is 10–15 mg/mL. Further monitoring, by checking the trough pre-dose, should be every 72 h, or earlier if renal function is a concern.

Aminophylline

Loading dose

A loading dose should not be given if the patient is already on oral theophylline. The loading dose in milligrams (mg) is 5 times the patient's weight in kilograms (kg), e.g. a 60 kg patient should be given a 300 mg loading dose. Note that in obese patients the dose should be calculated on the basis of ideal body weight (see Box 4.1, p. 115) rather than actual weight. The loading dose should be added to 50–100 mL normal saline or 5% dextrose and administered over 20 min IV.

Continuous infusion

Add 500 mg (2 × 10 mL vials of 25 mg/mL solution) to 500 mL normal saline or 5% glucose to make a 1 mg/mL solution. Give IV, using an infusion rate controlling pump, according to weight; the rate in mL/h is half the body weight in kg, i.e. 80 kg = 40 mL/h. Check plasma theophylline concentration 4–6 h after onset of infusion and daily thereafter. Note dose adjustment for obese patients, as per loading dose, above.

Amphotericin

This must be given as a test dose, which should be followed by an infusion of a gradually increasing concentration, assuming there is no adverse reaction. Reconstitute with sterile water shaking gently, before adding to glucose 5% infusion bag. The amount of water to mix, the test dose, the infusion preparation and dose escalation vary according to the preparation used: consult your local policy or pharmacist.

Digibind®

Digibind® is indicated for known or strongly suspected digoxin toxicity where measures beyond withdrawal of the digoxin and correction of electrolyte abnormality are felt to be necessary.

Acute ingestion

If patients present with life-threatening symptoms of digitalis toxicity and an estimate of the amount ingested is not available, 20 vials of Digibind® may be administered. This is enough to treat most life-threatening ingestions in adults and large children.

Where the amount ingested is known, the number of vials to be administered can be calculated by taking the total body load in milligrams and dividing by 0.5. The total body load in acute ingestion is the total amount of digoxin ingested multiplied by 0.8 (to account for incomplete absorption).

Chronic toxicity

In an adult in whom toxicity results from chronic digoxin use, an urgent digoxin level should be checked. The number of vials of Digibind® required = serum digoxin concentration (ng/mL) multiplied by the patient's weight (kg), divided by 100. When a steady-state concentration is not available, a dose of 6 vials will usually be adequate to reverse toxicity.

Table 4.4 Dobutamine infusion rate (mL/h) for 0.5 mg/mL concentration

Weight (kg)	Desired dose (μg/kg/min)			
	2.5	5	10	15
40	12	24	48	60
50	15	30	60	90
60	18	36	72	108
70	21	42	84	126
80	24	48	96	144

Dobutamine

Dilute a 20 mL vial (250 mg of 12.5 mg/mL) in 500 mL normal saline or 5% dextrose to achieve a concentration of 0.5 mg/mL. Infuse, through a large vein according to the patient's weight and the desired dose (Table 4.4). Note, dobutamine is incompatible with sodium bicarbonate. Patients should have cardiac monitoring while on dobutamine.

Phenytoin

If a patient with seizures is taking oral phenytoin, an urgent phenytoin level should be checked prior to phenytoin use (high phenytoin levels may be the cause of the fits). Otherwise, give loading dose of 15 mg/kg (0.3 mL/kg of 50 mg/mL vial) at a maximum rate of 50 mg/min, with BP and ECG monitoring. Infusions should be made using normal saline not glucose. Irrigate the venous access with saline after the infusion to prevent phlebitis.

Maintenance doses of 100 mg every 6–8 h can be given and adjusted according to measurement of plasma concentrations. Note, there is a logarithmic relationship between the dose administered and the final plasma concentration; therefore small dose increases can result in large increases in plasma concentration.

DRUG MONITORING

Drug monitoring can mean a variety of things, such as monitoring the physical or biological effects of an agent, e.g. antihypertensive and anticoagulant drugs, respectively. Alternatively, it may mean the regular monitoring of side-effects or adverse biochemical effects, e.g. checking renal function following the introduction of an ACE inhibitor. However, drug monitoring may involve regular measurement of serum levels of a drug. This is known as therapeutic drug monitoring.

Therapeutic drug monitoring

Therapeutic drug monitoring (TDM) is required for medications with a narrow therapeutic range. Guidelines regarding sampling times and the exact therapeutic ranges quoted may vary slightly from hospital to hospital.

Indications

TDM can be used to assess whether a patient has been given a sufficient loading dose and for monitoring of therapeutic drug concentrations. TDM is particularly important if factors influencing the drug concentration have changed such as addition or discontinuation of an interacting drug, a change in renal or hepatic function or dose adjustment. In addition, TDM may be used to identify when side-effects or treatment failure are due to elevated or low plasma concentrations, respectively.

Sampling

For TDM to be effective, a blood sample should be taken at a specified time after the latest dose that allows distribution of the medicine in the body before sampling. Sampling too soon could show higher than expected concentrations and lead to unnecessary concern about toxicity, e.g. digoxin. Some drugs require measurement of both peak and trough concentrations, e.g. gentamicin (see 'Dose calculation', p. 115). This establishes whether a therapeutic concentration has been achieved initially and whether it is followed by a period of lower drug levels. This minimizes side-effects and ensures safe re-dosing.

Sampling is best performed when drug concentrations are at a 'steady state', i.e. the amount taken into the body each day is equivalent to the amount of drug removed. The time taken to get to steady state varies depending on the drug being used and host factors, particularly renal and liver function.

DRUG USE IN SPECIAL CIRCUMSTANCES

In your prescribing, you should consider how a patient's other medical conditions will affect the way a drug is metabolized and its action.

Renal and liver impairment

Most medications are cleared by either renal or hepatic excretion. Where there is dysfunction in either one or both of these systems, serum drug concentrations can fluctuate leading to unexpected responses to standard dosing. For additional advice, see the appropriate appendices in the BNF.

Renal impairment

As renal function deteriorates there is a corresponding reduction in the clearance of many substances via the kidney; this includes drugs and their metabolites. In renal impairment:

- quantify the patient's renal function; see below
- avoid nephrotoxic drugs
- prescribe drugs that are not dependent on renal clearance
- consider reducing the dose or frequency of drugs being administered; the extent of any dose reduction should reflect the degree of renal impairment, the amount of the drug that is cleared by the renal route and the risk of toxicity
- remember that active metabolites can also accumulate and cause side-effects, e.g. opiates.

Quantifying renal function

To quantify renal function and guide prescribing, creatinine clearance should be measured via a 24 h urine collection or estimated using the Cockcroft–Gault equation (see 'Dose calculation', p. 115). Calculated creatinine clearance is acceptable for use in the majority of patients, but is not suitable where renal function is changing rapidly.

The estimated GFR (eGFR) is an alternative tool now quoted by many biochemistry labs. It uses serum creatinine, age, gender and race along with a measure for standard body surface area to judge the severity of chronic kidney disease. Like other values of calculated creatinine clearance it cannot be used accurately to assess acute renal insufficiency and should not be used to influence drug dosage adjustments in this context.

Liver impairment

There is no easy way to calculate the degree of liver impairment or predict how liver disease will affect drug clearance. For this reason, the advice given is often more general than that for renal impairment.

Impaired drug metabolism

Impaired liver function can lead to an increase in the bioavailability of drugs that have a high first-pass metabolism (metabolism of a medication by the liver before it reaches the rest of the body) and a marked rise in serum concentration. If possible, choose a drug eliminated by the kidney, rather than one dependent on the liver, and use the smallest dose possible to reduce the risk of toxicity.

Reduced plasma protein production

When hepatic synthetic function is depressed, suggested by a low serum albumin, the free serum concentration of drugs that are highly protein bound, e.g. phenytoin, may increase. This should be considered when interpreting the results of therapeutic drug monitoring assays, which often measure the total drug concentration rather than the free proportion.

Reduced production of coagulation factors

Coagulation factor production will be reduced when liver synthetic function is impaired. This will be reflected by an increased prothrombin time. Potential benefits of anticoagulant therapies should be weighed against the additional risk of bleeding.

Drug-precipitated hepatic encephalopathy

Sedative drugs can precipitate hepatic encephalopathy in patients with liver failure, e.g. benzodiazepines should be used with caution in patients with alcohol withdrawal and liver impairment.

Oedema and ascites

Oedema and ascites are common in chronic liver disease and can be worsened by drugs that cause fluid retention, e.g. NSAIDs.

Avoidance of hepatotoxic drugs

Numerous drugs are hepatotoxic (see the appropriate appendix in the BNF). Examples include amiodarone, erythromycin, methotrexate, rifampicin and valproate.

The elderly

Elderly patients are often on many different medications. The list of medications they are prescribed should be reviewed on a regular basis and kept as simple as possible. As the body ages, drug metabolism and clearance mechanisms become less efficient and a number of physiological changes occur, for example:

- plasma protein production is reduced resulting in greater availability of highly protein-bound drugs
- liver blood flow and metabolism are reduced, increasing bioavailability of drugs with a high 'first pass' metabolism
- renal function deteriorates reducing the elimination of drugs cleared by the kidney.

Elderly patients are also more susceptible to the effects and side-effects of drugs, for example:

- sensitivity to hypnotics is increased and standard doses should be reduced, e.g. zopiclone dose should be reduced from 7.5 mg to 3.75 mg
- a lower dose of digoxin may be necessary if renal function is impaired
- there is an increased risk of GI bleeding with NSAIDs.

Pregnancy

The possibility of pregnancy should be considered when prescribing for any female of child-bearing age. A significant number of pregnancies are not planned and there is a possibility that the patient may be pregnant and unaware of it.

Ideally, drug treatment should be avoided in pregnancy, especially during the first trimester. If a drug is necessary, it should only be prescribed when the benefit to the mother outweighs the risk to her and her baby. The mother should be informed of any possible risks to her fetus and the decision to initiate treatment should be a joint one. Drugs can have a harmful effect on a fetus at any stage of pregnancy (for a complete list, see the appropriate section of the BNF):

- first trimester treatment increases the risk of congenital malformations, e.g. ACE inhibitors, ibuprofen, quinolone antibiotics, statins, warfarin
- second and third trimester drug use may cause growth and development problems, e.g. ACE inhibitors, aminoglycosides, amiodarone, gliclazide, thiazide diuretics.

Most medicines are not directly tested in pregnant patients, but some medicines will be listed as 'not known to be harmful' and, by implication, thought to be safe. This listing is most commonly given to drugs that have been on the market for some time without reported problems in pregnancy. Newer drugs will have less information available about their use in pregnancy, and are best avoided.

Breast-feeding

When a mother is breast-feeding, the safety of the baby should be considered and non-essential medications avoided. Where treatment is necessary, inform the patient of the risks involved before initiating treatment. Potential problems may be seen with drugs that:

- affect milk production, e.g. bromocriptine, combined oral contraceptives and levodopa
- are secreted into breast milk, either at low concentration with low risk of clinical effects, e.g. diclofenac, paracetamol, penicillins, or at a higher concentration potentially resulting in the baby receiving a therapeutic or proportionally larger dose than the mother, e.g. cyclophosphamide, carbimazole, ciprofloxacin, clarithromycin.

Children

Children differ from adults in their handling and response to drugs and doses should not be calculated as if they were simply small adults. In addition, it is best to choose a drug licensed for children. Many drugs have not been formally tested in children and do not have a specific paediatric licence. Therefore, it cannot be assumed that a medication safe in adults is also safe in children. For detailed advice on prescribing in children, see the BNF for Children.

When prescribing for a child:

- seek advice from a senior or local pharmacist if you have not used the medicine before
- use the child's weight and age to determine an appropriate dose
- consider an appropriate formulation; this will be influenced by the dose required and their ability to manage tablets or capsules
- avoid certain medicines because of known incidence of particular side-effects, e.g. quinolones have been associated with arthropathy, aspirin has been associated with Reye's syndrome

- consider that the different stages of childhood development also affect drug handling
- use special caution in neonates due to the complicated dose calculations required.

PRESCRIBING FLUID AND BLOOD

Prescribing fluid

It is good practice to ensure that all of the patients under your care who need IV fluids overnight have them prescribed before you leave at the end of the day.

If you are called to prescribe fluids for a patient that you do not know, it is important to check what the aims and risks of the fluid treatment are. DO NOT simply write up the same fluid at the same rate as before. Establish as much as is practically possible about the patient's past and recent medical history, noting especially cardiac disease, diabetes, current creatinine, K^+ and Na^+. Assess the patient for signs of dehydration or shock and cardiac failure, and look for evidence of their recent fluid intake, including antibiotics and transfusion, and fluid output, including urine, diarrhoea and insensible losses. For further guidance on fluid management in patients with shock, see 'Shock', p. 250. Whether the patient is shocked or not, consider the following:

- the need for continued fluid administration
- the need for a change in rate
- the choice of fluid, including the proportion of saline to dextrose
- the need for potassium.

A standard short-term fluid regime in a young patient without shock or electrolyte disturbance could be:

- 500 mL 5% dextrose IV over 6 h
- 500 mL 5% dextrose IV over 6 h
- 500 mL 0.9% saline IV over 6 h.

In the elderly, infusing each bag over 8 h would be more usual, whereas, in those with evidence of recent acute fluid loss, e.g. diarrhoea, the initial bag might need to be over 2 h.

Blood products

Blood products are prepared from human blood and can be split into two categories:

- blood components: red cell concentrate, platelets, fresh frozen plasma (FFP) and cryoprecipitate
- plasma derivatives: prepared under pharmaceutical manufacturing conditions from large pools of human plasma, they include coagulation factors, immunoglobulin and albumin.

Transfusion of blood products can be life-saving, e.g. red cell concentrate, platelets and FFP are often all required in an acute variceal bleed. However, they are finite resources and transfusion reactions can occur. Blood products should not be used indiscriminately and all staff involved in their provision have a responsibility to ensure that the right patient gets the right blood product at the right time.

Blood groups

Blood group classification reflects antigen expression, the most clinically relevant of which is the ABO classification (Table 4.5). ABO matching ensures that

Table 4.5 ABO immunology

Patient's ABO blood group	Red cell antigens expressed	Serum antibodies	Compatible blood
O	None	Anti-A and anti-B	O
A	A	Anti-B	A, O
B	B	Anti-A	B, O
AB	A and B	Neither	A, B, O

the antigen expressed on the transfused red cells does not react with the patient's own serum antibodies. Hence, group O red cells do not express A or B antigens and may be transfused to all patients, independent of their ABO status. Therefore, group O negative (negative refers to Rhesus antigen negative; see 'Haemolytic disease of the newborn', p. 321) is termed the 'universal donor'.

Use of blood components

Consent

At present there is no legal requirement in the UK to gain formal consent for the transfusion of blood products. However, you should give the patient information on the benefits and risks (see below) of transfusion and discuss the reasons for recommending it. You should also mention any other options that may be available for an individual, e.g. oral iron therapy, and recognize that some patients, such as Jehovah's witnesses, will refuse transfusion.

Risk

The risks are small with 10–15 adverse events per 100000 issued components. They should be balanced against potential benefits.

Wrong blood

This is the commonest adverse event with 12 reported errors per 100000 components. You have a responsibility at the time of cross-matching and blood administration to ensure that the identification of the patient is correct.

Infection

Despite the concerns that exist about infection transmitted by blood component transfusion, the risk is very small. Transfusion-transmitted infection (including bacterial infection) accounts for only about 0.1 adverse events per 100000 components.

Reaction

Acute transfusion reaction and transfusion-related acute lung injury (TRALI) account for about 2 adverse events per 100000.

Ordering blood products

If a transfusion of red cells is indicated or the need anticipated in the near future, a sample of the patient's blood should be sent to the lab:

- group and save: used to determine blood group only; no blood is set aside
- cross-match: the blood group will be determined and the requested number of units set aside in the blood fridge; if the patient has had a transfusion in between the initial sample and the current episode, or if 72 h has elapsed since the initial sample, a repeat sample will be required
- if emergency blood is required, telephone the lab; you will most likely need to give O-negative blood in the first instance.

The use of most other blood products, including platelets and FFP, require prior discussion with a haematologist. Remember, when ordering FFP in the emergency situation, that it needs to thaw before it can be given.

Prescription of blood products

Some hospitals have specially designed ICPs for blood product transfusions which include an area for the nurses to document patient observations during the transfusion. Check that the patient is correctly identified and that you are prescribing the appropriate products. A unit of red cell concentrate should be infused within 4 h. Platelets and FFP should be given over 30 min. Be careful not to overload patients with a history of cardiac failure. Oral diuretic cover with furosemide 20–40 mg may be required.

Special circumstances

CMV-negative components must be used in patients with HIV, CMV-negative pregnant women and CMV-negative recipients of allogenic stem cell grafts. Gamma-irradiated components should be used in a variety of other situations, including:

- patients receiving purine analogues, e.g. fludarabine, cladribine, deoxycoformycin
- exchange transfusions
- any granulocyte transfusion
- all recipients of allogeneic haemopoietic stem cell (HSC) grafts
- allogeneic HSC donors before or during the harvest of their HSC
- autologous HSC grafting: any transfusion within 7 days of the HSC collection; any transfusion from the start of conditioning therapy until 3 months post-transplant or until 6 months post-transplant if conditioning total body irradiation has been given
- Hodgkin's disease, at all stages of the disease
- congenital immunodeficiency with defective cell-mediated immunity.

Reporting of adverse events and errors

An adverse event related to a blood product may result from a reaction to the product or be through error of administration. Blood transfusion practice is heavily regulated and national reporting mechanisms exist. If a patient is thought to be the subject of an adverse event, this must be brought to the attention of the laboratory staff.

SECTION 2
Symptoms and related acute presentations

Cardiac and chest 5

CHEST PAIN

Initial assessment

Delay in the diagnosis of ST-segment elevation myocardial infarction (STEMI) can result in serious morbidity and an increase in mortality. As with all acutely unwell patients, an ABC assessment is required. A 12-lead ECG should be performed as soon as possible, even before a full history is taken or complete examination performed. However, careful clinical assessment including a more detailed history and examination is then essential, as for those with other causes of chest pain (see 'Patients without STEMI', p. 128).

Patients with STEMI

Patients may present with angina pectoris. This is classically described as central chest discomfort, often described as a pressure, tightness or weight, extending like a band across the chest and radiating into the arms, left more often than right. There may be associated autonomic symptoms including nausea, vomiting and sweating (diaphoresis). Alternative presentations include unexplained pulmonary oedema, collapse, abdominal pain or arrhythmia.

STEMI is defined by typical ECG changes in one or more coronary artery territories (see p. 83). Reperfusion therapy should not be delayed in patients presenting within 12 h of symptom onset who meet the relevant ECG criteria:

- ST elevation ≥1 mm in two contiguous limb leads or ≥2 mm in two contiguous chest leads
- new or presumed new left bundle branch block (LBBB)
- posterior myocardial infarction (suggested by anterior ST depression in leads V1–V4 and confirmed by significant ST elevation in posterior chest leads).

Clinical assessment should be rapid and focused. Typical findings on history and examination are as for other patients presenting with myocardial ischaemia. However, look for evidence of shock, pulmonary oedema and arrhythmias (these may be the cause of, or result from, cardiac ischaemia). Enquire about previous cardiac disease and any potential contraindications to treatment, particularly thrombolysis. The management of STEMI, including appropriate reperfusion therapy, is discussed below. If ECG criteria for reperfusion therapy are not met on the initial ECG, but clinical suspicion remains, repeat the ECG 30 min later and re-assess.

Management

Oxygen and opiate pain relief should be given early. All patients should have continuous cardiac rhythm monitoring and be admitted to CCU. In patients presenting within 6 h of symptom onset, the ideal choice of reperfusion therapy is primary percutaneous coronary intervention (PCI, see below). However, thrombolysis is an acceptable alternative where this is not available. In patients presenting between 6 and 12 h after onset of symptoms, the risk:benefit ratio strongly favours primary PCI over thrombolysis, but this should still be offered where PCI is not available.

Percutaneous coronary intervention

Primary

The best treatment for STEMI is primary percutaneous coronary intervention (PCI), although availability is limited. It is associated with high infarct-related artery patency rates, reduced rates of re-infarction and reduced risk of stroke as compared with thrombolysis. Where PCI is anticipated, patients should receive aspirin 300 mg, clopidogrel 600 mg and be considered for a glycoprotein IIb/IIIa receptor antagonist, e.g. abciximab. If primary PCI cannot be performed within 90 min of diagnosis, patients should receive thrombolysis (unless contraindicated).

Rescue

Where patients given thrombolysis fail to reperfuse (see below), referral for rescue PCI should be considered.

Thrombolysis

The thrombolytic agent(s) available to you will depend on local protocols. Both fibrin-specific lytics and streptokinase (see below) are effective and reduce mortality. Specific administration regimes are given in Table 5.1 (also check your own unit's protocol and the BNF). Before offering thrombolysis, check for contraindications:

- active bleeding or bleeding diathesis
- recent haemorrhage, trauma or surgery, including dental extraction (1 month)
- coma
- stroke within past 3 months
- aortic dissection
- known structural cerebral lesion including neoplasm
- any prior intracerebral haemorrhage.

Relative contraindications include active peptic ulcer disease, uncontrolled hypertension, pregnancy, current use of anticoagulants, prolonged external chest compression, diabetic retinopathy, severe liver disease or oesophageal varices, heavy vaginal bleeding. Where any is present, discuss the patient with a senior.

Table 5.1 Thrombolytics

	Initial treatment	Co-therapy
Streptokinase (SK)	1.5 million units in 100 mL 5% dextrose or N saline over 30–60 min	Usually none[a]
Alteplase (tPA)	15 mg IV bolus, then 0.75 mg/kg over 30 min, then 0.5 mg/kg over 60 min. Total dose not >100 mg	IV heparin 24–48 h[a]
Reteplase (r-PA)	10 units IV bolus then further 10 units IV bolus 30 min later	IV heparin 24–48 h[a]
Tenecteplase (TNK-tPA)	Single IV bolus: <60 kg = 30 mg; 60–69 kg = 35 mg; 70–79 kg = 40 mg; 80–89 kg = 45 mg; ≥90 kg = 50 mg	IV heparin 24–48 h[a]

[a]Possibly LMWH in the future.

Reperfusion following thrombolysis is defined as a reduction in the extent of ST-segment elevation by >50% on an ECG, 90 min after the initiation of treatment.

Fibrin-specific lytics

These have greater efficacy than streptokinase, but are relatively short-acting agents and, therefore, there is a risk of re-occlusion. Anticoagulation is recommended for 48 h following administration. Commonly, an infusion of unfractionated heparin is used; however, there is increasing evidence for the use of LMWH (for administration and doses see 'Heparin', p. 109). While the efficacy of tenecteplase (TNK) and recombinant tissue plasminogen activator (r-tPA) are similar, TNK can be given as a single bolus. Therefore, it is often chosen because of its ease of administration, e.g. for use in out-of-hospital thrombolysis. Since the risk of stroke is increased in patients over 75 years old given fibrin-specific lytics, some centres advocate the use of streptokinase in this population (check your local protocol).

Streptokinase

Streptokinase has a more prolonged anticoagulant effect than the fibrin-specific lytics. Therefore, unfractionated heparin is often not given to patients treated with this form of thrombolysis. However, recent evidence suggests benefit from low molecular weight heparin as an adjunct to streptokinase. This has been added to many CCU protocols, but you should check your local guidelines.

Common side-effects of streptokinase include nausea, vomiting, hypotension and anaphylaxis. Streptokinase is a bacterial enzyme which can induce an antibody response; therefore, repeated administration beyond 4 days of the original dose is not advised due to an increased risk of anaphylaxis and reduced efficacy. Hypotension can be dangerous in unstable patients, but can be ameliorated by stopping the infusion temporarily and re-starting it at half the previous flow rate.

Anti-platelet agents

Aspirin

Many patients will have already received 300 mg in the ambulance. However, you should not assume that this is the case and always actively ensure that it has been given. If it has not, it should be given immediately after the ECG.

Clopidogrel

There is evidence that patients receiving thrombolysis, especially those within 12 h of the onset of their myocardial infarction, should also receive clopidogrel. 300 mg should be given at the time of thrombolysis (reduced to 75 mg in patients over 75 to reduce the risk of bleeding complications) and then continued at a daily dose of 75 mg, irrespective of age.

Other drugs

- intensive glycaemic control, e.g. sliding scale insulin, is indicated in patients with known diabetes or an admission blood glucose >11 mmol/L; however, avoid regimens that result in infusions of large volumes of fluid as this may cause pulmonary congestion
- an ACE inhibitor (at 36 h) should be considered
- statins should be considered, as in any patient with acute coronary syndrome (ACS).

Early coronary arteriography

For those patients who successfully reperfuse with lytic therapy, there remains the option of coronary arteriography with a view to follow-on PCI the next morning. You should check your local protocol.

Long-term treatment

- general: smoking cessation, cholesterol and weight reduction
- β-blockers, statins, ACE inhibitors and anti-platelet therapy should be considered

- patients with clinical or echocardiographic evidence of LV dysfunction (LV ejection fraction <40%) and those with diabetes should be considered for an aldosterone antagonist, e.g. eplerenone 25–50 mg daily and/or an implantable cardiac defibrillator (ICD)
- cardiac rehabilitation programmes with a step-wise return to normal function have been shown to improve long-term outcome.

Complications

The following complications may occur in any patient with myocardial ischaemia; however, they are more common in STEMI:

- arrhythmias and heart block: see 'Arrhythmias', p. 132
- pulmonary oedema: see p. 146
- shock: see p. 250
- mechanical complications: papillary muscle rupture resulting in mitral valve regurgitation (new pan-systolic murmur maximum at apex); septal rupture (new harsh pan-systolic murmur at right sternal border)
- Dressler's syndrome: fever, pericarditis and pleurisy post-MI; occurs weeks to months after the infarct, usually subsides after a few days; if prolonged, may respond to NSAID or corticosteroid therapy.

Patients without STEMI

History

Myocardial ischaemia

Myocardial ischaemia may present with classical angina pectoris (as above). Alternative presentations include isolated jaw or arm pain and exertional breathlessness without pain (particularly in patients with diabetes). This is sometimes referred to as an 'angina equivalent', i.e. when there is no underlying respiratory cause of breathlessness and subsequent investigation demonstrates obstructive coronary artery disease in the presence of preserved left ventricular systolic function.

Anginal pain should be characterized as stable or unstable. Unstable angina is defined by an increase in the frequency and/or severity of previously predictable (i.e. stable angina) symptoms or pain precipitated at a significantly reduced workload, including pain at rest. Unstable angina is important to recognize, as it indicates a potentially unstable atherosclerotic plaque which may rupture, causing coronary artery occlusion and myocardial infarction.

Oesophageal spasm

This can be similar in character to ischaemic cardiac pain, with similar radiation to the neck and shoulder and may also be relieved by GTN. However, there is usually no association with exercise and there may be a preceding history of heartburn. The ECG during severe pain remains normal.

Pulmonary embolism

This typically causes sudden breathlessness and may be associated with immediate central chest discomfort or pre-syncope. Pleuritic chest pain is typically worse on deep breathing or coughing and may not be present initially (see 'Presentation', p. 152). Patients with significant pulmonary embolism (PE) can sometimes present with syncope, shock and right upper quadrant abdominal pain, due to liver congestion.

Spontaneous pneumothorax

This can cause symptoms very similar to PE, but is less likely to cause hypotension (except with tension pneumothorax). It is often easily identified on a plain chest X-ray (see 'Investigation', p. 149).

Pericarditis

Pericarditis may be associated with a history of a recent viral illness, pharyngitis or connective tissue disease. Classically, the pain is described as sharp, central in location, exacerbated by lying flat and eased by leaning forward. The resting ECG may show concave-upwards ST elevation across more than one coronary territory (see 'ECGs', p. 83).

Aortic dissection

Aortic dissection is a life-threatening cardiothoracic surgical emergency. The diagnosis should be suspected in patients with sudden-onset 'tearing' inter-scapular back pain. Aortic aneurysms may also leak or rupture without dissection, leading to isolated neurological deficits, abdominal pain, acute MI or acute renal failure.

Physical examination

In addition to standard clinical assessment, it is important to identify specific concerning findings:

- abnormal pulse rate: tachy- and brady-arrhythmias may precipitate ischaemic cardiac chest pain in patients with underlying coronary artery disease
- hypotension: can cause additional cardiac ischaemia; a significant difference between right and left brachial blood pressures (>15 mmHg) may indicate an aortic dissection; in the context of pulmonary oedema and a low cardiac output, cardiogenic shock is considered to be present when the systolic BP is <80–90 mmHg
- pulmonary oedema, suggested by fine bi-basal inspiratory crepitations: this can result in hypoxia and precipitate angina in patients with stable coronary artery disease; alternatively it may develop secondary to myocardial ischaemia; pulmonary oedema should always prompt an early ECG to exclude acute MI
- heart sounds and murmurs: valvular dysfunction and heart failure can precipitate or result from myocardial ischaemia
- pericardial rub, often described as the sound of 'walking on snow': may be present in patients with pericarditis
- chest wall tenderness: suggests musculoskeletal pain, e.g. costochondritis
- neurological deficits: may occur as a result of carotid artery involvement in an aortic dissection

A description of the signs typically associated with 'pulmonary causes' of chest pain can be found in 'Breathlessness', p. 139.

Investigations

Electrocardiograph

It is vital to perform an early ECG in patients presenting with chest discomfort: see 'Initial assessment', p. 125. Remember that pericarditis can cause saddle-shaped ST elevation, often in more than one vascular territory.

Troponin

Troponins are specific tests of myocardial necrosis and should be performed in patients with suspected ACS. Troponin levels start to rise 3 h after myocardial injury. Therefore, the timing of blood samples in patients with ACS is crucial. A troponin level should be checked on admission and 12 h after the onset of pain to ensure a late rise in troponin is not missed.

The 12-h troponin concentration can be used to quantify infarct size in acute myocardial infarction and has been recently introduced as a means of classifying non-STEMI acute coronary syndromes. In patients with symptoms consistent with myocardial ischaemia but without ST elevation on their admission ECG, a troponin T concentration (μg/L):

- >1.0 indicates non-ST elevation myocardial infarction (NSTEMI)
- <0.01 indicates acute coronary syndrome (ACS) without myocyte necrosis

- between 0.01 and 1.0 indicates ACS with myocyte necrosis, according to the British Cardiac Society (European and American cardiac societies would characterize this as a NSTEMI).

Troponin levels will remain elevated for at least 1 week after myocardial injury; therefore, repeated sampling within this time is unhelpful and potentially confusing. Note, in the absence of coronary artery disease, elevated troponin levels can also occur in patients with cardiac failure, PTE, rapid atrial dysrhythmias and renal failure.

Troponin and cardiovascular risk in ACS

Patients with troponin-positive non-STEMI acute coronary syndromes (i.e. NSTEMI and ACS with myocyte necrosis) have a greater immediate cardiovascular risk, including that of readmission, infarction and death. However, troponin is only one of several variables that predict outcome in this setting.

Troponin-negative patients (i.e. ACS without myocyte necrosis) may be at a greater short-term risk than those with positive results if other risk factors are present, e.g. age, ST changes, known coronary disease. This concept is the basis of risk stratification scores such as GRACE and TIMI. GRACE scores are more accurate at predicting short-term outcome, but more complicated than TIMI scores (Tables 5.2 and 5.3) which can be calculated easily during an on-call shift. This risk stratification can identify those at greatest risk, in whom early investigation, e.g. arteriography, should be performed.

Table 5.2 The TIMI score

Factor	Score
Age over 65	1
>3 CAD risk factors (Fhx, HBP, high chol, DM, smoker)	1
Known CAD (stenosis > 50%)	1
Aspirin use in the past 7 days	1
Recent (<24 h) severe angina	1
Increased cardiac markers	1
ST deviation of more than 0.5 mm	1
Risk score = Total points (0–7)	

Table 5.3 Risk of cardiac events (%) in patients with ACS by 14 days

TIMI score	Death or MI	Death, MI or urgent PCI
0–1	3	5
2	3	8
3	5	13
4	7	20
5	12	26
6–7	19	41

Other blood tests

The following tests should be requested all patients presenting with chest pain:

- FBC to exclude anaemia
- lipids and LFTs: LFTs should be documented prior to commencement of statin therapy; patients with biliary colic can also present with chest pain (see 'Biliary colic', p. 161)
- TFTs to exclude hyperthyroidism
- WBC, CRP and viral titres in suspected pericarditis
- arterial blood gas analysis should be considered if SaO_2 <92%; avoid unnecessary arterial puncture in patients who may be considered for thrombolysis or PCI (right radial access is commonly required)
- D-dimer: should not be checked routinely (see p. 153).

Imaging

Chest X-ray

A chest X-ray should be considered in all patients with chest pain and performed urgently in those with symptoms or signs of pneumothorax. Patients with pulmonary thromboembolism may have a normal CXR. In those with an aortic dissection, the CXR may show mediastinal widening, with or without a pleural effusion.

Echocardiography

This is unnecessary in the acute setting, but should be considered in patients with myocardial infarction or suspected LV dysfunction. It may be diagnostic in acute thoracic aortic dissection and massive PTE (see p. 154).

Cross-sectional imaging

Urgent spiral CT should be performed if aortic dissection is suspected. Cardiac MRI can accurately quantify infarct size, using gadolinium contrast, in addition to LV function and myocardial viability. MRI can also differentiate acute myocarditis from myocardial infarction in patients with atypical chest pain and an elevated troponin. This difference can have significant long-term implications.

Management of chest pain without STEMI

Patients with ACS

These patients are at risk of further events in relation to plaque rupture. As with STEMI, initial management is dictated by 12-lead ECG findings. In the UK, standard therapy should include:

- oxygen and opiate analgesia
- aspirin 300 mg loading dose, followed by aspirin 75 mg daily indefinitely
- clopidogrel should be prescribed for all patients with ischaemic ECG changes or a subsequent rise in troponin; 300 mg should be given as a loading dose (some units use 600 mg loading doses to achieve more rapid platelet inhibition), followed by 75 mg daily for at least 12 weeks
- low molecular weight heparin should be prescribed for patients with ischaemic ECG changes and continued until pain free for 2 days, e.g. enoxaparin 1 mg/kg SC 12-hourly (reduce the dose in renal failure and elderly patients), or fondaparinux 2.5 mg daily (avoid fondaparinux in patients who may need inpatient angiography and PCI)
- nitrates: while there is no proven survival benefit, ongoing pain can be treated using IV nitroglycerin (0.6–1.2 mg/h), or IV isosorbide dinitrate (1–2 mg/h).

Small molecule IIb–IIIa glycoprotein antagonists

These drugs are short-acting but potent inhibitors of platelet aggregation. They are usually reserved for high-risk patients with ongoing chest pain or dynamic ECG changes, or those in whom early PCI is contemplated (see indications for further investigation below). Check your unit's protocol; if used, remember to adjust the dose in renal impairment.

Indications for further investigation

- high-risk patients, e.g. TIMI score of 5 or more, should be considered for early coronary arteriography with a view to follow-on PCI
- patients at moderate risk, e.g. TIMI score 3–4, can be considered for early coronary arteriography or non-invasive assessment prior to discharge, e.g. exercise tolerance testing or stress myocardial perfusion scanning
- low-risk patients, e.g. TIMI less than 2, who present with possible cardiac chest pain may be reassured by an exercise tolerance test; this strategy may reduce the rate of re-admission in this group.

Long-term treatment

In addition to aspirin (and clopidogrel for at least 12 months in patients with ECG changes on admission, or a rise in troponin), patients with ACS should be commenced on a statin before discharge, e.g. simvastatin (40 mg daily), along with a β-blocker and an ACE inhibitor, unless contraindicated.

Non-ischaemic causes of chest pain

Pericarditis

Standard treatment is with NSAIDs, although corticosteroids and colchicine have also been used. Patients should be considered for a follow-up echo to assess LV systolic function.

Pulmonary thromboembolism

See 'Breathlessness', p. 152.

Pneumothorax

See 'Breathlessness', p. 148.

Oesophageal pain

Antacids, alginates and proton pump inhibitors can be used to treat oesophageal reflux and oesophagitis. Sublingual nitrates can be useful in oesophageal spasm. Other measures include smoking cessation, weight and alcohol reduction.

Aortic dissection

Treat as for shock and seek immediate senior review and a cardiothoracic surgical opinion. Send blood for routine parameters and cross-match 10 units. Management depends on the type and size of dissection. Therefore, urgent spiral CT should be arranged and the patient transferred to ICU once stabilized.

ARRHYTHMIAS

The term arrhythmia is used to describe any cardiac rhythm other than sinus rhythm. Arrhythmias are classified on the basis of their rate, rhythm and likely origin.

- tachyarrhythmias (rate >100 b.p.m.) versus bradyarrhythmias (rate <60 b.p.m.)
- regular versus irregular
- narrow complex (supraventricular) versus broad complex (ventricular or supraventricular with aberrant conduction).

These ECG features should be used to broadly characterize any arrhythmia and generate a short list of possible underlying causes. This allows you to conduct a more focused examination of the ECG, identify the specific arrhythmia and initiate appropriate treatment. Detailed guidance on the identification of the arrhythmias discussed below is given in 'ECGs', p. 84.

Initial assessment and urgent management

The effect of the arrhythmia on the patient, and whether they have underlying cardiac disease, or other co-morbidities, will influence your initial actions. New symptoms of pain or breathlessness, or a fall in systemic BP from the patient's normal or previous measurements, should prompt immediate further assessment and management of the arrhythmia. Absolute indications for emergency electrical cardioversion of a tachyarrhythmia and the pacing of a bradyarrhythmia include:

- cardiogenic shock, suggested by a low BP, cool peripheries, elevated JVP and oliguria
- florid pulmonary oedema
- severe cardiac pain, unresponsive to standard treatment or untreatable by other means because of hypotension
- evidence of cerebral hypoperfusion, e.g. diminished conscious level.

Emergency DC cardioversion

You will need the help of an anaesthetist to sedate the patient and manage their airway. A synchronized DC shock should be delivered once the patient has been sedated or anaesthetized and may be repeated up to three times (see 'Cardioversion', p. 58).

Pacing

Emergency cardiac pacing is necessary in patients with haemodynamically unstable bradyarrhythmias and in certain specific rhythm disorders where the probability of cardiac arrest is high, e.g. complete heart block (see 'Temporary Cardiac Pacing', p. 54).

Narrow complex tachyarrhythmias

These are defined by a QRS duration <0.12 s and are supraventricular in origin. They are often well tolerated and have a good long-term prognosis; however, this may not be the case in patients with chronic heart disease or coronary artery disease.

Rhythm identification

Determine if the rhythm is regular or irregular; this will dictate immediate management. Look at the rhythm strip if one is available and refer to 'ECGs', p. 84. If you cannot convince yourself of the regularity of a narrow complex tachyarrhythmia, consider inducing AV block (see 'Interventions', below).

Vagal manoeuvres should be attempted first, e.g. carotid sinus massage (see below) or the Valsalva manoeuvre (ask the patient to hold their breath and bear down). If these have no effect intravenous adenosine can be used. The effect of successful AV block is outlined in Table 5.4.

Table 5.4 The effect of transient AV block on narrow complex tachyarrhythmias

Rhythm	Effect
Irregular	
Atrial fibrillation	Reveals chaotic fibrillation waves
Atrial flutter	Reveals 'saw-tooth' flutter waves
Regular	
AVNRT	Terminates
AVRT	Terminates
Atrial tachycardia	Reveals abnormal P wave morphology; PR<RP interval
Multifocal atrial tachycardia	Reveals abnormal, multiple P wave morphologies

Carotid sinus massage

The carotid sinus sits above the bifurcation of the common carotid artery and can be located midway between the angle of the mandible and the thyroid cartilage. Contraindications to CSM include carotid artery disease, recent CVA or previous MI.

Position the patient at 45° with their head stretched slightly towards the left; connect them to an ECG machine and begin a single lead recording; identify the right carotid sinus and massage firmly for 5 s; observe the ECG trace. If there is no effect try the other side, but never massage both simultaneously.

Adenosine

Intravenous adenosine induces transient AV block and has a half-life of around 30 s. Occasionally adenosine can produce transient ventricular standstill and it should be given in a monitored environment with continuous 12-lead ECG recording. It should be avoided in patients with a history of bronchospasm. The patient should be warned that they will experience transient symptoms of nausea, flushing and chest discomfort.

A 6 mg IV bolus should be given via a large-bore cannula (3 mg if given via a central line), followed by a rapid saline flush of at least 10 mL (ideally using a free flowing drip). This should induce transient AV block and reveal the nature of the arrhythmia; it may terminate certain arrhythmias as discussed in Table 5.4. The absence of symptoms suggests an inadequate dosage. If the first treatment is unsuccessful, try 12 mg (plus flush) and repeat if necessary after 1–2 min.

Irregular narrow complex tachyarrhythmias

This is most likely due to atrial fibrillation (AF), or atrial flutter with variable block. Patients with AF may present with palpitation, chest pain or breathlessness. Symptoms are more likely if the ventricular response rate is rapid, if the patient is older or has underlying cardiac disease. Collapse, hypotension and embolic complications, e.g. cerebrovascular accident, are less common presentations. Look for clinical evidence of an underlying cause:

- cardiac: ischaemic heart disease, myocardial infarction, valvular heart disease (particularly mitral), heart failure, hypertension, cardiomyopathy, post-cardiac surgery
- non-cardiac: electrolyte disturbance (e.g. hypokalaemia, hypocalcaemia, hypomagnesaemia), thyrotoxicosis, sepsis, acidosis, or drugs (such as digoxin, alcohol, β-agonists).

Investigation

Send blood for electrolytes (particularly hypo- and hyperkalaemia, hypomagnesaemia, hypocalcaemia), TFT (thyrotoxicosis), inflammatory markers, Coag and a digoxin level, if appropriate. In patients with suspected myocardial ischaemia a troponin level should be checked, 12 h or more after the onset of symptoms.

An echocardiogram should be performed once the ventricular response rate has been controlled. This allows assessment of cardiac structure, function and embolic sources. This information can be used to guide decisions regarding elective DC cardioversion in the future; see below.

Management of AF

Treat potential precipitants, e.g. hypokalaemia, digoxin toxicity, sepsis. Chemical or electrical cardioversion can be considered, but it is worth noting that there is no long-term survival advantage for rhythm control (i.e. cardioversion to sinus) over rate control (where the patient remains in AF) assuming effective anticoagulation.

Anticoagulation

Patients who have been in AF for >48 h may have developed atrial clot and are at risk of systemic embolization on reversion to sinus rhythm. In this situation, patients should be anticoagulated unless there is a contraindication, pending a decision between DC cardioversion and rate control. Note that LMWH is not licensed for use in AF; unfractionated IV heparin should be used. Initiate warfarin and discontinue heparin once the INR is over 2 (see also 'Warfarin', p. 110).

In patients with persistent AF, long-term anticoagulation should be considered. The benefit of this should be balanced against potential risks, e.g. GI bleeding, intracranial haemorrhage, especially in those prone to falls or in whom compliance may be a problem.

Electrical cardioversion

As with any tachyarrhythmia, AF causing significant haemodynamic compromise should be managed by emergency DC cardioversion (see also 'Defibrillation and cardioversion', p. 58). This should not be performed in patients with long-standing AF, and is unlikely to produce maintainable sinus rhythm if precipitants are not addressed.

Elective cardioversion, e.g. for persistent AF, requires at least 3 weeks of anticoagulation with warfarin and an interval transoesophageal echocardiogram to ensure that there is no intracardiac thrombus.

Chemical cardioversion

Immediate chemical cardioversion should only be attempted if, from the patient's history, the onset of AF clearly occurred <48 h ago and there is a haemodynamic advantage to be gained. Otherwise, elective DC cardioversion can be considered at a later date, once anticoagulation has been established and information on cardiac function is available.

If chemical cardioversion is desired, all patients should be anticoagulated as above. Success is most likely in those with AF of a short duration. If the patient is asymptomatic, with a normal blood pressure, consider rate control (see below), anticoagulation and management of any likely precipitant (see Table 5.4). Pharmacological options for chemical cardioversion include:

- amiodarone: 300 mg IV over 20–30 min, followed by 900 mg infusion over 24 h
- flecainide: 2 mg/kg IV over 10–30 min, maximum dose 150 mg (avoid if patient has ischaemic heart disease or LV dysfunction), then up to 600 mg infusion over 24 h.

Rate control

Rate control is the treatment of choice where cardioversion is not appropriate, e.g. in patients who have been in AF for more than 48 h. In patients with adequate left ventricular systolic function, a β-blocker should be considered first, e.g. atenolol (25–50 mg twice daily). If this fails, consider adding a rate-limiting calcium channel antagonist, e.g. diltiazem (60 mg 8-hourly) or amiodarone; see below. If this fails, or in patients unable to tolerate β-blockers or calcium channel antagonists, due to LV dysfunction or hypotension, use digoxin. The loading dose of digoxin is dependent on the volume of distribution; for a standard 70 kg male, 500 μg is given PO/IV and then again 6–8 h later; lower doses should be considered for smaller patients and the elderly. The maintenance dose needed, e.g. 125 μg PO daily, is dependent on renal function.

If the ECG shows δ waves, Wolff–Parkinson–White syndrome should be considered (see also 'ECGs', p. 85). In this condition, digoxin and verapamil are contraindicated; they may accelerate conduction down the accessory pathway leading to VT or VF. If rate control proves difficult, consider elective DC cardioversion (see above).

Paroxysmal AF

In patients who describe paroxysmal symptoms, and in whom periods of AF with a rapid ventricular response arise suddenly and without warning, useful treatments are sotalol (40–80 mg twice daily) and amiodarone (100 mg PO 8-hourly for 1 week, then 100 mg twice daily for 1 week, followed by a maintenance dose of 100 mg orally once daily). However, amiodarone has a large number of side-effects and the risk of developing them is dose dependent and cumulative.

Other irregular narrow complex tachyarrhythmias

Atrial flutter with variable block

See 'Atrial flutter', below.

Multifocal atrial tachycardia (MAT)

Commonly presents in advanced chronic lung disease. May appear similar to AF on ECG, but P waves are discernible and at least three different P wave morphologies are typical. The differentiation from AF is important, as digoxin will exacerbate MAT and DC cardioversion is ineffective.

The treatment of choice is anticoagulation and rate control, with a calcium channel antagonist or cardioselective β-blocker if no reversible airways disease is present, e.g. bisoprolol. Treatment of any underlying lung disease should be optimized.

Regular narrow complex tachyarrhythmias

Sinus tachycardia

This is a normal physiological response to exercise, emotion, pain and pregnancy and reflects increased sympathetic drive. It accompanies many acute medical problems including sepsis, hypovolaemia, myocardial ischaemia and hypoxia.

Specific treatment is rarely necessary and, in general, is not recommended. Instead, treat the underlying cause. β-blockers can be helpful if the patient is persistently symptomatic or anxious.

Atrial flutter

Where there is doubt about the presence of atrial flutter, CSM or administration of adenosine (see above) can produce transient AV block and reveal underlying atrial flutter waves. Management should be as for AF, but chemical cardioversion is less likely to succeed; elective DC cardioversion may be necessary.

AV nodal re-entrant tachycardia

Due to a re-entrant circuit within the AV node. Usually terminated by adenosine (see above), but, if contraindicated or unsuccessful, alternatives include flecainide (2 mg/kg IV over 10 min, maximum dose 150 mg, do not use if history of IHD) or verapamil (5 mg IV over 2 min, repeated after 5 min to a maximum of 20 mg). If episodes recur, consider referral to an electrophysiologist for catheter ablation.

AV re-entrant tachycardia

Caused by a re-entrant tachycardia conducted by an accessory pathway between atria and ventricles. The two commonest pathways are:

- the bundle of Kent (Wolff–Parkinson–White syndrome; associated with δ waves, see 'ECGs', p. 85; digoxin and verapamil contraindicated)
- the James pathway (Lown–Ganong–Levine syndrome; short PR interval, no δ wave).

Treatment should be immediate DC cardioversion if there is significant haemodynamic compromise; see above. Otherwise, IV flecainide (2 mg/kg IV over 10 min, maximum dose 150 mg, avoid in IHD) or disopyramide (2 mg/kg over 5 min under ECG monitoring, maximum total dose 150 mg) can be effective, in which case either drug bolus is followed by an infusion. Digoxin and verapamil are contraindicated. Adenosine may terminate an AVRT, but facilities should be available for immediate DC cardioversion if the rhythm deteriorates into a broad complex tachyarrhythmia. If recurrent symptoms develop refer to an electrophysiologist for catheter ablation.

Atrial tachycardia

Often due to sinoatrial disease or digoxin toxicity. Rapid ventricular response can be controlled with adenosine or other AV node blocking drugs. β-blockers are the treatment of choice for long-term rate control and catheter ablation should be offered in difficult cases.

Broad complex tachyarrhythmias

These are defined by a QRS duration >0.12 s and are likely to be ventricular in origin. However, an atrial dysrhythmia with pre-existing, or rate-related, aberrant conduction may produce a similar-looking ECG trace. Ventricular arrhythmias are often poorly tolerated, even in patients with a previously normal heart, and their long-term prognosis is less favourable.

Rhythm identification

Determine if the rhythm is regular or irregular. A regular trace is likely to be VT; ECG features that favour VT, rather than an SVT with aberrant conduction, are described in 'ECGs', p. 86. If these are not helpful, and the patient is clinically stable, consider administering a bolus of adenosine. An SVT with aberrant conduction will be terminated by this manoeuvre; atrial fibrillation or flutter will slow to reveal pathognomic atrial activity (see Table 5.4, p. 133); true VT will be unaffected. This assumes an adequate dose of adenosine has been given (suggested by the patient experiencing typical side-effects). If in doubt, treat as VT.

Regular broad complex tachyarrhythmias

VT

May be precipitated by ischaemia, cardiomyopathy, acidosis and electrolyte upset, particularly hypomagnesaemia (commonly associated with diuretics or a history of alcohol excess). VT is common post-MI (up to 40%) and of no prognostic importance immediately post-infarct, but late, persistent VT is a poor prognostic sign.

Check if the patient has a pulse; if not, manage as per ALS guidelines (see 'Cardiac arrest', p. 11). If the patient has a pulse, but is haemodynamically compromised as described above, proceed to emergency DC cardioversion (see 'Defibrillation and cardioversion', p. 58).

If the patient is haemodynamically stable, send urgent bloods for electrolytes and attempt immediate chemical cardioversion. The patient should be transferred to HDU/CCU. Amiodarone is the treatment of choice; 300 mg IV should be given over 20–60 min under ECG monitoring and a maintenance dose of 900 mg infused over 24 h. Intravenous lidocaine is an alternative (100 mg IV over a few minutes; 50 mg in smaller patients), but this should be avoided if the patient has a history of LV dysfunction. Intravenous magnesium (8 mmol bolus given over 5 min) should be given to all patients, followed by 60 mmol in 50 mL dextrose over 24 h, pending laboratory results. If VT is recurrent or persistent, DC cardioversion or overdrive pacing should be considered.

SVT and bundle branch block

The patient may have previous evidence of bundle branch block. Differentiation from VT can be difficult. Look for ECG features, described in 'ECGs', p. 86. Presentation and treatment are as for standard supraventricular narrow complex tachycardia (see p. 136).

Irregular broad complex tachyarrhythmias

AF and bundle branch block

An IV adenosine bolus will transiently slow the rhythm and reveal a chaotic baseline with no P waves. Treatment is as for narrow complex AF (see p. 134).

Ventricular ectopic beats

Ventricular ectopic beats (VEBs) may be seen in normal individuals and only require treatment (usually with β-blockers) if the patient has symptoms of palpitations. In this setting, VEBs may suggest subclinical disease and referral for basic cardiac assessment would be reasonable. Ischaemia, hypoxia, electrolyte imbalance, digoxin toxicity, drugs and stimulants can all cause VEBs and treatment should be directed to the underlying cause.

Persistent and frequent VEBs may occur post-MI or in chronic heart failure, in which case they are associated with a poorer prognosis. Suppression with drugs does not affect this.

Torsades de pointes

Literally translated as 'twisting of the points' (see also 'ECGs', p. 86). Causes include electrolyte disturbances, particularly hypomagnesaemia, congenital long QT syndrome and drugs, e.g. tricyclic antidepressants, disopyramide, macrolide antibiotics. Patients often present with collapse or are mislabelled as having seizures. Usually non-sustained, but may degenerate into VF.

Give IV magnesium sulphate (8 mmol over 5 min, then 60 mmol over 24 h) to all patients. Transvenous overdrive pacing will suppress the arrhythmia by shortening the QT interval. If unavailable, IV isoprenaline (see below) is a useful alternative, but this should be avoided in known long QT syndrome.

Long-term treatment may not be necessary if the precipitant is removed; otherwise β-blockers and an implantable cardiac defibrillator may be necessary.

Bradyarrhythmias

These are defined by a heart rate <60 b.p.m. Sinus bradycardia may be physiological in young athletic individuals, or those on certain drugs, particularly β-blockers and rate-limiting calcium channel antagonists.

Pathological bradycardia is suggested by symptoms, including collapse, palpitation, blackouts, chest pain or breathlessness, and may be caused by sinoatrial node disease or a delay in AV node conduction resulting in 1st, 2nd or 3rd-degree heart block.

Common causes include myocardial infarction or ischaemia, drugs, conduction system fibrosis (Lev and Lenegre syndromes), hypothyroidism, hypothermia, hypokalaemia, granulomatous cardiac disease (e.g. sarcoidosis), myocarditis and connective tissue disease.

Assessment

Where symptoms are present, give oxygen, cannulate a vein and record a 12-lead ECG. Immediate management is dictated by the effect of the arrhythmia on the patient. Therefore, look for the following:

- systolic BP <90 mmHg or a significant drop from previous recordings
- profound bradycardia (pulse <40 b.p.m.)
- ventricular escape arrhythmias
- clinical or radiological evidence of heart failure.

Management

Haemodynamically unstable

If any of the above is present, give a 500 μg IV bolus of atropine and seek senior help. If heart rate and blood pressure do not respond, continue to give atropine 500 μg IV boluses up to a maximum of 3 mg. Where there is no response, transcutaneous pacing should be commenced, irrespective of the underlying rhythm, and urgent transvenous pacing arranged (see p. 54).

Intravenous isoprenaline is another temporary measure that can be used while transvenous pacing is arranged. Start with a 0.2 mg IV bolus, followed by an infusion (1 mg in 100 mL of normal saline, start at 1 mL/min and titrate according to heart rate). Note, this often results in profound anxiety and may not be effective.

Haemodynamically stable

Even if the patient is not haemodynamically compromised, obtain IV access and have atropine ready in case things change. Transfer any symptomatic patient to CCU/HDU.

Examine the 12-lead ECG closely; look at a long rhythm strip if available. Determine the cause of the bradyarrhythmia; this will be either sinus bradycardia or 1st, 2nd or 3rd-degree heart block (see 'Heart Block', p. 87). Send bloods for urgent electrolytes, glucose and thyroid function. Organize a chest X-ray.

All symptomatic patients should be discussed with cardiology regarding the need for an immediate temporary pacing line. The higher the degree of AV block, the greater the risk of progression to asystole. Indications for early placement of a temporary wire include:

- recent asystole
- Mobitz type II 2nd-degree AV block and symptoms
- 3rd-degree (complete) heart block
- ventricular pause >3 s.

BREATHLESSNESS

Breathlessness, or dyspnoea, is a subjective term. It describes the uncomfortable and abnormal ventilatory drive that accompanies many acute medical problems. The physiological mechanism of breathlessness is complex and involves stimulation of stretch receptors in the respiratory muscles, fluid receptors in the juxtacapillary bed and the central chemoreceptors sensing hypoxia and hypercapnia.

Acute severe breathlessness can be terrifying for both the patient and the doctor charged with relieving it. Moreover, the appropriate identification and referral of patients with breathlessness to ITU can be a difficult and intimidating experience. This section provides a structured approach to the clinical assessment of breathlessness and explores the common reasons for acute dyspnoea.

General assessment

Enquire about the speed of onset of dyspnoea, associated symptoms and patterns of breathlessness in response to possible exacerbating factors.

Speed of onset of dyspnoea

Breathlessness due to pulmonary thromboembolism or pneumothorax is often instantaneous, especially in patients with pre-existing respiratory disease. The dyspnoea that accompanies most other conditions, including pneumonia or a lower respiratory tract infection, a developing pleural effusion, or an exacerbation of COPD, is often more subtle, developing gradually over a period of days or weeks.

Patients with chronic lung diseases, e.g. COPD and pulmonary fibrosis, may drift slowly into respiratory failure and the history of increasing dyspnoea may stretch back months or even years. Therefore, review of any available case-notes, ABGs or lung function is essential.

Associated symptoms and signs

Almost any condition in medicine can cause breathlessness. Identifying associated symptoms should allow you to narrow your differential diagnosis; the commoner ones include cough, sputum production ± haemoptysis, wheeze, chest pain and peripheral oedema.

Cough

Cough is extremely common and has numerous causes itself. In general terms, cough suggests endobronchial (e.g. COPD, asthma, bronchial malignancy) or upper airway disease, although parenchymal lung diseases such as pulmonary fibrosis are also associated with cough.

Sputum production

Mucoid (clear) sputum suggests fluid or inflammation. Purulent (green) sputum is more suggestive of infection.

Haemoptysis

The presence of blood in the sputum does not always mean it is coming from the lungs: check for a history of mouth, gum or nasal bleeding. Genuine haemoptysis is commonly associated with bronchial carcinoma, infection (including TB), bronchiectasis or PTE. More rarely it is due to cardiac disease (mitral valve or LVF), aspergilloma, vasculitis or primary bleeding disorders. The choice of investigation is shaped by other findings from the history and examination that suggest a possible cause. However, in general, check for hypoxia and, where indicated, take samples for FBC, LFT, U&E, Coag, ESR and autoantibodies (including ANCA ± anti-GBM). A CXR is required. In any smoker or recent ex-smoker, bronchoscopy ± CT scanning should be considered, even where the CXR is normal. All patients with haemoptysis should be referred for specialist respiratory assessment.

It is important to quantify the amount and frequency of the bleeding. Most patients with haemoptysis describe occasional mild amounts of blood within their sputum and can be investigated as an outpatient. However, massive haemoptysis (defined arbitrarily as >200 mL/day) can be life-threatening. Death is usually by asphyxiation rather than exsanguination. The patient should be transferred to HDU, cross-matched, two large-bore venous cannulae should be inserted and hypoxia treated. Opiate cough suppressants and (in the absence of PTE) tranexamic acid can be considered to suppress bleeding. If large amounts of bleeding occur suddenly, early aspiration and protection of the airway is vital. Investigation by bronchoscopy is usually not helpful until the acute bleeding has subsided. Pulmonary angiography and embolization is also sometimes used.

Wheeze

Wheeze is an expiratory sound that indicates narrowing of the small and medium-sized airways. It should be distinguished from stridor (see 'Stridor', p. 311), which is a harsh sound heard during inspiration and suggests proximal, large airway narrowing.

Wheeze is most frequently associated with COPD or asthma, but can also be heard in patients with pulmonary oedema (cardiac asthma) and bronchiolitis. Wheeze is usually polyphonic, reflecting diffuse disease in airways of varying calibre, resulting in variable pitch. Monophonic wheeze localized to one area of the chest is occasionally seen in patients with narrowing of a single medium-sized airway, usually by tumour.

Chest pain

Typical anginal pain preceding breathlessness suggests pulmonary oedema and should prompt exclusion of acute myocardial infarction (see 'Chest pain', p. 125). Pleuritic chest pain suggests injury or inflammation of the pleura and is most commonly seen in pneumonia, pulmonary embolism and viral infections.

Peripheral oedema

Gravitational oedema, be it pedal or sacral, suggests intravascular volume overload. However, remember that:

- some gravitational oedema is appropriate in normovolaemic patients with low oncotic pressure and is usually due to significant hypoalbuminaemia (<20 g/L)
- patients may have chronic lower limb oedema (suggested by skin thickening and haemosiderosis) unrelated to their acute dyspnoea (e.g. chronic venous insufficiency)
- lower limb oedema in patients with chronic respiratory failure is rarely due to cardiac dysfunction (despite the often used, but inappropriate, term cor pulmonale); oedema in this setting usually reflects secondary hyperaldosteronism and leaky capillaries, due to hypoxia and hypercapnia, not right ventricular failure.

It is essential to assess intravascular volume state carefully by looking at the jugular venous pressure, mucous membranes, skin turgor and fluid balance charts.

Patterns of breathlessness

Breathlessness of any aetiology can be exacerbated by exercise. However, variation in relation to other factors can suggest the likely underlying cause: lying flat (orthopnoea and paroxysmal nocturnal dyspnoea suggest pulmonary oedema); time of day (nocturnal symptoms are common in asthma); exposure to environmental conditions or allergens (change in ambient temperature, air quality, pet dander, etc. can trigger asthma).

ITU referral

Referral to ITU should be considered in critically ill patients who have a realistic chance of recovering and a worthwhile quality of life (QoL) to regain. A patient's QoL should always be reported as they have described it to you, not how you perceive it (see also 'Quality of Life', p. 349).

In all situations, it is essential to liaise with ITU early. This allows time for a thorough ITU assessment, a discussion with the patient and their family, and planning of an ITU bed if appropriate. The anaesthetist will need details of the patient's previous health, their level of activity and dependence on others.

Specific situations

Pneumonia associated with respiratory failure (PaO_2 <8 kPa) despite high flow oxygen should prompt ITU referral.

COPD is now a less common reason for ITU referral following the introduction of non-invasive ventilation (NIV). Patients who should be referred are those with severe hypoxaemia, good lung function and a good level of pre-admission function. Predictors of a poor outcome from invasive ventilation in COPD include multiple organ failure, poor pre-admission function, long-term O_2 therapy, low body mass index, low sodium, low albumin and co-morbid disease. Overall ITU mortality is 20–25% in patients with COPD. Age is not a useful prognostic variable.

Asthma

Asthma is becoming increasingly common in Western societies; current UK prevalence is estimated at 10–15%. Asthma is characterized by eosinophilic airway inflammation and reversible airflow obstruction. Typical symptoms include breathlessness associated with wheeze, and cough which is often worst at night. Trigger factors that precipitate bronchospasm can often be identified in asthmatics, especially those with atopic tendencies.

In the UK, death from acute severe asthma is thankfully rare, nevertheless, a small number of often-young people die tragically every year. Predictors of fatal asthma include repeated attendance at A&E, psychosocial instability, three or more asthma medications and previous near-fatal asthma. The clinical features of severe asthma exacerbations are shown in Table 5.5. Peak flow (PEFR), respiratory rate (RR), heart rate and SpO_2 should be recorded immediately during initial assessment.

Table 5.5 Markers of acute severe and life-threatening asthma

Acute severe asthma	Life-threatening asthma
PEFR 33–50% of best[a]	PEFR <33% of best[a] or unable to comply
RR ≥25/min	SpO_2 <92% or PaO_2 <8 kPa on any FiO_2
HR ≥110/min	Normal $PaCO_2$
Unable to complete sentence in 1 breath	Silent chest, falling respiratory effort, exhaustion, confusion, coma, arrhythmias

[a] Predicted peak flow values can be used when patients are unaware of their best value.

Investigation

- peak flow recording: serial peak flows should be recorded to track clinical course
- arterial blood gases: $PaCO_2$ should be low due to hyperventilation; a normal or high $PaCO_2$ is an ominous sign
- chest X-ray: to exclude a pneumothorax.

Management

Goals of therapy include maintaining tissue oxygenation, reversing bronchospasm, attenuating airway inflammation and treating any precipitating lung injury (e.g. infection, pneumothorax).

Oxygen therapy

High flow oxygen should be delivered, ideally with humidification. Hypercapnia in acute asthma indicates hypoventilation due to exhaustion. CO_2 retention due to reduced hypoxic drive is not a problem in asthma. Therefore, oxygen prescription should be liberal and a normal or raised $PaCO_2$ should prompt treatment intensification and referral to intensive care, not a reduction in inspired oxygen concentration.

Bronchodilators

Nebulized bronchodilators should be administered 1–4-hourly and driven by oxygen. Dosing frequency can be increased as required and can be continuous if necessary. β_2-agonist monotherapy (e.g. salbutamol 2.5–5 mg/dose) can be effective but many clinicians prescribe an anticholinergic agent in combination (e.g. ipratropium 0.5 mg).

In patients with little or no effective ventilation, IV salbutamol (initially 5 μg/min) should be started. Salbutamol causes hypokalaemia, tremor and tachycardia. Monitoring of serum potassium and the heart rhythm are recommended.

Steroids

Asthma is an inflammatory condition and oral steroids should be given as soon as possible (e.g. 40–50 mg prednisolone once off, then once daily). Intravenous steroids (e.g. 100–200 mg hydrocortisone bolus, then 6-hourly) should only be used when the oral route is compromised as they do not work any quicker.

Steroids are usually continued for at least 5 days or until the patient recovers (defined as a return of peak flow to normal for several days). Steroids can then be discontinued, or weaned back to a previous maintenance dose as appropriate. Inhaled steroids should be continued (or started) during an acute exacerbation.

Magnesium sulphate

Intravenous magnesium sulphate (1.2–2 mg) may produce additional bronchodilation in some patients and should be given to those with severe life-threatening asthma. Repeated doses can lead to hypermagnesaemia and respiratory muscle weakness.

Intravenous fluids

Patients with acute severe asthma have high insensible losses due to tachypnoea. Dehydration may exacerbate mucus plugging. Although there is no evidence to support their use, most clinicians prescribe 6–8-hourly IV fluids, until the patient is able to eat and drink comfortably again.

Antibiotics

Most infective exacerbations are caused by viruses. However, if there is clinical suspicion of a precipitating bacterial infection or radiological consolidation, empirical antibiotics can be prescribed pending sputum culture results; see also p. 245.

Monitoring of treatment

PEFR, RR, SaO_2, HR and BP should be recorded every 15 min initially; the frequency of observations can be reduced as the patient improves. Repeated arterial blood gas sampling is only necessary if the initial $PaCO_2$ was normal/high, or if the patient deteriorates. Otherwise maintain SaO_2 above 92% using high flow oxygen.

Indications for invasive ventilation

- deterioration despite maximum medical therapy, e.g. a falling peak flow, PaO_2 <8 kPa and falling, $PaCO_2$ >6 kPa and rising (usually associated with a rising $[H^+]$)
- exhaustion, drowsiness, coma
- respiratory arrest.

Liaise with ITU early. Most units would rather be made aware of a patient they can review than be faced with someone in extremis in the middle of the night.

COPD

Chronic obstructive pulmonary disease (COPD) is defined as an FEV_1 <80% predicted and an FEV_1/FVC ratio of <70%, without significant response to bronchodilators. COPD is caused by cigarette smoking in over 95% of cases and results in 30 000 deaths in the UK annually. Patients with COPD present particular problems to even experienced physicians and a logical approach to their care is essential. This section addresses:

- management of an acute exacerbation
- oxygen prescription in COPD
- non-invasive ventilation in COPD.

Acute exacerbation of COPD

Two or more of the following criteria define an acute exacerbation:

- an increase in sputum volume
- an increase in sputum purulence
- increased breathlessness.

Most exacerbations are caused by infection (viral > bacterial), or a change air temperature or quality. Exacerbations can be disabling in patients with significant COPD, resulting in respiratory failure and decompensated acid–base balance. Admission is mandatory in patients requiring oxygen therapy, intravenous treatment, or in those unable to cope at home.

Investigations

- FBC, U&E, CRP (with a theophylline level if appropriate)
- ECG
- CXR
- ABG, ideally on air: arterial $[H^+]$ is the best predictor of prognosis in an acute exacerbation
- sputum culture (and blood culture if febrile).

Treatment

Nebulized bronchodilators

Salbutamol 2.5–5 mg and ipratropium 0.5 mg 4-hourly: dosing frequency can be increased if necessary.

Steroids

Prednisolone 30–40 mg once daily (or IV hydrocortisone 100–200 mg 6-hourly if the oral route is compromised) has been shown to shorten the course of an exacerbation and should be given for 7–14 days. Steroids should be avoided if there are contraindications (e.g. active GI bleeding).

Antibiotics

These should only be prescribed if there is objective evidence of bacterial infection (purulent sputum, CRP elevated, radiological consolidation). Oral monotherapy is usually adequate (e.g. amoxicillin 500 mg 8-hourly or clarithromycin 500 mg 12-hourly), but should be modified by subsequent sputum culture results. If there is radiological consolidation, antibiotic choice should reflect local guidelines for community acquired pneumonia (CAP).

Oxygen

This is usually, but not always, necessary in patients with an acute exacerbation. Where dyspnoea is significantly increased and/or respiratory failure has developed, arterial blood gases should be checked and controlled oxygen therapy prescribed (see 'ABGs', p. 31, and 'Oxygen delivery', p. 66). ABGs should be monitored in patients with type II respiratory failure (see below).

Intravenous aminophylline

Historically, this has been used in patients with acute exacerbations who do not improve quickly with nebulizers and steroids. However, recent evidence suggests that it has no effect on lung function, symptoms or length of hospital stay. There is no evidence available regarding its effect on mortality. However, it may still be used in patients who are unwell where further therapeutic options are limited.

Aminophylline may precipitate cardiac arrhythmias and patients should have cardiac monitoring. Omit the normal loading dose in patients taking an oral preparation and check a serum level within 24 h of initiation.

Non-invasive ventilation (NIV)

This has an important role in COPD patients with decompensated type II respiratory failure and is discussed below.

Mucolytics

These reduce the viscosity of secretions and aid expectoration. There is some evidence that they can shorten the course of an exacerbation in patients treated with antibiotics; however, they are not prescribed routinely. Saline nebulizers are a useful alternative.

Oxygen prescription in COPD

In patients with chronic type II respiratory failure, permanent hypercapnia due to chronic alveolar hypoventilation alters the sensitivity of the chemoreceptor network responsible for ventilatory control. Hypoxia, not hypercapnia, becomes the main ventilatory stimulus and overzealous oxygen prescription can lead to loss of this 'hypoxic drive', worsening hypercapnia and a dangerous respiratory acidosis.

In COPD, you should not aim for a normal PaO_2 but a PaO_2 that is normal for the patient (see 'Oxygen delivery', p. 67). This can be estimated from previous ABGs; in many patients a PaO_2 of 6–8 kPa is adequate. If you cannot maintain an adequate PaO_2 without precipitating hypercapnia and a respiratory acidosis, ventilatory support should be considered to allow delivery of sufficient oxygen.

Non-invasive ventilation in COPD

Non-invasive ventilation (in the form of bi-level pressure support) has been shown to reduce mortality, the need for invasive ventilation, length of hospital stay and the cost of an admission with an acute exacerbation. NIV is indicated in patients with an exacerbation in whom a decompensated respiratory acidosis (H^+ >45 nmol/L, $PaCO_2$ >6 kPa) persists despite a period of controlled oxygen therapy and optimal medical management. Note that respiratory failure (PaO_2 <8 kPa) is not necessary for patients to meet NIV criteria, but if adequate oxygenation can only be achieved at the expense of a rising $PaCO_2$ and an uncontrollable respiratory acidosis, NIV is indicated.

The decision to start NIV

Discuss with a senior colleague first, then with the patient and their family. A contingency plan should be made at the outset regarding what to do if NIV fails and this should be documented in the notes. Is NIV to be the ceiling of treatment or would the patient be an appropriate candidate for ITU referral? Contraindications to NIV are listed below, but those marked (*) can be considered relative if NIV is the only treatment option.

- cardiac or respiratory arrest*
- severe facial trauma or burns*
- fixed upper airway obstruction
- inability to protect the airway*
- undrained pneumothorax*
- life-threatening hypoxaemia
- copious sputum production/secretions
- haemodynamic instability, confusion or reduced conscious level
- vomiting, recent upper GI surgery, bowel obstruction.

In practice, NIV is often prescribed by medical staff, but initiated and adjusted by nurses or physiotherapists. Most UK hospitals will have a non-invasive ventilation (NIV) protocol which you should read. The British Thoracic Society publish detailed guidelines on NIV on their website.

The ventilator

There are numerous machines available. Most modern systems deliver continuous bi-level pressure support which cycles between a peak inspiratory positive airway pressure (IPAP) and a lower expiratory positive airway pressure (EPAP). Pressure support is preferred as volume support can result in excessive airway pressures and an increased risk of pneumothorax. IPAP augments the tidal volume of each breath and off-loads the respiratory muscles. Expiratory positive airway pressure (EPAP) and positive end expiratory pressure (PEEP) reduce expiratory small airway collapse.

Each ventilatory cycle is triggered by the patient's own ventilation. The sensitivity of the triggers can be altered, but should usually be set at maximum. Most ventilators have a back-up rate that will initiate ventilation if the patient's respiratory rate falls. Typical ventilator settings in a spontaneous/timed mode are shown in Table 5.6.

The mask

Choosing a mask that fits the patient is essential. Full-face masks that cover both the nose and mouth are preferable. Try a few sizes on the patient, before you start the machine. If the mask is too big there will be a significant air leak; too small and it will be uncomfortable for the patient. Hold the mask over the patient's mouth before you start and reassure the patient constantly; an NIV mask can be claustrophobic in patients already struggling for breath.

Monitoring

RR, HR, SaO_2, and BP should be monitored. In addition, look for patient–ventilator synchrony, mask leaks and patient comfort. Check ABGs at 0, 1 and 4 h.

Table 5.6 Typical NIV settings in a spontaneous/timed mode

Variable	Initial setting	Optimization
EPAP	4 cmH_2O	May need to increase to 8–12 cmH_2O if obese/sleep apnoea overlap
IPAP	12 cmH_2O	Increase to a max. of 20 cmH_2O (2 cm increments) as tolerated by the patient
Back-up rate	15 breaths/min	May need to be reduced as patient improves
Trigger sensitivities	Maximum	None usually required
FiO_2	Be guided by O_2 requirements pre-NIV	Titrate O_2 flow rate to maintain SaO_2 between 85% and 90%

Improvements in RR and $[H^+]$ at 1 and 4h are associated with a better outcome. Consider withdrawing NIV, if no improvement is seen in RR, $PaCO_2$ or $[H^+]$ at 4h.

In patients who do improve, the optimum duration of NIV is unclear. If stability can be achieved this allows time for medical therapies to work and NIV can be weaned over a few days with breaks for nebulizers, meals and visitors.

Troubleshooting NIV

- If $[H^+]$ or $PaCO_2$ do not fall, check for patient–ventilator asynchrony or a mask leak; consider reducing the FiO_2 (SaO_2/PaO_2 inappropriately high), or increasing IPAP (as ventilation is insufficient).
- If there is a significant clinical deterioration, or the PaO_2 falls, ensure the patient is receiving optimal medical therapy and look for evidence of complications, e.g. pneumothorax, retained secretions/mucus plugging, aspiration; consider increasing the FiO_2 or increasing EPAP (as a means of further recruiting unventilated lung units); consider whether the patient is a candidate for invasive ventilation.
- If the systemic BP drops significantly, reducing IPAP can help.
- If the patient complains of dry, painful eyes, check for leaks from the top of the mask, tighten the mask or plug leaks with a swab.
- If pain or ulceration over the bridge of the nose is a problem, loosen the mask.
- If nasal congestion develops, use decongestant medication, e.g. pseudoephedrine 60mg 8-hourly, but continue with NIV.

Pulmonary oedema

Acute pulmonary oedema may be cardiogenic or non-cardiogenic in origin.

Cardiogenic pulmonary oedema

This develops when left ventricular end-diastolic pressure (LVEDP) rises, causing the hydrostatic pressure within the pulmonary veins and capillaries to exceed the oncotic pressure of the plasma. In a patient with a normal oncotic pressure (suggested by a normal serum albumin), pulmonary oedema develops at a pulmonary capillary wedge pressure (PCWP) above 18 mmHg, usually because of an insult that reduces the mechanical efficiency of the heart muscle (e.g. acute myocardial infarction).

Patients with acute cardiogenic pulmonary oedema present with severe, often frightening, breathlessness. The patient will be sweating, sitting forward and be clammy to the touch. Their peripheries will feel cool, reflecting reduced cardiac output and peripheral vasoconstriction due to excessive sympathetic drive. The jugular venous pressure is often elevated and crackles are usually audible at the lung bases (and may extend to the apices). Wheeze (cardiac asthma) is not uncommon.

Important points to note from the history and examination include:

- preceding chest pain: think MI, ACS and consider aortic dissection
- preceding palpitations: suggests arrhythmia, so look at an ECG and monitor rhythm
- heart rate: the heart rate (HR) should be high due to excessive sympathetic drive; an inappropriate HR may hint at a cause, e.g. a HR >150 or <60 should prompt careful examination of the ECG for evidence of a tachy- or brady-arrhythmia
- blood pressure: blood pressure (BP) is usually high in acute pulmonary oedema, for the same reason as HR; a low BP suggests cardiogenic shock, but might also be the patient's normal BP (this is more likely in patients with acute-on-chronic heart failure); look for old BP charts in the patient's notes.

Investigations

- FBC, U&E, LFT, CRP, Glu, TFT, obtain IV access at the same time
- ECG

- CXR
- arterial blood gas if SaO_2 is <92%, ideally on air
- troponin: check at 12h in patients with associated chest pain; if pain-free, timing is less well defined but should probably also be at 12h.

Treatment

Sit the patient up and administer high flow oxygen (if possible, check ABGs first: controlled oxygen therapy may be necessary in patients with COPD). Address any precipitants, e.g. myocardial ischaemia, arrhythmias.

Intravenous loop diuretic

Give a 50–120mg bolus of IV furosemide (1–2mg IV bumetanide). Patients with chronic renal impairment will need higher doses. Give a second bolus if diuresis is insufficient after an hour, and if diuresis remains poor consider:

- whether the diagnosis is correct
- whether the kidneys are being perfused (requires a mean arterial blood pressure ≥ 65mmHg, if less than this, consider inotropic support; see also p. 251)
- starting a continuous infusion of a diuretic (e.g. furosemide 10–20mg/h).

Intravenous opiate

Opiates act as analgesics, venodilators and anxiolytics, e.g. morphine (2.5–5mg) or diamorphine (1.25–2.5mg). They also reduce sympathetically driven vasoconstriction. However, consider the potential for respiratory depression and hypotension.

Nitrates

Nitrates produce venodilatation, reduce preload and lower LVEDP; however their use is limited by their tendency to cause or worsen hypotension. An infusion of IV nitrates should be considered in all patients with pulmonary oedema, assuming a systolic BP of ≥110 mmHg. Examples include GTN (Nitrocine®) or isosorbide dinitrate (Isoket®).

Inotropes

Should be considered in patients with cardiogenic shock (cardiogenic pulmonary oedema and a systolic BP <90mmHg). Dobutamine (2.5–10µg/kg per min) is the most suitable as it stimulates β_1 and β_2 adrenoreceptors resulting in an increase in myocardial contractility, cardiac output and BP, and a fall in systemic vascular resistance. However, it also increases myocardial oxygen demand and heart rate at higher doses.

Ventilatory support

Continuous positive airway pressure (CPAP) can help in cardiogenic pulmonary oedema with respiratory failure. Typically, it should be set at 5–10cm H_2O and the inspired oxygen concentration titrated to maintain SaO_2 >90%.

Non-cardiogenic pulmonary oedema

Also known as acute respiratory distress syndrome (ARDS), non-cardiogenic pulmonary oedema develops as a result of plasma leak from a damaged and over-permeable pulmonary capillary bed despite normal hydrostatic pressure in the pulmonary venous circulation. Patients usually present with progressive breathlessness and a risk factor for ARDS.

Causes

- *direct*: pneumonia, aspiration of gastric contents, inhalation of toxins, near drowning
- *indirect*: septicaemia, severe acidosis, pancreatitis, burns, transfusion reaction and drugs including streptokinase, IV β-blockers and aspirin (in overdose).

Diagnostic criteria

There are various definitions in use, most include:

- bilateral diffuse lung infiltrates on CXR
- hypoxaemia (most simply defined as a PaO_2 <8 kPa despite high flow oxygen)
- normal pulmonary capillary wedge pressure (<15 mmHg)
- reduced lung compliance (measured while ventilated).

Investigations

In practical terms, ARDS is a diagnosis of exclusion. The principal diagnoses to exclude are cardiogenic pulmonary oedema, a diffuse infective pneumonia (bacterial, viral or fungal) and diffuse alveolar haemorrhage. The following investigations should be considered in all patients:

- FBC, Coag, U&E, LFT, CRP, glucose, amylase
- blood cultures (and appropriate site-specific cultures)
- ECG and CXR
- ABGs should be updated regularly (consider an arterial line; see 'Arterial lines', p. 32): titrate FiO_2 to maintain a PaO_2 >8 kPa; consider ventilation if this cannot be achieved
- echocardiography should be performed to document LV function
- pulmonary artery catheterization may be used to confirm the diagnosis and distinguish between cardiogenic and non-cardiogenic oedema
- fibreoptic bronchoscopy and broncho-alveolar lavage should be considered in patients in whom infection is suspected, but has not yet been adequately excluded (e.g. those not expectorating).

Treatment

Patients with suspected ARDS should be managed in a medical HDU or ITU. Treatment is largely supportive; the underlying cause should be identified and treated, although in practice this may not possible. Intravenous antibiotics are often given empirically and there is conflicting evidence on the efficacy of steroid therapy.

Prognosis

The prognosis of ARDS has improved over recent years and survival is now >50%. This probably reflects better supportive care rather than any advance that modifies the disease process. ARDS with a primary pulmonary cause has the worst prognosis.

Pneumothorax

A pneumothorax (PTX) results from a spontaneous or traumatic tear in the visceral and/or parietal pleura. The resulting alveolo- or broncho-pleural fistula allows air to enter the pleural space, compromising lung function. Spontaneous pneumothorax is more common than traumatic pneumothorax and can be classified as primary (in patients with previously normal lungs) or secondary (in patients with underlying lung disease).

Classification

Tension pneumothorax

This is an uncommon but dangerous situation in which the offending pleural tear acts as one-way flap valve. Mediastinal structures, including the heart are displaced away from the PTX and cardiac output may be compromised, leading to death. If a tension PTX is suspected (tracheal deviation and displacement of the apex beat away from the affected side ± hypotension) the lung must be decompressed immediately by inserting a large IV cannula into the pleural space and aspirating air until the patient improves. Do not wait for an X-ray. An intercostal drain should then be inserted with the cannula still in place.

Spontaneous pneumothorax

Primary spontaneous pneumothorax (PSP)

Most common in young, tall men (male to female ratio is 5:1). Smoking increases the risk of PSP (by over 20 times in men) and a significant proportion of patients with PSP have subpleural apical blebs at thoracoscopy. These blebs are thought to rupture and create the necessary alveolo-pleural fistula. Sudden-onset ipsilateral chest pain may be the only symptom in PSP.

Secondary spontaneous pneumothorax (SSP)

More dangerous than PSP and carries a significant mortality risk (10%). Even a small PTX in a patient with severe pre-existing lung disease can cause severe dyspnoea and require urgent treatment.

Traumatic pneumothorax

This may result from any blunt or penetrating injury to the chest. Only 50% will be visible on plain X-ray and CT scanning should be considered if there is clinical suspicion. Associated chest wall and visceral injuries are common.

Clinical features

Symptoms include sudden ipsilateral pleuritic chest pain, a variable degree of breathlessness ± a dry cough. Clinical signs are often subtle, but may include a hyper-resonant percussion note, diminished chest expansion and reduced breath sounds on the affected side.

Investigation

Obtain IV access and send blood for FBC, Coag, U&E and CRP. Perform an ECG and order a CXR. If there is evidence of a tension PTX, treatment must not be delayed and you should not wait for the chest X-ray to be performed.

The British Thoracic Society (BTS) has simplified the classification of spontaneous PTX based on the appearance of the CXR, into small (<2 cm visible rim of air) or large (>2 cm visible rim of air). Small pneumothoraces may not be visible on a plain chest film and further imaging may be necessary.

A lateral decubitus chest film may improve diagnostic sensitivity, but a CT scan of thorax may be required. Expiratory CXRs do not increase diagnostic sensitivity.

Management

Oxygen therapy

All patients with a PTX should receive high flow oxygen (10 L/min) as this increases the rate of air re-absorption across the pleura. Patients with underlying COPD should have arterial blood gases checked first and may need controlled oxygen therapy.

Drainage

Follow the BTS guidelines, these are available on their website; key points include:

- if there is evidence of tension PTX, take immediate action (see above)
- consider conservative management of PSP if the patient is asymptomatic and otherwise fit
- aspiration should always be attempted before intercostal drain insertion in PSP
- patients who have had a successful aspiration can usually be discharged with early clinic review but should be considered for further observation overnight if they live alone, or the original pneumothorax was large
- a SSP should only be aspirated if is small, causing minimal symptoms and the patient is young (<50 years old); otherwise an intercostal drain should be inserted

- if the patient has had a PTX before, or their lifestyle or employment puts them at significant risk of developing a second one in the future (airline pilots, frequent flyers, divers), they should be referred to a chest physician regarding possible pleurodesis.

Persistent air leaks

Bubbling in the chest tube bottle during expiration or coughing indicates that the pleural tear responsible for the pneumothorax is patent and a connection exists between the tip of the drain and the interior of the lung. When this continues for >48 h after insertion of the drain it is known as a persistent air leak. If a drain is removed at this point the lung will deflate. In this situation consider suction, but thoracoscopy and definitive pleural repair may be necessary.

Traumatic PTX

Where a PTX results from trauma, other chest injuries are common and the patient should be managed with an intercostal drain and referred to a thoracic surgeon.

Pleural effusion

Normally, the pleura produce approximately 150 mL of lubricating fluid each day. Pleural effusions develop when the balance between pleural fluid secretion and resorption is disrupted. Depending on the underlying disease process, pleural fluid collections may contain serous or haemoserous fluid, pus (empyema), blood (haemothorax) or chyle (chylothorax).

Symptoms

Breathlessness is most common if the effusion is large or the rate of accumulation has been rapid. Small effusions may cause breathlessness in patients with pre-existing lung disease. Dull chest ache and pleurisy may also be reported.

Signs

Classical signs include reduced chest expansion, a stony dull percussion note, reduced air entry and diminished vocal resonance.

Investigation

The aim is to confirm the presence of pleural fluid and identify a likely aetiology.

CXR

Should be performed in all patients. Typical radiological features include homogenous opacification with a lateral meniscus. A completely straight superior border suggests a hydro-pneumothorax rather than a simple effusion. In massive effusions there may be a complete 'white out' and the mediastinum will be pushed away from the affected side; if it is not this suggests underlying lung collapse. Look for evidence of underlying disease that might explain the effusion:

- LV dysfunction: cardiomegaly, upper lobe venous diversion, bilateral effusions
- infection: evidence of pneumonia, e.g. lobar consolidation, cavitation or pleural empyema (suggested by a localized or lobulated pleural collection in a non-gravity dependent area such as the lateral chest wall)
- malignancy: intrapulmonary mass lesion, pleural-based mass, lymphangitis
- trauma: adjacent rib fractures.

Thoracocentesis

A 'pleural tap' should be performed in all patients with an unexplained pleural effusion (see 'Pleural aspiration', p. 38). The key information to be gained is the differentiation of transudative and exudative effusions (Table 5.7) and the exclusion of pleural infection. Samples should be sent for the following:

- biochemistry: protein, LDH, glucose, $[H^+]$ in non-turbid samples

Table 5.7 Causes of transudative and exudative pleural effusions

Transudates	Exudates
Reflect increased hydrostatic pressure or reduced oncotic pressure in the pulmonary venous circulation	Reflect localized lung or pleural disease leading to increased capillary permeability and reduced pleural resorption
Common	
Left ventricular failure Cirrhotic liver disease Nephrotic syndrome	Parapneumonic ± empyema Malignancy, including mesothelioma PTE Rheumatoid
Less common	
Constrictive pericarditis Meigs' syndrome (ovarian tumour) PTE (10–20% are transudates) Malignancy (5% are transudates)	TB Pancreatitis Other autoimmune diseases, e.g. SLE Post-cardiac injury (Dressler's syndrome) or surgery

- cytology: for examination for malignant cells and differential cell count
- microbiology: for Gram- and auramine-stain and culture (including AAFB).

See 'Pleural fluid', p. 76, for guidance on the interpretation of pleural fluid appearances and tests.

Thoracic ultrasound

If the effusion is difficult to detect clinically, ultrasound should be used to guide diagnostic thoracocentesis. Ultrasound can also be used to identify pleural-based mass lesions, pleural thickening and loculations within collections.

CT thorax

This should be performed in unexplained exudates after the majority of the pleural fluid has been drained. It is useful in distinguishing benign from malignant pleural disease and may reveal an intrapulmonary mass or other likely cause. Intravenous contrast improves depiction of the pleura surfaces.

Pleural biopsy

In unexplained exudative pleural effusions, further investigation to exclude malignancy and TB should be considered. Closed, or Abrams', pleural biopsy can be performed on the ward without referral to radiology or surgery. However, diagnostic sensitivity for malignancy is only 47% in the best published series compared with 87% for CT-guided cutting needle biopsy. Therefore, if malignancy is suspected, the latter is preferable if the patient is otherwise fit. Other alternatives include video-assisted thorascopic surgical (VATS) biopsy or medical thoracoscopy. Diagnostic yield from Abrams' biopsy is higher in suspected pleural TB, in which setting it may still be worthwhile.

Tuberculin testing

This should be performed in cases of unexplained lymphocytic effusion, particularly if there are other features of TB infection. The result must be interpreted in the context of previous BCG vaccination and current immune function. T-spot testing may change this practice.

Bronchoscopy

This should not be performed routinely unless the patient has new endobronchial symptoms or a parenchymal lung mass on imaging.

Management

The overriding principle in treating all pleural effusions, whether transudative or exudative, is 'treat the underlying cause'. Nevertheless, the immediate priority in patients who are breathless is to relieve symptoms. This can often be achieved by aspiration of up to 1 L of pleural fluid. If there are typical clinical and radiological features of heart failure, this should be treated first, as 75% of effusions in this situation will resolve within 72h. If symptoms persist, repeated pleural aspiration can be performed. However, specific indications for intercostal drainage include:

- massive symptomatic effusion: when aspiration of sufficient pleural fluid to provide sustained relief is felt impractical; be aware that rapid drainage of large volumes of pleural fluid can result in re-expansion pulmonary oedema or circulatory collapse (limit initial drainage to 1 L)
- malignant pleural effusion: where chemical pleurodesis is considered, the lung must be fully re-inflated and pleural fluid drainage <150 mL/24 h for this to be effective
- empyema: as indicated by frank pus on pleural aspiration or pathogenic organisms on Gram-stain or culture; pleural fluid with a pH of <7.2 is likely to progress to an empyema and should be drained.

Pulmonary thromboembolism

A pulmonary thromboembolism (PTE) is a sudden vascular occlusion within the pulmonary circulation. Over 75% of PTEs result from the transit of thrombotic material from the deep venous system in the legs, through the right heart, into the pulmonary vascular bed.

Classification

- massive PTE is associated with RV dilatation/dysfunction on echocardiography and a systemic arterial blood pressure <90 mmHg
- sub-massive PTE is associated with RV dilatation/dysfunction on echocardiography or biomarkers, but a normal systemic arterial blood pressure (≥90 mmHg)
- non-massive PTE is not associated with haemodynamic compromise.

Risk factors

Major risk factors

These increase the relative risk by a factor of 5–20:

- surgery: major abdominal or pelvic surgery, orthopaedic surgery (especially lower limb)
- obstetric: late pregnancy, recent caesarean section, pre-eclampsia
- malignancy: abdominal, pelvic or metastatic
- lower limb: fracture or varicose veins
- reduced mobility: hospitalization or institutional care
- previous proven PTE.

Minor risk factors

The following increase relative risk by a factor of 2–4:

- cardiovascular co-morbidity: congenital heart disease, heart failure, hypertension, central venous line in situ
- oestrogens: oral contraceptive pill, HRT
- miscellaneous: occult malignancy (present in approx. 10% patients with PTE/DVT), obesity, neurological disability, inflammatory bowel disease, dialysis and others.

Presentation

Massive PTE may present as syncope, collapse or cardiac arrest. More common symptoms include dyspnoea, which is often sudden in onset, chest pain and haemoptysis. Chest pain in large PTEs may be central, but is more typically pleuritic.

Physical signs are often absent in non-massive PTE. Common findings include tachycardia and tachypnoea. Central cyanosis indicates hypoxia and suggests a large PTE. Other concerning features are elevation of the jugular venous pressure, a parasternal heave and a split 2nd heart sound with a loud P_2, which suggest right heart strain. A low-grade fever (<38°C) is common. Also, look for signs of an associated deep venous thrombosis (DVT) and other risk factors.

Investigations

Diagnosis is difficult because the presentation of PTE is often non-specific. Accurate diagnosis, without resorting to extensive investigation of every patient with unexplained breathlessness, requires an understanding of the strengths and weaknesses of the diagnostic tests available and the importance of pre-test probability scoring.

Pre-test probability

The BTS suggests a simple pre-test scoring system based on the Wells and Geneva scoring systems. Consider first if the patient has clinical features compatible with a diagnosis of acute PTE, e.g. tachypnoea, pleuritic chest pain or haemoptysis.

If a diagnosis of PTE appears plausible look for: (1) a major risk factor (see above) and (2) the absence of any other reasonable explanation, e.g. pneumonia. A clinical probability score can then be assigned:

- high when both (1) and (2) are present
- intermediate when either (1) or (2) is present
- low when neither (1) or (2) is present.

ECG

May be normal, but sinus tachycardia is common. Signs of right heart strain (right axis deviation, anterior T-wave inversion, and right bundle branch block) may be present. The classic S1 Q3 T3 pattern is fairly uncommon.

CXR

May be normal or show an elevated hemidiaphragm, linear atelectasis, pleural effusion, wedge-shaped pulmonary infarction or localized pulmonary oligaemia (Westermark's sign).

ABG

May be normal, but commonly demonstrates hyperventilation (low pCO_2, low H^+). Hypoxaemia indicates a large PTE and may not respond well to increasing FiO_2 due to V/Q mismatch.

D-dimer

D-dimers are fibrin degradation products and are sensitive, but not specific, markers of acute venous thromboembolism (sensitivity 87–99%, but specificity only 60–70%). Any condition that results in fibrinolysis (including malignancy, infection, pregnancy, inflammatory disease) will lead to an elevated D-dimer and a false positive result. A positive D-dimer should never be the sole indication for a CT pulmonary angiogram (CTPA).

The performance of each D-dimer assay is different; therefore you need to know which test your hospital uses before interpreting the results. For example, no further imaging is necessary in patients who have a low or intermediate clinical probability and a negative ELISA D-dimer.

D-dimer testing does not improve diagnostic accuracy in patients with a high pre-test clinical probability. Therefore, in such a setting, a D-dimer should not be requested and appropriate imaging should be ordered instead. D-dimers should only influence clinical decision-making if they are negative and undertaken in the context of low or intermediate pre-test probability scoring, depending on the assay used.

Biomarkers

Troponin and NT-proBNP may be elevated due to acute right heart strain. Both markers are of proven prognostic value in acute PTE and may form part of future treatment algorithms.

Echocardiography

Echocardiography can be diagnostic of massive PTE and may show a proximal clot in the main pulmonary artery. However, the sensitivity of echocardiography is low and this limits its usefulness in the acute setting.

V/Q scanning

Ventilation and perfusion should be well matched throughout healthy lungs. A focal perfusion defect in an area of normally ventilated lung suggests a PTE; this will be reported as a high probability scan. V/Q scanning is difficult to interpret in chronic lung disease, which is often associated with a degree of V/Q mismatch. The test is most reliable in patients with previously normal lungs and a normal CXR. In this setting a normal V/Q scan reliably excludes a PTE and a low probability scan in a patient with low pre-test clinical probability scoring makes the odds of PTE very low. In patients with other pre-test scores, low and intermediate scans are essentially non-diagnostic and further investigation should be considered. A high probability scan is highly suggestive of PTE, but false positives can occur, especially where the pre-test probability is not high.

CTPA

CTPA is the current gold standard investigation. It has the advantage that alternative diagnoses can also be detected; however CTPA cannot completely exclude PTE as small subsegmental clots may be missed and the test is highly operator dependent. Therefore, in a patient with a high clinical probability and a negative CTPA, further imaging should be considered, e.g. leg ultrasound, invasive pulmonary angiography.

Management

Massive PTE

In massive PTE, there is acute haemodynamic disturbance due to RV outflow tract/pulmonary circulation obstruction. These patients are at risk of rapid death unless patency of the pulmonary circulation can be restored quickly. Give oxygen and, if not contraindicated, thrombolysis should be considered. Alteplase (10 mg IV over 2 min, then up to 90 mg over 2 h) is preferable to streptokinase as the latter can exacerbate hypotension. An IV infusion of unfractionated heparin should be started after thrombolysis.

Non-massive PTE

- oxygen if hypoxic
- low molecular weight heparin (LMWH) should be adjusted to weight and given to all intermediate and high-risk patients pending investigation (assuming there is no contraindication); LMWH should be continued until the patient is established on oral anticoagulation (see also 'Initiating warfarin', p. 111); it can be continued for the full period of treatment if oral anticoagulation is contraindicated
- oral anticoagulation with warfarin (target INR range of 2–3); 3 months' treatment is adequate for patients with a transient risk factor (e.g. postoperative or related to a fracture); indefinite treatment should be considered if a risk factor cannot be identified, or the risk of PTE is persistent, e.g. malignancy
- recurrent PTE should be treated with life-long anticoagulation.

Pneumonia

Pneumonia is defined as an acute respiratory illness associated with radiological evidence of consolidation.

Causes and classification

Pneumonia is most commonly due to bacterial infection, but may result from viral or fungal infections or non-infectious inflammatory stimuli. These include eosinophilic pneumonia and the acute 'idiopathic interstitial pneumonias', e.g. cryptogenic organizing pneumonia and acute interstitial pneumonia (see 'Pneumonitis and fibrosis', p. 158).

Infectious pneumonia is commonly classified based on the clinical circumstances in which the illness develops. This is highly suggestive of the likely causative organism and the empirical antibiotic treatment chosen should reflect this. The remainder of this section will focus on the infectious pneumonias.

Community acquired pneumonia

Community acquired bacterial pneumonia (CAP) is the commonest infectious cause of death. 40% of patients will require admission to hospital, 5–10% of these will require admission to ICU and 50% of those admitted to ICU will not survive. CAP is most commonly caused by *Streptococcus pneumoniae (Pneumococcus).* However, *Mycoplasma pneumoniae* and *Chlamydia pneumoniae* are more common in young patients. *Haemophilus influenzae* is common in older patients and those with chronic lung disease. A preceding viral infection predisposes to infection with *Staphylococcus aureus* and recent travel should prompt consideration of *Legionella pneumophila* infection.

The term 'atypical pneumonia' is often used to describe CAP due to *Mycoplasma, Legionella* or *Chlamydia.* These infections are more commonly associated with a preceding prodromal illness, extra-pulmonary manifestations and a discrepancy between the extent of clinical findings and radiological abnormalities. However, these clinical features are not reliable and the term has recently fallen out of favour.

Hospital acquired pneumonia

This is a pneumonia occurring 48 h or more after hospital admission. Gram-negative organisms, anaerobes or MRSA are the usual infective agents.

Aspiration pneumonia

Occurs following aspiration of material from the oropharynx or stomach due to vomiting, reflux, impaired swallowing or a depressed conscious level, e.g. alcoholism, general anaesthesia. Infection with anaerobes and/or Gram-negative organisms is typical.

Pneumonia in the immunocompromised

Most infections are caused by the same organisms that cause CAP in immunocompetent patients. However, infection with Gram-negative pathogens, e.g. *Pseudomonas aeruginosa*, or with low virulence 'opportunistic' organisms, e.g. *Pneumocystis carinii* (PCP; now called *P. jirovecii)* or environmental mycobacteria, may occur. Infection with multiple organisms is more common than in the immunocompetent.

Presentation

Pulmonary symptoms include cough and sputum production (rust-coloured sputum suggests pneumococcal infection), breathlessness and pleuritic chest pain. Haemoptysis can occur. Systemic symptoms may include anorexia, fever, rigors, upper abdominal pain (particularly if associated with hepatitis) and vomiting.

Typical clinical signs of lobar consolidation may be present (dull percussion note, reduced air entry, crackles and bronchial breathing), particularly with pneumococcal infection; there may also be a pleural rub. Look specifically for evidence of respiratory failure and shock.

Investigation

- FBC (including differential cell count), U&E, LFT, CRP, Glu±Coag should be checked in all patients
- ABGs should be checked if SaO_2 <92%, or there is evidence of shock

- CXR is necessary for the diagnosis (multilobe involvement, cavities or pneumothorax suggests *S. aureus* infection); may also identify complications, e.g. pleural effusion (parapneumonic or empyema), lung abscess
- ECG
- sputum (Gram-stain and auramine and/or Ziehl–Neelsen stain for AAFB) and blood cultures should be sent in all patients
- consider serological tests for specific organisms: acute and convalescent serum samples can be sent for *Mycoplasma, Legionella, Chlamydia* and viral titres (previously known as an atypical pneumonia screen); *Pneumococcus* and *Legionella* antigens can also be checked in urine
- other useful tests include sampling of pleural fluid, throat and nasopharyngeal swabs (especially in children) and cold agglutinins (positive in 50% of patients with *Mycoplasma* infection)
- in severe CAP, consider bronchoscopy and bronchoalveolar lavage, particularly if the patient is not expectorating or is immunosuppressed
- CT scanning is of no additional benefit in uncomplicated CAP, but may be useful in patients with empyema or suspected lung abscess
- non-infective causes of pneumonia should be considered in patients who do not respond to standard antibacterial therapy or in whom there are atypical features from the outset: consider CT scanning, bronchoscopy and transbronchial lung biopsy to exclude cryptogenic organizing pneumonia, PCP and eosinophilic lung disease.

Assessment of severity

CAP should be defined as severe or non-severe; this influences antibiotic choice. Severe CAP is characterized by the presence of two or more of the following adverse prognostic factors:

- respiratory rate ≥30/min
- age ≥65 years
- co-existing disease, e.g. diabetes, COPD, cardiac disease
- new or worsened confusion (defined as an AMT ≤8/10; see 'Scores in the acutely ill', p. 4)
- urea ≥7 mmol/L
- blood pressure ≤90 (systolic) or ≤60 (diastolic) mmHg
- hypoxaemia
- albumin ≤35 g/L
- WCC >20 or <4 × 10^9/L
- bilateral or multilobar radiological change
- positive blood culture, regardless of the organism.

These have been refined into the 'CURB-65 score', which accurately predicts mortality from CAP. One point is given for each of five core severity criteria (confusion, urea, respiratory rate, blood pressure and age). Mortality rate correlates linearly with the resulting score: 0 = 2.4%, 1 = 8%, 2 = 23%, 3 = 33%, 4 or more = 83%. Young patients (<50 years old) with a score of 0–1 and no other medical problems have a particularly low mortality rate and can be managed as an outpatient with oral antibiotics. ICU admission should be considered in patients with a CURB-65 score >4.

Management

Antibiotics

Cultures should be collected first, but this should not delay antibiotic administration. Empirical antibiotics should be given as soon as the clinical diagnosis is made. The choice of antibiotic should reflect the clinical setting and severity. Standard antibiotic treatment for CAP is summarized in Table 5.8.

Table 5.8 Antibiotic treatment of community acquired pneumonia

	Preferred treatment	Alternative (if allergic or intolerant)
Community treatment		
Non-severe CAP	Amoxicillin 500 mg–1 g 8-hourly	Clarithromycin 500 mg 12-hourly *or* erythromycin 500 mg 6-hourly
Hospital treatment		
Non-severe CAP	Oral treatment: Amoxicillin 500 mg–1 g 8-hourly ± clarithromycin 500 mg 12-hourly *or* erythromycin 500 mg 6-hourly IV treatment: Amoxicillin 500 mg 6-hourly *or* benzylpenicillin 1.2 g 6-hourly *plus* clarithromycin 500 mg 12-hourly *or* erythromycin 500 mg 6-hourly	Oral treatment: Clarithromycin 500 mg 12-hourly *or* erythromycin 500 mg 6-hourly *or* levofloxacin 500 mg daily IV treatment: Levofloxacin 500 mg daily IV
Severe CAP	Co-amoxiclav 1.2 g 8-hourly IV *or* ceftriaxone 1–2 g daily IV *or* cefuroxime 1.5 g 8-hourly IV *plus* clarithromycin 500 mg 12-hourly IV *or* erythromycin 500 mg 6-hourly IV ± flucloxacillin 2 g 6-hourly IV	Levofloxacin 500 mg daily IV *plus* benzylpenicillin 1.2 g 6-hourly IV

Oxygen

High-concentration oxygen therapy (FiO_2 >0.35) should be provided to all patients with hypoxaemia, acidosis or shock. Controlled oxygen therapy should be used in patients with chronic type II respiratory failure (e.g. COPD), but hypoxaemia must be corrected.

Fluids

Intravenous fluid replacement should be provided in patients with severe CAP, particularly if there is associated renal impairment. In normovolaemic patients, hypotension suggests shock and inotropic support may be required (see 'Shock', p. 250)

Analgesics and antipyretics

Unless contraindicated, NSAIDs should be prescribed for pleural pain, e.g. diclofenac (50 mg 8-hourly). This will aid expectoration but should be avoided if there is associated renal impairment. Paracetamol (1 g 6-hourly) may be given in addition, or as an antipyretic.

Additional therapy

- antifungal therapy is indicated in suspected or confirmed fungal pneumonia, e.g. IV amphotericin B (dose according to formulation; note test dose required first) or oral fluconazole (400 mg daily)
- PCP should be treated with high-dose co-trimoxazole (120 mg/kg in 4 divided IV doses); steroids should be added in patients with respiratory failure
- physiotherapy is commonly used but with little evidence to substantiate this practice.

Pneumonitis and fibrosis

Patients can present with acute breathlessness due to interstitial lung disease such as sarcoidosis, eosinophilic pneumonitis or allergic alveolitis. Alternatively, they may have hypoxia due to fibrosis that has caused breathlessness to develop over a matter of months. A detailed history can be helpful: in the case of alveolitis, there may have been contact with an allergic agent such as damp hay or pigeons; fibrosis may be associated with an occupational history of asbestos exposure; sarcoidosis may be associated with other clinical manifestations such as ophthalmic disease.

Fine inspiratory crackles can be heard, the patient may be hypoxic and a restrictive defect may be found on pulmonary function tests. Relevant blood tests should be considered, e.g. eosinophil count; levels of precipitating antibodies to a possible allergen; angiotensin converting enzyme levels; autoantibodies, including ANCA. High-resolution CT scanning is often helpful in establishing the extent of the disease and may show features that point to its aetiology. However, lung biopsy (transbronchial, CT-guided or surgical) may be needed to achieve a definitive diagnosis. Management usually involves oral corticosteroids ± immunosuppressants.

SECTION 2
Symptoms and related acute presentations

Abdominal 6

ACUTE ABDOMINAL PAIN

Acute abdominal pain is a common presentation to a variety of hospital specialties including A&E, surgery, medicine and O&G. The wide differential that needs to be considered reflects this variety, as summarized in Figure 6.1. It should be remembered that elderly patients may present with vague symptoms and often have non-specific findings on examination.

General assessment

History

Document the nature of the abdominal pain:

- site (including radiation of pain)
- time, mode of onset and duration
- severity and any progression over time
- character, e.g. constant, intermittent, colicky, burning, stabbing, sharp or dull
- exacerbating and relieving factors
- associated features, e.g. nausea, vomiting, weight loss, change in bowel habit, urinary symptoms.

Document when the patient last ate and drank. In all pre-menopausal females, record the date of last menstruation and ask about the possibility of pregnancy. Gynaecological causes of pain should always be considered (see p. 333).

Examination

If the patient is unwell, begin by assessing ABC and looking for evidence of shock (see 'Shock', p. 250). Then inspect, palpate, percuss and auscultate the abdomen. Remember to warm your hands before you touch the patient and look specifically for organomegaly, abnormal pulsations or evidence of:

- peritonitis, suggested by rigidity, guarding and absent bowel sounds (absent bowel sounds may also be seen in ileus)

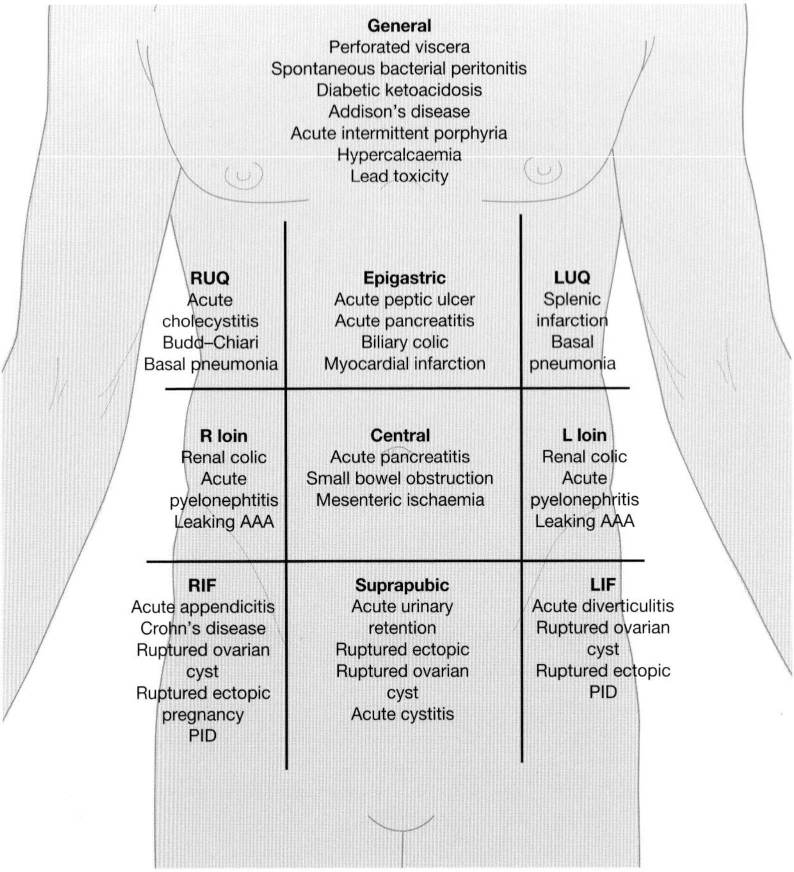

Figure 6.1 Causes of acute abdominal pain, by quadrant.

- visceral inflammation or localized peritonitis, suggested by local tenderness with or without rebounding
- obstruction, suggested by abdominal distension, generalized tenderness and tinkling bowel sounds.

Remember to examine hernial orifices and external genitalia in all patients and perform a per-rectal (PR) examination if GI bleeding or obstruction is suspected. Occasionally, it may also be possible to feel a tender appendix on PR.

Investigations

Investigations should be tailored to the clinical presentation, but the following initial tests should be considered in all patients:

- FBC (WBC may not increase in the elderly), Coag and a G+S
- U&E, LFT, glucose, calcium, amylase (minor elevations common), CRP
- blood cultures if febrile
- ECG
- erect CXR: look specifically for free air under the diaphragm
- supine abdominal film: look for renal calculi, bowel dilatation (>2.5 cm for small intestine and >6 cm for colon) and air in the biliary tree
- urinalysis, including pregnancy test in all females of child-bearing age.

Urgent surgical referral

Patients who are shocked require rapid and adequate fluid resuscitation (see 'Shock', p. 250). An urgent surgical opinion should be sought if visceral perforation, generalized peritonitis or bowel obstruction is suspected. All patients should be fasted pending surgical assessment.

Hepatobiliary and pancreatic causes of abdominal pain

Acute cholecystitis, biliary colic and acute cholangitis result from inflammation, infection or obstruction of the biliary tree, usually by gallstones. Gallstones and biliary obstruction can also cause acute pancreatitis. The aetiology, presentation and management of these conditions are outlined below.

Acute cholecystitis

Acute cholecystitis results from inflammation of the gallbladder wall and, in the majority of cases, is due to impaction of a stone in the neck of the gallbladder or cystic duct.

Presentation and investigation

Patients present with fever and persistent right upper quadrant pain. Murphy's sign (pain on palpation of the right subcostal region during inspiration) is a useful indicator and is sensitive, but not specific for acute cholecystitis. Acute inflammation of the gallbladder in the absence of biliary calculi (acute acalculous cholecystitis) may occur and is most common in children and adults who have recently undergone severe physical stress (e.g. severe trauma or burns) and are critically ill.

Liver function tests may show an elevated ALP (± bilirubin) and there may be evidence of an inflammatory response. Ultrasound scanning should be performed and may demonstrate the presence of gallstones, a sonographic Murphy's sign or thickening and dilation of the gallbladder wall.

Management

Appropriate analgesia, intravenous fluids, antibiotics and early referral for cholecystectomy.

Biliary colic

Biliary colic occurs when a gallstone blocks either the common bile duct or the cystic duct.

Presentation and investigation

There is severe, constant right upper quadrant or epigastric pain which usually increases over a 2–4 h period before settling. The pain may radiate to the right shoulder or through to the back and may be triggered by a fatty meal. Pain typically occurs a few hours after a meal and wakes the patient from sleep.

Associated symptoms include nausea, vomiting and fever, although fever with pain for over 24 h is more likely to be due to acute cholecystitis. Murphy's sign is usually positive during the attack. An ultrasound will identify the presence of gallstones with thickening of the gallbladder wall in the acute phase.

Management

Give appropriate analgesia until pain settles and refer for subsequent cholecystectomy once the acute episode has resolved.

Acute cholangitis

Acute cholangitis results from infection of the biliary tree. In the majority of cases, this is associated with common bile duct calculi, instrumentation of the biliary tree at endoscopic retrograde cholangiopancreatography (ERCP) or a structural abnormality, such as primary or secondary sclerosing cholangitis.

Presentation and investigation

The classic presentation is with 'Charcot's triad' of fever, jaundice and right upper quadrant pain, but these features may not always be present. Blood tests demonstrate elevation of WBC and CRP and derangement of LFT, often revealing a mixed pattern (see 'Abnormal LFTs', p. 178). Amylase may be elevated if there is associated calculi impaction at the ampulla of Vater. Blood cultures are positive in up to 50% of patients.

Management

This should include analgesia, intravenous fluid resuscitation, broad-spectrum IV antibiotics, e.g. ceftriaxone 2 g once daily and metronidazole 500 mg 12-hourly. In addition, patients with severe cholangitis and bile duct obstruction require endoscopic or percutaneous transhepatic biliary drainage.

Acute pancreatitis

This is defined as an acute inflammatory process of the pancreas. There are numerous potential causes, summarized by the mnemonic 'GET SMASHED': Gallstones and Ethanol (alcohol) excess explain 80% of cases; the others are Trauma, Steroids, Mumps (and other viral infections), Autoimmune disease (e.g. polyarteritis nodosa, SLE), Scorpion bites, Hypercalcaemia, Hyperlipidaemia, Hypothermia, ERCP and Drugs (e.g. sulphonamides, azathioprine, NSAIDs, diuretics).

Presentation

Patients present with severe periumbilical or generalized abdominal pain that often radiates through to the back. Pain may be eased by sitting forward and associated symptoms include nausea and vomiting. There may be fever and/or shock in severe attacks. Periumbilical or flank discoloration (Cullen's and Grey-Turner's signs, respectively) may also be seen.

Investigation

Diagnosis is made on the basis of typical clinical features and high serum amylase levels (3–4 times the upper limit of normal). The levels may decline quickly over 2–3 days. Therefore, if a patient presents late, serum amylase levels may be normal or only mildly elevated. However, urinary amylase levels are often high and should be checked. Hyperamylasaemia is not a specific marker of acute pancreatitis and may occur in other conditions, e.g. visceral perforation, small bowel obstruction or ischaemia, leaking aortic aneurysm and MI. Serum lipase is a more specific test and should be used if locally available. All patients should have an abdominal ultrasound performed to visualize the pancreas and biliary tree and exclude gallstones.

The severity of acute pancreatitis should be scored on admission using the modified Glasgow criteria (Table 6.1), Ranson score or APACHE (see p. 11). A CRP level >150 mg/L at 48 h is a reliable marker of a severe attack. Severe acute pancreatitis is associated with acute pancreatic necrosis and may lead to multiple organ failure and/or local complications such as fluid collections, pseudocyst formation, pancreatic abscess, haemorrhage or venous thrombosis. Therefore, in this context, a CT abdomen should be performed.

Management

Adequate fluid resuscitation is essential, especially in patients with evidence of shock (see 'Shock', p. 250). All patients should be catheterized to allow accurate monitoring of fluid balance, and central venous monitoring is often helpful. In addition, all patients should be managed in a high dependency environment and ICU referral should be considered in severe cases. Pain should be controlled using opiates. A nasogastric tube should be passed if the patient has protracted vomiting, especially if there is an associated ileus. Early nutritional support is recommended for all patients with severe pancreatitis.

Table 6.1 Modified Glasgow criteria

Variable	Level to meet criteria
Age (years)	>55
WBC	>15 × 10^9/L
Glucose (if not diabetic)	>10 mmol/L
Urea	>16 mmol/L
Arterial oxygen partial pressure	<8.0 kPa
Calcium	<2.0 mmol/L
Albumin	<32 g/L
Lactate dehydrogenase	>600 U/L

≥3 present within 48 h of admission indicate severe disease.

Spontaneous bacterial peritonitis (SBP)

This is defined as an acute bacterial infection of ascitic fluid and may occur in any patient with ascites, regardless of the underlying aetiology. It is associated with a poor long-term outcome in patients with ascites due to liver cirrhosis.

Presentation and investigation

Presentation is variable and approximately one-third of patients are asymptomatic. Fever, mild abdominal discomfort and worsening confusion may be present. However, SBP should be suspected in any patient with liver disease, who presents with an acute deterioration without any obvious precipitant. For this reason, all patients admitted to hospital with ascites should have a diagnostic paracentesis (see 'Ascitic tap', p. 46, and 'Ascitic fluid', p. 78).

Examination findings vary from normal to overt peritonitis. In severe cases, patients may be haemodynamically compromised and pyrexial. The presence of any stigmata of chronic liver disease or evidence of encephalopathy should be documented. A PR examination should be performed to exclude gastrointestinal bleeding as an additional cause for hepatic decompensation.

Management

Broad-spectrum IV antibiotics should be administered, e.g. ceftriaxone (2g once daily), metronidazole (500mg 8-hourly). Careful assessment of intravascular volume state is essential. If there is evidence of shock, treat as advised in 'Shock', p. 250. In patients with chronic liver disease and profound hypoalbuminaemia, the use of IV salt-poor albumin should be considered. Antibiotic regimes should be modified once formal bacteriology results are known.

Prophylaxis with norfloxacin (400mg once daily) is recommended for patients once they have recovered from an acute episode of SBP; however, some gastroenterologists advocate its use in all patients with ascites.

Gastrointestinal causes of abdominal pain

Acute peptic ulcer

This is defined as a break of 3mm or greater in the mucosa of the stomach or duodenum. It occurs due to an imbalance of damaging factors (e.g. acid secretion, NSAIDs, *Helicobacter pylori*) and mucosal protective factors (e.g. mucus, bicarbonate, prostaglandins).

Presentation

Peptic ulcers are very common and may be asymptomatic. More commonly they present with epigastric or more generalized abdominal pain; gastric ulcers tend to cause pain while eating, whereas duodenal ulcers tend to cause pain between meals or during the night. A minority of patients present with complications such as haematemesis, melaena or perforation.

Investigation and management

If perforation is suspected, patients should be fasted, receive adequate intravenous fluid resuscitation and early surgical review.

Upper GI endoscopy allows confirmation of the diagnosis, biopsy of potential malignant lesions and testing for *H. pylori* (CLO test). This should be performed as an inpatient if there as symptoms suggestive of active GI bleeding (e.g. significant haematemesis, or melaena) or malignancy (e.g. weight loss, a palpable abdominal mass or dysphagia).

In other patients, a decision must be made between outpatient endoscopy and an empirical trial of acid suppression therapy. Current guidelines recommend that all patients should be given a trial of acid suppression therapy. If this is unsuccessful they should have non-invasive testing (serological or urea breath testing) for *H. pylori* infection as a first-line test.

Those with a positive test should receive eradication therapy. Various regimes are available; these generally consist of a high-dose proton pump inhibitor, clarithromycin and metronidazole, or amoxicillin for 1 week. Eradication should be confirmed, after completion of a course of treatment, by a urea breath test.

Those with a negative test over the age of 55 should have endoscopy, reflecting the higher incidence of stomach cancer in this population (see 'Stomach cancer', p. 359).

Bowel obstruction

Bowel obstruction may occur in the large or small bowel. The latter can be classified as complete or partial, and simple (non-strangulated) or complicated (strangulated). Strangulated obstructions are surgical emergencies, as any delay in the diagnosis may lead to bowel ischaemia.

Small and large bowel obstructions differ in regard to their principal causal conditions. The majority of small bowel obstructions occur secondary to herniae or post-surgical adhesions: hernial orifices must be examined thoroughly. Large bowel obstruction is more commonly caused by colonic neoplasms or diverticular disease. However, conditions that can result in either type of obstruction include volvulus, inflammatory bowel disease and impaction with a foreign body (small bowel) or faeces (large bowel).

Presentation

Patients may present with abdominal pain, distension, vomiting and/or constipation. The most prominent features of the history may point to the approximate level of the obstruction, e.g. vomiting alone is a feature of high obstruction. Small bowel obstruction tends to present with colicky abdominal pain, vomiting and, depending on the level of obstruction, constipation. Large bowel obstruction has a similar presentation. However, vomiting is less prominent and, if present, may be faeculant. Suprapubic pain may be associated with constipation.

Investigation

Check FBC, U&E, LFT, Ca^{2+} and order an AXR. A supine abdominal X-ray may be helpful in the diagnosis of bowel obstruction and in determining the level of obstruction; see 'AXR', p. 101. However, differentiation between strangulation and simple obstruction should be made using clinical parameters, not on abdominal X-ray findings. The level of obstruction can be determined on CT, which may also help to determine the aetiology. Further investigation for large bowel obstruction may include sigmoidoscopy or colonoscopy.

Management

Intravenous fluids should be given and electrolyte disturbances corrected. All patients require broad-spectrum IV antibiotics, e.g. ceftriaxone (2 g once daily) and metronidazole (500 mg 8-hourly), and should have a nasogastric tube passed to decompress the bowel. The nasogastric tube should be left on continuous gentle suction. Additional management is dependent on the type of obstruction.

Small bowel obstruction

In cases of partial or simple obstruction, non-operative supportive treatment is sufficient: the obstruction will resolve in the majority of patients within 72 h. Urgent surgical intervention is required for those who fail to respond to non-surgical treatment or where a complete obstruction is present, as the risk of strangulation is high. In cases with an incarcerated hernia, manual reduction should be attempted and, if successful, an elective hernia repair should be arranged as soon as possible.

If obstruction occurs in patients with known inflammatory bowel disease, e.g. Crohn's disease, initial management should be conservative and include IV steroids (see 'Crohn's disease', p. 166). A barium follow-through or MRI should be performed to fully stage the extent of disease. Surgical input is required if resolution is not rapid, or if long or multiple strictures are present. Treatment options include small bowel resection, with or without stricturoplasty, in combination with immunosuppressive therapy.

Large bowel obstruction

Treatment of large bowel obstruction depends on the cause: neoplastic lesions will need surgical resection or endoscopic stenting. Sigmoid volvulus can be reduced by rigid sigmoidoscopy.

Acute appendicitis

This is defined as an acute inflammatory process within the appendix.

Presentation

The classical presentation is with periumbilical pain which subsequently localizes to the right iliac fossa. Associated symptoms may include anorexia, nausea and vomiting (vomiting generally follows the onset of the abdominal pain). Diarrhoea, constipation or urinary symptoms may also be reported.

Examination findings can be non-specific; however there may be rebound tenderness in the right iliac fossa and voluntary guarding. If perforation has occurred, generalized peritonitis may be present. Other 'classical' signs to note are:

- Rovsing's sign: right iliac fossa pain on palpation of the left iliac fossa
- obturator sign: right iliac fossa pain induced by internal rotation of the flexed right hip.

Investigation

Routine blood tests may reveal a neutrophilia, and CRP will usually be raised. Urinalysis may be abnormal and the diagnosis should not be discarded because of this. Investigation findings may be normal and the diagnosis is often made on clinical grounds. However, if there is diagnostic doubt abdominal imaging, e.g. ultrasound, should be performed. This is particularly the case in women of child-bearing age.

Management

All patients should be fasted until specialist surgical review, while intravenous fluids, antiemetics and analgesia are administered, according to individual requirements. For preoperative wound prophylaxis, metronidazole IV (500 mg 8-hourly) should be used. If the patient is felt to be at risk of abscess or perforation, a broader approach to antibiotic cover is required and ceftriaxone (2 g IV daily) should be added.

Crohn's disease

Crohn's disease is a chronic inflammatory disease of the gastrointestinal tract that can affect any mucosal membrane from the mouth to the anus. Unlike ulcerative colitis (see p. 171), Crohn's is characterized by segmental involvement and involves all layers of the bowel wall.

Presentation

Presenting symptoms in Crohn's vary considerably and depend on which parts of the bowel are affected. The classical presentation is with fatigue, weight loss, abdominal pain and diarrhoea. An acute presentation may signify a complication, e.g. perforation or abscess formation. A flare of ileo-colic disease may present with fever, right iliac fossa pain, nausea and vomiting (i.e. mimicking acute appendicitis), with or without signs of small bowel obstruction. Occasionally, patients may also present with complications relating to malabsorption, malnutrition or bleeding.

Examination findings may be normal. Low-grade fever and tachycardia are suggestive of active disease. More commonly, there may be mild abdominal tenderness or peritonism. Localized peritonitis may occur; however, generalized peritonitis suggests bowel perforation. Signs of bowel obstruction may also be present. A PR examination should be performed in all patients as perianal disease may be apparent.

Investigation

All patients should have routine haematological and biochemical tests. Elevated WBC and inflammatory markers may signify luminal disease or indicate abscess formation or perforation. Hypoalbuminaemia is a consistent predictor of poor outcome. An AXR should be performed in all patients to exclude colonic dilatation or perforation. An abdominal US is useful to view thickened bowel loops and to localize abscesses.

Management

Acute flares should be treated with IV hydrocortisone (100 mg three times daily) and, if the large bowel is affected, 5-ASA, e.g. mesalazine (400 mg 6-hourly). If patients fail to settle, consider early surgical referral or immunomodulatory therapy such as infliximab. Patients are at an increased risk of thrombosis and, unless otherwise contraindicated, should be commenced on LMWH, e.g. enoxaparin (40 mg SC daily). Once control is achieved, steroid sparing agents such as azathioprine or 6-mercaptopurine should be considered. For the management of Crohn's disease complicated by bowel obstruction, see p. 165.

Acute diverticulitis

Diverticular disease is very common and usually affects the sigmoid colon. Diverticulae are herniations or 'out-pouchings' of the mucosa and submucosa through the muscularis layer and are thought to result from high intra-luminal pressures. Diverticular disease is generally asymptomatic until local inflammation develops (diverticulitis), in response to faecal obstruction of the diverticular neck. Other complications of diverticular disease include pericolic abscess formation, fistula formation (generally occurs between the colon and bladder, uterus, vagina or small bowel), perforation and rectal bleeding.

Presentation

Acute diverticulitis may present with abdominal pain (predominantly left iliac fossa pain), altered bowel habit, PR bleeding, fever, nausea and vomiting. If associated fistulae are present, symptoms may also include pneumaturia, faeculent vaginal discharge or malabsorption.

On examination, patients are often febrile and tender in the left iliac fossa; signs of perforation with or without peritonitis may also be present. Rectal examination may be tender and fresh blood may be seen; a mass may also be palpated.

Investigation

The WBC may be normal or elevated; haemoglobin may be reduced secondary to PR bleeding. Blood cultures should be taken before intravenous antibiotics are given but should not delay their administration. AXR should be performed to exclude associated ileus or perforation. CT abdomen (rather than barium enema) should be performed in patients who present acutely and allows identification of complications, e.g. abscess or fistula formation. Colonoscopy should be performed after the acute episode in all patients who have PR blood loss, to exclude underlying carcinoma.

Management

Fluid resuscitation should be given where the patient is haemodynamically compromised, in addition to analgesia, antispasmodics and broad-spectrum IV antibiotics, e.g. ceftriaxone (2g once daily) and metronidazole (500mg 8-hourly). Patients should be advised of the potential benefits of a high-fibre diet. Surgical input is required if the patient fails to respond to medical therapy, or if complications are present.

Vascular causes of abdominal pain

Mesenteric ischaemia

Although this is relatively rare, it is associated with high morbidity and mortality. Acute mesenteric ischaemia may be thrombotic or embolic in origin. Chronic mesenteric ischaemia is usually related to atherosclerosis. Risk factors include those classically associated with vascular disease, e.g. smoking, diabetes, AF.

Presentation

Acute mesenteric ischaemia classically presents with severe, but poorly localized, abdominal pain, of gradual onset, with vague or no abdominal findings on examination. The pain may be of sudden onset if secondary to arterial emboli.

Chronic mesenteric ischaemia typically results in non-specific abdominal pain, which occurs half an hour after eating. Patients often have associated weight loss, reflecting their reluctance to eat because of pain.

Investigations

In acute mesenteric ischaemia biochemical findings may be non-specific, but patients may have elevated amylase, WBC and a lactic acidosis (particularly associated with infarction). Plain AXR is frequently normal, but may demonstrate mucosal thumb-printing or 'pneumatosis intestinalis'.

CT abdomen should be considered in patients who are haemodynamically stable. However, mesenteric angiography is often diagnostic and also allows selective thrombolysis.

Management

Treatment options depend on the haemodynamic status of the patient and the underlying suspected aetiology. General measures include oxygen, adequate fluid resuscitation, broad-spectrum IV antibiotics, e.g. ceftriaxone (2g once daily) and metronidazole (500mg 8-hourly), and opioid analgesia. A nasogastric tube should be passed if there is an associated ileus and abdominal distension. Early ICU referral should be considered in patients who are haemodynamically unstable.

The surgical team should be involved early; if the patient has signs of peritonitis, urgent laparotomy should be considered. For cases of chronic mesenteric ischaemia, treatment options include angioplasty, stent insertion or formal surgical revascularization.

Ruptured or leaking abdominal aortic aneurysm

An abdominal aortic aneurysm (AAA) results from atherosclerotic degeneration of the lining (tunica media) of the arterial walls. Patients are usually asymptomatic until the aneurysm enlarges to such an extent that it causes symptoms related to compression of adjacent structures or ruptures.

Presentation

Expanding AAAs tend to cause progressive symptoms such as abdominal or back pain (severe, constant low back or flank pain), groin pain (due to compression of femoral nerve), claudication or syncope. An AAA should always be considered in patients presenting with loin pain and haematuria (resulting from dissection of renal artery), especially those over 50 years of age, with a history of atherosclerosis or hypertension. Patients with ruptured AAA present with cardiovascular collapse.

Examination findings may be normal if the leakage or rupture has been contained by the tamponade effect of a retroperitoneal haematoma. Classical findings of shock and a pulsatile abdominal mass are seen in less than a third of patients.

Investigation

Abdominal CT scanning accurately defines the extent and type of aneurysm and allows assessment of arterial structures involved.

Management

Two large-bore intravenous cannulae should be inserted. Aim for a systolic blood pressure of 100 mmHg. If the patient is hypotensive, fluid resuscitation should be aggressive (see 'Shock', p. 251). Where the patient is hypertensive, consider IV β-blockers unless contraindicated. Adequate analgesia should be given and all patients catheterized. Early surgical evaluation is imperative. Treatment should not be delayed for CT scanning.

Renal causes of abdominal pain

Renal colic

Presentation

Renal calculi affect up to 3% of the population. Patients classically present with colicky loin pain, which may radiate to the groin. Associated symptoms include nausea, vomiting, urinary frequency and dysuria.

Abdominal examination may be unremarkable or reveal flank tenderness; bowel sounds may be reduced if there is an associated ileus. In patients over 50 years of age presenting with loin pain, a leaking abdominal aortic aneurysm should be actively excluded (see AAA, above).

Complications include ureteric obstruction with renal failure, infected hydronephrosis, pyonephrosis, perinephric abscess and overwhelming sepsis (often with Gram-negative organisms).

Investigations

Urinalysis, MSU (for microscopy and culture) and KUB radiograph should be performed in all patients. In addition to standard haematological and biochemical tests, urate, calcium and phosphate should also be checked. A 24 h urinary measurement of calcium, urate and phosphate is also useful. If there is a family history of renal calculi, cystinuria should be excluded.

Management

Ensure adequate hydration and analgesia (diclofenac 100 mg PR initially, then opiates). Antiemetics and antispasmodics may also be helpful. Most stones pass spontaneously, but referral to urology is indicated where there is uncontrolled pain, associated renal failure, previous renal transplantation or where infection or obstruction is suspected. Where infection is suspected, broad-spectrum antibiotic therapy should be started, e.g. ceftriaxone (2 g IV daily) and metronidazole (500 mg IV 8-hourly), or see local guidelines.

Stone analysis and a detailed metabolic assessment are useful in patients who present with recurrent calculi. In this setting, lithotripsy or resection may be necessary.

Acute pyelonephritis

This is defined as an acute bacterial infection of the renal parenchyma. It is commoner in females and may, if recurrent, result in chronic renal failure. Other complications include abscess formation (perinephric or nephric) and septic shock.

Presentation

Classically, patients present with urinary symptoms (e.g. frequency, urgency, dysuria or haematuria), flank or back pain (generally unilateral but can be bilateral) and are often systemically unwell (e.g. fever, nausea, vomiting). However, this is extremely variable and the presentation may be vague, particularly at the extremes of age. Examination may reveal shock, fever and costovertebral angle or suprapubic tenderness.

Investigation

Most patients with pyelonephritis have significant pyuria; proteinuria is also common, but when it exceeds 3 g (in 24 h urine collection) glomerulonephritis should be suspected. The WBC is usually elevated; however, blood cultures are only positive in 20% of patients. Imaging of the kidneys is indicated to assess any anatomical variation, which may predispose to infection, and to exclude complications. Detailed imaging is required when response to treatment is slow, or if the patient's condition deteriorates.

Management

Fluids should be given to ensure adequate hydration, along with analgesia and IV broad-spectrum antibiotics. These should aim to cover Gram-negative organisms, particularly *E. coli* which is responsible for approximately 50% of cases. An appropriate regime would be ceftriaxone (2 g IV once daily) and ciprofloxacin (500 mg IV 12-hourly) ± gentamicin (3–5 mg/kg IV). Referral to urology is required if imaging suggests cortical or perinephric abscess, as drainage may be required.

Gynaecological causes of abdominal pain

Gynaecological pain may be physiological or pathological, e.g. ruptured ectopic pregnancy, ovarian cyst torsion/rupture, fibroids (see p. 333).

DIARRHOEA, VOMITING AND CONSTIPATION

Diarrhoea

Diarrhoea can be defined as an increase in stool frequency, relative to that which is normal for the patient. Usually the stools are of a more liquid consistency. Diarrhoea commonly occurs acutely, but may be chronic. Some causes are listed in Table 6.2.

History

Determine the onset of the diarrhoea and the stool characteristics such as consistency, volume, colour and frequency. In chronic diarrhoea, a stool chart can be helpful. Ask specifically about associated symptoms such as abdominal pain, weight loss, fever, PR blood or mucus, nausea or vomiting. Enquire if any family members or close contacts have been affected and document any recent change in diet. An occupational, drug and travel history should also be taken.

Table 6.2 Causes of diarrhoea

Aetiology	Onset	Examples
Infective	Acute	Bacterial: *Salmonella, Campylobacter, Escherichia coli, Staphylococcus aureus, Clostridia, Shigella, Yersinia enterocolitica* Viral: Rotavirus, Norwalk virus, adenovirus Parasites: *Cryptosporidia, Giardia, Entamoeba*
Inflammatory	Acute or chronic	Ulcerative colitis, Crohn's disease, pseudomembranous colitis
Endocrine	Acute or chronic	Thyrotoxicosis, diabetes mellitus
Pharmacological	Acute	Antibiotics, digoxin, PPIs, laxatives, metformin, methyldopa
Neoplasm	Acute or chronic	Colonic neoplasm, pancreatic neoplasm, carcinoid syndrome, VIPomas
Gastrointestinal	Acute or chronic	Malabsorption, pancreatic disease, diverticular disease, coeliac disease, ischaemic colitis, irritable bowel syndrome, faecal impaction with overflow, bacterial overgrowth, lactulose intolerance
Surgical causes	Acute	Appendicitis, short bowel syndrome

Fresh blood mixed in with the stool is suggestive of inflammatory bowel disease or certain intestinal infections, e.g. *Campylobacter*. Bowel cancer should be actively excluded in older patients. Bloody diarrhoea associated with abdominal pain after eating is suggestive of ischaemic colitis. Pancreatic disease should be actively excluded in patients with chronic diarrhoea associated with abdominal pain, pale stools (suggesting steatorrhoea) and weight loss.

Examination

General examination should include an assessment of hydration and nutritional status. Document HR, BP and temperature. Full abdominal examination, including a rectal examination, should be performed in all patients. The stool should be inspected where possible.

Investigations

- U&E, LFT (including albumin), Coag, random Glu, TFT, CRP and FBC; in patients with inflammatory bowel disease, interpret CRP and WCC with caution as elevated levels may suggest perforation, rather than infection
- blood cultures should be taken if the patient is febrile, or if salmonella infection is suspected
- three stool samples for microscopy, culture and sensitivity should be taken in all patients
- if there has been recent hospitalization or antibiotic administration, ask for *Clostridium difficile* toxin; up to 10% of patients with inflammatory bowel disease are *C. difficile* positive

- faecal calprotectin should be sent, if locally available; this is a reliable means of identifying intestinal inflammation and can be used to differentiate organic bowel pathology (e.g. inflammatory bowel disease) from irritable bowel syndrome; false positives can occur with infection which should be excluded first
- if there has been recent travel, send a 'hot' stool sample for cysts, ova and parasites; contact your microbiology team prior to sending the sample
- arrange a plain AXR to exclude toxic dilatation of the bowel (transverse colon >5.5 cm or caecal pole >9 cm with loss of haustration); where there are ongoing symptoms the AXR may need to be repeated daily
- sigmoidoscopy or colonoscopy should be carried out if inflammatory bowel disease or colorectal malignancy is suspected
- further abdominal imaging, including ultrasound, CT or barium studies may be helpful.

Management

General management

Isolate and barrier nurse all patients in whom you have a strong suspicion of an infective cause. Liaise early with the local infection control team.

Early and adequate rehydration is essential. In mild cases, oral rehydration may suffice. If IV fluids are required, the rate and volume of fluid administered should be titrated against clinical parameters and balanced against the risk of fluid overload. If the patient is shocked, treat as suggested in 'Shock and fluid balance', p. 251. Electrolyte replacement should be guided by biochemistry results. Close monitoring of fluid balance is required. Avoid the use of anti-diarrhoeal drugs, as most cases of infective diarrhoea are self-limiting and these agents may prolong the illness.

Management of specific conditions

Infective diarrhoea

Most forms of acute infective diarrhoea are self-limiting, but may be associated with considerable morbidity and mortality in certain patient groups, e.g. children, elderly, immunosuppressed or malnourished patients.

If bacterial infection is confirmed on stool culture then appropriate antibiotics should be commenced if the patient is still symptomatic. Liaise with the microbiology team regarding local protocols. Depending on the organism grown, the local Public Health team may also need to be informed.

Patients with active *C. diff* infection should be treated initially with oral metronidazole 400 mg 8-hourly for 7 days. If resistant, oral vancomycin 125 mg 6-hourly should be used. There is a high risk of perforation with toxic dilatation, so early input from the surgical team is important.

Inflammatory bowel disease (ulcerative colitis)

Both ulcerative colitis (UC) and Crohn's disease may present with acute, often bloody, diarrhoea. Although it may be impossible to distinguish between the two clinically, diarrhoea is more common in UC. This reflects the fact that UC, in contrast to Crohn's, is always confined to the large bowel and invariably affects the rectum. Crohn's more commonly presents with symptoms of abdominal pain and, therefore, its management is discussed in that section (see p. 166).

Acute flares of UC should be managed by a multidisciplinary team including a physician and surgeon. First-line medical treatment should be with IV steroids, e.g. intravenous hydrocortisone (100 mg 6-hourly for 72 h), and thereafter a reducing dose of oral prednisolone. Patients should also be given oral 5-aminosalicylates if they can tolerate them, e.g. Asacol® (800 mg 8-hourly) or Pentasa® (2 g twice daily). All patients should be given thromboembolic prophylaxis, e.g. enoxaparin (40 mg daily), and early parenteral nutrition should be considered.

The need for second-line medical therapy should be assessed on day 3; options include IV ciclosporin or infliximab. These are effective in approximately 30% of patients, and colectomy can be avoided. Indications for urgent colectomy include colonic dilatation (>6cm: toxic megacolon); deteriorating clinical or laboratory measurements at any time; failure to respond to maximum medical therapy after 7–10 days.

Vomiting

Vomiting is usually an acute, self-limiting phenomenon. However, some conditions are associated with chronic symptoms. The aetiology is often multifactorial; common causes are listed in Table 6.3.

Table 6.3 Common causes of vomiting

Aetiology	Examples
Infective	*S. aureus, B. cereus, V. parahaemolyticus* and viruses, e.g. Norwalk (norovirus)
Gastrointestinal	Hiatus hernia, GORD, oesophageal motility disorders, oesophageal compression or stricture, gastroenteritis, gastritis, peptic ulcer disease, cholecystitis
Renal	Renal colic, UTI, renal failure
Surgical	Pyloric stenosis, gastric volvulus, pancreatitis, bowel obstruction, incarcerated hernia, appendicitis
Pharmacological	Alcohol, antibiotics, chemotherapy agents, opiates, codeine, digoxin
Psychological	Bulimia
Intracranial	Meningitis, brainstem stroke, raised intracranial pressure (e.g. space occupying lesion), middle ear disease, e.g. Ménière's disease, labyrinthitis
Metabolic/endocrine	Pregnancy, Addison's disease, diabetic ketoacidosis, hypercalcaemia, uraemia
Miscellaneous	Acute myocardial infarction, severe infection

History

Ask specifically about associated symptoms, e.g. weight loss, diarrhoea, abdominal pain, headache, urinary or respiratory symptoms. Determine the circumstances around the vomiting, e.g. whether preceded by nausea, associated with eating, worse in the early morning (suggestive of pregnancy, alcohol abuse or raised intracranial pressure). Determine the colour of the vomit, e.g. bile or blood stained, or faeculent.

In females of child-bearing age, specifically ask the date of their last period and the possibility of pregnancy. A detailed drug history may also identify the aetiological agent.

Examination

Assess hydration and nutritional status. Perform a full abdominal examination, including a search for lymphadenopathy, assessment of the hernial orifices, and a PR. Examine closely for signs of sepsis and, where possible, examine the vomit.

Investigations

- U&E, LFT, glucose, Ca^{2+}, amylase and FBC
- consider a pregnancy test in females of child-bearing age
- sepsis screen: urinalysis, stool culture and CXR
- further investigations should be tailored to the most likely diagnosis, e.g. AXR, abdominal ultrasound, upper GI endoscopy, CT abdomen, CT brain.

Management

General management involves parenteral administration of an antiemetic and rehydration with IV fluids, if necessary. All patients in whom a surgical cause is suspected should be kept fasted until a decision on surgical management is made. In other patients, management is directed towards the underlying cause, e.g. treatment of diabetic ketoacidosis or sepsis.

Antiemetics

There are a variety of antiemetics available. These act by different pathways and, therefore, are best suited to specific clinical settings:

- cyclizine (50 mg PO/IM/IV 8-hourly) is an antihistamine and is effective in a variety of settings including vertigo and labyrinthine disorders
- prochlorperazine, or Stemetil (20 mg PO acutely, followed by 10 mg PO after 2 h; prevention 5–10 mg PO 8-hourly), is a centrally acting dopamine antagonist and acts by blocking the chemoreceptor trigger zone (CTZ); it is particularly useful in the treatment of nausea related to neoplasia, radiation or drugs
- metoclopramide, or Maxolon (10 mg PO/IM/IV 8-hourly), has similar central effects to prochlorperazine, but also increases gastrointestinal motility; this prokinetic action makes it effective in nausea related to gastroduodenal, hepatic and biliary disease; metoclopramide should be avoided in children and young adults in whom it can cause severe dystonic reactions
- domperidone (10–20 mg PO 6–8-hourly) does not cross the blood–brain barrier, reducing the risk of side-effects such as dystonic reactions or sedation
- $5HT_3$ antagonists (e.g. ondansetron; 4–8 mg 12-hourly) block receptors both centrally and in the GI tract; they are effective in postoperative nausea and that related to cytotoxic drug therapy.

Constipation

Constipation encompasses a wide range of symptoms from infrequent bowel motions, change in stool consistency and difficulty in evacuation. It may be due to disorders of the large bowel and rectum, or secondary to other conditions. Some causes are listed in Table 6.4 overleaf.

History

Document normal bowel habit (consistency + frequency). Determine the patient's definition of constipation and enquire whether it is acute or chronic. Enquire about associated symptoms, e.g. weight loss, fresh blood loss PR, and any recent change in diet or lifestyle, new drugs and relevant psychosocial factors. Consider associated conditions, e.g. diabetes mellitus, hypothyroidism, Parkinson's disease.

Examination

Assess their general condition and look for clinical evidence of dehydration, cachexia, anaemia or hypothyroidism. Abdominal and PR examination should be performed in all patients. Consider pelvic examination in females if there are associated gynaecological symptoms.

Table 6.4 Causes of constipation

Aetiology	Examples
Gastrointestinal	Anatomical outlet obstruction, e.g. rectal neoplasm or prolapse, rectocele Functional outlet obstruction, e.g. pudendal nerve damage, external sphincter spasm Colonic, e.g. left-sided colonic disease (volvulus, inflammatory stricture, cancer), colonic ileus, reduced colonic motility (chronic laxative abuse), Chagas' disease, Hirschsprung's disease
Neurological	Spinal cord injury, head injury, CVA, Parkinson's disease
Dietary factors	Reduced fibre or fluid intake
Pharmacological	Opiates, ferrous sulphate, calcium antagonists, phenothiazines, tricyclic antidepressants
Endocrine	Hypothyroidism, panhypopituitarism, MEN type 2, diabetes mellitus (autonomic neuropathy)
Miscellaneous	Depression

Investigations

Investigations should be guided by the history and examination:

- U&E, LFT, Glu, Ca^{2+}, TFT and FBC
- faecal occult blood testing should be performed, especially in middle-aged or elderly patients presenting with chronic constipation
- all patients over 50 years with a family history of bowel cancer should have a colonoscopy.

Not all patients need further imaging (ultrasound, CT, Gastrografin/barium studies) or colonoscopy. These should be reserved for patients with sinister symptoms (such as weight loss and anaemia) or persistent symptoms despite simple measures, e.g. dietary changes or a trial of laxatives.

Gastrografin, rather than barium, contrast studies are preferable in patients who present acutely and who may have a bowel perforation. Gastrografin is an osmotic laxative, which may be an advantage in patients with constipation.

Management

Although the most important facet of management should be to treat the cause of constipation, medical therapy is invariably required. Commonly prescribed laxatives include:

- bulk-forming: Fybogel® (ispaghula), 1 sachet twice daily after food
- stimulant: glycerol suppositories; senna, initially 1–2 tablets at night
- osmotic: lactulose, initially 15 mL twice daily; Movicol®, 1–3 sachets daily increased to 8 sachets daily for faecal impaction.

GASTROINTESTINAL BLEEDING

Acute gastrointestinal (GI) bleeding is common and is associated with significant morbidity and mortality. It is important to distinguish between upper and lower GI bleeding as their management, following fluid resuscitation, is different.

Upper GI bleeding

This is defined as bleeding proximal to the ligament of Treitz, i.e. proximal to the duodenojejunal junction. Most patients present with melaena or haematemesis, which can be red, dark red, brown or 'coffee ground' in colour. Other symptoms may include syncope or abdominal pain. Occasionally fresh blood may be passed per rectum if there is torrential bleeding from an upper GI source. Causes include: peptic ulcer (duodenal > gastric); gastric or duodenal erosions; Mallory–Weiss tear; inflammation of the oesophagus, duodenum or stomach; neoplasm (gastric > oesophageal); vascular malformations and general causes of bleeding diathesis.

History

- determine the circumstances surrounding the bleed and document the volume of blood lost
- ask about associated symptoms such as syncope, abdominal pain, weight loss, diarrhoea or change in bowel habit
- take an accurate drug history: ask about recent NSAID (including aspirin), corticosteroid or anticoagulant use
- check for co-morbid disease, e.g. cardiac, renal or respiratory disease
- always document alcohol intake and smoking history.

Examination

If the patient is shocked, manage as per 'Shock and fluid balance', p. 251. Stigmata of chronic liver disease indicate a high probability of variceal haemorrhage. The following signs suggest a major bleed:

- history of syncope
- tachycardia: HR >100/min
- systolic BP <100 mmHg
- cool peripheries
- confusion or reduced GCS.

Investigations

Two large-bore cannulae should be inserted and blood sent for U&E, LFT, glucose, FBC, Coag. Between 4 and 10 units of blood should be cross-matched, depending on the size of the bleed. An ECG should be performed in all patients over 40 years. Patients should be classified into high and low risk groups by calculating their Rockall score (Table 6.5); a score <3 is associated with an excellent prognosis, a score >8 indicates a high risk of death. Most units would advise that patients with a score >3 should be considered for early endoscopy. This allows identification of the bleeding source, local control in some circumstances and planning of further treatment.

Table 6.5 Rockall score

Variable	Score			
	0	1	2	3
Age (years)	<60	60–79	>80	–
Shock	None: systolic BP ≥100, HR <100	Systolic BP ≥100 but HR >100	Systolic BP <100	–
Co-morbidity	None	All other diagnoses	Heart disease	Malignancy, renal or liver failure

General management

- begin by assessing ABC
- restoration of the circulating volume is essential; fluid resuscitation should be early and aggressive (see 'Shock', p. 251); be more cautious in patients

with known cardiac disease and consider central venous access and invasive monitoring
- in patients with evidence of a major bleed, urgent transfusion may be required; use O-negative blood until cross-matched blood becomes available
- correct any coagulopathy or thrombocytopenia with FFP and platelet transfusion; this requires early liaison with haematology
- arrange admission to the high dependency unit if the patient remains unstable after initial fluid resuscitation; keep the patient nil by mouth and repeat heart rate and BP observations every 15 min.

Specific management

This can only be planned with confidence once endoscopy has identified the source of bleeding. Therefore, early endoscopy is essential in patients with a large bleed, haemodynamic instability or high Rockall scores (see above).

Peptic ulcer disease

Endoscopic therapy

Oesophageal, duodenal (Fig. 6.2) or gastric ulcers can be injected with 1:100 000 IU adrenaline (epinephrine) or diathermied using a heater probe. If specific re-bleeding risks are identified during endoscopy (e.g. adherent clot or a visible vessel) or if the endoscopist is not happy that haemostasis has been achieved, the upper GI surgical team should be informed. Gastric ulcers should be re-scoped within 6 weeks to ensure healing and all persistent ulcers should be biopsied.

Pharmacological therapy

- proton pump inhibitors: clot formation and therefore haemostasis is pH dependent; therefore an 80 mg IV bolus of omeprazole should be given at presentation in known or suspected peptic ulcer bleeds and continued at a rate of 8 mg/h for the next 48–72 h (Hong Kong protocol); this can then be converted to oral therapy
- *H. pylori* eradication: prescribe triple therapy (see p. 164) if the CLOtest® is positive.

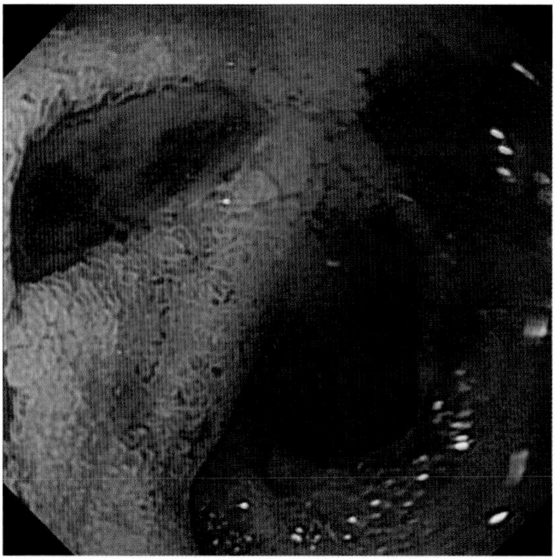

Figure 6.2 Duodenal ulcers.

Variceal haemorrhage

- urgent endoscopy should be arranged for all patients with suspected variceal bleeding; endoscopic band ligation is preferred for bleeding oesophageal varices (Fig. 6.3); injections of thrombin or Histoacryl® glue are used for gastric varices

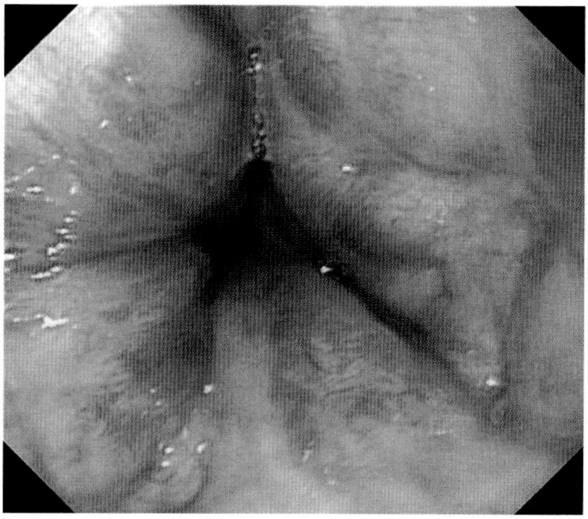

Figure 6.3 Oesophageal varices at endoscopy.

- intravenous terlipressin (2mg bolus, 1–2mg 6-hourly) should be considered, especially when endoscopy is not immediately available or if haemostasis could not be achieved at endoscopy; be cautious in patients with documented cardiac disease
- if haemostasis is difficult to achieve, or endoscopy is not immediately available, a Sengstaken–Blakemore tube should be inserted by an experienced operator; only inflate the gastric balloon (using 250–350mL of air), and maintain traction using wooden tongue depressors taped together across the tube at the mouth
- all patients with cirrhosis should received broad-spectrum antibiotics for 7 days
- re-bleeding from oesophageal varices within days to weeks is common; repeat endoscopic band ligation should therefore be planned, and/or patients commenced on secondary prophylaxis with propranolol (40–80mg 12-hourly)
- when the bleeding is uncontrolled, especially if the bleeding has been torrential, a transjugular intrahepatic portosystemic stent shunt (TIPSS) should be arranged.

Oesophagitis, gastritis, duodenitis, gastric or duodenal erosions

Give an oral proton pump inhibitor and eradicate *Helicobacter pylori*, if CLOtest® is positive. Stop NSAIDs or corticosteroids. If biliary gastritis is present, consider the use of sucralfate.

Mallory–Weiss tears

Generally, no treatment is necessary. If there is bleeding at the time of endoscopy, the bleeding point can be injected with adrenaline.

Lower GI bleeding

This is defined as bleeding distal to the ligament of Treitz. Common presenting symptoms are the passage of fresh or dark blood PR, abdominal pain, cramping or syncope. Blood loss may be occult and patients may present with symptoms of anaemia. Causes of lower GI bleeding include the following:

- gastrointestinal: diverticular disease, inflammatory bowel disease, polyps, bowel cancer, portal colopathy and rectal varices, benign anorectal disease (e.g. haemorrhoids, anal fissures)

- infective: *Campylobacter*, *E. coli*
- vascular: ischaemic colitis, angiodysplasia/AV malformations
- miscellaneous: coagulopathy, systemic vasculitis affecting the colon, radiation-induced enteritis, endometriosis.

History and examination

As for upper GI bleeding; see above.

Investigations and general management

- see upper GI bleeding above
- AXR: to look for dilated loops of bowel or bowel wall oedema
- rigid/flexible sigmoidoscopy: will identify any anorectal disease or any colitis affecting the sigmoid colon
- colonoscopy: should be performed in all patients at some stage to exclude an occult colonic lesion
- CT angiography: can be used to identify the bleeding site; this may be required urgently if the patient is unstable with signs of shock despite fluid resuscitation
- barium and other studies: if occult lower GI bleeding is suspected, barium studies or capsule studies can be helpful.

Specific management depending on aetiology

Diverticular disease

If bleeding is uncontrollable, segmental bowel resection may be required.

Angiodysplasia

Treatment options include segmental bowel resection, selective mesenteric embolization or argon plasma endoscopic therapy.

Rectal varices

Endoscopic intravariceal injection with thrombin is often helpful, but specialist measures may be required if bleeding is severe.

ABNORMAL LIVER FUNCTION

Abnormalities of liver function tests are very common. The individual assays commonly checked are bilirubin, the aminotransferases (AST and ALT), alkaline phosphatase (AlkP) and gamma-glutamyltranspeptidase (GGT). Although these tests are normally described as 'liver function tests', they are neither sensitive nor specific for liver function and, in fact, more accurately reflect liver damage. Albumin and prothrombin time are better indicators of synthetic liver function. Nevertheless, particular LFT patterns are useful in determining a likely aetiology and directing further investigation.

Assessment

History

- patients are often asymptomatic; however, they may complain of abdominal pain, weight loss, itch, fatigue, dark urine or pale stools; abdominal pain, if present, is most common in the right upper quadrant and strongly suggests biliary disease
- ask about specific risk factors for hepatitis, e.g. a history of jaundice or blood transfusions, intravenous drug use, high-risk sexual activity and contact with jaundiced persons or recent foreign travel
- check for a history of previously abnormal LFT and evaluate the past medical history for potential causes of abnormal liver function, e.g. diabetes, gallstones or cancer

- document recent drug history, including over-the-counter and herbal medication
- record alcohol intake in units/week.

Examination

- make a general assessment of the patient, paying particular attention to the presence of jaundice, cachexia, lymphadenopathy and stigmata of chronic liver disease
- look for signs of encephalopathy (confusion, flap/asterixis, impaired psychometric tests such as drawing pentagons); this is particularly important in patients with known or suspected chronic liver disease or fulminant hepatic failure (see below).

Initial investigations and general management

In patients with known liver disease check glucose, U&E, FBC, Coag and continue to monitor these. An abdominal ultrasound should also be performed; this will help to guide further tests and may reveal an obvious cause, e.g. gallstones, liver metastases. Otherwise, further tests should be guided by the pattern of LFT abnormality observed; this is described in detail below.

Patients should be closely monitored; look specifically for evidence of developing encephalopathy, coagulopathy, bleeding or hypoglycaemia. If the PT is prolonged, intravenous vitamin K should be given to reverse any contributing dietary deficiency. If the patient is actively bleeding, fresh frozen plasma can be used to rapidly correct the coagulopathy (see 'Blood products').

Patterns of LFT derangement

If an ultrasound scan of the upper abdomen does not reveal an obvious cause, the pattern of derangement should be used to direct further tests and narrow the differential diagnosis. The common patterns described are a transaminitis, an obstructive pattern, a mixed pattern and an isolated rise in bilirubin.

Transaminitis

This pattern may also be described as hepatitis. There is a predominant rise in AST and ALT, indicating hepatocellular injury or death. Patients may or may not be jaundiced. The extent of the abnormality correlates with the severity of the liver injury. Common causes are listed below and can be split into mild, moderate and severe categories:

Mild transaminitis (<100 U/mL)

Consider the following causes:

Drug reaction

Can be caused by medications such as statins, antibiotics or NSAIDs.

Chronic viral hepatitis

Check hepatitis A, B, C and E serology; if B positive, also check for hepatitis D.

Fatty liver

This a reactive pathological response to a variety of conditions, e.g. drugs (tamoxifen, methotrexate, amiodarone), viruses (hepatitis C, HIV), or toxins (alcohol, petrochemicals, phosphorus poisoning). In general, it is self-limiting and reversible; however, a minority will progress to cirrhosis, see below. There may be hepatomegaly and GGT may be very high; jaundice is unusual. Ultrasound examination will reveal a bright liver.

Non-alcoholic fatty liver disease (NAFLD)

This is an extremely common and under-recognized disorder associated with insulin resistance. It is common in obesity, the metabolic syndrome and type 2 diabetes mellitus. LFT abnormalities are usually mild. Factors associated with more advanced disease, i.e. non-alcoholic steatohepatitis (NASH), rather than simply fatty liver include an AST:ALT ratio greater than 1, a more cholestatic pattern, positive anti-smooth muscle or nuclear antibodies. Patients with NAFLD may progress to cirrhosis, and investigation and treatment of precipitants is therefore important.

Alcoholic hepatitis

Characterized by jaundice, an AST > ALT, progressive cholestasis, coagulopathy and high WBC. It may occasionally be associated with haemolysis (Zieve's syndrome). Bilirubin rises as the condition progresses and may exceed 500 U/mL in severe cases. The Glasgow alcoholic hepatitis score (GAHS) can be used to predict adverse outcomes (Table 6.6). Patients with a score ≥9/12 are at a greater risk of early death and should be prescribed corticosteroids or pentoxiphylline; e.g. oral prednisolone 20–60 mg daily, assuming no contraindication.

Table 6.6 The Glasgow alcoholic hepatitis score

Variable	Score		
	1	2	3
Age	<50	≥50	–
Urea (mmol/L)	<5	≥5	–
WCC ($\times 10^9$)	<15	≥15	–
PT ratio	<1.5	1.5–2.0	>2.0
Bilirubin (μmol/L)	<125	125–250	>250

Alcoholic cirrhosis

This may be associated with normal or mildly elevated transaminases (AST > ALT). Bilirubin and GGT are usually elevated, in association with a low albumin, high MCV, prolonged PT and low platelets.

The prognosis of a patient with cirrhosis can be assessed using the Child–Pugh score (Table 6.7), which grades the disease into three categories: A, <7; B, 7–9; C, >9. Survival in grade C is likely to be under 12 months without transplantation. Patients should also undergo surveillance for complications: upper GI endoscopy to look for oesophageal varices and abdominal ultrasound and serum α-fetoprotein for hepatocellular carcinoma (see below). If varices are absent, endoscopy should be repeated every 1–2 years.

Table 6.7 The Child–Pugh score

Variable	Score		
	1	2	3
Encephalopathy	None	Mild	Marked
Bilirubin			
μmol/L	<34	34–50	>50
in PBC/PSC	<68	68–170	>170
Albumin (g/L)	>35	28–35	<28
PT (seconds prolonged)	<4	4–6	>6
Ascites	None	Mild	Marked

Moderate transaminitis (100–500 U/mL)

Consider the following causes:

- flare of chronic hepatitis (B or C)
- flare of autoimmune chronic hepatitis
- drug toxicity
- non-alcoholic steatohepatitis (NASH)
- Wilson's disease: characterized by episodes of acute hepatitis, although can present with fulminant hepatic failure or more insidious chronic hepatitis; it is an autosomal recessive disorder of copper metabolism, reflected in a low serum caeruloplasmin; treatment is usually with penicillamine, but transplantation should be considered.

Severe transaminitis (>1000 U/mL)

Consider the following causes:

- acute viral hepatitis (A, B, C and non-A–E, EBV, CMV)
- drug toxicity, e.g. paracetamol (see below) or ecstasy overdose
- shock liver, may be secondary to hypotension, e.g. sepsis or haemorrhage, or hypoxia
- presentation of autoimmune chronic hepatitis: check antinuclear (ANA) and smooth muscle (SMA) antibodies.

Obstructive pattern

There is a predominant rise in alkaline phosphatase and GGT. These are canalicular enzymes and this pattern suggests cholestasis, which may be due to obstruction within the pancreatobiliary tree. If suspected, further investigation should include an early abdominal ultrasound with or without ERCP or MRCP. The severity of the enzyme rise does not correlate with the degree of obstruction and patients may or may not be jaundiced. Common causes of this pattern include:

Pancreatobiliary disease

- biliary calculi
- pancreatic disease: carcinoma of the head of pancreas, pancreatic pseudocyst,
- primary or secondary sclerosing cholangitis and biliary strictures
- cholangiocarcinoma.

Liver disease

Primary biliary cirrhosis

This is a chronic and progressive cholestatic condition of the liver which results in destruction of the intrahepatic bile ducts. It is an autoimmune disease which predominately affects females, mainly in their 5th or 6th decade. Patients may be asymptomatic or complain of non-specific symptoms, such as fatigue or itch.

Diagnosis is suggested by cholestatic LFTs, and confirmed by the presence of anti-mitochondrial antibodies (AMA). Jaundice, ascites or encephalopathy (i.e. hepatic decompensation) indicates advanced disease. Treatment is aimed at controlling symptoms, but liver transplant should be considered in patients with poor quality of life or liver failure. Ursodeoxycholic acid improves the LFTs, but no effect has been reported on disease progression.

Others causes of an obstructive pattern

- cholestatic variant of NAFLD
- hepatocellular carcinoma (see p. 183)
- metastatic liver disease
- pharmacological: antibiotics, androgens, anabolic steroids, OCP.

Mixed pattern

A mixed cholestatic/hepatitic pattern is common. Causes include sepsis, drug reactions, cholangitis, congestive cardiac failure, alcoholic liver disease.

Isolated rise in bilirubin

Gilbert's syndrome

Affects 5% of the population and is due to reduction in the function of UDP glucuronyltransferase, which results in slow conjugation of unconjugated bilirubin. It is asymptomatic and entirely benign.

The diagnosis is suggested if bilirubin is higher in fasting, as compared with postprandial, samples (as ketones displace unconjugated bilirubin from albumin). The diagnosis can be confirmed by a genetic TATA box sequence test.

Haemolysis

Patients generally present with symptoms of anaemia (breathlessness, fatigue or worsening angina) rather than with jaundice (see 'Haemolytic anaemia', p. 278). Treatment is tailored to the underlying cause.

Fulminant hepatic failure

This is said to be present when patients with severe acute liver injury develop encephalopathy within 8 weeks of their first symptoms, in the absence of pre-existing liver disease. The commonest causes in the UK are paracetamol poisoning (see 'Poisoning', p. 239) and acute viral hepatitis. Unless there is active bleeding, administration of clotting factors should be avoided as this negates the prognostic value of PT. If paracetamol toxicity is confirmed, or suspected, *N*-acetylcysteine should be administered without any delay (see 'Paracetamol', p. 239).

Criteria for liver unit referral

Early discussion with a liver unit is imperative, even if the patient does not meet official referral criteria. Criteria that are associated with a high mortality and mandate referral to a liver unit for intensive management and/or liver transplantation are as follows:

Paracetamol related

- arterial pH <7.3 or H^+ >50 following resuscitation
- PT >100 s, creatinine >200 and significant encephalopathy, hypoglycaemia.

Non-paracetamol related

- PT >100 s
- Three or more of: age <10 or >40 years; cause being non-A–E hepatitis, halothane or drug reaction; duration of jaundice before encephalopathy >7 days; PT >50 s; bilirubin >300.

Hepatic encephalopathy

This is a reversible neuropsychiatric syndrome that may complicate acute or chronic liver failure. The diagnosis is essentially clinical, with patients presenting with a variety of clinical features from life-threatening coma with cerebral oedema (almost exclusively seen in acute or fulminant liver failure) to subclinical, occult or mild confusion/disorientation. Examination findings may include asterixis (liver flap), hepatic fetor, brisk tendon reflexes, constructional apraxia and a slow mentation. Factors which precipitate encephalopathy include:

- increased protein load (e.g. ingestion of large protein meal or upper GI haemorrhage)
- decreased excretion of ammonia (e.g. renal failure or constipation)
- electrolyte disturbance (sometimes precipitated by diuretics)
- drugs (especially sedatives)
- sepsis.

The aim of treatment is to ensure adequate hydration with specific treatment targeted towards removal of precipitants.

Hepatocellular carcinoma

In Western society, hepatocellular carcinoma generally occurs as a complication of cirrhosis, and is more common in males than females. In cirrhotic patients, the risk of developing HCC is 2–3% per year. Although small tumours can be cured, HCC is rarely symptomatic at this stage and most patients present late. Therefore, all patients with cirrhosis should undergo screening every 6 months with liver ultrasound and serum α-fetoprotein measurement. However, patients with hepatitis B should be entered into a HCC surveillance programme after the age of 40, irrespective of their stage of liver disease.

NUTRITION

Approximately one-third of patients are malnourished on admission to UK hospitals. Despite this, formal nutritional assessment is commonly overlooked. Malnutrition leads to muscle weakness, poor wound healing and an increase in hospital mortality and length of stay. Therefore, it is essential that patients with risk factors are recognized early. These include:

- persistent nausea and vomiting
- malabsorption, e.g. IBD, bowel resection, pancreatic disease
- psychological disorders, e.g. anorexia nervosa
- an inability to chew or process food, e.g. elderly, previous stroke, ill-fitting dentures.

In addition, any process that results in increased energy requirements increases the risk of malnutrition, for example:

- sepsis, cancer, trauma, major burns, postoperative state
- excessive physical activity, e.g. marathon runners
- cardiac, respiratory, liver or renal failure.

Nutritional assessment

History and examination

Assess the patient's nutritional status and their nutritional needs:

- document any change in body weight and the time period over which this occurred
- ask about food intake and pay particular attention to food and meal-time preferences
- ask if the patient has any feeding difficulties, e.g. swallowing
- record the general functional capacity/activity level of the patient
- calculate body mass index (BMI); see below
- examine for loss of subcutaneous fat, muscle wasting or presence of oedema
- examine for evidence of underlying causal diseases.

BMI

BMI = weight/height^2 and is expressed in kg/m^2. A normal BMI is 18.5–24.9; 25.0–29.9 is overweight and over 30.0 defines obesity. A BMI of <18.5 suggests malnutrition.

Investigations

Patients with risk factors for malnutrition should have a nutritional screen which includes U&E, LFT (including albumin), FBC, coagulation screen, glucose, lipid profile, TFT, calcium, zinc, phosphate and vitamin B_{12} and folate. These should be repeated weekly in patients receiving supplementary feeding.

Further specific investigations should be tailored to symptoms. Specialist investigations of body mass or body fat/water compartments are usually reserved for research.

General management of nutrition

In simple cases, dietary advice and snacks between meals can improve nutritional intake. If this approach fails, or if there are more specific nutritional problems, e.g. swallowing dysfunction or malabsorption, some form of nutritional support may be necessary.

The support available ranges from high-calorie oral supplementation to more involved liquid enteral feeding regimes using a nasogastric/nasoduodenal/nasojejunal tube or an endoscopically placed gastrostomy/jejunostomy tube. The decision regarding the route of enteral feeding is generally based on the patient's wishes, their current medical state, duration of feeding and risk of aspiration.

Where long-term feeding is contemplated a percutaneous endoscopic gastrostomy (PEG) tube should be used. Regardless of the route chosen, all liquid enteral feeds must be introduced slowly, initially using water, followed by increasing volumes and concentrations of feed. Vomiting and diarrhoea may develop initially and close liaison with a dietician is required to calculate and monitor the correct feeding regime. Legal and ethical considerations may also emerge where a patient who is otherwise physically and mentally incapacitated can be kept alive with supportive feeding.

Occasionally, parenteral intravenous feeding using a central venous catheter may be required. However, this approach introduces a significant risk of both line infection and venous thrombosis. Electrolytes must be monitored daily during feeding.

Cachexia

Cachexia is a term often used to describe the weight loss experienced by patients with cancer. However, a similar process may occur in states of severe stress or organ dysfunction, e.g. burns, cardiac or respiratory failure.

Cachexia occurs because of an altered physiological state of metabolism. Resting energy consumption is increased and changes in body biochemistry occur. In particular, circulating levels of inflammatory cytokines increase, whereas those of vitamins (e.g. vitamin A) and trace elements (e.g. zinc) fall. In addition, there is increased protein turnover with muscle catabolism, reduced albumin synthesis and increased production of 'acute phase' hepatic proteins such as CRP and fibrinogen. Moreover, both lipid and carbohydrate metabolism are affected, with increased gluconeogenesis, increased lipid, glucose and fatty acid oxidation, and reduced lipogenesis.

Cachexia in cancer

This altered metabolic state appears to relate directly to the presence of the tumour, since it can return to normal when the tumour is removed. However, it does not always correlate with disease stage.

Since cachexia is an active physiological state, feeding alone is unhelpful. However, reduced food intake occurs in over 80% of patients with advanced cancer. Cancer-related anorexia is partly due to the development of altered taste sensation: patients prefer high levels of salt and sugar and often dislike red meat. In addition, nausea, constipation and depression play a part.

Although steroids (e.g. prednisolone 20 mg daily, reducing to 10 mg daily after 2 weeks) can improve mood and appetite, they do not have any effect on cachexia metabolism, or produce any improvement in muscle mass. Some studies suggest the use of megestrol acetate (160 mg twice daily) together with NSAIDs (such as ibuprofen 400 mg 8-hourly) or eicosapentaenoic acid may have some impact on the cachectic process. It is also important to treat nausea, constipation and pain.

Anorexia

In addition to cancer and other severe disease states, anorexia may develop as part of an eating disorder (anorexia nervosa). It usually occurs in adolescent girls and is suggested by weight loss of at least 25% of ideal body weight, avoidance of high-calorie foods, distorted body image, and amenorrhoea.

In addition to emaciation, physical changes may occur, such as development of lanugo hair, hypotension, bradycardia and peripheral cyanosis. Biochemical signs of vomiting or laxative abuse may be present. Psychotherapy is an essential part of management. Approx. 20% make a full recovery, but death occurs in 5% due to suicide or complications.

Obesity

Excess weight carries an increased risk of cardiorespiratory, cerebrovascular and malignant disease. A BMI >30 is used to define obesity, but the relationship between waist and hip circumference provides additional information regarding the pattern of adiposity. A waist measurement of >35 inches in women and >40 in men, or a waist to hip ratio of >0.8 in women and >0.95 in men reflects a centripetal pattern of body fat distribution, typical of the 'metabolic syndrome'.

In such patients, excess abdominal girth is associated with hyperlipidaemia, insulin resistance, glucose intolerance and a greater risk of diabetes, hypertension and cardiovascular disease. There may be a genetic predisposition to this syndrome; however, poor diet and a sedentary lifestyle undoubtedly contribute. Health risks can be modified by reducing fat and refined carbohydrate intake, increasing fibre intake and the amount and frequency of aerobic exercise.

HAEMATURIA AND URINARY RETENTION

Haematuria

Presentation

Haematuria can be frightening for patients and concerning for doctors. It usually stops spontaneously and most patients can be referred to a rapid access haematuria clinic. However, those with clot retention, symptomatic anaemia or shock require urgent assessment and admission to hospital. Up to 30% of patients with haematuria will have significant underlying pathology.

Investigation

Check FBC, U&E, LFT, calcium, phosphate, coagulation, urinalysis and MSU. Consider upper urinary tract imaging, e.g. renal ultrasound. Bladder ultrasound can be performed, although it has a low specificity, and cystoscopy is the gold standard test.

Fibreoptic cystoscopy can be performed using local anaesthetic gel, avoiding general anaesthesia in this predominantly elderly group. The procedure takes about 5 min, although the patient will be hospitalized for around 2 h.

If a tumour is identified at cystoscopy, regional or general anaesthesia can be arranged to permit deeper biopsies for tumour staging and to allow bi-manual palpation to assess the depth of spread.

Causes

The most common causes are urinary tract tumours, stones and infection. However, genital examination may also reveal a prolapse, vulvitis or ulcerating phimosis.

Tumours

See 'Bladder cancer', p. 367, and 'Renal cancer', p. 368.

Stones

Stones in the ureter or kidney cause haematuria, often in the absence of significant pain. Pain and fever suggest stone obstruction (see 'Renal causes of abdominal pain', p. 168).

Infection

Urethritis, cystitis or prostatitis can all cause haematuria, often associated with lower urinary symptoms, e.g. frequency, urgency, dysuria. Treat with antibiotics according to local policy.

Nephritis

Nephritis (see p. 215) can cause haematuria and should be suspected if cystoscopy and urinary tract imaging are negative. The patient should be referred to the renal team for further assessment.

Urinary retention

Presentation and investigation

Common features include failure to pass urine and a painful lower abdominal swelling. Consider other causes for these symptoms, including renal failure or a leaking abdominal aortic aneurysm; check for shock, a pulsatile mass, poor femoral pulses and a history of hypertension.

Acute retention is usually painful or uncomfortable and should be managed by catheterization. Patients can have significant prostatic enlargement without symptoms, or retention without palpable enlargement. Urinary retention may be precipitated by constipation, acute prostatitis, or a glass or two more alcohol than the individual's usual intake. If renal function is unimpaired and there is no pain, catheterization (with its risks of introducing infection) need not be immediate for the continent patient.

After any acute retention is treated, examine the prostate for size, hardness, irregularity and tenderness. Send a CSU for culture and arrange a KUB to look for subtrigonal calculi (which can trigger bladder symptoms, including retention), followed by bladder US.

Chronic retention often presents with frequency or incontinence, and the bladder can be painless, floppy, and difficult to palpate. Ultrasound can show retention of fluid and prompt the diagnosis.

Treatment of acute urinary retention

Treatment is normally by urethral catheterization (see 'Urinary catheterization', p. 34), although this may not be technically possible in all patients.

Where an experienced surgeon has failed to pass a urethral catheter, or such failure is anticipated from the patient's previous history, a suprapubic catheter should be inserted by a suitably experienced clinician (see p. 36).

After catheterization, monitor the volume of urine drained, as 1 L or more suggests chronic retention. Renal impairment requires hourly urine output measurement rather than 'free' drainage. If post-obstruction diuresis (of >200 mL/h) follows in a patient with renal impairment, intravenous fluids should be administered to match output and prevent pre-renal failure. Shock from sepsis or haemorrhage are not prevented by clamping catheters. A 'trial without catheter' can be arranged as an outpatient or inpatient. In patients with prostate enlargement, α-blockade is sometimes used to maximize success.

SECTION 2
Symptoms and related acute presentations

7 Endocrine, electrolyte and renal

DIABETES MELLITUS

Diabetes mellitus (DM) is a common disorder with a UK prevalence of approximately 4%. This figure is expected to increase as the population ages and obesity becomes more common.

Modes of presentation

Routine blood testing

This is now the commonest presentation. If a random plasma glucose is >14 mmol/L in a patient without hyperglycaemic symptoms, a fasting plasma glucose concentration should be checked. If this is >7 mmol/L, on two separate occasions, then the WHO criteria for diagnosis are met.

Symptoms

Polyuria with nocturia, thirst, balanitis or pruritus vulvae, weight loss, tiredness, visual upset and cramps should prompt urine testing for glucose and ketones and estimation of plasma glucose and electrolytes. A 2-h post-prandial plasma glucose >11 mmol/L confirms the diagnosis. Associated ketonuria and a venous bicarbonate <24 mmol/L suggest that insulin treatment will be necessary.

Ketoacidosis

Some 15–20% of patients with DM aged <15 years first present as medical emergencies with life-threatening ketoacidosis (see p. 189). This can of course present at any age and life-long insulin treatment is mandatory.

Incidental evidence of complications

Patients not known to have diabetes may present to optometrists for eye testing with signs of diabetic retinopathy. Similarly, patients with proteinuria, or symptoms and signs of peripheral neuropathy should be investigated for undiagnosed DM. If this is confirmed, it is likely that the patient has had untreated DM for over 10 years.

Management of established DM

DM is essentially a self-managed condition and most patients will have received advice from healthcare professionals at the time of diagnosis. This advice may be forgotten or ignored. Therefore, hospital admissions present valuable opportunities to re-engage patients and update their knowledge. Most hospitals have diabetes healthcare teams to support this. Primary healthcare teams also have a key role in the education of patients with DM, especially those not requiring insulin.

Dietary measures

Dietary discretion is the cornerstone of good glycaemic control, whether medication is used or not. Patients should be encouraged to look closely at food labelling; avoiding products that have glucose or sugar as one of the first three ingredients. A refresher consultation with a dietician can also be beneficial.

Monitoring

Three measures are available: urine glucose testing, blood glucose testing and glycated haemoglobin.

Urine glucose self-testing

This is not as popular as blood glucose self-testing because of concerns regarding accuracy and cleanliness. However, persistently negative fasting urine glucose, checked once or twice a week, is a reasonable target for patients with type 2 DM if they would rather test urine than blood.

Blood glucose testing

Bedside or self-testing with blood glucose strips and meters is now exceedingly common in hospitals and the community. Boehringer Mannheim made the most widely used strips in the 1970s and 1980s. Hence the term BM is still used to describe bedside or self-testing with blood glucose strips. If used properly, these are exceedingly accurate, except when the blood glucose concentration is very low (<3.0 mmol/L).

It is crucial that patients understand that blood testing should be used to facilitate treatment adjustment and the optimization of their glycaemic control.

Glycated haemoglobin

Glycated haemoglobin (HbA1c) is a measure of glycaemic control over the preceding 2 months. The HbA1c is the main tool used to assess longer-term glycaemic control, but should not be thought of as simply an average blood glucose. Keeping it below 7% minimizes future microvascular complications and reduces morbidity and mortality. It reflects compliance with treatment, including diet, but can also be affected by stressful life events. Time trends are as important as one-off measurements.

Medication

You should be aware of the indications, side-effects and potential problems related to each of the drug classes used in the management of DM.

Metformin

This drug is used as first-line therapy in type 2 diabetics who are overweight or obese. Diarrhoea is the most common side-effect, but can be minimized by taking the tablets with food. The starting dose is 500 mg once daily, titrated to a maximum daily dose of 1 g 8-hourly, aiming for a fasting plasma glucose of 4–6 mmol/L. Metformin can be used in combination with both a sulphonylurea and glitazone if necessary, but should be stopped if the eGFR falls below 60 mL/min.

Sulphonylureas

These include gliclazide and glibenclamide and they are often used in non-obese type 2 diabetics with hyperglycaemic symptoms. The starting dose should be low, but then titrated to achieve a fasting plasma glucose of 4–6 mmol/L, e.g. gliclazide (40 mg daily titrated to 160 mg twice daily). Symptomatic hypoglycaemia (<3.0 mmol/L) usually necessitates a dose reduction and is an indication for treatment withdrawal in elderly patients with renal impairment.

Glitazones

Both rosiglitazone and pioglitazone are insulin-sensitizing agents used in type 2 DM. These drugs are usually added to metformin or a sulphonylurea when fasting plasma glucose levels remain >6 mmol/L at the maximum tolerated dosage. Glitazones should be started in low dose and, because it takes 6 weeks for the drug to achieve its optimal effect, dose titration should not be considered before then.

Glitazones should be avoided in patients with heart disease. Fluid retention is common. Liver function tests may become abnormal and should be monitored in the early stages of therapy.

Insulins

There are a variety of insulins available for use in the UK. These are life-saving treatments in type 1 diabetes, although more patients with type 2 diabetes are having insulin added to their regime to achieve better glycaemic control.

The choice of insulin for each patient is influenced partly by patient preference and partly by the duration of action. The normal daily starting dose of subcutaneous insulin in type 1 DM is 0.5 units/kg with a usual maintenance dose of 0.8 units/kg. Twice-daily dosing of an intermediate-acting insulin is commonly used, e.g. Mixtard 30®. Basal-bolus regimes combine a once-daily dose of long-acting insulin, e.g. Lantus®, and three pre-prandial doses of short-acting insulin, e.g. Novorapid®. In type 2 DM, patients are insulin resistant and may require higher doses.

Hypoglycaemia, both symptomatic and asymptomatic, is the most common side-effect and is an indication for specialist diabetic review. In general terms, insulin should never be stopped completely in patients with type 1 diabetes because of the risk of life-threatening ketoacidosis.

Complications of DM

Patients with type 1 and 2 DM have difficulty controlling blood glucose levels due to insulin deficiency and insulin resistance, respectively. This difficulty is exacerbated during intercurrent illness when stress-related insulin resistance develops, insulin doses may be omitted and the patient may be unable to eat and drink normally due to anorexia, nausea, vomiting or altered consciousness.

Diabetic ketoacidosis (DKA)

Type 1 diabetics are at risk of developing life-threatening ketoacidosis if insulin is omitted, or if insulin dosage is not increased during intercurrent illness. Patients with type 2 diabetes do not generally develop DKA, even if they have been started on regular insulin therapy because of poor glycaemia control.

Presentation

Patients may present with features of an intercurrent illness. Hyperglycaemic symptoms (polyuria, polydipsia) are often prominent, in addition to vomiting (due to gastroparesis), hyperventilation (Kussmaul's, reflecting acidosis), significant dehydration and confusion. Abdominal pain is present in approximately 10% and is particularly common in children.

Assessment

An accurate assessment of intravascular volume is essential (see 'Shock and fluid balance', p. 250). Smell the patient's breath for the 'sweet' odour of ketones. Look for evidence of a precipitating infection or other illness, e.g. chest or urine infection, MI, recent CVA. Request the following investigations in all patients with suspected DKA, but do not delay management; see below:

- FBC and Coag: a stress-related leucocytosis may occur in the absence of infection
- U&E and LFT: note Na^+, K^+ and renal function; remember that severe hyperglycaemia produces a technical error in Na^+ measurement; corrected Na^+ = measured $Na^+ + 1.6 \times$ ([plasma glucose (mmol/L) − 5.5]/5.5)

- glucose: may not be very high; see below
- ABG: determine the severity of any acidosis; severe cases (pH<7) should have early senior input
- urinalysis: ketones should be strongly positive; weak positive may reflect recent starvation
- ECG: look for evidence of myocardial infarction or arrhythmias, the latter may reflect electrolyte abnormalities; treat as per 'Arrhythmias', p. 132
- septic screen: CRP, blood cultures, CXR and urine cultures; other investigations should be directed by symptoms
- amylase: acute pancreatitis can accompany DKA in around 10%; amylase may be slightly elevated without pancreatitis.

Diagnosis

The diagnosis of DKA requires evidence of both:

- acidosis: as indicated by an elevated arterial hydrogen ion concentration (>50 nmol/L) or reduced arterial blood pH (<7.3), or a reduced venous bicarbonate (<15 mmol/L)
- ketosis: on either urinalysis or blood testing; beware other causes of acidosis in patients with diabetes, including lactic acidosis and salicylate poisoning.

Hyperglycaemia is very likely to be present, but is not essential for the diagnosis. DKA can occur with blood sugars as low as 10 mmol/L and the blood sugar may also be lowered if the patient has suspected the diagnosis themselves and administered a bolus of subcutaneous insulin recently. However, this will be insufficient to reverse the acidosis because of profound dehydration.

Management

The cornerstones of DKA management are intravenous fluid rehydration, insulin therapy and potassium replacement.

Fluids

Osmotic diuresis and insensible losses, largely related to hyperventilation, result in significant intravascular depletion; the average fluid deficit in DKA is around 10% of total body water (3–6 L). This should be replaced over the first 24 h; an appropriate regime is as follows:

- start with normal saline and switch to 5% dextrose once blood glucose falls below 12 mmol/L
- if the blood glucose rises after this switch, do not change back to saline; simply adjust the dose of insulin
- give the first and second litres of IV fluid over 1 h, the third litre over 2 h and all subsequent litres over 4 h, taking into consideration the risks of fluid overload and clinical response.

Insulin

Start an infusion of soluble insulin, e.g. 50 IU of Actrapid® insulin added to 50 mL of normal saline, as soon as the diagnosis is confirmed. An appropriate insulin prescription is provided in Table 7.1. This can be modified according to clinical response; aim for a fall in blood glucose of 3–6 mmol/L per hour. More rapid correction of blood glucose can lead to cerebral oedema.

Improvement of glycaemic control should be accompanied by an improvement in acidosis. Intravenous insulin should be continued until the patient is eating and drinking normally and the acidosis and ketosis have resolved; SC insulin can then be restarted or introduced.

Potassium

All patients with DKA will be significantly K^+ depleted. Acidosis promotes H^+/K^+ exchange in the kidney and loss of the K^+ in the urine; K^+ is also lost during vomiting. Despite this, intravascular K^+ may appear normal or elevated initially. This

Table 7.1 An example insulin prescription for use in DKA

Blood glucose (mmol/L)	Insulin infusion rate (units/h)
>12	6
8.1–12	3 and change IV fluid to 5% dextrose
4.1–8	2
2.1–4	1 and contact doctor
<2	Stop and contact doctor

reflects profound dehydration and catabolism of protein and glycogen stores, with or without renal impairment. K^+ replacement should be guided by serum electrolytes (Table 7.2). Omit K^+ from the first, rapidly infused, litre of normal saline, until serum levels are known.

Table 7.2 K^+ replacement in DKA

Serum K^+ (mmol/L)	Amount of KCl (mmol/L) to add to each litre
>5.0	0
3.5–5	20
<3.5	40

Other general measures

- regular monitoring: DKA is a medical emergency and the patient should be transferred to the HDU, if available
- venous access: large-bore venous access should be obtained; if peripheral access is poor (common if recurrent admissions with DKA), the patient is shocked or has co-existing cardiac disease, consider whether a central line is required
- urinary catheter: if the patient is oliguric or has renal impairment, is old or has another disease that could make fluid overload a problem, consider inserting a urinary catheter and measuring hourly urine volumes
- conscious level: monitor GCS (see 'GCS', p. 11)
- anticoagulation: dehydration increases blood viscosity, and sepsis or other acute illness will result in fibrinolysis; all patients with DKA should receive prophylactic doses of LMWH, e.g. enoxaparin 40 mg SC (reduce to 20 mg if eGFR <60 mL/min)
- antiemetics: gastroparesis is common; give parenteral antiemetics, e.g. metoclopramide 10 mg 8-hourly, and keep the patient NBM for the first 6 h; consider the use of a NG tube if vomiting is persistent or conscious level is reduced
- antibiotics: should be given if there is evidence of infection; remember that a leucocytosis is common and does not necessarily reflect sepsis.

Monitoring

Rapid normalization of biochemistry, particularly sodium and glucose, can be dangerous. Therefore, careful monitoring is essential:

- check U&E, including venous bicarbonate, at baseline and again at 1, 2, 4, 6 and 12 h
- capillary blood glucose, using BM strips, should be measured hourly
- laboratory glucose should be measured 4-hourly
- an ABG should be checked at baseline, but needs to be checked again only if the patient's clinical condition appears to be worsening.

Hyperosmolar non-ketotic coma

HONC occurs in type 2 diabetics; patients are often elderly and the mortality is much higher that than of DKA (approx. 40%). Blood glucose rises slowly and is often extremely high (>50 mmol/L). Severe dehydration and pre-renal failure are common, but ketoacidosis does not occur. Mortality correlates best with serum osmolality and there is a high frequency of thrombotic complications.

Presentation

The patient is usually known to have type 2 DM and will often present with confusion, polyuria, polydipsia and severe dehydration. Thrombotic complications (e.g. CVA, MI, DVT) and seizures are less common.

Diagnosis

Secured by significant hyperglycaemia in association with a calculated plasma osmolality >350 mmol/kg. Calculated osmolality = [2 × (calculated Na^+ + K^+) + urea + glucose]. For calculated Na^+, see p. 189.

Assessment

Look for evidence of precipitating infection or thrombotic complications, including a full neurological assessment; record the GCS. Check the following:

- glucose: usually >50 mmol/L
- U&E and LFT: remember hyperglycaemia will interfere with Na^+ measurement; see DKA section above for guidance on calculating corrected Na^+ concentration; otherwise, Na^+ may be underestimated, producing pseudohyponatraemia or masking significant hypernatraemia associated with dehydration
- calculate serum osmolality
- ABGs and urinalysis: ketoacidosis will not be present; lactic acidosis, a poor prognostic marker, may be present if the patient is grossly volume deplete or in renal failure
- FBC and Coag: leucocytosis may be present in the absence of infection
- ECG: look for evidence of myocardial infarction or arrhythmias; the latter may reflect electrolyte abnormalities (see 'Arrhythmias', p. 132)
- CXR
- septic screen, including CRP, blood and urine cultures; other cultures should be dictated by symptoms.

Management

The most important measures are cautious IV fluid rehydration, IV insulin therapy and thrombosis prophylaxis. In contrast to DKA, blood glucose should be normalized very slowly.

Fluids

The average fluid deficit is 8–10 L. Aim to replace this over 2–3 days. Avoid fluid overload, and in elderly patients or those with a history of cardiac disease consider inserting a central venous line to guide fluid prescription.

An appropriate IV fluid regime is as follows: give the first litre over 1 h, the second and third over 2 h and all subsequent litres over 6 h, until rehydrated. Also take into consideration the risk of fluid overload and the clinical response. If the plasma Na^+ concentration is >160 mmol/L, consider using 0.45% saline for the first 3 L. Switch to 5% dextrose once the blood glucose is <15 mmol/L.

Insulin

Insulin prescription should aim to reverse hyperglycaemia slowly; therefore use a modified version of the DKA protocol, as provided in Table 7.3. Insulin can be stopped and oral hypoglycaemic agents restarted, or introduced, once the patient is eating and drinking again.

Table 7.3 An example insulin prescription for use in HONC

Blood glucose (mmol/L)	Insulin infusion rate (units/h)
>22	6
17.1–22	4
15.1–17	3
11.1–15	3 and change fluid to 5% dextrose
7.1–11	2
4–7	1
<4	Stop and contact doctor

Potassium

Potassium will tend to fall as insulin moves it into cells. Replace K^+ as per management of DKA (Table 7.2).

Other measures

As indicated above, all patients should receive thrombosis prophylaxis, e.g. enoxaparin (40mg SC daily; use 20mg if eGFR <60mL/min). Vomiting is common: manage with parenteral antiemetics, e.g. metoclopramide (10mg 8-hourly). Where there is persistent vomiting, consider inserting a NG tube. Keep NBM for at least 6h. Antibiotics should be given if there is evidence of infection. If there is confusion or a reduced GCS that does not improve with therapy, consider a CT brain scan to look for evidence of a recent CVA.

Hypoglycaemia

Hypoglycaemia is common in diabetics receiving insulin. Symptoms occur when the blood glucose falls below 3.0mmol/L and are commonly categorized into:

- adrenergic symptoms: sweating, tachycardia, pallor and hunger
- neuroglycopaenic symptoms: morning headache, incoordination, inappropriate behaviour, confusion and coma.

Most patients will be able to easily recognize mild hypoglycaemia and reverse it by taking a sweet drink or item of food. If more severe hypoglycaemia develops despite this, or the patient has a poor awareness of hypoglycaemia, increasing neuroglycopenia will make it less likely that the patient will be able to take appropriate steps to manage the problem.

Without prompt intervention irreversible cognitive impairment can result. Therefore, family members or healthcare professionals will be required to administer mucosal glucose solutions, e.g. Hypostop®, or glucagon (SC, IM or IV). Where available, e.g. in hospitalized patients, an IV bolus of 50mL of 20% dextrose should be given. Fifty per cent dextrose should be avoided because of the risk of extravasation-associated skin necrosis.

Common reasons for hypoglycaemia include poor carbohydrate intake, excessive insulin or unaccustomed exercise. The onset of renal impairment, hypothyroidism or hypopituitarism should also be considered.

Following a significant episode of hypoglycaemia the patient and healthcare team should attempt to modify any factors that contributed to the event. This might include withdrawal of a long-acting sulphonylurea in an elderly patient, or a reduction in the dose of subcutaneous insulin in a young type 1 patient.

Microvascular complications

These include diabetic retinopathy, nephropathy and neuropathy which all result from a diffuse microvascular injury affecting the retina, glomerulus and intraneural capillaries, respectively. The hallmark of this process is thickening of the capillary basement membrane and increased vascular permeability. The risk of developing microvascular complications is closely related to inadequate glycaemic control.

Diabetic retinopathy

This represents a common cause of adult blindness in developed countries. Patients are often asymptomatic until the condition is advanced or maculopathy develops. Therefore, regular screening by either fundoscopy or retinal photography is essential as early retinal photocoagulation is an effective treatment; see below. Diabetic retinopathy is classified as follows:

- background (or non-proliferative): venous dilatation and microaneurysms, blot haemorrhages and exudates (leakage of plasma from abnormal capillaries)
- pre-proliferative: venous beading and increased tortuosity (indicating capillary non-perfusion), clusters of microaneurysms, multiple cotton wool spots (these are important to identify, being representative of areas of retinal ischaemia due to arteriolar occlusions) and macular, or perimacular, exudates or haemorrhages
- proliferative: visible new vessel formation on the retina (neovascularization); may be associated with pre-retinal haemorrhage, gliosis (deposition of fibrous tissue anterior to the retina) and retinal detachment
- maculopathy: exudates, haemorrhage, oedema or cotton wool spots on, or around, the macula.

The prognosis and need for specialist referral is dependent on the stage and extent of the process (Table 7.4). Retinal photocoagulation is indicated for severe non-proliferative retinopathy and all proliferative retinopathies. This has been shown to reduce visual loss by 85% (reduced to 50% if maculopathy present).

Table 7.4 Prognosis and indication for specialist referral in diabetic retinopathy

Type	Prognosis	Management
Background	No immediate threat to sight	Optimize glycaemic, BP and lipid control and other risk factors, e.g. smoking, alcohol; fundoscopy surveillance every 6 months; refer if rapid progression
Pre-proliferative	Sight-threatening	Optimize risk factors and refer; avoid rapidly lowering blood glucose as this may worsen retinopathy
Proliferative	Sight-threatening	Optimize risk factors and refer
Maculopathy	Sight-threatening	Optimize risk factors and refer

Diabetic nephropathy

This is a common cause of end-stage renal failure (ESRF). Renal abnormalities progress from thickening of the glomerular basement membrane and expansion of matrix material in the mesangium to nodular deposits in the glomeruli and eventual glomerulosclerosis and heavy proteinuria. The chance of a type 1 diabetic developing nephropathy over 20 years is approximately 30%. Particular risk factors include poor glycaemic control, long duration of diabetes, associated hypertension, ethnicity (more common in Asians) and the presence of other microvascular complications.

Treatment of established nephropathy is often unrewarding and frequently requires renal replacement therapy. Therefore, screening and prevention, or at least amelioration, are essential. Microalbuminuria (urinary albumin 3–30 mg/24 h) is an important predictor of progression to diabetic nephropathy, especially in type 1 diabetics in the first 10 years following diagnosis. After this, and in type 2 diabetics (who tend to be older), microalbuminuria may be explained by other vascular diseases. Progression to albuminuria (urinary albumin 30–300 mg/24 h), especially if associated with hypertension, is likely to reflect diabetic nephropathy.

The following should be considered in patients with progressive proteinuria or established diabetic nephropathy:

- tight glycaemic, BP and lipid control
- institution of either an ACE inhibitor or angiotensin II receptor antagonist, whether the patient is hypertensive or not, renal function permitting (both have been shown to delay the development of nephropathy)
- discontinuation of metformin once serum creatinine >150 mmol/L, due to an increased risk of lactic acidosis
- changing long-acting sulphonylureas, e.g. glibenclamide, to short-acting agents, e.g. gliclazide, to reduce the risk of hypoglycaemia due to poor clearance
- renal replacement therapy for ESRF: may be of benefit earlier on in diabetic nephropathy, as compared with other conditions
- renal transplantation: there is rarely enough time for nephropathy to recur in the grafted kidney; can be combined with pancreatic transplantation, but organ supply is limited.

Diabetic neuropathy

This affects 30% of diabetics and, like other microvascular complications, is more likely in patients with poor glycaemic control and a long history of diabetes. Pathological features include axonal degeneration and demyelination, thickening of the basement membrane and thrombosis in intraneural capillary blood vessels. The most frequent clinical manifestations are found in the peripheral nervous system, resulting in neuropathic phenotypes affecting sensory, motor and autonomic nerves.

Symmetrical sensory polyneuropathy

Frequently asymptomatic, but may present with paraesthesiae in the feet, or less commonly hands, pain in the legs or a burning sensation in the feet. The earliest clinical sign is often diminished vibration sense distally, followed by glove and stocking sensory loss and absent reflexes. Overt muscle weakness, wasting and motor dysfunction are rare. A diffuse small-fibre neuropathy may result in altered pain and temperature sensation and can result in foot ulcers and Charcot arthropathy.

Treatment involves tight glycaemic control with insulin and symptomatic management. Therapeutic options include oral amitriptyline, gabapentin, carbamazepine or opiate analgesics, topical capsaicin and IV lidocaine.

Asymmetrical motor neuropathy

This presents with severe, painful and progressive wasting of the proximal muscles of the limbs, usually the legs. Sometimes referred to as diabetic amyotrophy, it is thought to reflect acute infarction of the lower motor neurones of the lumbosacral plexus. CSF protein may be raised. Treatment is largely supportive, using similar therapies to those used in sensory neuropathies, and recovery usually occurs within 1 year. However, some patients may be left with a permanent disability.

Mononeuropathy

This most commonly affects the 3rd and 6th cranial nerves and the femoral and sciatic nerves. The onset is acute, but recovery is common and often spontaneous. Presentation involving more than one nerve is termed mononeuritis multiplex.

Autonomic neuropathy

This is less clearly correlated with glycaemic control and is an ominous sign; 30–50% of patients will be dead within 10 years of developing autonomic neuropathy, commonly due to sudden cardiac arrest. Clinical features depend upon the visceral system affected but include:

- cardiovascular: postural hypotension, resting tachycardia
- gastrointestinal: dysphagia due to oesophageal dysmotility, gastroparesis, constipation
- genitourinary: urinary incontinence, atonic bladder, erectile dysfunction
- sudomotor: gustatory sweating, anhidrosis
- pupillary: diminished pupil size, delayed or absent light reflex.

Macrovascular complications

These are responsible for significant morbidity and most of the excess mortality associated with diabetes mellitus; 70% of all deaths in diabetic patients occur because of myocardial infarction or stroke. The pathogenesis of macrovascular disease is similar to that in non-diabetic patients, but atherosclerosis occurs prematurely and is more aggressive. The influence of other risk factors, e.g. smoking, is also amplified in diabetes.

Randomized controlled trials have shown that the risk of macrovascular complications can be reduced by tight BP control (<140/80 mmHg) and treatment with both a statin for hyperlipidaemia and an ACE inhibitor. Coronary, cerebrovascular and peripheral arterial disease should be treated as they are in non-diabetic patients. There is some evidence that tight glycaemic control (using an IV insulin infusion) immediately after myocardial infarction improves long-term outcome, but this has yet to be proven in large studies.

Managing DM in hospital inpatients

Nutrition

Nutrition and energy delivery can become complicated in diabetic patients who are unable to eat as a result of altered consciousness, anorexia, or specific gastrointestinal pathology. 500 mL 10% dextrose intravenously will provide 50 g of carbohydrate and, if given 6-hourly, will supply 200 g daily and avoid ketosis in type 1 diabetics. In prolonged postoperative catabolic states, protein and fat intake will also need to supplemented, using parenteral nutrition if the gut cannot be used.

Monitoring

Additional blood glucose monitoring is essential in diabetic patients in hospital. It will often be your responsibility to determine the frequency of these and the target blood glucose. These should be tailored to the clinical situation, for example:

- a pregnant type 1 diabetic in labour will require hourly blood glucose monitoring to allow adjustment of an IV insulin infusion; this would aim to maintain blood glucose around 4 mmol/L, thus avoiding neonatal hypoglycaemia
- an elderly type 2 diabetic on metformin, convalescing after total hip replacement, might only need a blood glucose checked daily.

Alterations in diabetic control

Hyperglycaemia

Mild hyperglycaemia is common in diabetic and non-diabetic patients during any acute illness. This is because conditions such as myocardial infarction, sepsis or trauma result in insulin resistance and 'stress hyperglycaemia'. If the glycaemia is mild, short-lived and asymptomatic, it is reasonable simply to observe the situation and regularly monitor blood glucose, electrolytes and urinalysis.

If the patient is symptomatic, or the illness is likely to be prolonged, the dose of insulin or oral hypoglycaemic agent should be increased. In certain severe illnesses, including myocardial infarction and multi-organ failure, tight control of blood glucose levels has been shown to reduce mortality and a sliding scale insulin infusion is often used.

Hypoglycaemia

Hypoglycaemia may also develop in diabetics with intercurrent illnesses. It is most commonly due to nausea, vomiting or other GI symptoms that preclude patients from eating normally. Management is as described on p. 193, but where eating patterns are not normal the dose of insulin or oral hypoglycaemics may have to be reduced or a sliding-scale insulin infusion started until the patient can eat normally.

Fasting for a procedure

Hospital inpatients are commonly required to fast for diagnostic procedures, surgery, or because of GI pathology. This poses particular problems for diabetics who must be switched onto an IV infusion of soluble, short-acting insulin and dextrose. Use the sliding-scale insulin prescription, suggested earlier for use in HONC, in Table 7.3, p. 193. This should be completed by the prescribing doctor and placed with the patient's cardex. The initial insulin dose per hour can be determined as follows:

- type 1 diabetes: simply sum the total subcutaneous insulin dose (units) and divide by 24 (hours)
- type 2 diabetes: see Table 7.5 for the approximate insulin equivalence for oral agents; if the patient takes additional subcutaneous insulin, add the total daily insulin dose to the equivalence figure and divide by 24 (hours).

Table 7.5 Approximate insulin equivalence for oral agents

Agent and dose	Equivalent insulin dose
Metformin 500 mg	4 IU
Gliclazide 80 mg	6 IU
Rosiglitazone 4 mg	5 IU

General anaesthesia

Intravenous 10% dextrose is used ± a short-acting soluble insulin intravenously. This can be stopped and the usual diabetes regime restarted once the patient has eaten their first meal postoperatively. Before elective surgery, diabetic control should be optimized via the surgical pre-assessment clinic and liaison with the diabetes team.

THYROID AND ADRENAL PROBLEMS

Thyroid disorders

Thyroid disorders may present with classical biochemical symptoms, localized symptoms due to neck swelling (goitre) or direct complications of thyroid hormone imbalance. Occasionally, they may be discovered incidentally when thyroid function tests are included in 'routine' blood tests done for other reasons.

History

Important features in the history include:

- symptoms of hypothyroidism: tiredness, weight gain, dry skin, hair loss, constipation, hoarseness, cold intolerance, symptoms related to bradycardia, menorrhagia, infertility, depression

- symptoms of hyperthyroidism: agitation, weight loss, diarrhoea, heat intolerance, palpitation, weakness, dyspnoea, amenorrhoea, loss of libido
- neck swelling: note first appearance and change in size and any associated pain, change in voice
- family and drug history, e.g. amiodarone, lithium
- recent pregnancy, thyroid surgery
- previous neck irradiation.

Examination

- general: weight, hair for thinning and dryness, agitation or mental slowness
- hands: skin for dryness or sweating, tremor, pulse, thyroid acropachy (clubbing in association with thyroid disease)
- eyes: proptosis, exophthalmos, lid retraction and lid lag, gaze palsies, conjunctival irritation
- legs: pretibial myxoedema, proximal myopathy, hyper-reflexia or delayed relaxation of reflexes, peripheral neuropathy
- neck: inspect while swallowing for goitre; palpate for diffuse enlargement or a solitary nodule; check for tenderness and lymphadenopathy (increases the chance of thyroid malignancy); percuss for retrosternal goitre; auscultate for a bruit.

Investigations

Thyroid function tests

This usually means TSH and T4. T3 can be requested in specific circumstances, e.g. suspected isolated T3 toxicosis, but often requires specialist input. TFT will reveal one of three patterns and any abnormality should be confirmed by a second test, given the likelihood of long-term medical therapy or ablative treatment.

- euthyroid (both free T4 and TSH are normal)
- hyperthyroid (free T4 is elevated; primary if TSH suppressed, secondary if TSH raised)
- hypothyroid (free T4 is low; primary if TSH raised, secondary if TSH low or normal).

Further investigations are rarely required in patients with hypothyroidism, but are necessary in hyperthyroidism to identify the underlying aetiology and potential complications. These may include:

Blood tests

Thyroid peroxidase (TPO) antibodies and TSH receptor antibodies are likely to be positive in patients with Graves' disease.

ECG

Will reveal atrial fibrillation in 10–40% of patients presenting with hyperthyroidism; incidence increases with age and male sex.

Uptake studies

These identify sites of increased iodine uptake within the thyroid gland and are used in hyperthyroid patients to differentiate toxic adenomas (single focus) from toxic multinodular goitre (several distinct foci) and Graves' disease (diffusely enhancing). Radio-iodine has been largely superseded by 99m-technetium scintigraphy which is quicker, uses a lower radiation dose and yields a higher-resolution image.

Radiology

If a mass is suspected in the gland, ultrasound and CT scanning should be considered.

Biopsy

Fine needle aspiration (FNA), or core tissue biopsy, of any mass identified can be performed under ultrasound guidance.

Hypothyroidism

Aetiology

- without goitre: most likely due to primary atrophic hypothyroidism or acquired hypothyroidism, e.g. secondary to previous thyroid surgery or radio-iodine treatment
- with goitre: most likely due to Hashimoto's thyroiditis (autoimmune condition, thyroid peroxidase (TPO) antibodies often strongly positive) or lithium-induced goitre.

Treatment

Regardless of the cause, treatment is with levothyroxine in a dose titrated to keep free T4 and TSH in the middle of the local laboratory range. Dose adjustments should not be made at intervals of <3 weeks. In elderly patients and those with cardiac disease, the starting dose of levothyroxine should be low, e.g. 25 or 50 μg; higher doses may precipitate angina. In patients with suspected hypopituitarism, hypothyroidism should not be treated until any adrenal dysfunction has been corrected; see p. 200.

In Hashimoto's thyroiditis, the goitre usually shrinks as the dose of levothyroxine increases. Treatment with oral prednisolone can expedite this, but is rarely required. Lithium-induced goitre regresses when lithium is stopped.

Hyperthyroidism

This is most likely due to Graves' disease (76%), toxic multinodular goitre (14%) or viral (de Quervain's) thyroiditis (3%).

Graves' disease

There are often florid thyrotoxic symptoms; however, older patients may present with atrial fibrillation or weight loss alone. There may be an associated goitre (± a bruit) and other features, including ophthalmopathy. Thyroid peroxidase (TPO) antibodies and TSH receptor antibodies are likely to be positive. There is a high 4-h radio-iodine uptake.

Treatment is with carbimazole in reducing doses, which offers a 40% chance of remission after 18 months. A 'block and replace' regime (high-dose carbimazole with later added levothyroxine) is an alternative with similar results. Radio-iodine (^{131}I) can be used for relapse. However, there is a 75% chance that the patient will develop hypothyroidism within 25 years. In younger patients, near total thyroidectomy with thyroxine replacement, as necessary, is an alternative. Propranolol (40 mg 6-hourly) can be used to control the tachycardia, unless contraindicated.

Toxic multinodular goitre

Patients are often only intermittently thyrotoxic. Thyroid antibodies are rarely present and the 4-h radio-iodine uptake is normal. Treatment with low-dose carbimazole is often successful, but radio-iodine is an effective alternative. Subsequent hypothyroidism can occur, but is unusual. In some patients the goitre may be predominantly retrosternal.

Viral thyroiditis

This is a painful goitre with often positive inflammatory markers and very low 4-h radio-iodine uptake. Patients will initially be hyperthyroid, later becoming hypothyroid, before thyroid function recovers.

Management is with non-steroidal anti-inflammatories and β-blockers for hyperthyroid symptoms. TFT must be carefully monitored as levothyroxine may be necessary in the hypothyroid phase.

Goitre

There are numerous causes of thyroid swelling. It is important to determine if the goitre is diffuse, or if there is a solitary thyroid nodule. TFT will reveal if there is any associated biochemical upset. Causes of a diffuse goitre include:

- simple goitre: often seen between ages 15–25 or during pregnancy; TFT normal; usually regresses spontaneously
- thyroid cyst, treated conservatively unless airway threatened
- toxic multinodular goitre (see p. 199)
- autoimmune (Hashimoto's thyroiditis; see p. 199).

Solitary thyroid nodules, identified by clinical examination, imaging or uptake studies are likely to require FNA to exclude malignancy. Causes of a solitary nodule include:

- thyroid adenoma: identified by uptake studies; treatment with radio-iodine is effective
- thyroid carcinoma: papillary, follicular, medullary or anaplastic
- thyroid lymphoma.

Thyroid malignancy is commonly treated by surgery ± radiotherapy or chemotherapy, depending on tissue type. Following this, life-long replacement therapy with levothyroxine is usually required.

Adrenal gland disorders

Each adrenal gland is really three glands in one:

- central adrenal medulla: secretes catecholamines and functions as part of the sympathetic nervous system
- surrounding adrenal cortex: secretes cortisol and androgens and functions as part of the hypothalamic–pituitary system
- outermost zona glomerulosa: secretes aldosterone under the influence of the renin–aldosterone system.

Hypersecretory adrenal gland disorders

These can be classified using the above anatomical boundaries.

Adrenal medulla

Phaeochromocytoma

This is extremely rare. Classical features include episodic hypertension and paroxysms of palpitations, pallor, sweats, headache and severe anxiety (so-called angor animi). Patients may also present with complications such as MI, left ventricular hypertrophy, accelerated-phase hypertension or associated syndromes, e.g. von Hippel–Lindau, MEN type 2, neurofibromatosis.

The diagnosis is confirmed by elevated metadrenalines (metabolites of adrenaline and noradrenaline) on a 24-h urine collection. Beware of false negatives as hormone surges are paroxysmal. Tumours can be localized by MRI, CT or scintigraphy using meta-iodo-benzyl-guanidine (MIBG). The rule of 10s applies: 10% are extra-adrenal, 10% are malignant, 10% familial.

Management is by surgical resection, after at least 6 weeks of medical treatment. A non-competitive α-blocker, e.g. phenoxybenzamine, should be started first followed by a β-blocker. Never start the β-blocker first as unopposed α-blockade can lead to vasoconstriction and severe hypertension.

Adrenal cortex

Cushing's syndrome

This results from excessive stimulation of glucocorticoid receptors. The commonest cause is iatrogenic Cushing's syndrome due to exogenous steroids although there are other causes:

- ACTH-dependent: pituitary tumour secreting ACTH (Cushing's disease); ectopic ACTH syndrome (e.g. lung cancer); iatrogenic (ACTH therapy)
- non-ACTH-dependent: iatrogenic (exogenous steroid administration); adrenal adenoma or carcinoma
- pseudo-Cushing's: results from cortisol excess secondary to another illness, e.g. alcohol excess, depression, obesity.

Clinical features include hypertension, myopathy, abdominal striae, acne, osteoporosis and the classical appearance of a moon face, buffalo hump and central obesity.

An accurate drug and alcohol history is essential. Cushing's syndrome is confirmed by an elevated 24-h urinary free cortisol and a positive low-dose dexamethasone suppression test (failure to suppress plasma cortisol to <60nmol/L). In situations other than pseudo-Cushing's, plasma ACTH will then reliably differentiate between ACTH-dependent and ACTH-independent causes. In the latter, CT scanning should be performed; in the former, pituitary MRI should be requested. If a pituitary tumour (Cushing's disease) is not demonstrated, ectopic sources of ACTH should be sought, e.g. lung and other malignancies.

Medical therapy can reduce the effects of Cushing's syndrome, e.g. metyrapone and ketoconazole inhibit corticosteroid synthesis, but definitive treatment depends on the underlying cause:

- iatrogenic Cushing's syndrome can be treated by drug withdrawal, where possible
- Cushing's disease is treated by transphenoidal resection of the responsible pituitary adenoma
- adrenal tumours are treated by laparoscopic resection, tumour bed irradiation and use of the adrenolytic drug mitotane ± chemotherapy
- ectopic ACTH secreting tumours should be resected if possible.

Zona glomerulosa

Conn's syndrome

This describes a syndrome of hypertension and hypokalaemia, due to secretion of aldosterone from an adrenal adenoma. It is an exceedingly rare cause of hypertension (approx. 0.5%), but refractory hypertension, presentation at a young age and hypokalaemia should prompt measurement of renin (will be low) and aldosterone (will be high) levels. Conn's adenoma can be differentiated from bilateral adrenal hyperplasia (found in up to 5% of patients with hypertension) by measuring the response to furosemide administration, or standing up. In Conn's, aldosterone levels will not rise further. The treatment of Conn's syndrome is surgical resection.

Adrenal insufficiency

This results in inadequate secretion of some or all of the hormone products of the adrenal glands. Symptoms and signs are extremely variable and detection requires a high index of suspicion. Classical presentations include:

- chronic symptoms of fatigue and abdominal pain with hypotension and hyponatraemia
- adrenal crisis; see overleaf.

The commonest cause is ACTH deficiency (secondary adrenal failure), due to abrupt withdrawal of exogenous steroids or the mass effect of a pituitary tumour. Addison's disease (primary adrenal failure) may be associated with increased buccal and skin pigmentation, reflecting stimulation of melanocyte stimulating hormone receptors by high levels of ACTH. Other causes of primary adrenal failure include tuberculous disease (look for adrenal calcification on AXR), congenital adrenal hyperplasia and the use of certain drugs, e.g. metyrapone, ketoconazole and etomidate.

Random plasma cortisol levels may be within the normal range during an acute illness and are not a reliable indicator of adrenal function. Therefore, the diagnosis must be confirmed by a short Synacthen test (SST), which can be performed at any time of the day:

- insert a butterfly needle or venous cannula
- using this, take a blood sample and administer 250 µg $ACTH_{1-24}$ (Synacthen) IM
- wait 30 min and take a second sample from the cannula
- send the samples taken at 0 and 30 min for analysis of plasma cortisol
- the sample taken at 0 min can also be sent for ACTH analysis (if so, must be sent on ice) to differentiate primary from secondary adrenal failure.

A 'normal' SST depends on your own laboratory's reference ranges. In general, patients with normal adrenal function will be able to generate a plasma cortisol concentration >460 nmol/L (170 µg/dL) at 0 or 30 min; the absolute increment is less important.

All patients will need glucocorticoid replacement therapy; some will also need mineralocorticoid replacement:

- glucocorticoid replacement: hydrocortisone 15 mg on waking, 5 mg around 1800 h; titrate dose according to response – excessive weight gain suggests too high a dose; persistent lethargy or hyperpigmentation suggest too low a dose
- mineralocorticoid replacement: fludrocortisone 0.05–0.1 mg daily; titrate according to electrolytes and plasma renin and aldosterone levels.

Adrenal crisis

This is a medical emergency and should be suspected in any patient presenting with unexplained hypotension, hyponatraemia, hyperkalaemia and hypoglycaemia. There may, or may not, be a history of adrenal failure (check a regular drug prescription if available) and evidence of a precipitating intercurrent illness or recent surgery.

Treatment is with hydrocortisone (100 mg IV 6-hourly) and rapid intravenous fluids (normal saline and 10% dextrose if hypoglycaemic). Exercise caution if there is profound hyponatraemia, as rapid correction of plasma sodium concentration can precipitate central pontine myelinolysis (see 'Hyponatraemia', p. 204).

ELECTROLYTE IMBALANCE

Electrolyte imbalance is commonly encountered in almost every clinical environment. This section provides a rapid review of the presenting features, investigation and immediate management of the most common electrolyte disturbances.

Hypernatraemia

Hypernatraemia is almost always due to water depletion. In normal individuals even a small rise in serum sodium (Na^+) concentration results in a powerful sensation of thirst. Therefore, significant hypernatraemia most commonly occurs in confused, elderly or physically disabled patients who are unable to access, or ask for, drinking water.

Hypernatraemia can also result from excessive water loss, e.g. burns or diarrhoea, mineralocorticoid excess, e.g. Cushing's or Conn's syndromes, or consumption of a massive Na^+ load, e.g. ingestion of seawater. Diabetes insipidus (DI), which can be either central or nephrogenic, usually presents with polyuria and polydipsia; hypernatraemia only develops if the patient's thirst mechanism is abnormal or their access to water is limited.

Symptoms

Patients may be asymptomatic or complain of lethargy, weakness, irritability or ankle swelling (due to oedema). Seizures and coma may develop when the serum Na^+ concentration rises above 158 mmol/L.

Clinical assessment and investigation

Look for clinical signs of hypovolaemia (dry mucous membranes, skin turgor, postural BP deficit) and associated co-morbidities, e.g. confusional states, dysphasia, physical disability. Enquire about regular medications, e.g. lithium can cause nephrogenic DI. Serum and urine osmolality should be high in dehydrated patients; an inappropriately low urine osmolality suggests DI.

Management

If the patient is clinically well, they should be allowed to drink to correct the water deficit. Patients who are hypovolaemic and unstable should be started on an appropriate IV fluid regime which has a lower Na^+ concentration than the serum, e.g. 0.9% saline IV or alternating bags of 0.9% saline and 5% dextrose.

Rapid correction of hypernatraemia is to be avoided unless the patient has neurological sequelae. This results in osmotic fluid shifts within the brain and can cause permanent neurological damage, e.g. central pontine myelinolysis. Shocked patients should be admitted to a high dependency unit and patients with suspected DI should be referred to an endocrinologist. Treatment of DI usually involves removal of any precipitating drugs and administration of desmopressin, if central, or indometacin ± a loop diuretic, if nephrogenic.

Hyponatraemia

Symptoms

Mild hyponatraemia (Na^+ 130–135 mmol/L) is common in hospital patients and does not usually cause symptoms. Where symptoms do occur, patients may complain of weakness, lethargy, confusion or headache and this should prompt investigation and appropriate management. Severe hyponatraemia (Na^+ <120 mmol/L) or a rapid fall in serum levels may be associated with seizures and coma and requires emergency intervention.

Clinical assessment

Use the history to identify possible causes, e.g. drugs, GI symptoms, existing medical problems. Clinical examination should focus on a thorough assessment of intravascular volume. Look at the mucous membranes, skin turgor, JVP and erect and supine BP for evidence of hypovolaemia. Peripheral oedema and ascites suggest hypervolaemia.

Causes

Causes are grouped according to the patient's intravascular volume status:

- hypovolaemic, where total body Na^+ is depleted but total water is depleted further: thiazide diuretics, hypoadrenalism (e.g. Addison's), diarrhoea and vomiting
- euvolaemic, where total body water is normal or mildly increased, also known as 'dilutional hyponatraemia': SIADH (see below), hypothyroidism, primary polydipsia, excess dextrose infusion
- hypervolaemic, where total body Na^+ is increased, but total body water is grossly increased: CCF, cirrhosis, nephrotic syndrome.

Investigations

The purpose of investigations is to identify the aetiology and monitor the response to therapy. Check:

- renal, liver, thyroid function and lipids: hyperlipidaemia can lead to pseudohyponatraemia
- blood glucose: hyperglycaemia is the cause in 10–15% of cases
- serum osmolarity as compared with the calculated value ($2 \times (Na^+ + K^+)$ + urea + glucose): if the resulting 'osmolar gap' is high (>10) consider ethylene glycol poisoning, severe hyperglycaemia or mannitol toxicity.

'Spot' urine Na^+ and correlation with volume state can be useful:

- low (<10 mmol/L) plus hypovolaemia suggests extra-renal Na^+ loss, e.g. diarrhoea, burns, fluid sequestration
- low (<10 mmol/L) plus hypervolaemia suggests inappropriate renal Na^+ retention, usually due to low renal perfusion and secondary hyperaldosteronism, e.g. CCF, cirrhosis, nephrotic syndrome
- high (>20 mmol/L) plus hypovolaemia suggests renal Na^+ loss, e.g. diuretics, intrinsic renal disease, hypoadrenalism, hypothyroidism
- high (>20 mmol/L) plus euvolaemia suggests SIADH.

Management

Treatment is only necessary in a very small minority of cases and should only be initiated after senior review. Mild asymptomatic hyponatraemia will usually respond to treatment of the underlying cause, which is also the mainstay of management in all individuals.

Patients with acute hyponatraemia and severe symptoms (e.g. coma or seizures) require more aggressive intervention. However, there is a risk of serious and irreversible CNS consequences, including central pontine myelinolysis, if the serum Na^+ level is corrected too rapidly. Do not aim to restore normal serum Na^+, but rather to achieve a safe level above 125 mmol/L, at a correction rate of no more than 2.5 mmol/L per hour:

- 1.8% (hypertonic, twice normal) saline 500 mL over 2–4 h may be given, and repeated as necessary; regular monitoring of U&E is essential
- furosemide (40 mg) should be administered during this treatment to avoid the risk of fluid overload; cardiovascular status must be carefully monitored.

SIADH

The syndrome of inappropriate ADH secretion (SIADH) results from renal water retention in response to an endogenous source of ADH. Causes include:

- tumours, e.g. brain, small-cell lung cancer
- CNS disease, e.g. stroke, infection
- lung disease, e.g. pneumonia
- drugs, e.g. carbamazepine, haloperidol, amitriptyline, cyclophosphamide
- pain, stress, nausea.

Patients are characteristically euvolaemic and therefore have no oedema. Appropriate investigations are given above. Management is usually conservative with treatment of the underlying cause and fluid restriction, e.g. 1.5 L/day. If unsuccessful, demeclocycline (300 mg 8-hourly) can be effective, with close monitoring of fluid balance and serum urea and electrolytes to avoid dehydration.

Hyperkalaemia

The majority of the body's potassium is intracellular. Although extracellular potassium only accounts for 2% of total body potassium, it has a major effect on the intracellular:extracellular ratio and, therefore, affects cellular resting membrane potentials. Plasma potassium is normally regulated around a narrow range of 3.5–5.0 mmol/L.

Symptoms and clinical effects

Patients may complain of progressive muscular weakness, but symptoms may be absent. Mortality is increased in patients with serum K^+ >6.0 mmol/L and there is a significant risk of cardiac arrhythmias when the serum K^+ is >7.0 mmol/L, particularly if there is a rapid increase in serum levels. Typical ECG changes include tented T waves, flattened P waves and QRS widening. The latter indicates an increased immediate risk of ventricular arrhythmias.

Causes

- artefact, e.g. in vitro haemolysis, thrombocytosis, delay in specimen processing or contamination from an EDTA containing bottle, e.g. FBC bottle
- drugs, e.g. K^+ supplements, potassium sparing diuretics, NSAIDs, ACE inhibitors, angiotensin receptor antagonists
- renal impairment, either acute or decompensated chronic
- hypoadrenalism, e.g. primary adrenal failure (Addison's disease); look for postural hypotension and pigmentation; consider a short Synacthen test.

Management

Perform an urgent ECG. The absolute serum concentration of K^+ is less important than the effect, if any, on cardiac conduction. If serum K^+ is >7 mmol/L or there are associated ECG changes, urgent treatment is required:

- discuss with seniors early and consider transfer to HDU for cardiac monitoring
- 10 mL 10% calcium gluconate IV over 10 min (20–30 min if taking digoxin) stabilizes membrane potential, reducing the potential for arrhythmias, but does not lower K^+; repeat every 20–30 min until ECG changes resolve
- 10 units of Actrapid® insulin added to 50 mL of 50% dextrose, given IV over 15–30 min, should lower K^+ for several hours (monitor BMs)
- regular nebulized salbutamol (5 mg) drives K^+ into cells
- consider IV bicarbonate if the patient is acidaemic, e.g. 50–100 mL 8.4% sodium bicarbonate given via a central line; do not mix this with calcium salts as precipitation will occur
- loop diuretics increase renal K^+ loss
- refractory hyperkalaemia is an indication for urgent haemodialysis, especially in the context of acute renal failure and oliguria.

Less acute measures include:

- calcium resonium to reduce K^+ absorption: give a 30 g enema initially followed by 15 g orally every 8 h; takes 24 h to work
- treat the underlying cause, e.g. rehydration in patients with pre-renal failure.

Hypokalaemia

Hypokalaemia is relatively common. Symptoms, if present, are often subtle and include fatigue and general weakness. Potential consequences include:

- cardiovascular: typical ECG changes, i.e. flattened T wave, ST depression, U wave; ventricular arrhythmias; relative digoxin toxicity (due to reduced competition with potassium at the Na^+–K^+-ATPase)
- muscular: weakness, myalgia, paralysis
- GI: functional paralytic ileus
- renal: polyuria due to acquired nephrogenic diabetes insipidus
- metabolic alkalosis.

Causes

- redistribution: insulin, β-agonists, theophylline and IV dextrose all cause K^+ influx into cells (therefore, be aware that hypokalaemia can occur during treatment of diabetic ketoacidosis)
- extra-renal K^+ loss (especially from the GI tract): associated alkalosis suggests vomiting or nasogastric aspiration; acidosis suggests diarrhoea, laxative abuse or GI fistula
- renal K^+ loss associated with hypertension: hyperaldosteronism (primary, Conn's syndrome or secondary, e.g. renovascular disease), Cushing's syndrome, steroid treatment
- renal K^+ loss associated with normal BP or hypotension: diuretic use (may be associated with an alkalosis), hypomagnesaemia and renal tubular acidosis.

Management

The dosage, route and duration of treatment depends upon the severity of the hypokalaemia and whether there is continuing potassium loss. Caution should be used in patients with renal insufficiency and those receiving ACE inhibitors or potassium sparing diuretics.

Serum K^+ 3.0–3.5 mmol/L

With mild hypokalaemia, oral potassium supplements are usually sufficient. Effervescent tablets, e.g. Sando-K®, are preferable despite the unpleasant taste since solid tablets such as Slow-K® may cause gastrointestinal ulceration. The suggested dose is 40–80 mmol/day: Slow-K® and Sando-K® tablets contain 8 and 12 mmol K^+, respectively; therefore, supplementation using 2 tablets 8-hourly of either is often adequate. K^+ should be monitored twice weekly, until the serum concentration is normal and stable. In addition, if the cause of the hypokalaemia has been treated, the need for supplementation should be regularly reassessed. If hypokalaemia is diuretic induced, try a potassium sparing diuretic instead.

Serum K^+ <3.0 mmol/L

High-dose oral or intravenous replacement will be necessary. Intravenous replacement is given using pre-prepared infusion bags. The choice of dose (20 or 40 mmol) will depend on the severity of hypokalaemia. Seek specialist advice if you need to give large amounts of potassium, e.g. at a concentration above 40 mmol/L or a rate of infusion above 10 mmol/h. Where oral supplementation is considered instead, the maximum dose that can be tolerated is 100–120 mmol/24 h, e.g. Sando-K® 3 tablets 8-hourly. K^+ should be monitored daily until the level is >3.0 mmol/L.

Hypercalcaemia

Clinical features

Mild hypercalcaemia is often asymptomatic. Clinical features are more frequent when serum calcium is above 3.0 mmol/L. These include confusion, polyuria, polydipsia and dehydration, nausea and vomiting, constipation and stupor.

Causes

- malignancy, due to either bony metastases or secretion of PTH-related peptide
- primary or tertiary hyperparathyroidism
- elevated 1,25 $(OH)_2$ vitamin D (vitamin D intoxication, sarcoidosis, TB)
- hyperthyroidism
- Paget's disease, if the patient is immobilized
- thiazide diuretics.

Investigation

- PTH: elevated or normal PTH is inappropriate and suggests hyperparathyroidism
- renal and thyroid function
- alkaline phosphatase: elevated in hyperparathyroidism, malignancy and Paget's disease
- unexplained hypercalcaemia should prompt further investigation for malignancy: breast examination, chest X-ray, serum and urine protein electrophoresis and renal ultrasound should be considered in all patients, with symptoms guiding additional investigation
- vitamin D can be checked; however, toxicity is unlikely to occur unless very large doses of cholecalciferol or 1-hydroxylated vitamin D derivatives have been consumed.

Management

Although there is a view that active treatment of mild to moderate hypercalcaemia is unnecessary, there is evidence of clinical improvement where serum calcium is lowered to normal. Active therapy with bisphosphonates can also reduce bone pain and skeletal events in patients with bony metastases.

Hypercalcaemia results in polyuria. Patients with serum calcium >3.2 mmol/L will be significantly dehydrated. A rapid IV infusion of 0.9% saline will actively promote calcium excretion. 4–6 L may be required; therefore patients with cardiac insufficiency should be closely monitored.

- record fluid balance and aim for an IV input at least 1L greater than output
- furosemide has been advocated to help prevent cardiovascular complications and promote calcium excretion, but may cause falls in serum potassium and magnesium and is not generally used in the routine management of hypercalcaemia.

Bisphosphonates

Intravenous pamidronate often effectively lowers serum Ca^{2+}. The dose given should reflect the degree of hypercalcaemia and the patient's renal function, e.g. 30–60 mg infused over 2–4 h in 0.9% saline via a large vein, often effectively lowers serum calcium; its effect becomes evident after 24 h and peaks at 48–72 h. Zoledronate has a longer duration of action than pamidronate and, although more expensive per dose, may be more cost-effective if repeated infusions are required.

Blood samples should be taken daily for the first 4–5 days following bisphosphonate therapy. Depending on the clinical and biochemical response, further doses may be required. Remember that the peak effect of bisphosphonate therapy may not be evident for 72 h. Additional doses of pamidronate can be considered after at least 48 h have elapsed, up to a total episode dose of 90 mg. Once normocalcaemia is achieved, oral bisphosphonates may be used to maintain serum calcium and reduce the risk of skeletal events in patients with bony metastases or myeloma, e.g. clodronate (800 mg twice daily).

Hypocalcaemia

Background

Total serum calcium concentration is often low in ill patients. Most commonly this is due to hypoalbuminaemia, reflecting the fact that approximately 50% of serum calcium is bound to albumin. Laboratories use a formula to allow for this, resulting in the 'adjusted' or 'corrected' serum calcium. Acidosis causes an increase in free calcium and alkalosis results in a fall. It is the free, ionized, calcium concentration that is physiologically active.

Clinical features

Mild hypocalcaemia is often asymptomatic, but may result in non-specific CNS signs. Chronic hypocalcaemia may cause cataracts, calcification of the basal ganglia and epilepsy. Symptoms may include:

- paraesthesiae, particularly around the mouth and lips
- muscle spasms, particularly of the hands, feet and face; tetany develops when hypocalcaemia is severe, or acute, or when an associated alkalosis increases neuromuscular irritability.
- rarely: laryngospasm, seizures and arrhythmia.

The following classical clinical signs indicate latent tetany:

- Trousseau's sign: carpal spasm within 3 min of inflating a BP cuff on the upper arm
- Chvostek's sign: twitching of the facial muscles induced by tapping over the parotid gland (branches of facial nerve).

Causes and investigations

Typical biochemical patterns for the common causes listed below are shown in Table 7.6.

- alkalosis: commonly due to hyperventilation, in which $PaCO_2$ will also be low
- hypoparathyroidism: most commonly due to surgical damage to the parathyroid glands following parathyroid, thyroid or neck surgery; other causes include autoimmune disease or infiltrative processes, e.g. haemochromatosis
- pseudohypoparathyroidism: due to a genetic PTH receptor signalling defect; serum PTH concentration is paradoxically high and there is a characteristic phenotype
- vitamin D deficiency: commonly due to poor diet and lack of exposure to sunlight; alkaline phosphate may be high; PTH should be high and leads to increased resorption of calcium from the skeleton and osteomalacia
- renal impairment: due to failure of vitamin D hydroxylation in the kidney (into the active form: 1, 25-dihydroxycholecalciferol); high PTH, alkaline phosphatase and phosphate indicate secondary hyperparathyroidism
- hypomagnesaemia: see below.

Table 7.6 Biochemistry of hypocalcaemia

	Total serum calcium	Ionized serum calcium	Serum phosphate	Serum PTH
Alkalosis	N	↓	N	N or ↑
Hypoparathyroidism	↓	↓	↑	↓
Pseudohypoparathyroidism	↓	↓	↑	↑
Vitamin D deficiency	↓	↓	↓	↑
Chronic renal failure	↓	↓	↑	↑

Management

Tetany

If there is associated hyperventilation, patients should be instructed to re-breathe air using a paper bag. Otherwise, 10 mL of 10% calcium gluconate should be given over 5–10 min. More rapid infusion of calcium leads to cardiac arrhythmias. Subsequent doses should be guided by serum calcium concentration and can include a continuous infusion.

Chronic hypocalcaemia

- oral calcium supplements containing 1–2 g of calcium per day may be used, e.g. calcium carbonate 1.25 g daily, and may be combined with vitamin D if indicated, e.g. Adcal D3®
- calcitriol (1,25-dihydroxycholecalciferol) is active vitamin D and may increase serum calcium in a matter of days, even in renal impairment.

In all patients, hypomagnesaemia or malabsorption should be treated. Serum calcium levels should be monitored in all patients on calcium supplements, especially if combined with oral vitamin D.

Hypomagnesaemia

Background

The majority of the body's magnesium (Mg^{2+}) is stored within cells. Normal serum Mg^{2+} concentration is 0.7–1.0 mmol/L. Approximately 30% of Mg^{2+} in the plasma is bound to albumin and, therefore, hypoalbuminaemia is associated with hypomagnesaemia. Significant hypomagnesaemia may result in hypocalcaemia and/or hypokalaemia.

Clinical features

Mild to moderate hypomagnesaemia is often asymptomatic. Symptoms that may occur include paraesthesiae, muscle cramps, irritability and confusion. Common causes include:

- alcoholism: by multiple mechanisms
- inadequate intake: including prolonged nasogastric suction
- gastrointestinal disorders: e.g. malabsorption, ileostomy, prolonged diarrhoea
- renal Mg^{2+} loss due to medication: e.g. aminoglycosides, cisplatinum, ciclosporin.

Management

Mild to moderate hypomagnesaemia (0.4–0.7 mmol/L) is common in sick, hypoalbuminaemic patients and may not require active intervention, especially if the underlying cause can be addressed.

- if there are associated clinical or biochemical disturbances, consider a single daily infusion of IV Mg^{2+} sulphate 16–32 mmol over 8 h (in saline or dextrose); several days of therapy may be required
- rapid Mg^{2+} infusions can be given in some arrhythmias, eclampsia and asthma, but these are largely independent of serum Mg^{2+} concentration and should be given as guided by local protocol.

RENAL DYSFUNCTION

Normal renal function requires adequate renal perfusion pressure and oxygen delivery, intact glomeruli and tubules, no obstruction to urine flow and the absence of sepsis or nephrotoxins. Renal impairment is suggested by a reduction in urine flow. Oliguria is defined as 100–400 mL urine/day and anuria as <100 mL/day.

Acute renal failure

There is no universally agreed definition of acute renal failure (ARF); however, the approximate incidence of patients with ARF requiring dialysis is 203 per million per year. Acute renal failure complicates 7% of hospital admissions and approximately 25% of oliguria in hospital is due to correctable pre-renal factors.

Despite significant advances in the management of ARF, mortality has changed very little over the last few decades. Uncomplicated ARF has a relatively good prognosis with a mortality rate of 5–10%, whereas the mortality of acute renal failure requiring dialysis is 50–75%. This probably reflects the fact that patients with ARF have multiple co-morbidities.

Causes of ARF

ARF is more likely where there is co-existing diabetes mellitus, chronic renal failure, jaundice or cardiovascular disease including hypertension. Certain procedures may also precipitate ARF, e.g. contrast radiography, angiography or vascular surgery. Patients with diabetes or pre-existing renal failure are particularly at risk and, where possible, other imaging techniques should be used in such patients. In addition, anticoagulation may precipitate cholesterol emboli syndrome, causing ARF.

The causes of acute renal failure are usually classified as pre-renal, intrinsic-renal and post-renal. Pre-renal failure usually presents with oliguria; intrinsic and post-renal failure may present with anuria, oliguria or polyuria.

Pre-renal ARF

Pre-renal failure may be due to:

- hypovolaemia associated with haemorrhage or volume depletion, including intravascular volume depletion associated with hypoalbuminaemia and oedema
- renal hypoperfusion, including that due to ACE inhibitors, angiotensin receptor blockers (ARBs) and non-steroidal anti-inflammatories (NSAIDs)
- hypotensive states, e.g. septic shock, cardiogenic shock, anaphylactic shock.

Both increases and decreases in arterial pressure are offset by the powerful effects of an autoregulatory mechanism that maintains glomerular filtration rate (GFR). As blood pressure falls, the afferent arterioles dilate while the efferent arterioles constrict, thus maintaining glomerular capillary pressure and filtration pressure. However, autoregulation is severely impaired at mean arterial pressures <70 mmHg. Therefore, severe systemic hypotension causes a reduction in GFR.

Drugs that interfere with autoregulation can cause pre-renal acute renal failure in patients with other risk factors such as pre-existing renal failure, hypovolaemia and atherosclerosis. Examples include:

- NSAIDs which inhibit prostaglandin-mediated afferent vasodilatation
- ACE inhibitors and ARBs, which inhibit angiotensin-mediated efferent vasoconstriction.

Delayed presentation or inadequate treatment of pre-renal failure will result in damage of the renal parenchyma, causing intrinsic renal failure, due to acute tubular necrosis (ATN).

Intrinsic ARF

Intrinsic renal failure may be due to damage to glomeruli, tubules, interstitium or blood vessels. ATN can be caused by a variety of renal insults, but ATN secondary to ischaemia or nephrotoxins is the most common cause; together, pre-renal failure and ischaemic ATN account for 75% of ARF.

Post-renal ARF

Post-renal failure due to obstruction is less common, but should always be considered, particularly in elderly men with prostatic symptoms or in patients with intra-abdominal malignancy. Prompt relief of the obstruction with a bladder catheter or a nephrostomy is essential.

Clinical assessment

History in ARF

Symptoms in acute renal failure are often non-specific and, in some patients, may be absent. A detailed assessment is essential and should include:

- urinary symptoms, e.g. dysuria, frequency, reduced urine flow: a history of complete anuria requires urgent ultrasonography to detect dilatation of the collecting systems
- recent illnesses, injuries or falls that could cause rhabdomyolysis
- symptoms of dehydration, e.g. thirst, postural dizziness, or fluid overload, such as breathlessness, ankle swelling
- new medication: ask specifically about ACE inhibitors and angiotensin receptor antagonists, NSAIDs, antibiotics, recreational drugs and over the counter medications including homeopathic or herbal remedies.

Examination in ARF

Assessment of any acutely ill patient should start with 'ABCDE'. Clinical examination should include an assessment of intravascular volume status: check capillary refill time, JVP and blood pressure, look for peripheral oedema, assess skin turgor and look at the fluid balance chart. Also look for signs of precipitating illness, including:

- a palpable bladder, suggesting urinary tract obstruction
- signs of infection
- evidence of a compartment syndrome, suggesting rhabdomyolysis
- muscle tenderness and a typical rash, suggesting vasculitis
- a vasculitic-like rash associated with an eosinophilia suggests cholesterol emboli.

Investigation of ARF

The kidneys have a role in many physiological processes and therefore ARF results in a variety of problems including abnormal biochemical homeostasis and problems with fluid balance. Apart from a rise in urea and creatinine, ARF also results in hyperkalaemia (which can be life threatening) and metabolic acidosis. Hyperphosphataemia and hypocalcaemia may also occur, as may a drop in haemoglobin. ARF has a direct negative impact on myocardial function and also suppresses the immune system.

Appropriate investigations are necessary to identify both the aetiology of the renal impairment and its potential sequelae:

- review the case-notes for previous creatinine and urinalysis, angiographic procedures (cholesterol emboli may develop many months later), anaesthetic records for intraoperative blood pressure
- ABG, U&E, creatinine, calcium, phosphate, LFT, CK (if indicated), glucose, CRP, urate, FBC, differential WCC (eosinophilia may be present in vasculitis, cholesterol emboli and acute interstitial nephritis) and coagulation screen
- autoimmune screen (if indicated): RF, ANA, ANCA, C3, C4, anti-GBM antibodies
- ASO titre if streptococcal infection suspected
- myeloma screen including urinary electrophoresis if appropriate
- urinalysis: proteinuria and haematuria suggest an acute glomerulonephritis (GN)
- urine microscopy may reveal cells, casts or crystals
- urine osmolality and urine sodium are seldom helpful (some patients with pre-renal failure have normal urine sodium and osmolality and many patients are on loop diuretics which will affect the urine results); the decision to give or to withhold fluids should be based on the clinical findings and not on urine biochemistry
- microbiology samples as indicated
- urgent ultrasound scan of the renal tract
- if acute interstitial nephritis is suspected: urine for eosinophils

- if rhabdomyolysis is suspected: urine for myoglobin
- CXR: for cardiomegaly, interstitial oedema or infection
- ECG
- in patients who may require dialysis, blood-borne virus status should be checked, e.g. hepatitis B, hepatitis C, HIV; this is usually done by renal unit staff.

Management of ARF

The management of oliguric/anuric ARF is supportive and consists of preventing and treating the sequelae of the condition:

- insert a bladder catheter and measure hourly urine volumes
- if the patient appears hypovolaemic or is hypotensive, give a fluid challenge, e.g. 250 mL of colloid over 30 min; be cautious in patients with evidence of cardiac failure
- if the blood pressure remains low after a fluid challenge ask for senior help; consider central venous pressure (CVP) monitoring and titrate fluids to maintain an appropriate CVP (normal CVP is 5–10 cmH_2O)
- loop diuretics are contraindicated and potentially harmful unless there is a clear indication such as fluid overload, although they may not cause a diuresis in this situation
- if blood pressure remains low despite adequate filling, inotropic support should be considered
- low-dose dopamine should not be used as it does not improve the outcome of ARF and may have an adverse effect in critically ill patients
- monitor fluid balance carefully: once the patient is adequately filled, the fluid input should replace the previous hour's urine output plus other losses, e.g. diarrhoea, plus insensible losses (approximately 20 mL/h, but may be more in warm environments, or if the patient is pyrexial); patients able to take oral fluid should have a fluid restriction of 400 mL plus previous day's urine volume; patients should be weighed daily
- treat hyperkalaemia: potassium can rise dramatically where cells are being broken down and dialysis may be required, e.g. tumour lysis syndrome or rhabdomyolysis
- treat acidosis: if the acidosis is due to bicarbonate loss from the gut or renal tubules and the patient is not overloaded, replace with 1.26% $NaHCO_3$; severe acidosis may contribute to hypotension and is an indication for dialysis
- stop nephrotoxins and drugs likely to cause hyperkalaemia, e.g. trimethoprim
- treat infection but remember to reduce the dose of antibiotic if appropriate
- use a prophylactic H_2 blocker, but reduce dose by half, or use a proton pump inhibitor
- consider DVT prophylaxis, but reduce dose by half
- consider the need for dose modification of all other prescribed therapy
- ensure adequate enteral nutrition and use phosphate binders for hyperphosphataemia
- use, on the advice of the renal unit team, specific therapies for specific diseases, e.g. steroids and immunosuppression for vasculitis.

Referral to the renal unit

After discussion with senior colleagues, referral should be considered early rather than late, as it can improve outcome. Prompt referral is especially important in the following patient groups:

- suspected acute GN
- patients with no obvious cause for their renal failure

- patients with immediate indications for dialysis, including life-threatening hyperkalaemia with ECG changes, severe acidosis, pulmonary oedema and uraemic pericarditis or pericardial effusions
- patients in whom dialysis is not thought to be appropriate, but advice regarding the best conservative approach is required.

Prevention of ARF

There are a variety of theoretical strategies for renal protection: increasing renal perfusion and oxygen delivery; reducing tubule energy requirements; avoiding nephrotoxins and manipulating the renal response to injury. The most effective preventative therapy is adequate volume expansion, although controversy exists over whether to use crystalloid or colloid. In practice, an appropriate volume is more important than the type of fluid used.

Care must be taken to avoid volume overload in the oliguric or anuric patient. Patients at risk should be identified, blood pressure and circulating volume maintained and nephrotoxins stopped. A large number of other agents have been used to prevent ARF in specific situations:

- adequate hydration with 0.9% saline has been shown to reduce the incidence of contrast nephropathy in patients with chronic renal failure undergoing essential contrast imaging studies. Concomitant administration of oral *N*-acetylcysteine may be beneficial
- allopurinol and rasburicase may help prevent urate nephropathy and tumour lysis syndrome (TLS) in patients with haematological malignancy given chemotherapy
- forced alkaline diuresis may help prevent tubule obstruction in TLS and is also used to prevent/attenuate ARF in rhabdomyolysis, although there is little evidence to support this practice.

Recovery from acute renal failure

Recovery from ARF is heralded by increasing urine volumes. Serum creatinine may not fall initially, although the rise will be less each day as the creatinine starts to plateau before falling. At this point the patient may become polyuric and it is essential to keep up with the urine output and other fluid loss to prevent pre-renal failure. Urinary loss of potassium and bicarbonate may also need to be replaced. Remember to correct potassium deficits before giving sodium bicarbonate. The majority of patients with ARF will recover completely. However, in 5% of patients ARF is irreversible and this figure rises to 16% in elderly patients. Patients left with residual damage may develop progressive chronic renal failure.

Acute on chronic renal failure

Patients with chronic renal failure (CRF) may present with an acute deterioration in their renal function. Investigation and management is essentially the same as in patients with ARF. Pay particular attention to new medication, any recent increases in drug doses, angiographic procedures within the last year, and infection. An urgent ultrasound should be arranged to exclude obstruction. Other investigations, listed in the ARF section, should be performed as indicated by the clinical picture. Management is as for acute renal failure.

Nephrotic syndrome

Nephrotic syndrome is characterized by proteinuria >3.5 g/24 h, hypoalbuminaemia, oedema and hyperlipidaemia. Protein loss occurs because of glomerular pathology and the causes include minimal change disease, focal segmental glomerulosclerosis, membranous nephropathy, mesangiocapillary

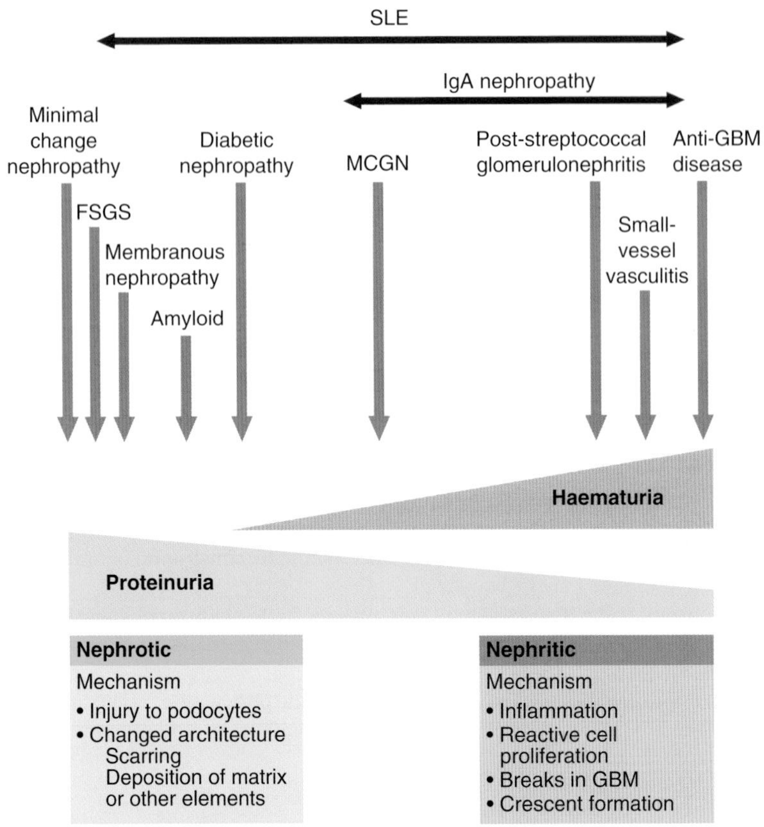

Figure 7.1 Spectrum of glomerular diseases. FSGS, focal and segmental glomerulosclerosis; GBM, glomerular basement membrane; MCGN, mesangiocapillary glomerulonephritis; SLE, systemic lupus erythematosus.

glomerulonephritis, diabetes mellitus and amyloidosis (Fig. 7.1). Investigation should include an immunology screen as above, quantification of the urine protein and an ultrasound scan of the kidneys. A renal biopsy will almost certainly be required.

Long-term treatment is largely supportive and includes diuretic therapy and a low sodium diet. Lipid lowering therapy and anticoagulation should be considered for patients with chronic or severe nephrotic syndrome. Pneumococcal vaccination should be considered, especially in children.

ARF in nephrotic syndrome

ARF may develop as a consequence of primary renal disease, renal vein thrombosis or hypovolaemia due to over-diuresis. Glomerular permeability is reduced due to foot process fusion and the tubules have changes similar to those found in acute tubular necrosis. In nephrotic syndrome, urinary sodium is low, but rises with the development of ARF due to acute tubular necrosis.

The commonest cause of nephrotic syndrome occurring in combination with ARF is minimal change disease (ARF is present in 18% of patients), e.g. due to NSAIDs. The risk of ARF is higher in males, older patients and those with more marked hypoalbuminaemia and proteinuria.

Occasionally, patients with nephrotic syndrome related to a chronic glomerulonephritis, e.g. IgA nephropathy, mesangiocapillary GN, membranous GN, develop crescents in the glomeruli resulting in ARF due to rapidly progressive glomerulonephritis (RPGN).

The treatment of ARF associated with nephrotic syndrome is aimed at the underlying cause. In all cases, nephrotoxins should be stopped. If the ARF is due to hypovolaemia, diuretics should be stopped and IV fluid should be given. Minimal change disease with ARF is treated with steroids. Patients with RPGN will require treatment with steroids and immunosuppression.

Nephritic syndrome

Nephritic syndrome is classically due to post-streptococcal glomerulonephritis, the incidence of which is decreasing in the Western world. Other diseases such as vasculitis, cryoglobulinaemia and mesangiocapillary GN may present with similar features (Fig. 7.1). The classical presentation is of oedema, haematuria, hypertension and oliguria with ARF. The disease is usually self-limiting, although microscopic haematuria may persist for some time after the acute episode. The prognosis is good when due to classical post-streptococcal GN. Occasionally patients may present with massive proteinuria and associated nephrotic syndrome.

Patients with ARF and nephritic syndrome should be investigated as for ARF. In particular, an autoimmune screen (see p. 211), complement levels, and an ASO titre should be sent. A renal biopsy can be considered, but may not be necessary as the disease may be self-limiting. Unusual features such as persistently low complement levels or massive proteinuria would justify a renal biopsy.

The management is similar to that for all causes of ARF described above. Infection and hypertension should be treated and diuretics should be given for massive oedema. Haemodialysis should be started early, if required for uraemia or fluid overload unresponsive to diuretics.

SECTION 2
Symptoms and related acute presentations

Neurological and psychiatric

8

THE UNCONSCIOUS PATIENT

Consciousness and coma, respectively, may be defined as 'a state of awareness of self and the environment' and the absence of such awareness. Consciousness is dependent on the proper functioning of the ascending reticular activating system, a complex functional grouping of structures in the brainstem, thalamic and sub-thalamic regions.

Terms such as 'drowsy' and 'obtunded' are often used clinically, but are imprecise and liable to variable interpretations. Instead, the Glasgow Coma Scale (GCS) should be used to describe the level of consciousness (see 'Acute scores', p. 9). The scale is also valuable when monitoring the clinical course of an unconscious patient.

Coma and coma-like states

Classification of coma

The appearance of coma can be categorized, on clinical grounds, into three distinct groups. This classification is useful, as it can be used to determine the likely underlying pathology:

- *coma with focal signs*: stroke; intracranial tumour
- *coma without focal signs but with meningism*: subarachnoid haemorrhage; meningoencephalitis
- *coma without focal signs or meningism*: anoxic–ischaemic brain damage; metabolic, toxic or drug induced; meningitis; post-ictal.

Non-coma but coma-like appearance

In these states, the patient may be aware of their surroundings but, when examined, they appear to be in a coma.

Akinetic mutism

Classically seen in those patients who have suffered diencephalic damage, e.g. frontal tumours; encephalitis; end-stage CJD. These patients are immobile (akinetic), do not vocalize (mutism) and may not open their eyes.

Vegetative state

These patients appear at times to be wakeful, with cycles of eye closure and eye opening that resemble sleep. However, close observation reveals that they are not aware and that there is no evidence of a functioning mind. In most cases, the patient can breathe spontaneously and has a stable circulation. A vegetative state may be transient or persist until death. It may follow a variety of severe brain insults, most commonly traumatic or hypoxic events.

Locked-in syndrome

This is a condition of tetraplegia and facial paralysis, with sparing of voluntary eye opening and vertical eye movements. It is usually caused by a pontine stroke.

Catatonia

This state is usually associated with psychiatric disease, but may also be seen with metabolic causes or with drug toxicity. The eyes are usually open with significantly reduced blinking. Passive limb movements may be associated with 'waxy flexibility'.

Assessment

The assessment of any comatose patient should begin with ABCDE (see 'Assessment of the acutely ill patient', p. 8). Thereafter, take a history, asking the family or other contacts, as necessary, for information regarding recent events, past medical and drug history. A detailed neurological examination is essential. However, this should always be preceded by a general physical examination; specifically, look for rash, cyanosis, jaundice, fetor hepaticus and signs of chronic liver disease.

Neurological examination

Additional guidance is given on, p. 5.

Pupillary responses

A strong light source should be used. The pupillary responses are normal in toxic and metabolic coma. Opiates and atropine are among certain medications that will interfere with the physiological response.

Eye movements

Abnormal reflex eye movements (the oculocephalic or doll's eye reflex) strongly suggest brainstem disease. Roving eye movements suggest a toxic/metabolic cause for the coma. Eye deviation, conjugate or dysconjugate, can also be useful in localizing the site of the structural lesion in coma.

Motor examination

Examination of the motor system is an essential part of the assessment in a patient with coma. Decerebrate rigidity refers to bilateral upper and lower limb extensor posture, usually the result of bilateral brainstem lesions. Decorticate posture refers to bilateral flexion of the upper limbs with extension of the lower limbs, usually suggesting an upper brainstem lesion. Asymmetry of signs can be very helpful as it suggests a structural cause of coma rather than a toxic or metabolic cause. Myoclonic jerks may occur in anoxic–ischaemic encephalopathies.

Investigations and management

Investigations

Initial investigations should focus on determining the underlying aetiology. These include BM and lab glucose, toxicology screen, liver function, CT brain ± EEG and

LP. Potential complications should then be evaluated, e.g. aspiration (CXR) and intracranial pressure-induced bradycardia (ECG ± cardiac monitoring).

Management

The patient's safety, the cause of their unconscious state (as above) and their longer-term support should all be considered.

When patients become unconscious suddenly, pay particular attention to their ability to protect their airway. Where their GCS drops below 8, they are likely to need airway support and ICU referral may be appropriate.

Where the period of unconsciousness is prolonged, nutrition and hydration will need to be considered. Initially, hydration can be maintained using intravenous fluids. Nutritional support should be instituted early and can be provided using a NG tube. Where long-term enteral feeding is required, insertion of a PEG tube may be more appropriate (see also 'Nutrition', p. 183)

When prescribing medication, consider the route that is most appropriate. Medications can be given IV where intravenous access has been obtained. If a NG or PEG tube is in situ, medication may be delivered by this route (check with a pharmacist or the BNF first).

Patients who are unconscious for any length of time are at increased risk of pressure sores and should be nursed appropriately; they should be turned regularly and their skin examined for early signs of pressure damage. They are also at risk of limb contractures and a physiotherapist should be involved early.

HEADACHE

Headache is a symptom that can have many causes. It can occur in isolation, as part of a primary headache syndrome, (e.g. migraine), or as a component of an evolving symptom complex suggestive of a secondary headache (e.g. brain tumour or meningitis).

Assessment

Initial assessment should aim to identify patients with clinical features suggestive of a secondary cause (see 'Secondary causes of headache', overleaf). In these patients, cranial imaging and further investigation should be considered.

History

Enquire about the following:

- onset and duration
- location, severity and quality of the pain
- frequency and timing of episodes
- associated features, aggravating and relieving factors
- past headache history.

Examination

In addition to a standard examination, the following features should be examined and documented:

- skin: for evidence of rash
- temporal artery: for tenderness and pulsation
- eye examination: including extraocular movements, pupils and fundi
- muscle power
- deep tendon reflexes and plantars
- coordination tests and gait.

Causes, investigation and management

Primary causes of headache

Further investigation is not usually required if a confident clinical diagnosis can be made.

Tension-type headache

Bi-temporal and/or occipital headache of gradual onset. Can be due to stress-related neck and scalp muscle tension. Relaxation and simple analgesics should be used.

Migraine

Recurrent headaches which are throbbing in nature, associated with nausea, vomiting, light or sound sensitivity and which get worse with physical exertion are likely to be migraine headaches. Focal neurological symptoms, particularly visual symptoms, are characteristic.

The treatment of migraine involves consideration and avoidance of precipitants, e.g. caffeine, fasting, alcohol, cheese, chocolate. Stress and cyclical hormonal levels are also factors. Pharmacological management involves simple analgesics, such as aspirin or paracetamol, often in a combination preparation with an antiemetic, such as metoclopramide. Moderate to severe attacks of migraine can be treated with a triptan, such as sumatriptan given orally (50–100 mg), as a nasal spray (10 mg) or, if necessary, as a subcutaneous injection (6 mg). In recurrent migraine, β-blockers can be used for prophylaxis, e.g. propranolol 80–160 mg daily.

Cluster headaches

Patients suffering from cluster headaches are more likely to be male and give a history of short-lasting nocturnal headaches. These occur in a cyclical manner, are often retro-orbital and associated with redness and watering of the ipsilateral eye and restlessness. The attacks can occur repeatedly over several weeks.

Acute attacks can be alleviated by inhalation of high oxygen flow for 15 min ± sumatriptan 6 mg SC (for further dosing and cautionary notes, see the BNF). Verapamil can be used as a preventive agent (80–120 mg orally three times daily).

Secondary causes of headache

Cranial imaging ± further tests should be considered in patients with secondary causes of headache. These may present with the following clinical syndromes.

Thunderclap headache

A sudden-onset headache that reaches its peak within 1 min is termed a thunderclap headache. A 'first or the worst' headache should always be investigated. Important causes include:

- subarachnoid haemorrhage
- meningo-encephalitis
- internal carotid artery dissection
- cerebral venous sinus thrombosis
- acute hypertension
- pituitary apoplexy
- acute glaucoma
- benign orgasmic headache.

Subarachnoid haemorrhage

This typically presents as a thunderclap occipital headache, often described as 'a massive blow to the back of the head'. Nausea and vomiting is commonly associated and signs of meningeal irritation, for example neck stiffness and Kernig's sign, or an alteration in consciousness may be present.

If subarachnoid haemorrhage is suspected, a non-contrast CT scan of the brain should be performed immediately. If this test is normal, a lumbar puncture should be performed at least 12 h after the onset of the headache to look for xanthochromia (see 'Lumbar puncture', p. 37, and 'CSF', p. 74).

Management may involve surgical intervention or be conservative, including the use of nimodipine to reduce vasospasm in cerebral arteries. Urgent neurosurgical referral is advised in all patients.

Headache associated with raised intracranial pressure

Raised intracranial pressure (ICP) is suggested by a headache that occurs predominantly in the morning and gets worse with physical exertion, coughing and bending, or is associated with nausea and vomiting. Causes include brain tumours and idiopathic intracranial hypertension.

Signs associated with raised ICP include altered consciousness, papilloedema, III and VI nerve palsy. Hypotension and bradycardia suggest coning. Treatment should be directed towards the cause.

Headaches associated with CSF hypovolaemia

These typically get worse within 30 min of sitting up and get better promptly on lying down. CSF hypovolaemia is most commonly seen after a lumbar puncture, but can also occur spontaneously.

Medication overuse headaches

It is well recognized that overuse of any medication used for the acute treatment of headache can itself cause a rebound headache. This is true not only of opioid-containing analgesics, but also for over-the-counter analgesics and triptans. The only definitive treatment is withdrawal from the offending medication.

Others

If clinical features suggestive of any of the following diagnoses are present, appropriate investigation should be considered:

- head injury (with or without a haematoma)
- vascular event
- infection, including meningo-encephalitis and brain abscess
- vasculitis, e.g. temporal arteritis
- hypertensive encephalopathy
- trigeminal neuralgia.

FITS AND FAINTS

Seizures are short-lived, usually stereotyped events, caused by a burst or several bursts of electrical activity from the central nervous system. Awareness may or may not be impaired. Epilepsy (a tendency to have recurrent seizures) is a common neurological disorder with a prevalence of about 1 in 200. The social and medical consequences of a diagnosis of epilepsy mandate accurate and prompt diagnosis, appropriate classification and treatment.

Emergency assessment and management of seizures

Clinical assessment

It is often not possible to elicit a history from the patient since they will be either actively fitting or post-ictal. Ask any witnesses or family members for information regarding recent events, past medical and drug history. Enquire specifically about any prior history of fits, alcohol or drug ingestion. Common seizure presentations include:

- generalized tonic–clonic seizures: these are the most common seizure type noted in adults and consist of a tonic phase (stiffness, cry out and cyanosis), followed by a clonic phase consisting of alternating movements reducing in

frequency and amplitude over several minutes, with subsequent confusion and drowsiness
- partial seizures: these result from an epileptic discharge that is restricted in distribution and can be subdivided into simple partial (with no alteration in awareness) or complex partial, where awareness of the environment is impaired and the patient has no recall of their activities.

More detailed clinical assessment is often not possible at this stage and emergency management should be initiated while simple investigations are performed; see below.

Investigation

Check BM and take bloods for FBC, U&E, LFT, Ca^{2+}, Glu and, if appropriate, blood cultures. If there is a concern about compliance with treatment, serum levels of any current antiepileptics should be measured.

Management

General measures

- assess ABC
- place in the recovery position and, if necessary, insert a nasopharyngeal airway
- if the patient has been fitting for >5 min, call for senior assistance
- give high flow oxygen and obtain venous access
- if BM is <3.5 mmol/L give 100 mL of 20% dextrose IV
- monitor pulse, BP, temperature and heart rhythm.

Control of seizures

Local protocols may be available and should be consulted. In general, benzodiazepines should be used first-line:

- lorazepam 2 mg IV over 4 min, repeated if necessary after 10 min, or
- diazepam 10 mg PR if no IV access
- if the patient is malnourished or alcoholic, give Pabrinex®, two pairs of vials IV over 10 min.

If one dose of benzodiazepine does not control the seizures (remember that this may have been given already by paramedical staff), then senior assistance should be called and IV phenytoin should be administered (15 mg/kg at 50 mg/min unless already taking oral phenytoin). In some hospitals, intravenous valproate can be used either first-line, or where the patient is on phenytoin. If these strategies fail to control the seizures, then the patient will most likely have been fitting for >30 min and has status epilepticus.

Status epilepticus

Status epilepticus is defined as a seizure lasting >30 min, or successive seizures with no recovery of awareness in between. It can arise either as a complication of recognized epilepsy (brought about by poor compliance, alcohol use, or illicit drug use) or as an initial presentation of epilepsy (secondary to encephalitis, trauma, drug use, or alcohol withdrawal). Status epilepticus is a medical emergency with a mortality of around 30%. Adequate diagnosis of any primary cause and appropriate treatment is vital in speeding recovery and minimizing complications.

Clinical features, investigation and treatment

Remember that while clonic movements may predominate in the early stages, these will become less pronounced with time. Recovery from status should not be assumed because movement has stopped. Where impairment of consciousness continues, an EEG should be performed to confirm that the ictal activity has stopped.

Whether there is pre-existing epilepsy or not, patients with status should have cranial imaging and, if there is a suspicion of encephalitis, a lumbar puncture. All patients should be referred to ICU and considered for ventilation and administration of a general anaesthetic to control seizures.

Elective assessment of a possible first fit

This is a frequent presentation to medical clinics, GP surgeries, and A&E departments. Do not assume that the cause is epilepsy, since approximately 50% of patients referred to a 'first seizure' clinic will have another explanation which becomes apparent with time.

Clinical assessment

The most important step is to differentiate seizure from syncope (Table 8.1). 'False positive' clinical diagnoses of seizure can result from a description of short-lived jerking movements that are not uncommon with syncope.

Table 8.1 Differential diagnosis of epilepsy

	Syncope	Seizure
Prodrome	Precipitants are common Hypotensive Visual disturbance Nausea Palpitations Hyperventilation Ringing in ears	Unprovoked Occasionally focal positive neurological symptoms
Eye witness account	Pallor, sweating Short-lived (<1 min) Intermittent jerking of limbs	Cyanosis Jerking limb movements of reducing frequency and severity
Recovery	Rapid recovery (<5 min) Brief disorientation (seconds) Urinary incontinence Tongue bitten (tip) 'Washed out'	Sleepy afterwards Confused Urinary incontinence Tongue bitten (sides) Dysphasia or other negative neurological symptoms

Specific enquiry should be made about general health (especially cardiac, diabetic, renal or hepatic disease), previous 'fits' in adult life or childhood, possible pregnancy, alcohol intake or recreational drugs (including the timing of last intake) and a family history of epilepsy or seizure.

When taking a history from a patient who has previously lost consciousness, it is important to ask about other potential seizure events, e.g. nocturnal episodes, myoclonic jerks, partial versus generalized seizures (see above). This information can help with the diagnosis and classification of any epilepsy.

Investigation

All patients should have an ECG carried out following an episode of blackout. Patients who have had a definite single seizure should have cranial imaging (CT, or ideally MRI) to exclude an intracranial lesion. An EEG will not help differentiate seizure from syncope, but may help in giving the patient advice about prognosis.

Treatment

In the UK, patients presenting with a possible first seizure, who have no risk factors for the development of epilepsy, are not routinely prescribed anticonvulsants. Patients without neurological deficit do not need admission provided they have someone at home to look after them. However, all patients with suspected first seizure should be given advice regarding driving eligibility (see 'Driving', p. 411).

Management of established epilepsy

The diagnosis of epilepsy has long-term ramifications and should only be made by a specialist with adequate training in the disorder. Approximately two-thirds of patients will be fully controlled with the first or second drug used. The others will require manipulation of drug combinations and possibly access to special programmes for surgical consideration.

Treatment

Long-term treatment for epilepsy should not be started by non-specialists. The dangers of inappropriate treatment, lists of pharmacokinetic interactions and recommendations for optimal dosage and combinations are complex and best considered in conjunction with national guidelines (SIGN 70 and NICE). Admission and driving concerns should be addressed as described above.

STROKE

A stroke may result from embolism from a distant site (usually cardiac), arterial thrombosis or haemorrhage into the brain substance. Stroke is the third most common cause of death in developed countries and is one of the most important causes of severe disability.

Recent advances in neuroimaging techniques have increased our understanding of cerebrovascular disease and enabled decisions regarding treatment to be made early. The development of stroke units has been another important step in ensuring provision of the best available care. Nevertheless, clinical history and examination remain the most important tools in the assessment of patients with stroke.

Diagnosis

Presentation

The sudden onset of focal neurological symptoms is the hallmark of a vascular event such as a transient ischaemic attack (TIA) or stroke. Therefore, it is useful to ask patients what they were doing at the time. At least half of all TIAs or strokes occur in the morning and patients often wake with a neurological deficit. Table 8.2 lists focal neurological symptoms that may suggest a TIA or a stroke.

The duration of symptoms is of paramount importance in differentiating stroke from other neurological conditions (Table 8.3, overleaf). A TIA is classically defined as a focal neurological deficit lasting <24 h and a stroke as a deficit lasting >24 h. However, neuroimaging techniques have blurred this distinction. Moreover, the advent of thrombolysis for some patients may require a revision of these criteria.

The diagnosis of stroke is usually straightforward, as the patient has a persisting neurological deficit at the time of presentation. A TIA, however, can pose considerable diagnostic difficulty because, in many patients, the symptoms resolve completely within 1 h. Migraine and epilepsy can be mistaken for a TIA and a careful history is essential.

Neuroimaging in stroke

Various clinical parameters, e.g. the presence or absence of headache and the consciousness level, have been proposed as a means of differentiating between ischaemic stroke and primary intracerebral haemorrhage. However, it is now universally accepted that no clinical scoring method can make this distinction reliably. Haemorrhage into the brain is immediately visible on a CT or MRI scan and, therefore, neuroimaging should be performed as soon as possible in patients presenting with symptoms suggestive of a stroke. In most patients 'as soon as possible' usually

Table 8.2 Presenting focal neurological symptoms of TIA/stroke

Type of injury	Symptoms
Motor	Weakness or clumsiness of one side of body (mono/hemiparesis) Bilateral weakness Swallowing problems Unsteadiness
Sensory	Altered feeling on one side of the body (para/quadriparesis)
Speech and language	Difficulty in understanding or expressing speech (dysphasia) Reading difficulties (dyslexia) Writing difficulties (dysgraphia) Slurred speech (dysarthria)
Visual	Loss of vision in one eye Visual field defect: hemi or quadrantanopia Double vision
Others	Vertigo Amnesia Visuospatial symptoms

Table 8.3 The timing of neurological presentations

Timing	Pathology	Associated features
Abrupt onset	Vascular: Infarction Haemorrhage	 Risk factors Pain, space occupying effects
Variable or fluctuating course (days to weeks)	Demyelinating	Previous minor neurological symptoms Temperature sensitivity L'hermitte's sign
Progressive (days to weeks)	Neoplastic Degenerative	Focal neurological symptoms or features of raised ICP Systemic features of neoplasm Onset in late or middle age
Static or progressive from early life	Congenital or genetic	Positive family history

means the next available slot or first thing in the morning. However, urgent neuroimaging (usually CT) should be performed in the following circumstances:

- where facilities for thrombolysis exist and patient presents within 3 h of symptom onset; see below
- a depressed or falling conscious level
- patients on warfarin or with a known coagulopathy
- clinical features of alternative diagnoses that would require alternative treatment, e.g. meningism, fever, a history of trauma.

Ischaemic stroke

Aetiology

Important factors include:

- large artery atherosclerosis: risk factors include age over 50 years, hypertension, diabetes mellitus, cigarette smoking and hypercholesterolaemia

- cardioembolic disease
- small artery disease: usually in patients with hypertension or diabetes
- others: e.g. arterial dissection, venous sinus thrombosis, vasculitis, AVM.

Clinical syndromes

Clinical features at presentation can be used to distinguish between anterior circulation (carotid), posterior circulation (vertebrobasilar) and lacunar strokes. Examples of these clinical syndromes include:

- TACS (total anterior circulation syndrome): hemiplegia, hemianopia, disturbance of higher cerebral function; associated with the greatest likelihood of death or serious disability
- PACS (partial anterior circulation syndrome): motor or sensory deficit with hemianopia or cortical dysfunction
- posterior circulation syndrome: ipsilateral cranial nerve and contralateral motor or sensory deficit; bilateral deficit (motor/sensory); eye movement disorder/hemianopia; cerebellar dysfunction
- lacunar syndrome: may result from occlusion of a single deep perforating artery; not associated with either visual field defects or any disturbance of higher cerebral function; examples include pure motor stroke, pure sensory stroke, ataxic hemiparesis, sensorimotor stroke.

Investigation

First-line investigations

All patients should have blood sent for FBC, U&E, ESR, Glu and cholesterol, an ECG, urinalysis and a non-contrast CT brain scan. A CT brain can exclude a primary intracerebral haemorrhage and will occasionally identify other pathology that mimics stroke symptoms, e.g. brain tumours. It also enables the physician to plan treatment, including thrombolysis.

MRI can be useful in certain situations, e.g. posterior fossa syndromes. Advanced neuroimaging techniques including MR or CT angiography, diffusion and perfusion weighted MRI, MR spectroscopy or functional MRI are available in specialized centres and are useful in specific scenarios.

Second-line investigations

Some 95% of ischaemic strokes and TIAs are caused by atherothrombotic disease, small vessel disease or cardioembolism. In the elderly and in patients with a known risk factor for stroke, second-line investigations may be restricted to carotid Doppler and echocardiography to look for evidence of large vessel atherosclerosis and a cardioembolic source, respectively.

The history may be used to guide further investigations. For example, a CT or MR angiogram of the neck vessels would be indicated in a patient presenting with a posterior circulation stroke who also has significant neck pain (suggesting a diagnosis of a vertebral dissection). In younger patients presenting with a stroke, additional investigations that may be appropriate include autoantibodies, thrombophilia screen, blood cultures, serum homocysteine, serum lactate, toxicology screen, CXR and CT or MR angiogram of the neck vessels.

Immediate management

TIA

Patients who have had a TIA do not always need to be admitted to hospital since, by definition, their symptoms have resolved. However, all should be referred to a rapid access TIA clinic for further investigation and management including the introduction of appropriate secondary prevention therapy; see overleaf.

Ischaemic stroke

Start with ABCDE. Most units will have an acute stroke protocol which should be consulted. Supportive IV fluids should be prescribed, and the patient fasted pending an urgent swallowing assessment. Pyrexia and infection should be controlled. Hypertension is common in the first 24h; treatment is not usually required and may precipitate a fall in cerebral perfusion with further ischaemic damage.

There is clear evidence that patients managed in stroke units have a better outcome. Therefore, a direct referral to the stroke team should be made. Nursing, physiotherapy and nutritional support should be provided as appropriate

Thrombolysis

The number of patients with ischaemic stroke being thrombolysed remains low. If facilities are available regionally, patients presenting within 3h of the onset of the stroke/TIA should be directed to the regional thrombolysis centre.

Secondary prevention

All patients with confirmed, non-haemorrhagic stroke should receive an antiplatelet drug such as aspirin immediately, unless there is a clear contraindication. There is growing evidence that the addition of dipyridamole to aspirin further reduces the risk of recurrence. Anticoagulation with warfarin is indicated in cardioembolic stroke and strokes associated with arterial dissection or cerebral venous sinus thrombosis.

Intracerebral haemorrhage

Presentation

Headache, nausea and vomiting are common. Neurological symptoms and signs will depend on the site of bleeding. The commonest cause of an intracerebral haemorrhage is hypertension and the commonest sites of a 'hypertensive bleed' are the basal ganglia and thalamus. Hypertension is also the commonest cause of a 'lobar haemorrhage', but a bleed in these areas should alert the clinician to the possibility of an AVM or an intracerebral aneurysm as the underlying cause. Anticoagulant and antiplatelet treatments are other important causes of a primary intracerebral bleed and a careful drug history should be taken.

Prognosis

A low GCS (<9) at presentation, a large haematoma or blood in the ventricular system on CT are all predictors of a poor outcome.

Management

Ensure ABC are maintained. Surgical evacuation of haematomas can be life-saving and an urgent neurosurgical opinion should be sought. Seizures should be treated with IV anticonvulsants (see 'Seizures', p. 221). Treatment of hypertension is controversial and should be discussed with a senior colleague. If signs of raised ICP (papilloedema, falling GCS, rising BP, bradycardia) are present, consider treatment with IV mannitol, after discussion with neurosurgery.

FOCAL NEUROLOGY

In the majority of cases, the cause of a focal neurological deficit can be elicited by a careful history and clinical examination.

Limb weakness

The anatomical site of the lesion (muscle, peripheral nerve, spinal cord, brain) can be inferred from the pattern of weakness (Table 8.4). If a neurological cause seems likely, determine whether there are associated changes in muscle tone or

Table 8.4 Patterns of weakness and associated disorders

Pattern of distribution	Localization	Associated symptoms	Special associated pathologies
Proximal	Skeletal muscle	Muscle pain or tenderness	Myopathies, e.g. alcohol, thyroid, polymyositis, drugs, dystrophies
Distal	Peripheral nerve	Sensory loss	Guillain–Barré
Unilateral (usually upper motor neurone)	Cortical	Visual	
	Midbrain	Sensory	
Paraparesis (affecting the legs)	Spinal cord	Sphincter problems	
	Parasagittal	Sensory loss	
Quadriparesis	High cervical spine	Neck pain; Sphincter problems	
Cruciate (one arm and contralateral leg)	Medulla		Vascular event
Pyramidal (strongest muscle groups predominate in each limb)	Upper motor neurone in affected limb		

reflexes. This allows differentiation between upper and lower motor neurone lesions:

- lower motor neurone weakness: flaccid and areflexic with wasting and fasciculation
- upper motor neurone weakness: spastic with increased reflexes and upgoing plantars.

Some disorders may present with weakness and a mixed picture of upper and lower motor neurone signs, e.g. motor neurone disease, cervical myelopathy.

Muscular and neuromuscular weakness

Myopathy

Myopathies are often endocrine (diabetic, thyroid disease), metabolic (alcohol) or inflammatory in origin resulting in weakness ± tenderness. Check Glu, LFT, TFT, B_{12}, folate, CK and consider autoantibodies, electromyography and muscle biopsy.

Myasthenia gravis

This disorder of neuromuscular transmission often presents with features of limb weakness, but also affects other muscle groups, e.g. bulbar, facial and ocular. The characteristic feature of myasthenia is fatigability: weakness worsening as the day progresses or with exertion that responds, at least in part, to rest.

Investigation and treatment

Check for acetylcholine receptor antibodies and refer for electromyography. Look for evidence of respiratory and bulbar dysfunction in patients presenting acutely. Symptomatic relief may be achieved with acetylcholine esterase inhibitors. However, immunosuppression is often required to prevent further antibody formation.

Lower motor neurone weakness

Direct nerve injury produces weakness and wasting of innervated muscles, resulting in hypotonia, hyporeflexia and fasciculation. Causes include trauma, acute polio infection, transverse myelitis and Guillain–Barré syndrome (see below).

Guillain–Barré syndrome

Often post-infectious, this results in neural inflammation with a progressive, ascending limb weakness ± respiratory muscle weakness (in the Miller–Fisher variant there is a descending pattern of weakness and early involvement of the ocular muscles is common). Identifying respiratory muscle involvement is crucial and forced vital capacity should be monitored closely. Treatment is with intravenous immunoglobulin or plasmapheresis, and intubation and ventilation may be necessary.

Upper motor neurone weakness

Lesions between the spinal cord and the cerebral cortex cause weakness with increased tone and hyper-reflexia. An abrupt onset suggests a vascular cause. Others include spinal cord injury, cerebral palsy, anoxic brain damage and demyelination, e.g. multiple sclerosis.

Multiple sclerosis

Demyelination may occur at any location in the CNS and produce a wide range of neurological symptoms. Weakness is usually of an upper motor neurone type on account of lesions in the cerebral cortex, brainstem or spinal cord. Sensation, cranial nerve function (particularly eye movements), bladder function (urgency, frequency) or cerebellar function (ataxia, dysarthria) may also be affected.

Investigation and treatment

An MRI of brain ± spinal cord, visual evoked responses and lumbar puncture should be considered (see 'Lumbar puncture', p. 37 and 'CSF', p. 74). In acute flairs, treat any precipitating cause, such as infection or dehydration, and consider high-dose corticosteroids, e.g. IV methylprednisolone (1 g daily for 3 days). If there are frequent or prolonged relapses immunomodulatory treatments, e.g. interferon, should be considered.

Mixed upper and lower motor neurone weakness

Mixed upper and lower motor signs, e.g. wasting with normal reflexes and upgoing plantars, are usually due to motor neurone disease (MND). In this progressive degenerative condition, sensory changes are absent or at worst minimal.

Investigation and treatment of MND

Structural causes and other neuropathies (metabolic and toxic as per myopathy above) should be excluded. Electromyography and nerve conduction studies may be diagnostic. There is no effective cure, but treatment with riluzole may prolong life.

Altered sensation

This is often described as 'numbness', which means different things to different people. Patients should be encouraged to clarify whether they mean the absence of sensation, altered sensation, weakness or paraesthesia. There are various important clinical patterns.

Distal limb numbness

Peripheral neuropathy is the most common pattern of numbness, possibly because metabolic or toxic processes preferentially affect the long axons. These may also produce motor effects such as weakness and loss of reflexes in a distal distribution. While diabetes mellitus is the most common cause, other metabolic, endocrine, toxic and inflammatory causes should be considered.

Isolated areas of numbness

The distribution of sensory loss may identify the particular root or peripheral nerve involved; see the dermatome map (see p. 7). Guidance on how to differentiate between radicular and peripheral neuropathies is given in Table 8.5. Processes affecting the root or peripheral nerve will often produce concomitant local lower motor neurone symptoms.

Table 8.5 Differentiation between peripheral and radicular neuropathy

Site	Nerve	Description
Arm	Ulnar nerve	Sensory loss, medial aspect of the hand Motor loss, intrinsic muscles of the hand (except thenar eminence)
	C8/T1 root	Sensory loss, medial aspect of the hand and forearm Motor loss of most of the intrinsic muscles of the hand
Leg	Peroneal nerve	Sensory loss, lateral shin and dorsum of the foot Weakness of ankle dorsiflexion
	L5 root	Sensory loss, lateral shin and dorsum of the foot Weakness of ankle dorsiflexion and ankle inversion

Dissociated sensory loss

This describes a situation where there is an unequal loss of the different modalities of sensation, occurring when the spinothalamic and dorsal column pathways are affected disproportionately by a pathological process:

- spinothalamic tracts (pain, temperature and some light touch): affected by lesions in central or anterior spinal cord, midbrain or thalamus
- dorsal column (light touch, vibration, proprioception): selectively involved in posterior cord lesions or by lesions at the dorsal root ganglia.

Sensory level

Numbness below a specific point on the trunk constitutes a sensory level, and suggests a lesion at the relevant level of the spinal cord. It is important to consider this at an early stage, as cord compression will require emergency surgical assessment.

Any cord lesion producing a sensory level may be associated with upper motor neurone weakness in areas supplied by the cord caudal to the lesion. Bilateral cord lesions may also produce sphincter dysfunction. Lesions in the central spinal cord can cause a sensory level with 'sacral sparing' since the centripetally arranged sensory fibres are unaffected by a central pathology.

Unilateral sensory deficit

This is rare but will be caused by an extensive lesion in the contralateral cortex or a small lesion in the subcortical sensory tracts. Mapping the distribution of any motor effects can help to localize the lesion.

Ataxia

Ataxia describes a loss of balance which can result either from lack of input (sensory ataxia) or failure to execute movements properly (cerebellar ataxia). Simple examination can help differentiate these:

- sensory ataxia: loss of proprioception with or without loss of vibration, light touch and pinprick sensation; positive Romberg's test and movement of fingers when eyes are closed with outstretched arms
- cerebellar ataxia: may be associated with poor heel–toe walking, poor finger–nose testing, dysdiadochokinesis and other cerebellar signs.

Special senses, sphincter function and cranial neuropathies

Special senses

- vision: check whether monocular or binocular visual loss (Table 8.6)
- hearing: the difference between conductive and sensorineural causes is best distinguished using an audiogram
- taste: it is rare for taste to be affected in isolation when the cause is neurological; the trigeminal and glossopharyngeal nerves supply the anterior two-thirds and posterior third of the tongue, respectively
- speech: distinguish between dysarthria (poor motor processing of speech) and dysphasia (poor central processing of language).

Table 8.6 Visual loss presentations

Source	Clinical findings	Identification
Retina: peripheral	Scotoma	Visual fields and retinal changes may be visible on fundoscopy
Retina: central (macula)	Central scotoma Poor acuity	
Optic nerve	Poor acuity Poor colour vision	Damage to nerve may be visible on fundoscopy
Optic tract	Homonymous hemianopia or quadrantanopia	Visual fields
Temporal optic radiation	Superior quadrantanopia	Visual fields
Parietal optic radiation	Inferior quadrantanopia	
Occipital cortex	Homonymous field defect but often macular sparing	Visual fields

Sphincter function

Unilateral neurological lesions do not tend to cause sphincter disturbance, so any associated bladder instability is likely to be caused by a lesion in the spinal cord or cauda equina (below L1). Lower motor neurone lesions cause difficulty with micturition (initiation or incomplete emptying), while upper motor neurone lesions tend to cause 'spastic bladder' (incomplete filling and frequent emptying). Both types of bladder dysfunction may present with the same symptoms (frequency, dysuria, nocturia, incontinence) and to distinguish these bladder ultrasound may be required to measure the residual volume (see also 'Urinary retention', p. 186).

Common cranial neuropathies

Bell's palsy

An isolated unilateral 7th nerve lesion is a common presentation. The weakness involves both the upper and lower face and may be accompanied by pain over the ipsilateral mastoid process, hyperacusis or loss of taste. Evidence supports steroid use to expedite recovery (the majority will recover fully with or without steroids).

Trigeminal neuropathy

Intermittent sharp electric shock-like pain, often triggered by touch or temperature, occurs over the distribution of one or all branches of the 5th cranial nerve.

Treatment with antiepileptic drugs may help reduce the frequency and severity of symptoms, e.g. carbamazepine (100 mg orally 1–2 times daily). However, as the aetiology often involves nerve compression by an arterial loop, some patients will require surgery.

FALLS AND IMMOBILITY

Falls

Falls are very common in older people and affect 30% of those over 65 each year. Around 10% of falls cause serious injury. Other serious consequences include loss of confidence, increased risk of dependency and institutionalization. Falls are partly preventable and it is important to address potential risk factors:

- abnormalities of gait and balance
- postural hypotension
- cognitive impairment
- visual impairment
- acute illness
- environmental factors
- drugs, e.g. benzodiazepines, antidepressants (especially tricyclics), antipsychotics, diuretics, antihypertensives, nitrates; polypharmacy (≥4 drugs) is an independent risk factor.

Assessment after a fall

Make a note in the case-sheet of your assessment and complete an incident report form if the fall occurred during an inpatient stay.

History

Take a careful history from the patient and any witnesses:

- enquire if they remember falling or when they were first aware of being on the ground
- enquire about preceding symptoms, e.g. loss of consciousness (syncope or seizure), light-headedness, aura, chest pain or palpitations
- look for evidence of causes of syncope (e.g. micturition, cough, stress) or vertebrobasilar insufficiency (e.g. neck movement)
- ask about pain that might suggest injury
- ask what happened after the fall, e.g. lying trapped for a prolonged period might result in rhabdomyolysis
- ask about previous falls and their circumstances
- further history is aimed at describing co-morbidities: acute illnesses can present with falls, e.g. a urinary tract infection
- document chronic illnesses, e.g. parkinsonism or diabetes and disabilities, drugs, and other risk factors as mentioned above
- see also the assessment of fits, p. 222.

Examination, investigations and initial management

Examination and investigations should be directed towards identifying acute causes and deficits that increase subsequent risk:

- assess neurological function, gait, balance, vision and cognition
- look for evidence of a postural drop in blood pressure: defined as a decrease in systolic pressure > 20 mmHg or diastolic drop of > 10 mmHg; patients should be supine for at least 2 min before measuring supine blood pressure, then remain standing for at least 1 min before measuring standing blood pressure
- look for injuries, particularly to the head, especially if the patient is on warfarin

- first-line investigations include ECG, blood glucose or BM and CK (rhabdomyolysis)
- second-line investigations might include a CT brain if there is evidence of structural brain disease or seizures, tilt table testing, or 24 h tape if there is unexplained syncope, or an echocardiogram if there is evidence of aortic stenosis.

The management of an acute fall involves the treatment of any acute precipitants and the consequences of the fall, e.g. analgesia for a vertebral fracture. Then, where possible, the risks of future falls and their consequences should be reduced.

Prevention and future management

It is best to address all the modifiable factors rather than simply deal with the presumed 'cause'. Multidisciplinary assessment is essential because assessment and modification of gait/balance and the patient's environment requires the expertise of a physiotherapist and an occupational therapist. Deciding on the modification of medical factors is complex and has to be tailored to specific patients. Therefore, in most cases it is best to ask for a specialist 'Care of the elderly' opinion: if in doubt, refer.

Immobility

Immobility resulting from acute or chronic illness and related disabilities is very common in hospitals. It is associated with many adverse effects including the rapid loss of muscle mass and cardiovascular deconditioning. Some older patients never recover from prolonged immobility.

Assessment and management

The first step is recognition. Although common in hospital, prolonged inactivity and bed rest is an abnormal state. It is important to document immobility as a problem, just as you would any other condition. Then consider potentially reversible factors, such as undiagnosed acute illness, pain, postural hypotension, side-effects of drugs (e.g. opiates), depression, hypothyroidism, parkinsonism and hypoactive delirium. Involvement of the 'Care of the elderly' team in assessment and management can be helpful.

Management

- address modifiable factors
- maintain health as far as possible by making sure nutrition is optimal and that complications of immobility, such as pressure sores, are avoided
- rehabilitation: early assessment and management by a physiotherapist is particularly important.

'Off legs'

This term tends to be used where someone who was previously mobile develops problems with balance, gait or falls acutely. Gait and balance problems are more prevalent than falls (which should be considered as already described). Their aetiology can be categorized into three groups:

- disordered limb coordination or power: cerebellar dysfunction, e.g. MS and other degenerative conditions; stroke; toxins; drugs
- unilateral or bilateral limb weakness or reduced sensation: stroke; Guillain–Barré; motor neurone disease; cerebral tumour; cord compression
- systemic illness, e.g. UTI or chest infection, hyponatraemia, hypokalaemia, uraemia, hypercalcaemia, thyroid disease, recent MI, anaemia, hypoactive delirium.

Investigation and management will depend on the suspected cause. However, if there is no evidence of acute bacterial infection or new drugs and basic laboratory tests are all normal, consider CT or MRI brain imaging ± lumbar puncture or nerve conduction studies.

DELIRIUM AND ALCOHOL WITHDRAWAL

Delirium

Delirium is defined as an acute confusional state. Cognitive impairment is the core deficit, but altered arousal, delusions, hallucinations and sleep/wake cycle disturbance are also common. Delirium is one of the most common disorders in hospital medicine, affecting about one in five of older inpatients.

Causes

Delirium is often due to a combination of predisposing and precipitating factors, rather than a single cause. Patients with a greater number of predisposing factors are more likely to develop delirium as a result of an apparently minor insult, e.g. urinary tract infection.

Predisposing factors include old age, cognitive and sensory impairment and alcohol abuse. Precipitating factors include acute illness, surgery or trauma; new or abrupt withdrawal of drugs or alcohol; metabolic disturbance.

Diagnosis

The central cognitive deficit in delirium is inattention. This can be assessed by determining if the patient is distractible, cannot consistently follow commands and loses the thread during a conversation. This is in contrast to a patient with dementia who may exhibit disorientation, but is usually able to maintain a conversation for several sentences. Formal assessment can be made by using either AMT or MMSE (see 'History and examination', p. 5).

Other features of delirium include disorganized thinking, altered level of arousal (ranging from hypervigilance to apathy, drowsiness or stupor), or psychotic features such as paranoia or hallucinations. It is important to note that >50% of patients with delirium never show agitation. In fact, where there is altered arousal, patients are most commonly hypoactive and these patients probably have a worse prognosis than patients with hyperactive delirium.

Prevention

All older people in hospital should be considered at risk of delirium. This is especially true of those with cognitive impairment and other co-morbidities. There is good evidence to suggest that the following measures are effective in preventing delirium:

- stop or reduce predisposing or precipitating drugs, e.g. anticholinergics, opioids, corticosteroids, β-blockers
- if possible, avoid benzodiazepines unless there is a clear history of alcohol abuse (see overleaf); however, do not withdraw benzodiazepines suddenly
- treat pain, constipation and electrolyte abnormalities
- screen for and treat visual, hearing and nutritional impairment
- avoid frequent ward transfer or bed relocation
- provide regular clear communication regarding the patient's reason for being in hospital, what is happening to them, the time and date, etc.

Investigation

Check a BM and oxygen saturation, routine bloods, urinalysis, blood cultures if there is evidence of infection, CXR and ECG. Further investigations should be directed by clinical findings. Consider CT brain ± LP if delirium persists and no cause is obvious.

Management

Management involves treating possible precipitants and controlling agitation. Patients should be nursed in quiet, well lit rooms, ideally by staff that they know. Avoid unnecessary physical contact as this may be misinterpreted as aggression.

Pharmacological management of agitation

- haloperidol 0.5–1mg PO or IM, at intervals of 20 min until acceptable change; do not over-sedate the patient as this can prolong the delirium
- after 3–4 doses, if there is no effect, consider lorazepam 0.5 mg PO or IM
- in patients with Parkinson's disease, or Lewy body dementia, avoid haloperidol and use lorazepam instead, 0.5 mg PO or IM at 20 min intervals
- for alcohol withdrawal, see below.

Persistent delirium

Delirium persists for weeks or months in around one-quarter of patients. It is very important to recognize and treat this appropriately. Misdiagnosing such patients as having depression or dementia can lead to the wrong treatments being administered or, worse, patients being inappropriately institutionalized. If there is any doubt as to this diagnosis, seek an opinion from geriatrics or psychiatry.

Alcohol intoxication and withdrawal

Acute alcohol intoxication

Alcohol intoxication is an extremely common problem. Assessment and management are aimed at preventing early complications and detecting and addressing possible alcoholism and its sequelae. Specific intervention in acute alcohol intoxication is rarely required; however, severe intoxication may cause respiratory depression and compromise the airway.

Assessment

In inebriated patients, consider all causes of impaired consciousness, not just those related to alcohol, e.g. hepatic encephalopathy, hypoglycaemia, traumatic haemorrhage and Wernicke's encephalopathy (thiamine deficiency causing ophthalmoplegia, ataxia and cognitive impairment).

Document consumption levels (may need informant) and look for evidence of liver disease, e.g. deranged LFT, cirrhosis of the liver.

Alcohol withdrawal

Alcohol withdrawal forms a spectrum from mild tremor and anxiety to delirium tremens. Patients who drink >60 units/week are at high risk of developing symptoms of withdrawal, although withdrawal can occur with lower levels of consumption. Symptoms may emerge between 6 and 72h after the patient's last drink. However, cases of delirium tremens have been reported as late as 10 days after the last intake of alcohol.

Delirium tremens is characterized by confusion, aggression, hallucinations, fever, tachycardia and hypertension. It is associated with a significant mortality rate and patients should be reviewed promptly and managed in a HDU, or at least in a well-staffed acute ward with monitoring and 24h medical staffing.

Management

- all patients should receive oral thiamine or IV Pabrinex®
- those with mild anxiety and irritability but no physical signs such as tremor or tachycardia may simply be observed
- those with physical manifestations (e.g. tachycardia, tremor or sweating), seizures, a history of alcohol withdrawal or whose regular intake is >60 units, should be commenced on benzodiazepines

- benzodiazepines use (e.g. diazepam 10–40 mg four times daily) should be titrated according to a recognized assessment score, e.g. CIWA (see below); the dose can be reduced in older patients
- benzodiazepine treatment can be reduced gradually over a few days according to the clinical state of the patient
- patients should not be discharged whilst still requiring benzodiazepine treatment.

Clinical Institute Withdrawal Assessment for Alcohol

The CIWA score stratifies the assessment of symptoms and signs of alcohol withdrawal to produce a cumulative score. The parameters assessed include nausea and vomiting, tactile disturbance (itch, paraesthesiae, burning, crawling sensation under skin), tremor, auditory hallucinations, sweating, light sensitivity or visual hallucinations, anxiety, headache, agitation and disorientation. CIWA monitoring can be discontinued when the score is <10 on three consecutive assessments.

ACUTE PSYCHOSIS

Psychosis refers to a mental state in which the patient has lost touch with reality and finds it difficult to think clearly, to communicate or to respond with appropriate emotions and behaviour. It is manifest by hallucinations, delusions, thought disorder and a lack of insight. There are many possible causes, but in the general hospital setting psychosis is mostly seen as part of delirium, alcohol withdrawal, medication (e.g. opiates, steroids, levodopa), drug abuse or dementia. In addition, it may be due to the onset of schizophrenia, affective or puerperal psychosis, or to an underlying neurological disorder (e.g. temporal lobe epilepsy).

Assessment

Consider delirium and dementia

Patients with psychotic symptoms should first be assessed for delirium (see p. 233). Psychotic symptoms occur in 30–50% of cases of delirium. Features that suggest delirium include:

- hallucinations and delusions that are poorly formed and transient in comparison to those seen in acute schizophrenia
- visual rather than auditory hallucinations
- an acute onset and fluctuating course.

Psychotic symptoms are also common in dementia. Hallucinations are more commonly visual and less well formed than in schizophrenia or bipolar illness. However, in Lewy body dementia, complex visual hallucinations can be seen. Patients with dementia may also have paranoid delusions, for example voicing concerns about theft of property.

General history, examination and investigation

When assessing the acutely psychotic patient, remember to consider your own safety and avoid seeing them alone. Adopt a calm, non-threatening stance and avoid physical contact where possible.

Enquire about recent major life events, alcohol or substance abuse, family history of mental illness and evidence of social isolation. Look for symptoms of affective disorders: psychological (low mood, reduced self-esteem, negative thoughts, loss of interest or pleasure, feelings of worthlessness, suicidal ideation) and physiological (reduced concentration, fatigue, early wakening ± insomnia, reduced appetite ± weight loss, constipation, loss of libido, amenorrhoea).

Specifically look for the 'first rank' symptoms of schizophrenia (one first-rank symptom is highly suggestive of the diagnosis):

- auditory hallucinations (voices referring to the patient in the second or third person)
- thought 'broadcasting', withdrawal or insertion
- passivity/being controlled externally
- delusions.

Other symptoms, such as apathy or loss of drive may also occur, although these tend to be found in chronic rather than acute schizophrenia.

Examination may show signs of personal neglect or flattened affect. Alternatively, in affective psychosis associated with bipolar disorder there may be agitation. In addition, there may be signs of compulsive behaviour.

Investigations should focus on excluding potential underlying aetiology: LFT, TFT, syphilis serology, HIV, urine drug screen, CT brain (see also 'Delirium', above).

Management

Patients with acute psychosis often lack insight and require admission in order to receive treatment and to prevent them harming themselves or others. Patients with delirium should be managed as above and any underlying medical conditions should be treated.

Schizophrenia is managed with antipsychotics (Table 8.7). These can take a few weeks to become effective and are associated with anticholinergic and extrapyramidal side-effects including tardive dyskinesia (involuntary chewing, grimacing, chorea which may respond to oral tetrabenazine 50–200 mg daily). In addition, they may result in corneal or lens opacities, photosensitive dermatitis, cholestatic jaundice, gynaecomastia and blood dyscrasias.

Serious side-effects can occur with prolongation of the QT interval (and subsequent VT ± sudden death) and neuroleptic malignant syndrome. This presents with fever, confusion and rigidity accompanied by raised WBC and CK. Treatment includes cessation of all antipsychotics, IV fluids and cooling. Consider the use of dantrolene sodium or bromocriptine.

Acute manic depressive psychosis relating to bipolar disorder are also managed with antipsychotics. However, long-term treatment to prevent recurrences includes lithium, carbamazepine and sodium valproate. Lithium can also be used for acute mania. It has a narrow therapeutic range requiring blood monitoring

Table 8.7 Antipsychotic medication

Group	Drug	Usual dose
Phenothiazines	Chlorpromazine Trifluoperazine Fluphenazine	100–1500 mg daily 5–30 mg daily 20–100 mg fortnightly
Butyrophenones	Haloperidol	5–30 mg daily
Thioxanthenes	Flupentixol	40–200 mg fortnightly
Diphenylbutylpiperidines	Pimozide	4–30 mg daily
Substituted benzamide	Sulpiride	600–1800 mg daily
Dibenzodiazepine	Clozapine	25–900 mg daily
Benzisoxazole	Risperidone	2–16 mg daily
Thienobenzodiazepines	Olanzapine	5–20 mg daily

and dose adjustment accordingly. Toxicity should be suspected in the presence of blurring of vision, ataxia, tremor or drowsiness. With long-term use, lithium can also result in nephrogenic diabetes insipidus, hypothyroidism and renal failure. U&E and TFT should be checked every 6 months.

SELF-INJURY AND SELF-POISONING

Presentation

The terms self-poisoning, self-harm, parasuicide and attempted suicide are used interchangeably to describe similar clinical presentations. Most cases involve 15–50 year olds and self-poisoning and self-harm often occur together. Self-laceration is by far the most common form of self-harm. Other presentations include injury to hands or head from self-induced trauma, attempted hanging, the swallowing of an object, exposure to carbon monoxide, stabbing, jumping, traffic-related episodes and drowning. Motivations for self-harm include relief or escape from a state of mind or situation; demonstration of love or feelings of rejection; seeking help; influencing or frightening someone.

Individuals presenting in this way may present again with self-harm or self-poisoning. Repeated attempts are associated with substance abuse, unemployment or social class 5, a personality disorder, living alone, a history of violence or a criminal record, recent bereavement or previous episodes.

History and examination

In some cases, a history will not be available. The patient may have a reduced conscious level; may be under the influence of alcohol or drugs, or may have been so when they took the substance; or they may not wish to declare what happened. Additional sources of history should be explored, e.g. accompanying friends or relatives, medicine containers and other evidence collected by paramedics at the scene. A conventional history should be taken (see 'History and examination', p. 3), but specific points that should be covered include:

- why the substance was taken: listen to the explanation as it will impact on your assessment of the likelihood of the event happening again
- what, how much and when the substance was taken: specific timing and quantity is important to assess the risk of clinical complications; great care should be taken to ensure there is clarity over what history is certain as compared with what is assumed; specific drugs should be identified using packets or drug identification aids
- how the event took place: look for signs of premeditation, e.g. a Beck's score of >4 suggests further risk of self-harm (Table 8.8)
- if any alcohol was involved, this may suggest that the event was impulsive rather than planned, but the clinical effect of the substance may also be magnified, e.g. paracetamol poisoning.

Assess ABCDE. Perform a full examination (see 'History and examination', p. 8, and 'Unconscious patient', p. 217). Pay particular attention to pupil size, temperature, sweating, respiratory and heart rates, GCS, skin for signs of injection or previous self-harm, and weight (to calculate dose of antidotes).

Investigation

Investigation will be influenced by any poison ingested, previous medical history and clinical examination findings. In cases of suspected self-poisoning or self-harm, patients should routinely have blood taken for FBC, U&E, Glu, LFT, Coag, paracetamol and salicylate levels and, where unconscious, ABG.

Table 8.8 Beck's scale for suicidal intent

Parameter	Score	Criteria
Isolation	0 1 2	Someone present Someone nearby or in vocal (incl. telephone) contact No-one nearby or in visual/vocal contact
Timing of event in relation to sources of intervention	0 1 2	Intervention probable Intervention not likely Intervention highly unlikely
Precautions against discovery or interruption	0 1 2	None Avoiding others but doing nothing to prevent intervention Active precautions, e.g. locking door
Action to gain help after the event	0 1 2	Notified a potential helper about event Contacted but did not specifically notify a potential helper Did not contact or notify any helper
Final acts in anticipation of death	0 1 2	None Thought about or made some arrangement for death Definite plans made, e.g. changing will
Active preparation for event	0 1 2	None Minimal Extensive
Suicide note	0 1 2	None Note thought about or written but torn up Note present
Overt communication of intent within 1 year before event	0 1 2	None Equivocal communication Unequivocal attempt

An ECG should be performed in all cases, and a CXR in those at risk of aspiration, or where foreign body ingestion or cardiorespiratory disease is suspected.

A urine drug screen can identify benzodiazepines, cocaine, ecstasy, opioids and cannabis, but may miss fentanyl derivatives, tramadol and other synthetic opioids. Consider, especially where the patient is seriously unwell, saving urine and serum for later analysis.

Management

In all cases, it is advisable to consult an on-line poisons database, e.g. TOXBASE®. Patients who appear to be at risk of further attempts should be referred for psychiatric evaluation. Consider the following specific interventions:

Poison removal

Eye or skin contamination

Remove any contact lenses and wash with saline or water and consider ophthalmology referral (see ophthalmic presentations, p. 313).

Ingestion

Gastric lavage

This should only be performed if a potentially life-threatening amount has been ingested within the past hour. Avoid if acids, alkalis or petroleum distillates have been ingested.

Activated charcoal

An adult dose of 50 g should be given if the toxin can be absorbed by charcoal (examples include carbamazepine, quinine and theophylline) and a toxic amount has been ingested within the past hour. Administer via a nasogastric tube in patients who cannot swallow, or who are at risk of aspiration. Repeated doses may be necessary, in which case a laxative should also be prescribed.

Bowel irrigation

Polyethylene glycol (1 L every hour) can be useful in toxic cases of iron, lithium and theophylline ingestion, or to clear packets of opiate drugs that have been swallowed. Its use is contraindicated in gastrointestinal haemorrhage or obstruction.

Urinary alkalinization

A dose of 1 L of 1.26% sodium bicarbonate IV over 3 h enhances salicylate and pesticide excretion by increasing urinary pH to between 7.5 and 8.5. This may cause hypokalaemia and volume overload.

Haemofiltration or haemodialysis

This is used in severe cases of salicylate, theophylline, ethylene glycol, methanol, lithium and carbamazepine overdose.

Supportive management

Poison inhalation

Give high flow oxygen ± nebulized salbutamol if there is wheeze. Further respiratory support, including ventilation, may be required.

Seizures

These are common in cases involving theophyllines, NSAIDs, anticonvulsants and tricyclic antidepressants. Use diazepam 10 mg IV initially in adults (see also 'Seizures', p. 221).

Shock and Impaired consciousness

See also 'Shock and fluid balance', p. 250, and 'The unconscious patient', p. 217. In poisoning, acidosis and electrolyte disturbance may produce an altered level of consciousness; high volumes of fluid ± inotropes may be required to treat shock and maintain the perfusion of vital organs.

Specific substances

Paracetamol

Paracetamol causes liver failure and renal failure (see also p. 182). A plasma paracetamol concentration (PPC) should be checked at least 4 h following ingestion to determine the need for *N*-acetylcysteine administration (either Parvolex IV or methionine PO) (Fig. 8.1). This antidote is most effective when given within 10 h of overdose. Therefore, if a patient presents >8 h after ingestion, treatment should not be delayed pending a paracetamol level. It can be stopped later, if the result is below the treatment line.

A sample for Coag, LFT and U&E should be checked after completion of the infusion and treatment continued beyond 24 h if the results are abnormal and until any derangement in liver or renal function improves.

Patients with a history of excess alcohol, malnutrition and those taking enzyme-inducing drugs, such as anticonvulsants, will be at greater risk of toxicity (Fig. 8.1). Likewise, in those with staggered ingestion over several days, the PPC will not predict outcome and you should have a low threshold for starting *N*-acetylcysteine. Equally, those in whom the history of dose or timing is not clear should be treated irrespective of their PPC.

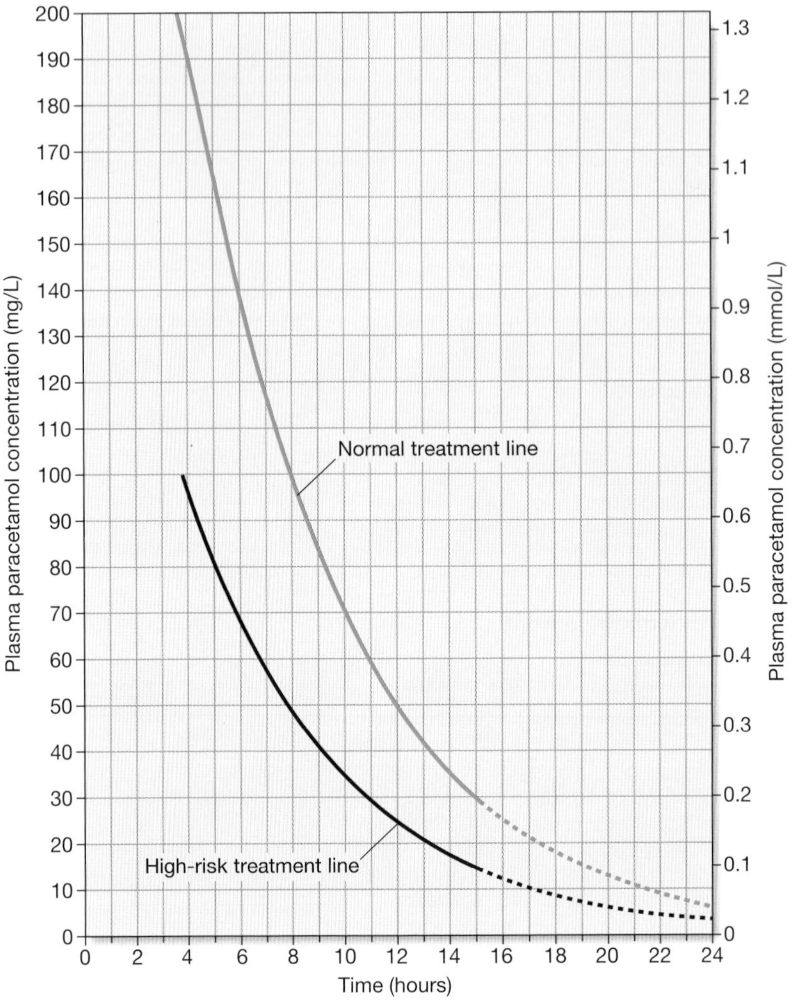

Figure 8.1 Paracetamol treatment graph. All patients with a plasma paracetamol concentration (PPC) above the normal treatment line should be treated. In addition, patients on enzyme-inducing drugs, including alcohol, and those who are malnourished should be treated if their PPC is above the high-risk treatment line.

In patients presenting over 15 h after ingestion, check the Coag, LFT and U&E, initiate treatment and consider discussing the case with your regional liver unit.

Adverse reactions to N*-acetylcysteine*

It is not always necessary to stop *N*-acetylcysteine treatment in the event of a reaction to the drug, as this is usually anaphylactoid rather than anaphylaxis. Manage the reaction with antihistamines and bronchodilators, but continue the therapy.

Salicylates

Salicylate overdose can produce nausea, tinnitus, deafness, hyperventilation, vasodilatation, sweating, petechial haemorrhages and, in severe cases, acidosis, renal failure, agitation, confusion, fits and coma. Rarely, pulmonary and cerebral oedema can develop.

Plasma concentrations should be measured at least 6 h after ingestion and interpreted in association with a clinical and acid–base assessment. Metabolic acidosis should be treated with IV sodium bicarbonate 8.4% and titrated to give an arterial pH of 7.4–7.5 (H^+ 32–40). Dehydration is often a problem and high-volume fluid replacement may be necessary; consider central venous access and invasive monitoring in patients with a history of cardiac disease.

Benzodiazepines

Drowsiness can be accompanied by cerebellar signs and confusion. Mild hypotension can occur as can respiratory depression. In isolated benzodiazepine overdose, a GCS <10 is rare. The specific antagonist, flumazenil, is only rarely required and must not be used as a 'diagnostic test'. It is also contraindicated in those with a history of convulsions, cardiac disease, overdoses involving drug combinations or those on tricyclic antidepressants or cocaine. When given, it should be administered slowly, 1 mg at a time, under ECG monitoring. If flumazenil is used, note that its half-life is shorter than that of most benzodiazepines and an infusion may be necessary to maintain any beneficial effects.

Opioids

Pin-point pupils are suggestive of opioid toxicity. Naloxone (0.8–2 mg IV in adults) can be given as a bolus and repeated every 2 min as necessary. Up to 20 mg may be required in some cases, but excessive dosing can precipitate acute opioid withdrawal with fits and sweating: therefore, careful dose titration is necessary. Consider an infusion of naloxone if the effect wanes, as its half-life is shorter than that of most opioids.

Amphetamines and ecstasy

These can cause cardiac arrhythmias, hyponatraemia, trismus, muscle pain, dilated pupils, blurred vision, dry mouth, sweating, hallucinations and psychosis. Hypertension and convulsions may occur and a hyperthermic syndrome can develop with rigidity, hyper-reflexia and hyperpyrexia resulting in shock, acidosis, rhabdomyolysis, renal and liver failure and ARDS. Therefore, a CK should be checked. Cooled fluids and dantrolene can help in hyperthermic cases, but paralysis and ventilation may be necessary. β-blockers should be avoided in the treatment of associated hypertension as they allow unopposed α stimulation and paradoxical worsening of the hypertension.

Tricyclic antidepressants

The risk of arrhythmias and fits is dependent on the duration of the QRS complex on ECG. Therefore, serial 12-lead ECGs should be monitored closely. The administration of 200 mL 8.4% sodium bicarbonate should be considered where the QRS complex is >120 ms, or 100 ms in the presence of a reduced conscious state.

SECTION 2
Symptoms and related acute presentations

9 Sepsis, shock and trauma

SEPSIS AND INFECTION

Definitions

All febrile patients require careful clinical evaluation for evidence of infection and any resultant haemodynamic effects. This requires an understanding of the different terms used to describe and classify patients with infection.

- systemic inflammatory response syndrome (SIRS): this often accompanies infection but may also be caused by non-infectious stimuli (e.g. pancreatitis, burns); it is defined by two or more of the following: temperature >38°C or <36°C, heart rate >90/min, respiratory rate >20/min or $PaCO_2$ <4.3 kPa, WBC >12 000/mm^3 or <4000/mm^3
- sepsis: SIRS plus a proven or suspected focus of infection
- severe sepsis: sepsis associated with organ dysfunction (e.g. renal or respiratory failure), hypoperfusion (e.g. lactic acidosis, oliguria, altered mental status) or hypotension (systolic <90 mmHg or a drop of 40 mmHg from baseline)
- septic shock: severe sepsis refractory to adequate fluid resuscitation.

This classification is important because severe sepsis and septic shock are life-threatening emergencies that can progress rapidly to multi-organ failure and death.

Clinical assessment and immediate management

Start by assessing ABC. Thereafter, take a brief history of recent events, past medical and drug history (including allergies) from the patient and/or relatives. Look for clinical evidence of a source of infection and any haemodynamic disturbance or hypoperfusion. Patients with sepsis tend to be vasodilated (warm, bounding peripheral and forearm pulses ± hypotension).

All patients with hypotension and/or evidence of organ hypoperfusion must be treated aggressively with immediate oxygen therapy (see 'Oxygen delivery', p. 66) and early, aggressive intravenous fluid resuscitation (see p. 251). In all patients:

- look for obvious clues to the source of the infection: this will help target subsequent investigations and guide empirical antimicrobial prescribing

- take blood cultures if infection is suspected, ideally before antibiotic administration, provided this does not result in treatment delay
- if the patient is unwell, administer appropriate broad-spectrum intravenous antibiotics as soon as possible (take blood cultures just before the first dose, if not already done); see 'Antibiotics' below for advice on the choice of empirical agent
- speed is important: call for senior help early including HDU or ICU input in patients with severe sepsis, septic shock or dangerous infections such as meningitis
- consider inotropic support in patients with septic shock (see p. 252).

Secondary survey

A more detailed assessment, focusing on possible sources of infection, can be undertaken once you are confident that the patient is stable. Aspects of the initial history and examination may need to be expanded. Friends and relatives may give you important additional information. Important pointers in this evaluation are summarized in Table 9.1, overleaf.

Investigations

The following investigations should be performed in all patients, but should not delay resuscitation and immediate management, if the patient is unwell:

- FBC, Coag, U&E, glucose, LFT, CRP, lactate
- ABG if SaO_2 <92%, if shocked or evidence of hypoperfusion
- blood cultures, urinalysis and MSU, together with other site-specific samples, e.g. throat swab, sputum and stool
- CXR and ECG
- in returning travellers, thick and thin blood films for malaria or an antigen blood test (for *P. falciparum*) should be sent; the test available will depend on local laboratory policy; other conditions to consider and relevant investigations are summarized in Table 9.2 on p. 245
- other tests may be appropriate in certain clinical settings, e.g. echocardiography in suspected endocarditis.

Antimicrobial therapy

Most hospitals have a site-specific prescribing policy for empirical antimicrobial therapy that incorporates national guidelines and local drug resistance data. An example is provided in Table 9.3 (see p. 245), but you should refer to local advice, where available.

Always ask about drug allergies and only use IV treatment if the patient has specific indications for this, e.g. inability to swallow or severity criteria. If IV therapy is commenced, aim to switch to oral therapy within 24–48 h where possible. Prolonged IV antibiotic therapy will be required in some situations, e.g. endocarditis, meningitis. Empirical therapy may require modification once culture and sensitivity results are obtained. Do not hesitate to seek senior advice from microbiology or infectious diseases departments.

Infection in the immunocompromised

Immunocompromised patients are susceptible to infection with organisms that would not normally cause disease in healthy individuals. Such 'opportunistic' infection can occur because of dysfunction or failure of the host's immune system, or reflect a breach in the body's normal physical barriers to infection. The identification of immunodeficiency, of what ever kind, allows appropriate investigations to be undertaken and adequate broad-spectrum antimicrobial treatment to be prescribed, pending culture results.

Table 9.1 Diagnostic pointers for patients with acute community-acquired sepsis

Presentation	Consider	Comments
Sore throat ± cervical lymphadenopathy	Bacterial or viral pharyngitis; glandular fever	Consider streptococcal bacteraemia if very unwell
Acute watery diarrhoea	Viral infection or salmonella, campylobacter, *C. difficile*	Ask about food and travel history, contact with young children or animals, recent antibiotics, achlorhydria or PPI therapy
Acute bloody diarrhoea	Campylobacter, *E. coli* 0157, shigella or acute diverticulitis	
Abnormal LFTs ± rigors and RUQ tenderness	Ascending cholangitis; malaria if travel history; hepatitis	Ask about travel; viral hepatitis unlikely if febrile
Headache, otherwise reasonably well	Common with viral infections and many others, e.g. sinusitis	Common symptom but consider possibility of neurosepsis
Headache with photophobia ± neck stiffness, vomiting and confusion	Meningitis	Seek senior help early. Rash suggests meningococcal septicaemia. Meningitis and encephalitis are difficult to distinguish – empirical treatment for both often needed. Follow local protocol
Headaches with fits and confusion rather than meningism	Viral encephalitis; severe bacterial meningitis; cerebral malaria if travel history	
Loin pain ± rigors	Pyelonephritis	Renal ultrasound ± KUB
Erythema, heat, swelling of skin and soft tissues	Cellulitis	Can be difficult to distinguish from DVT
As above, but with marked pain ± septic shock	Necrotizing fasciitis	Rare but serious; urgent surgical review required
New murmur, cutaneous signs, e.g. splinter haemorrhages, risk factors present	Endocarditis	Ensure 3 sets of blood cultures are obtained plus echo, ESR and CRP
Acute mono-arthritis or back pain	Septic arthritis	Look for signs of cord compression if spine involved
Rash	Meningococcal infection, streptococcal infection, viral exanthems	Remember non-infectious causes, e.g. drug rash

HIV-infected individuals

HIV infection causes a progressive defect of cell-medicated immunity and opportunistic infection may develop. This has become less common since the introduction of highly active antiretroviral therapy (HAART). However, HIV infection should always be considered in patients with risk factors, particularly those with unusual infections (Table 9.4, p. 246). Infection in HIV patients is a complex area, so seek senior advice early.

Table 9.2 Fever in a patient who has travelled overseas recently

Presentation	Consider	Comments
Headache ± rigors and CNS symptoms	Malaria	Send blood for thick and thin films ± antigen
Headache, abdominal symptoms; occasionally a faint rash ('rose spots')	Typhoid/ paratyphoid	Difficult to distinguish from malaria; send blood cultures
Cough and dyspnoea	Legionnaires' disease, viral RTI, avian influenza	Avian 'flu must be considered if returning from an endemic area
Haemorrhagic features	Viral haemorrhagic fever	Very rare; major clinical and infection control challenge

Table 9.3 A guide to empirical antibiotic therapy for adults

Clinical presentation	Treatment	Dose	Days of therapy
Mild to moderate infection (all doses are for oral therapy)			
Cellulitis	Flucloxacillin + penicillin V	1–2 g 6-hourly 500 mg 6-hourly	7–14
Cystitis	Co-amoxiclav	375 mg 8-hourly	3
Exacerbation of COPD	Amoxicillin *or* clarithromycin	500 mg–1 g 8-hourly 500 mg 12-hourly	5–7
CAP	Amoxicillin + clarithromycin	500 mg–1 g 8-hourly 500 mg 12-hourly	7
Severe infection (all doses are for IV therapy[a])			
Cellulitis	Flucloxacillin + benzylpenicillin	1–2 g 6-hourly 1.2–2.4 g 6-hourly	10–14
Pyelonephritis	Ciprofloxacin ± gentamicin (if severe)	500 mg 12-hourly Local guidelines[b]	7–14
Intra-abdominal sepsis	Amoxicillin + metronidazole + gentamicin	1 g 8-hourly 500 mg 8-hourly Local guidelines[b]	7–14
Meningitis	Ceftriaxone[c] + amoxicillin[d] ± aciclovir (in encephalitis)	2 g 12-hourly 2 g 6-hourly 10 mg/kg TDS	7–14
Sepsis, uncertain source	Amoxicillin + metronidazole + gentamicin	1 g 8-hourly 500 mg 8-hourly Local guidelines[b]	7–14
CAP	Augmentin + clarithromycin ± flucloxacillin	1.2 g 8-hourly 500 mg 12-hourly 1–2 g 6-hourly	7–14
Postoperative or aspiration pneumonia	Ceftriaxone[c] + metronidazole	2 g once daily 500 mg 8-hourly	7–10

[a]For many patients on IV therapy, a switch to oral administration after 24–48 h is appropriate.
[b]Many hospitals now use a once-daily gentamicin regimen.
[c]There is an increasing trend to use alternatives to cephalosporins.
[d]Omitted if the patient is not immunocompromised and is <55 years of age.

Table 9.4 Medical conditions potentially related to HIV infection

System	Condition(s)
Respiratory	Atypical pneumonia (consider *Pneumocystis*), TB
GI	Unexplained weight loss, chronic diarrhoea, oesophageal candidiasis
Haematological	Lymphadenopathy, lymphoma, thrombocytopenia
Dermatological	Kaposi's sarcoma, seborrhoeic dermatitis, severe molluscum contagiosum
Oral	Candidiasis, oral hairy leukoplakia
Others	Acute HIV seroconversion, unusual infections, tumours or neurological

Acute primary HIV infection

Patients present with fever, lymphadenopathy, rash, oral ulceration ± neurological symptoms. Opportunistic infections may also be present in undiagnosed and untreated advanced HIV infection.

Secondary infection

The incidence of secondary infections correlates closely with the patient's CD4 count. Patients with early disease and relatively normal counts usually present with infections due to 'common' organisms or those found in patients with non-HIV immunocompromise, e.g. pneumococcal infection, TB, syphilis (and other STIs), VZV (shingles), recurrent HSV.

Patients with more advanced disease and lower CD4 counts are susceptible to infection with a wider spectrum of low-virulence opportunistic organisms:

- <500 cells/mm^3: oral candidiasis
- <200 cells/mm^3: PCP (see below), invasive candidiasis, cerebral toxoplasmosis
- <100 cells/mm^3: chronic diarrhoea (cryptosporidiosis), fungal meningitis (cryptococcal)
- <50 cells/mm^3: CMV retinitis, *M. avium intracellulare* (MAI).

Pneumocystis pneumonia

Pneumocystis jirovecii pneumonia (previously *Pneumocystis carinii* pneumonia, hence the acronym PCP) usually presents sub-acutely with a dry cough, dyspnoea, fever and bilateral, often subtle, CXR changes. Diagnosis requires a high index of suspicion, confirmed by PCR ± immunofluorescence performed on induced sputum or BAL fluid (see also 'Breathlessness', p. 157).

Neutropenic sepsis

Patients undergoing chemotherapy frequently develop drug-induced neutropenia. The risk of infection is increased when the neutrophil count falls below 1.0×10^9/L. A variety of infections may occur, including unusual and drug-resistant bacteria, fungi (e.g. candida, aspergillus) and viruses (e.g. VZV, CMV).

Neutropenic patients may become very unwell if treatment is delayed, so early empirical antimicrobial treatment should be started if there are features of sepsis (see above) or if the temperature rises above 38.5°C once or 38°C twice in 2h. Figure 9.1 shows an example of a typical management protocol. Neutropenia without sepsis is managed differently and may not require either antibiotics or admission. Prophylactic antibiotics (e.g. ciprofloxacin) may be used along with further FBC monitoring.

Previous splenectomy

Following splenectomy, patients are at an increased risk of invasive bloodstream infections, particularly from *S. pneumoniae* and other encapsulated organisms such

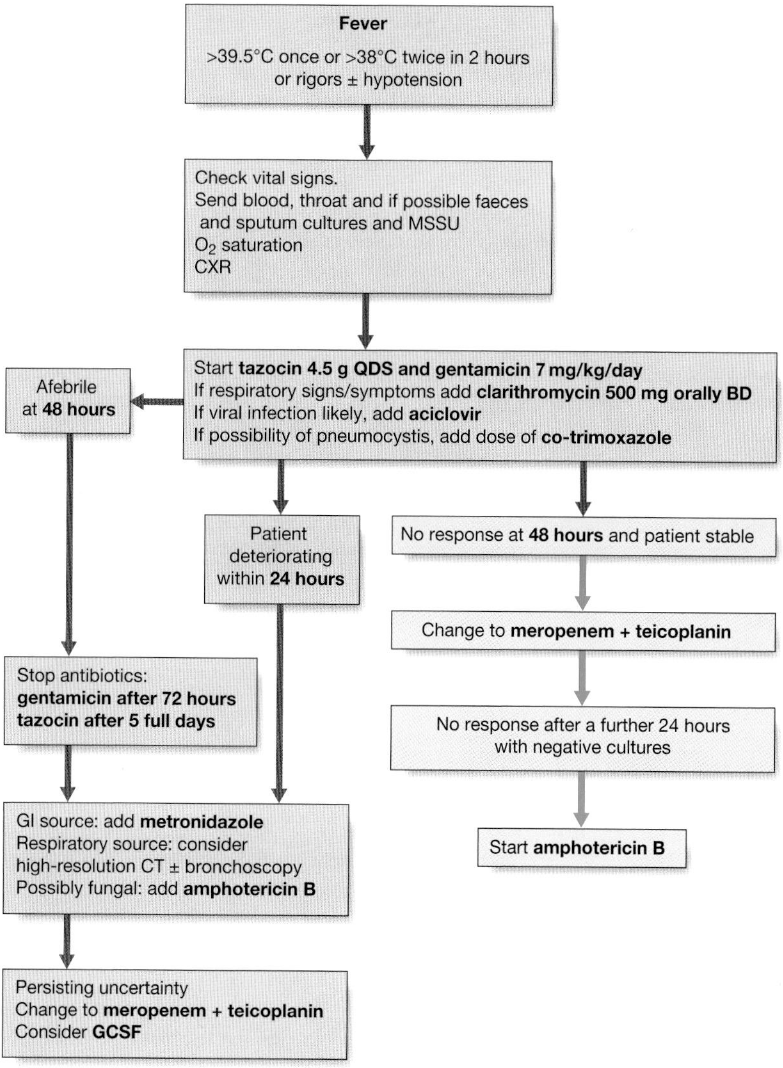

Figure 9.1 Management protocol for neutropenic sepsis.

as *N. meningitidis* and *H. influenza*. Vaccination is usually offered, e.g. Pneumovac®, and many patients are prescribed low-dose penicillin prophylaxis. They are also at increased risk of severe malaria.

Intravascular devices

Intravascular devices, e.g. peripheral and central lines, constitute a breach of the normal host defences and predispose the patient to skin infection and bacteraemia. Insertion sites should be looked after carefully and inspected regularly. If infection develops, consider *S. aureus* (including MRSA) and coagulase-negative staphylococcal infection as potential causes. Empirical use of a glycopeptide antibiotic, such as vancomycin, may be indicated for suspected infection if the patient is unwell (refer to local protocol). If an infection develops when a line is already in situ, it may have to be removed.

Pyrexia

Normal body temperature is around 37°C and elevation above 38°C is almost always pathological. Minor elevations in body temperature may be physiological, e.g. during menstruation or exercise.

The commonest cause of pyrexia is infection, although there are numerous other possible explanations, including drug reactions, malignancy and connective tissue disorders. Conversely, some patients with an infection may not develop a fever, particularly the elderly or immunosuppressed. Indeed, hypothermia is a well-recognized manifestation of severe sepsis.

Pyrexia of unknown origin

Pyrexia of unknown origin (PUO) is defined as a persistent fever, of at least 2 weeks, which remains undiagnosed despite appropriate initial investigations. Potential causes are given in Table 9.5.

Table 9.5 Potential causes of a pyrexia of unknown origin

Infectious	Non-infectious
TB (pulmonary or non-pulmonary)	Drug reactions
Bacterial endocarditis	Malignancy: lymphoma, leukaemia, solid organ (e.g. renal, GI)
Intra-abdominal abscesses	Thyrotoxicosis and other endocrine diseases
Bone and joint sepsis	Connective tissue disorders, e.g. RA, SLE, Still's disease
Infected implanted medical device	Thromboembolic disease
Syphilis	Alcoholic liver disease
Lyme disease	Inflammatory bowel disease
Brucellosis	Granulomatous disorders, e.g. sarcoid
Certain viral infections – HIV; CMV	Hypothalamic dysfunction
Fungal infections	Factitious fever
Imported infections – malaria; amoebic liver abscess	

PUO can pose a significant diagnostic challenge. Repeat the history and examination carefully since new findings may emerge. Further investigations should be guided, where possible, by the clinically suspected source, but they are likely to include:

- repeat blood cultures
- samples for AAFB and mycobacterial culture, including sputum, urine and any biopsy material
- serology: chlamydia, mycoplasma, CMV, HIV ± others, e.g. Q-fever, bartonella, brucella
- ANA, RF, ANCA screen
- echocardiogram (transoesophageal if available)
- imaging (US, CT or MRI) ± organ biopsy
- others, where indicated, e.g. lumbar puncture; liver biopsy; bone marrow biopsy; bronchoscopy and lavage; upper and lower GI endoscopy; labelled WBC scan.

Treatment should ideally be guided by the results of these investigations, but empirical antimicrobial therapy may need to be commenced if the patient is deteriorating and/or endocarditis is suspected.

Fluid balance

Safe intravenous fluid prescription requires an understanding of physiological principles and the effect of disease processes on normal homeostasis.

Fluid compartments

Total body fluid is approximately 60% of body weight, meaning that an average 75kg male contains 45L of water. This water is contained within distinct fluid compartments within the body. Intracellular fluid (ICF) accounts for two-thirds of body water (30L). Extracellular fluid (ECF) accounts for one-third of body water (15L) and is composed of:

- interstitial fluid (ISF) comprises three-quarters of the ECF; surrounds cells and does not circulate
- intravascular fluid comprises one-quarter of the ECF; circulates as the extracellular component of blood
- transcellular fluid accounts for fluid outside normal compartments, e.g. CSF, mucus.

Factors that influence the movement of water between these fluid compartments include pressure, tonicity and the permeability of the barriers in between. The most important site of fluid exchange between fluid compartments is the vascular capillary bed, a schematic of which is presented in Figure 9.2. The structures and physiological factors involved at this level influence fluid balance management in both healthy individuals and those with disease:

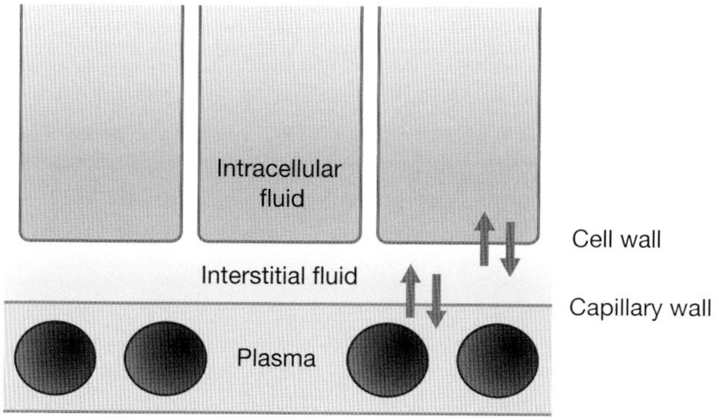

Figure 9.2 The capillary bed.

Capillary wall

The capillary wall acts as a filter through which water and solutes pass freely; larger molecules including plasma proteins and lipids are unable to pass through. Flow across the capillary wall is determined by the balance between hydrostatic pressure (forcing fluid out of intravascular space; determined blood pressure) and oncotic pressure (sucking fluid back in; generated by plasma proteins). In healthy individuals, the net effect is a small flow of fluid into the interstitial space, producing lymph. However, this balance can be altered in disease causing capillaries to leak protein, e.g. sepsis, resulting in a net loss to the interstitial space and oedema.

Cell wall

Although water moves freely across the cell wall, the movement of solutes is selective. Sodium, the main extracellular cation, is pumped out of cells in exchange for potassium (potassium and magnesium are the main intracellular cations).

Osmolality

Osmolality describes the concentration of osmotically active particles in solution (normally 280–290 mmol/kg serum) and is similar in ECF and ICF. However, this equilibrium can be disrupted by illness or IV fluid administration, e.g. if plasma becomes hypotonic, water will flow into cells to equalize the osmolality gradient, causing cell swelling and possibly lysis.

Clinical relevance

A basic understanding of the fluid compartments of the body and the way in which fluid is likely to 'shift' is important when managing fluid balance. For example, an IV infusion of any fluid will initially increase the intravascular ECF, but the composition of the fluid will dictate its ultimate distribution:

- dextrose is quickly metabolized to water, passing freely throughout the total body water
- normal saline is isotonic with ECF and will increase the volume of interstitial fluid and plasma
- colloid solutions will be less able to diffuse across the capillary membrane and will stay in the intravascular space longer.

Normal maintenance requirements

Normal water requirements are estimated at 20–40 mL/kg per day. In healthy individuals this is achieved by drinking (approx. 1200 mL), eating (1000 mL) and water oxidation (300 mL). Fluid losses are comprised of urine (1500 mL) and insensible losses from skin and lungs (850 mL). The GI tract produces between 6–8 L of fluid/day, but most of it is reabsorbed with only 150 mL lost in faeces.

Fluid resuscitation

Intravenous fluid prescription should be regarded like any other type of prescribing and, where possible, patients should be encouraged to drink. Maintenance requirements and replacement fluids should be considered separately. Consider the following:

- urine output and daily weights are the best monitors of fluid balance
- for every 1°C rise in temperature give an extra 1 L/day
- 1 L normal saline and 2 L 5% dextrose is a common maintenance regime
- avoid excessive saline infusion as this can cause hyperchloraemic acidosis
- GI secretions are electrolyte rich, so replace with saline like for like
- after surgery K^+ may rise due to cell damage, so check before supplementing.

See also the general guidance on prescribing fluids, 'Prescribing blood and fluids', p. 122.

Shock

Shock is defined as inadequate organ perfusion and tissue oxygenation. While profound shock is easy to recognize, earlier signs can be subtle.

Early signs

- tachycardia: an attempt to preserve cardiac output, reduced in the elderly or those who are β-blocked
- cool or pale peripheries: vasoconstriction reduces blood flow to non-essential organs; in distributive forms of shock (see overleaf) the peripheries may be warm due to vasodilatation
- narrow pulse pressure: diastolic pressure rises to maintain preload and, therefore, cardiac output
- reduced urine output: renal blood flow is reduced and ADH secretion is increased.

Late signs

- falling blood pressure: this occurs once compensatory mechanisms have been overwhelmed
- reduced consciousness: autoregulation of cerebral blood flow is unable to compensate adequately
- tachypnoea: may indicate metabolic acidosis or ARDS
- negligible urine output.

Mechanisms and causes

Shock can be classified into hypovolaemic, cardiogenic and distributive forms depending on the underlying mechanism.

Hypovolaemic shock

In hypovolaemic shock, there is insufficient circulating blood volume. This may be due to haemorrhage, dehydration, burns or fluid sequestration, e.g. acute pancreatitis.

Cardiogenic shock

This results from primary cardiac pump failure, which may be due to acute myocardial infarction, cardiomyopathy or dysrhythmia.

Distributive shock

The primary problem is diminished systemic vascular resistance (SVR), which may occur for several reasons:

- septic shock: vasodilatation in response to any severe infection (most commonly, Gram-negative endotoxin-secreting bacteria)
- anaphylactic shock: due to vasodilatation as a result of histamine release in response to an allergen, e.g. bee sting
- neurogenic shock: due to loss of vascular autonomic stimulation following spinal cord or brain injury.

Treatment

The general treatment of shock must be aggressive and begin early. Remember the ABCDE approach (see 'Assessment of the acutely ill patient', p. 8). Establish a patent airway and ensure adequate oxygenation (>92%): this helps to reverse anaerobic metabolism and metabolic acidosis. Ensure adequate IV access is available (at least two green cannulae) and start IV fluids; see below.

Treat the underlying cause: consider broad-spectrum antibiotics if there is evidence of sepsis (fever, rash, signs of peripheral vasodilatation). If the patient is bleeding, transfuse O-negative blood initially, pending cross-match, and consider definitive intervention to stop bleeding, e.g. laparotomy or urgent endoscopy. Cardiogenic shock and pulmonary oedema should be managed as described in 'Breathlessness', p. 146.

Fluids

Fluid resuscitation increases intravascular volume, venous return and cardiac output, but can be detrimental in patients with co-existing cardiac dysfunction or primary cardiogenic shock. Therefore, it is essential to assess intravascular volume state (mucous membranes, skin turgor, JVP, lung bases, oedema) accurately, early and regularly. Facilities should be available for invasive monitoring if bedside assessment of clinical parameters is not felt to be sufficient.

Fluid challenge

Where the patient appears hypovolaemic, give a fluid challenge:

- in adults, run in 250 mL of fluid as rapidly as possible (20 mL/kg in children)
- the speed and volume of the fluid are more important than its composition
- be more cautious in patients with co-existing cardiac disease, in whom central venous access and CVP monitoring should be considered
- it is essential to assess the effect of the challenge as soon it is complete; look at HR, BP, urine output and other measures of tissue perfusion.

Monitoring

Pass a urinary catheter and measure hourly urine volumes. Regularly re-assess vital signs to monitor response to treatment. Minimum treatment goals include achieving a urine flow of >0.5 ml/kg/h and a mean arterial BP (MABP) of >65 mmHg; MABP = DBP + $\frac{1}{3}$(SDP–DBP). However, restoration of an 'adequate circulation', as defined by satisfactory end-organ perfusion and resolution of acidosis, is more important than achieving an arbitrary numerical target MABP. Consider early invasive monitoring in shocked patients who clinically appear hypervolaemic or have evidence of cardiac failure. Inotropic support is more appropriate than aggressive fluid administration in patients with cardiogenic shock. Patients with distributive forms of shock may require a balanced regime of fluids and vasopressor agents.

Inotropes and vasopressors

Patients who remain hypotensive despite adequate filling should be considered for inotropic or vasopressor support. Therefore, by definition, all should have invasive monitoring of central venous pressure, ideally in a high dependency or intensive care environment. Inotropes (e.g. adrenaline, dobutamine) directly affect cardiac performance and have a variable effect on systemic vascular resistance. Vasopressors (e.g. noradrenaline) increase vascular tone and systemic vascular resistance and have relatively little direct effect on cardiac pump function. The pharmacological properties of the commonly used agents are listed in Table 9.6.

The principal goal of inotropic or vasopressor support is to improve tissue perfusion and restore normal aerobic metabolism. This is achieved by manipulating cardiovascular physiology in a way that seeks to reverse the processes that have resulted in shock. The differing haemodynamic profiles of the agents available allow some tailoring of inotropic support to the presumed mechanism(s) of shock.

Table 9.6 Physiological effects of inotropes

Inotrope	HR	SVR	MAP	CO
Dobutamine	++	±	±	++
Noradrenaline	–	++	++	±
Adrenaline	+	+	+	++

Adrenaline

Adrenaline (epinephrine) may be used in patients with multifactorial shock, e.g. sepsis in a patient with heart failure. It causes both an increase in cardiac contractility and output (β_1 inotropic effect) and a moderate increase in SVR (SVR increased by α_1 stimulation, slightly offset by β_2 stimulation in skeletal muscle beds).

Dobutamine

Dobutamine is commonly used in patients with cardiogenic shock because it increases myocardial contractility and cardiac output (β_1 effect) but has little effect on SVR. β_2 stimulation in skeletal muscle beds can lead to significant vasodilatation in patients with sepsis in whom it can exacerbate hypotension and should be avoided.

Noradrenaline

Noradrenaline (norepinephrine) is a vasopressor. It is commonly used in patients with distributive forms of shock, e.g. septic shock. It results in peripheral vasoconstriction and an increase in SVR (α_1 effect). This increased afterload is beneficial in pure distributive shock but can adversely affect cardiac output in patients with significant LV dysfunction.

Intervention in hypovolaemic shock

The response to fluid resuscitation in hypovolaemic shock can be used to determine the need for emergency surgical or endoscopic intervention. Therefore, close monitoring is essential, as described above. Patients can be classified as follows:

- rapid responders: if the parameters return quickly to baseline then resuscitation has been adequate; fluid infusion rate can be slowed to maintenance and response can be monitored
- transient responders: parameters deteriorate when fluids are slowed, suggesting ongoing blood loss or inadequate resuscitation; increased IV fluids and definitive treatment are required
- non-responders: if resuscitation is unable to keep up with losses then definitive treatment must be undertaken immediately, e.g. ruptured AAA.

Outcome of shock

The mortality rate in septic shock is high and ranges from 30% to 50%. The prognosis of cardiogenic shock is poorer still. The outlook is best in hypovolaemic shock, assuming the cause of fluid or blood loss can be identified and treated.

Anaphylaxis

Anaphylaxis is an acute life-threatening reaction, triggered by an immunological mechanism and resulting in a release of histamine and other vasoactive mediators. Symptoms usually develop within minutes of exposure to the stimulus, but may be delayed by up to 30 min. They may include: cutaneous features (e.g. pruritus, flushing, urticaria, angio-oedema); gastrointestinal features (e.g. nausea, vomiting or diarrhoea); wheeze and respiratory distress; vasomotor symptoms (e.g. syncope, hypotension, dizziness, tachycardia).

Management of an acute attack

An ABCDE approach should be adopted (see 'Assessment of the acutely ill patient', p. 8). If the patient is shocked, proceed as suggested on p. 251. The patient should be laid flat with their legs elevated. Give adrenaline (epinephrine) 1:1000, 0.2–0.5 mL IM or SC; this can be repeated after 5 min (in children 0.01 mg/kg, maximum 0.3 mg). Inhaled adrenaline can also be used for laryngeal oedema. Chlorphenamine (10–20 mg IV) should also be given. In prolonged reactions, or in the presence of hypoxaemia, oxygen should be given. In patients with bronchospasm not responsive to adrenaline, nebulized salbutamol 5 mg should be used. Corticosteroids should be started in all patients: IV hydrocortisone (100 mg every 6 h) should be used in severe attacks; oral prednisolone (30–40 mg) can be used in less severe episodes. If the patient is taking β-blockers, glucagon should be given (1–5 mg IV over 5 min ± infusion). Severe or prolonged cases should be managed in an HDU setting. A reaction that has been successfully treated may recur up to 8–12 h later, and patients should remain as inpatients for at least this period to allow adequate monitoring.

Attempts should be made to prevent future attacks and distinguish between an anaphylactic reaction and disorders that may mimic anaphylaxis. Identify possible precipitants from the history: drugs, bites or stings, foodstuffs (especially nuts, shellfish, packaged food dyes), skin contacts (e.g. latex), preceding activities (e.g. exercise, seminal fluid). RAST, skin testing and specific challenge tests can be used to identify clinically relevant allergens, under specialist supervision.

Patients with confirmed anaphylaxis should be given education on the avoidance of possible future allergens, the wearing of MedicAlert® jewellery, and when and how to self-administer pre-loaded adrenaline injection syringes. In some patients, specialist allergen immunotherapy or desensitization can be helpful (e.g. in insect venom anaphylaxis).

MAJOR TRAUMA

Death following traumatic injury occurs in three 'peaks'. The first of these occurs at the time of injury or within minutes of the event. Such patients die at the scene or en route to hospital. The second peak occurs during what is called the 'golden hour'. Deaths during this period may be preventable as they are generally attributable to exsanguination from major abdominal organs, arterial injuries or severe pelvic fractures, or rapidly expanding intracranial haemorrhage.

It is now recognized that inadequate resuscitation during this so-called 'golden hour' allows propagation of a generalized immunological cascade, which culminates in the systemic inflammatory response syndrome (see 'Pyrexia', p. 248), multi-organ failure and a third peak of death in the days and weeks that follow. Therefore, rapid assessment and high-quality emergency care are essential in trauma patients and may prevent avoidable deaths.

Structured assessment and management

Each patient should be assessed and then managed according to the following scheme:

- primary survey to identify and treat injuries which may cause death within minutes with simultaneous resuscitation
- AMPLE history: Allergies, Medications, Past medical/surgical history, Last meal and Events pertaining to mechanism of injury
- emergency imaging
- secondary survey: to identify less rapidly fatal injuries as well as all other injuries
- definitive care: to treat identified injuries, i.e. surgery, intensive care observation.

Due to the accelerated pace of activity, the risk of needle-stick injury and splashes is significantly higher. For this reason, protective aprons, eye protection and single or double layered gloves should be worn. It is important for those performing surgical procedures to be aware of unexpected sharps, e.g. broken ribs, bone fragments or retained foreign bodies. Care must also be taken when removing patients' clothing as fragments of glass or offensive objects, e.g. needles or knives, may be concealed. Where possible, the team should maintain a calm environment to reduce patient anxiety and promote clarity of instructions.

Primary survey

Use the ABCDE approach:

- A: Airway + cervical spine control
- B: Breathing: ensure effective ventilation
- C: Circulation: identify shock and life-threatening haemorrhage
- D: Disability: brief central and peripheral neurological examination
- E: Exposure/environment: remove all clothing, keep patient warm.

Airway and cervical spine control (A)

Maintaining a patent airway is paramount in all patients. In those with potential neck injuries, the cervical spine must be immobilized.

C-spine immobilization

- lie the patient flat with a C-collar in situ
- approach the patient from the top of the trolley (i.e. not the left or right side of the trolley); immobilize the C-spine by holding the trapezius muscles bilaterally and stabilizing the head with your forearms, if sandbags are not in situ

- attempt to establish eye contact with the patient by leaning forward so that you are directly over the patient's face; talk to them so that they do not try to turn their head to speak to you.

Airway management

Unless there are contraindications, provide high flow oxygen (15 L/min) via a non-re-breathing ('trauma') mask. Airway management is described in 'Cardiac arrest', p. 11, but the following points should be considered in trauma cases:

- frequent suctioning may be required to prevent aspiration of blood or vomit
- avulsed teeth should be removed using McGill's forceps; 'blind finger sweeping' of the oropharynx should be avoided in trauma patients
- nasopharyngeal airways should not be used if you suspect a basal skull fracture
- facial injuries may cause upper airway obstruction.

Intubation

Endotracheal intubation by rapid sequence induction is indicated for:

- A: apnoea
- E: exhaustion or expected clinical course
- I: increased ICP
- O: obstructed airway (actual or impending)
- U: unconscious (GCS <8)/uncooperative combative patients.

Breathing (B)

For guidance regarding the assessment and management of conditions that result in dyspnoea, see 'Breathlessness', p. 139. Traumatic causes include:

Traumatic pneumothorax

An 'open' pneumothorax is suggested by a 'sucking' chest wound. When the diameter of a chest wound exceeds two-thirds of the diameter of the trachea, air will preferentially enter through the deficit in the chest wall which may function as a one-way valve and can result in tensioning. Management should be as follows:

- apply a 3-sided non-occlusive dressing (i.e. a square piece of gauze taped on three sides over the wound) until definitive drainage is possible to prevent further extension of the pneumothorax
- insert a chest drain as soon as possible, away from the chest wound
- lavage and dress the wound
- administer IV antibiotics and tetanus prophylaxis (see 'Wounds and burns', p. 272).

Pulmonary contusions

Caused by blunt trauma, these result in ventilation:perfusion mismatch, hypoxia and infiltrates on CXR. They are commonly associated with rib fractures, but may occur in the absence of fractured ribs in younger patients due to pliability of the ribcage.

Flail segment

Defined by two or more fractures in three or more adjacent ribs, resulting in paradoxical movement of the chest wall on inspiration. A flail segment is invariably associated with pulmonary contusions ± traumatic pneumothorax. Ventilatory support may be required if respiratory failure develops.

Circulation (C)

Management of the shocked patient is described in detail in 'Shock and fluid balance', p. 251. In trauma patients, a variety of injuries may result in shock through different mechanisms.

- hypovolaemic: the most common form of shock; haemorrhage may be from an obvious external wound or occult and contained within chest, abdomen or pelvis
- neurogenic: caused by damage to the sympathetic chain which lies adjacent to the spinal cord; the consequent loss of vasomotor tone causes peripheral vasodilatation. Patients who sustain an injury to the upper cervical cord (i.e. above C5/6) may lose sympathetic innervation to the heart and be unable to mount an appropriate compensatory tachycardia. Transfer to a spinal unit should be considered in all patients with neurogenic shock once they have been stabilized.
- cardiogenic: can be due to direct cardiac injury (e.g. a contusion resulting in a dyskinetic ventricular segment); myocardial ischaemia due to hypotension (more likely if there is pre-existing coronary disease); impaired ventricular filling due to either tamponade or tension pneumothorax which causes torsion of the superior or inferior vena cava.

Assessment

Identify potentially life-threatening sources of haemorrhage and shock. Remember that the elderly and patients on β-blockers may not be tachycardic. Look specifically for:

- haemothorax: a patient lying flat may collect a large volume of blood in the hemithorax before it is detectable by percussion
- abdominal fullness or tenderness
- pelvic fracture: massive pelvic bleeding may occur from tearing of the venous plexus; carefully perform a pelvic spring test (see 'Pelvic injury', p. 263).

Immediate investigations

Immediate investigations should reflect the patient's injuries and general condition. In trauma patients, care should be taken to interpret the initial full blood count results in the context of the veno-dilution effect of administered fluids. The haematocrit is a readily available, but underused test. In addition, serum lactate is a very useful indicator of tissue perfusion and should be requested.

Intravenous access

While assessing the circulation, you (or a member of your team) should simultaneously obtain intravenous access. If a peripheral line cannot be secured in the upper limbs, an 8 F (rapid infuser) line should be placed in the femoral vein. If this is unsuccessful, a greater cephalic vein cut-down should be performed, 1 cm superior and 1 cm anterior to the medial malleolus. In children <6 years of age who have difficult peripheral access, intraosseous needle insertion and infusion is recommended.

It is often difficult to secure IV lines in place to moist, clammy skin and they should be taped and then secured with cling bandage. Cling bandage should be placed over the whole cannula and access to the cannula should be obtained by cutting down through the bandage.

Fluid resuscitation

Hartmann's is the preferred crystalloid fluid for trauma resuscitation. Colloid should be initiated in any hypotensive patient while blood products are sought (see p. 251).

Severe continued bleeding

Scalp wounds bleed profusely and patients may exsanguinate from them; rapid closure of these wounds may be achieved with staples and, if necessary, revised with conventional sutures if CT is required following stabilization of the patient. In addition, severe epistaxis may be catastrophic and threaten the airway (see 'ENT', p. 309).

Disability (D)

The identification of new 'disability', either mental or physical, requires careful neurological examination; see p. 5. Formally document neurological status using the GCS; see p. 9. Pupils should be assessed for equality (where pupil size difference of 1 mm is acceptable), reactivity and accommodation. A unilateral dilated pupil suggests compression of the 3rd cranial nerve on the affected side, which can occur with an expanding extradural haematoma (an indication for immediate neurosurgical intervention).

Patients with evidence of blunt spinal cord injury require high-dose steroids. Liaison with regional spinal unit should be sought early: steroids should be started within 8 h of injury. This may lower the level at which neurological dysfunction occurs and, in the context of C2/3/4 injury, may make the difference between spontaneous breathing and ventilator dependence.

Exposure/environment (E)

Jewellery and contact lenses should be removed. All clothing should be cut with trauma shears to enable full inspection of the patient and avoid missing less obvious injuries.

Great care must be taken to prevent hypothermia by inadvertent exposure of the patient for prolonged periods of time or the administration of cold fluids. Blankets and re-warming apparatus (such as a 'bear hugger') should be used and all IV fluids and blood products should be warmed prior to administration. Note that:

- a decrease of 1–2°C may cause coagulopathy, decreased renal and gut perfusion and reduced myocardial contractility
- elderly patients have reduced glycogen stores and may, therefore, be unable to mount a physiological response to the cold
- patients who are paralysed and ventilated are unable to generate a shivering response.

Completing the primary survey

- perform a log roll and remove the patient from the spinal board
- inspect the whole back for evidence of injury, e.g. entry or exit wounds, bruising
- perform a PR and document anal tone and prostate position
- examine external orifices and consider urinary catheter insertion (unless there is a urethral injury) and NG tube insertion if there is a significant risk of aspiration
- consider a pregnancy test in all woman of child-bearing age irrespective of any denials of potential for pregnancy
- 'AMPLE' history should be obtained (see p. 254), from paramedics or relatives if not available from the patient.

Emergency imaging

Comprehensive CT scanning is often used; however, initial investigation may include:

- CXR: subphrenic air, lower rib fractures
- erect/decubitus and supine abdominal films: absent psoas shadow
- pelvic X-rays: fractures
- ultrasound should be used to exclude testicular rupture if this is suspected clinically.

Secondary survey

The secondary survey is a thorough 'top-to-toe' examination which should be performed when life-threatening injuries have been excluded or definitively treated. General examination of these areas is as described in 'History and Examination', p. 1. Occasionally, it may not be possible to perform a secondary survey in the emergency department if the patient has a circulatory issue that requires immediate intervention. If so, this must be documented clearly in the notes, so that the team looking after the patient can perform one.

Head

- general inspection: palpate for the presence of a skull fracture; it may be necessary to log roll the patient to examine the posterior aspect of the head
- scalp lacerations: should be examined under local anaesthetic
- face: CSF rhinorrhoea or CSF otorrhoea suggest a basal skull fracture; periorbital bruising (raccoon eyes) and mastoid bruising (battle sign) are late signs; the patient may have an area of reduced sensation on the cheek due to compression of the infra-orbital nerve
- eyes: see also p. 318; ensure that contact lenses have been removed
- ears: examination of the tympanic membrane may reveal haemotympanum (a purplish discoloration) which also suggests basal skull fracture
- mouth: re-examine for any evidence of loose teeth and/or malocclusion of the bite.

Neck and chest

- trachea: check for deviation
- in the context of penetrating injury, auscultate the neck for any bruits and palpate for thrill
- examine the C-spine
- subcutaneous emphysema may be palpable; look for other evidence of pneumothorax or pneumomediastinum
- inspect the chest for any external signs of injury, e.g. seatbelt sign: traumatic chest injuries are associated with significant mortality
- palpate the sternum and thoracic cage for tenderness: a flail chest denoting underlying contusion and potentially compromising ventilation may be found at this time
- penetrating chest wounds below the nipple line are considered thoraco-abdominal wounds, as approximately 40% have both abdominal and thoracic components.

Abdomen and pelvis

- re-inspect the abdomen for adequacy of movement on inspiration and expiration
- look for any evidence of distension
- note any bruising or wounds; look especially for the presence of a seatbelt mark as this suggests an increased risk of intra-abdominal injury
- enquire about shoulder-tip pain and check for tenderness, guarding, rigidity or fullness which may suggest an underlying haematoma or fluid collection: failure to pass urine or haematuria may indicate urethral, renal or bladder injury
- check for AP and lateral stability of the pelvis (see 'Pelvic injury', p. 263); note that excessive rocking of the fracture site may increase bleeding from the sacral venous plexus
- peritoneal lavage may be considered to look for evidence of bleeding.

Back

- log roll and carefully examine the spine for deformity or tenderness
- check again for any small penetrating wounds.

Extremities

- look for wounds or deformities: bruising may indicate an underlying fracture
- examine ankles and knees, wrists and elbows for range of movement and stability
- hip and shoulder examination cannot be fully performed until you are satisfied there is no spinal injury.

Definitive management

This will depend on the nature of the patient's injuries. Laparotomy should be considered where there has been a gun-shot wound or a penetrating wound of unknown depth. Other indications include shoulder-tip pain, a large return of blood on peritoneal lavage, air under the diaphragm, developing peritonitis, persistent shock or a non-functioning kidney on IVU. An expanding testicular haematoma will need evacuation. Excision of an infarcted testis is sometimes necessary.

Fractures

All fractures occurring in trauma patients should be immobilized at this stage, if not before. This reduces analgesic requirement and helps control haemorrhage. Immobilization also reduces potential for fat embolus and prevents further damage to neurovascular structures. Open fractures should be dressed with gauze soaked with Betadine®. Where possible, tension on skin should be relieved by reduction.

- unstable pelvic fractures require urgent reduction and immobilization (see 'Pelvic injury', p. 263)
- femoral shaft fractures require reduction under femoral nerve block (see 'Femoral fractures', p. 262)
- trimalleolar fractures of the ankle require immediate reduction (see 'Ankle fractures', p. 261).

Clinical examination of the compartments adjacent to a fracture should also be performed and documented. A low threshold for measurement of intra-compartmental pressure should be maintained, in order to prevent the catastrophic consequences of compartment syndrome.

FRACTURES AND MINOR TRAUMA

General approach

Assessment

In addition to a full medical history, establish how the injury was sustained, and any predisposing risks such as osteoporosis, fits, recurrent falls, arrhythmias or drug ingestion. In the case of an assault or accident, remember that you may be called on to give evidence in court (see 'Wound assessment', p. 272).

Enquire about numbness or loss of function, e.g. the inability to weight-bear or move a distal appendage. Check for symptoms that could suggest other internal injury, e.g. haematuria.

Examine for signs of shock (see 'Shock and fluid balance', p. 250). Inspect for obvious deformity, shortening of long bones; palpate for bony landmarks, overlying swelling, heat, crepitus at fracture ends, peripheral pulses and capillary refill; and examine for disruption to motor or sensory function. Always test for 'active' joint movement first to avoid causing unnecessary pain. Useful tests for specific fractures can be found in the sections below relating to each body area. X-ray (usually two films taken at right angles to each other) is the usual initial radiological investigation, but CT and MRI may be used in specific circumstances, e.g. base of skull fracture. Document the region of the bone that has been fractured (proximal, midshaft, distal) and whether it:

- involves an intra-articular surface or joint dislocation
- is displaced, rotated, impacted or angulated
- involves >2 sections of bone (comminuted)
- is transverse, oblique or spiral in direction
- is simple or compound (open)
- is associated with neurovascular damage.

Management principles

Sprains and strains

Sprains and strains (swelling and pain over ligaments or ligamentous insertion points) can be managed with analgesia and RICE: rest, ice packs within a cloth for 10–15 min at a time, compression (removing the bandage at night) and elevation. However, recent studies suggest that compression does not improve healing time significantly.

Fractures

Analgesia

Analgesia alone may be sufficient for certain fractures which require no other intervention, e.g. single rib or coccyx. Start with simple analgesics and anti-inflammatories. Opiate analgesia may be required for severe pain (see also 'Common prescribing', p. 108).

Fracture reduction

This can be achieved by closed (e.g. manipulation under anaesthesia or traction) or open (also known as direct) means. The method used will be specific to the individual injury; each is described in the relevant section below.

Fracture immobilization

A back-slab or sling can be used following reduction for minor and stable fractures. Alternatively, traction can be used to maintain reduction, i.e. skin (adhesive strapping), bone (using a pin through a bone) or fixed (e.g. Thomas splint). Internal fixation, e.g. with plates and screws, 'K' wires, intramedullary nails or tension band wiring, is indicated for the following:

- intra-articular fractures
- fractures requiring nerve or vessel repair
- patients with multiple injuries or injury to long bones
- pathological fractures
- failure of conservative treatment, e.g. non-union.

Complications

These may include:

- local complications of the injury, e.g. bleeding, ischaemia, infection, skin necrosis
- systemic complications of the injury, e.g. fat embolism (suggested by confusion, breathlessness, fits, fever, a petechial rash) or crush syndrome (soft tissue ischaemia triggering DIC and toxin-mediated acute tubular necrosis)
- complications resulting from immobilization of a limb or person, e.g. PTE, pneumonia, renal stones
- failure of the fracture to heal: this is more likely in comminuted or pathological fractures, if there has been an avulsed fragment, or where the patient's general health is poor.

Ankle and foot injuries

These are the most common types of musculoskeletal injury.

Ligamentous injuries

Commonly known as ankle sprains, these affect the lateral talofibular ligamentous complex. Rupture of the anterior tibiofibular ligament (ATFL) is the commonest form of ankle sprain. Pain and swelling along the lateral aspect of the ankle joint are typical, usually following an inversion injury. For treatment see 'Management: sprains and strains' above. If there is a lot of swelling, an X-ray should be performed to exclude a fracture of the lateral malleolus.

Malleolar fractures

Lateral malleolar fractures are most common; these are described using the Webber classification which distinguishes fractures based on their position in relation to the distal tibiofibular syndesmosis:

- type A fractures: distal to the syndesmosis
- type B fractures: involve the syndesmosis
- type C fractures: proximal to the syndesmosis.

Significant trauma and twisting of the talus within the ankle mortice can result in fracture of both the medial and lateral malleoli. If this is associated with fracture of the posterior segment of the distal tibia, known as 'off-ending', a trimalleolar fracture results.

Investigation

The Ottawa ankle rules should be followed: X-ray imaging is indicated if the patient is unable to take two steps unaided *or* if there is tenderness over any of the following:

- the base of the 5th metatarsal (MT)
- the navicular
- the posterior aspect of the distal 1.5 inches of the lateral or medial malleolus
- the proximal fibula.

Treatment

Undisplaced fractures of the medial malleolus may be treated conservatively; see 'Management: fractures' above. Displaced fractures require open reduction and internal fixation (ORIF) to prevent malunion. Opening of the medial joint space (on an AP projection of the ankle joint) implies rupture of the deltoid ligament and fracture instability; this also requires ORIF. Trimalleolar fractures require urgent reduction to ensure the integrity of the skin and neurovascular supply.

Talar fractures

The most important is the talar neck fracture which follows forced dorsiflexion of the foot and may result in avascular necrosis of the talus. Manipulation, plaster fixation and/or wires may be required.

Calcaneal fractures

These are crush fractures that occur after a fall from a significant height. They may be bilateral or associated with a talar fracture. A lumbar spine fracture should also be excluded. Treatment may be conservative or involve ORIF depending on the fracture site and any associated injuries, particularly talar fracture.

Tarsal dislocation and metatarsal fractures

Mid-tarsal dislocation results in pain and swelling and requires early manipulation and plaster stabilization. The Lisfranc dislocation of the tarso-metatarsal joint causes significant swelling and pain on weight bearing and can impair blood supply to the medial foot. It may not be visible on the initial X-rays and stress views (under GA) may be required. It requires reduction and screw fixation. Metatarsal injuries (often crush) are usually treated conservatively, but can be associated with compartment syndrome or neurovascular damage. A 'march' fracture of the second metatarsal is seen after prolonged walking/running; a plaster cast should be applied for 6 weeks.

Knee injury

Patellar dislocation

Predominantly occurs in young sports players who present with pain and an inability to flex their knee. Lateral dislocation is more common than medial dislocation. Both should be reduced and managed with analgesia, RICE (see 'Management principles', p. 260) and subsequent physiotherapy.

Ligament injury

Cruciate ligament tears commonly result from twisting of the femur in relation to the tibia, e.g. a sudden change in direction with the foot fixed on the ground. Pain, effusion and haemarthrosis may result. Clinically, the 'drawer' test may be useful: sit on the foot of the flexed, affected leg and test whether it can be drawn anteriorly (anterior cruciate injury) or pushed back (posterior cruciate injury); neither movement is normal. Treatment involves 3 weeks' rest and plaster support. Surgical repair is indicated if the patient wishes to return to sporting activities.

Collateral ligament tears result from varus or valgus stress at the knee joint. They present with pain and tenderness over the affected ligament and may also cause an effusion ± haemarthrosis. Treatment involves immobilization (usually with a knee brace), RICE (as above) and, after a period of convalescence, muscle strengthening exercises.

Meniscal tears

These often result from a twisting injury. Extension of the knee is limited and it may 'lock' when the displaced fragment blocks the femoral/tibial condyle plane. Joint line tenderness is common. Arthroscopy to remove the displaced fragment is often necessary.

Leg injury

Tibial fractures

These follow rotational/torsional stress or direct trauma to the long axis of the bone. Oblique or spiral fractures are common. Proximal tibial fractures may result in damage to the popliteal artery at the junction of the proximal one-third and distal two-thirds. A minimally displaced fracture may be immobilized in a long leg cast under mild sedation. More significant disruption requires intra-medullary nailing.

Fibular fractures

The fibula is a non weight-bearing bone. However, it is susceptible to direct trauma to the lateral aspect of the leg. Isolated fractures of the fibular shaft do not require immobilization. All long bone fractures have the potential to create a compartment syndrome; however, fractures of the shaft of the fibula are also susceptible to acute or chronic microvascular compromise, due to raised lateral compartment pressures. The patient may re-attend complaining of pain that is disproportionate to the severity of the mechanism of injury or examination findings. There may also be loss of sensation in the first web space and pain on resisted or passive dorsiflexion of the foot.

Femoral fractures

Significant force is required to cause fracture of the femoral shaft. Therefore, look carefully for other injuries. Femoral shaft fractures may be associated with a loss of 750 mL to 1 L of blood in the region of the fracture site.

Treatment

A femoral nerve block can be used in the case of fractures that lie within the middle and proximal one-third of the femur. Morphine analgesia should also be provided as required. The fracture should be immobilized and reduced using a Thomas splint at the earliest opportunity. This reduces the potential space into which bleeding may occur, decreases the risk of fat embolus and reduces further pain. Definitive fixation with an intramedullary nail may then be performed.

Hip injury

Fractured neck of femur

More common in the elderly female population, in which osteoporosis is a predisposing factor. There is a significant associated mortality (30% at 1 year) due to the high incidence of co-morbid disease. Such fractures are broadly classified into intracapsular or extracapsular. Avascular necrosis of the femoral head is a serious potential complication resulting from damage to the blood supply to the femoral head as it is reflected back up the neck of the femur.

Assessment

Classically, hip fractures cause external rotation, adduction and limb shortening due to the unopposed action of the psoas muscle (which inserts distal to the fracture site). Pain on internal or external rotation of the hip is highly suggestive of an undisplaced fracture.

Treatment

Surgical options include replacement of the femoral head by hemiarthroplasty or total hip replacement. Intertrochanteric fractures (along the base of the femoral neck between the trochanters) should be fixed using a dynamic hip screw. Patients who are not fit for theatre will require traction and supportive management.

Dislocation of the hip

Some 90% are posterior and classically result from a dash-board injury to the knee during a road traffic accident. The leg is flexed, shortened and adducted. There may be damage to the sciatic nerve and avascular necrosis of the femoral head may develop if the hip is not reduced promptly.

Management of a posterior dislocation

The head of the femur can usually be lifted back into the joint under anaesthetic but requires adequate training and competence. Ask an assistant to hold the pelvis; flex both the hip and knee joints to 90° and correct any adduction or internal rotation; hold the patient's lower leg between your knees and grasp the patient's knee with both hands; lean back and lever the knee up, pulling the patient's hip upwards until a clunk is heard.

Pelvic injury

Major pelvic injury

Significant force is required to disrupt the pelvic ring, e.g. a road traffic accident or a fall from a significant height. This typically results in an 'open book' fracture, characterized by disruption of the anterior aspect of the pelvis at either the pubic symphysis or ipsilateral superior and inferior pubic rami. There may be associated damage to the urethra or sacral venous plexus; the latter may result in low-pressure slow bleeding into the pelvis, hypovolaemia and a risk of death. Therefore, major pelvic trauma is an orthopaedic emergency.

Assessment and management

The patient should be assessed carefully and regularly for signs of shock. Fluid resuscitation should be aggressive and commenced early (see 'Shock and fluid balance', p. 251).

Perform a pelvic spring test by gently pressing on the anterior superior iliac spines bilaterally. The test is positive if pain is provoked and you should stop immediately. If the test is negative, repeat it by applying lateral pressure to the iliac crests. It is essential to take care when testing the pelvis, as a naturally occurring physiological tamponade and clot may be disrupted by careless manipulation. If the patient can pass urine, perform a urinalysis. Gross haematuria or blood at the urethral meatus is highly suggestive of urethral or bladder injury; microscopic haematuria is a less reliable sign. If urethral injury is suspected, a cystourethrogram should be performed prior to urinary catheterization and an urgent urology opinion sought. Look for evidence of associated abdominal or thoracic injuries and consider urgent ultrasound examination, peritoneal lavage and appropriate imaging.

Major pelvic fractures require urgent reduction, ideally by external fixation by the on-call orthopaedic team. This is not complicated and can be accomplished in the emergency department. If application of an external fixator is unduly delayed, consider use of a pelvic sling, which involves wrapping a sheet around the pelvis to minimize movement at the fracture site. Open surgical repair of bleeding pelvic vessels is no longer favoured because of inevitable loss of pelvic tamponade. Instead, angiography and arterial embolization should be performed.

Minor pelvic injury

The commonest form of pelvic injury is an isolated fracture of the inferior pubic ramus. This typically occurs in elderly patients following a fall backwards onto their bottom. These are painful injuries which resolve with conservative management.

Upper limb injury

Hand injury

Thumb fractures

These are most common at the base of the first metacarpal and may be intra-articular (Bennett's). The latter is very unstable and requires internal K-wire fixation. Otherwise, thumb fractures can usually be managed by reduction and plaster support.

Metacarpal fractures

These usually occur after punching something. Neck fractures are more common and can be managed by 'buddy-strapping' to an adjacent finger. Shaft fractures are more unstable and may require ORIF.

Mallet finger

This results from hyperflexion of the extensor tendon to the terminal phalanx, e.g. following impact of a ball onto the tip of an outstretched finger. It may be associated with an avulsion fracture of the terminal phalanx. A hyperextension splint (e.g. Stack) is used for 6–8 weeks unless there is large bone fragment or joint subluxation (when internal fixation may be necessary).

Wrist and distal radius fractures

These injuries are commonly due to a fall on an outstretched hand (FOOSH).

Scaphoid fracture

Often due to forced dorsiflexion of the wrist which may look normal, but movements, especially dorsiflexion, are often limited. Typically, hyperextension of the thumb and gripping are painful and examination reveals anatomical snuff box and volar scaphoid tenderness (tenderness along the palmer aspect of the scaphoid bone). Scaphoid fractures may result in avascular necrosis of the proximal segment of bone.

The fracture may not be visible on the initial X-ray and MRI may be required for early definitive diagnosis. Where this is not available, the patient should be treated on the basis of clinical suspicion. The wrist should be immobilized in a cast that extends from below the elbow to beyond the knuckle (including the thumb to the base of the nail). This is principally for comfort and has not been proven to reduce the incidence of avascular necrosis of the proximal segment. Repeat X-rays should then be performed at 10–14 days. Internal fixation will be required if there is evidence of avascular necrosis or non-union.

Colles' fractures

These usually occur in elderly females following a fall on an outstretched hand. This may result in the classical 'dinner-fork' wrist deformity. Radiological features include dorsal angulation and radial deviation of the distal fragment.

Undisplaced or stable fractures should be manipulated under anaesthesia (e.g. Bier's block, regional or general), otherwise the patient may lose the ability to supinate and pronate the forearm. Internal fixation is used for unstable or intra-articular fractures or those with volar displacement (Smith's fractures).

Manipulation of a Colles' fracture

Adequate training and competence is required. With an assistant holding the elbow, traction is applied to pull the distal fragment forwards and towards the ulnar side. Apply a back-slab cast up to the knuckles. Provide the patient with a sling and organize for a check X-ray in 10 days; if the fracture is in a satisfactory position the cast can be completed. The fracture will take approximately 6 weeks to heal.

Elbow injuries

Radial head fractures

These also commonly result from a fall on an outstretched hand. The force of the fall is transmitted through the long axis of the radius to the head, which impacts against the lateral epicondyle of the distal humerus. The patient will complain of pain, especially on pronation and supination, and there may be limited extension of the elbow joint.

Management

Aspiration of any fracture haematoma and injection of long-acting analgesia greatly reduces pain. Patients may then benefit from a short period of immobilization in a long arm cast and oral analgesia. If there is associated dislocation of the radio-ulnar joint, internal fixation will be required.

Supracondylar fractures

These can be extension or flexion (less common) and may be associated with damage to the brachial artery. Secondary ischaemia and fibrosis of the forearm muscles may result in Volkmann's ischaemic contracture. All but minor fractures without neurological or vascular compromise should be referred for surgical repair.

Thereafter, the arm should be immobilized in a long arm cast flexed at the elbow. The degree of flexion that can be achieved will be dependent on neurovascular function. While the cast is being applied, check if the pulses are absent. If they are, extend the elbow until they return and complete the cast.

Elbow dislocation

This usually occurs in young people after a fall onto an extended elbow. Presentation is with a painful swollen, flexed and deformed elbow. It is often associated with brachial artery and nerve injury: check distal neurovascular function. AP and lateral elbow X-rays will confirm dislocation and allow exclusion of any associated fracture.

Management

Prompt reduction is essential and should usually be performed under IV sedation. The procedure depends on the type of dislocation and requires adequate training and competence.

- posterior: provide countertraction to the upper arm while applying traction longitudinally at the wrist and forearm; continue traction as the elbow is flexed, providing downward pressure on the proximal forearm

- anterior: provide anterior pressure from behind the distal humerus while applying posterior and downward pressure to the forearm.

After reduction, test mobility, stability and neurovascular function; repeat the X-ray and place in a collar and cuff or back slab for 3 weeks.

Humeral fractures

Humeral shaft

These fractures occur when lateral forces are applied, e.g. falling to the side. Shaft fractures may be transverse or oblique (from direct injury) or spiral (from rotational force). They are often treated conservatively with a U-slab and sling. Surgical treatment, by ORIF, is necessary if there are multiple injuries or injury to the radial nerve. These fractures have significant potential for malunion which may compromise limb function.

Humeral head or neck

These occur more frequently in the elderly population and, if undisplaced, should be treated conservatively. They are painful; however the risk of malunion and compromised upper limb function is much less than with shaft fractures. These are best immobilized in a Polysling® which enables the arm to be bound to the body, reducing movement at the shoulder joint and fracture site and allowing the weight of the limb to maintain the reduction. Displaced fractures require ORIF.

Shoulder injuries

Dislocation

The shoulder is the most commonly dislocated joint in the body. About 95% of shoulder dislocations are anterior. Reduction requires adequate training and competence.

Anterior

These occur following a fall onto the arm or shoulder. The arm is often held at the side of the body in external rotation. The shoulder looks flat and the head of the humerus may bulge anteriorly and may be palpable in the axilla. Axillary nerve damage can lead to deltoid paralysis and loss of sensation below the shoulder (regimental badge distribution).

X-ray the joint (AP and axillary lateral) to exclude a fracture before attempting reduction. Reduction should be performed with analgesia and sedation, e.g. morphine 10mg and midazolam 5–10mg with appropriate monitoring. A variety of techniques may be used including traction–countertraction or forceful leverage. However, these traditional methods are painful and potentially traumatic. The external rotation method is an alternative:

- use appropriate analgesia and sedation to achieve shoulder muscle relaxation
- stabilize the elbow against the trunk with the elbow flexed at 90°
- gradually externally rotate the forearm as permitted by muscle relaxation
- abduct the arm slightly as it is externally rotated
- the shoulder should reduce before the forearm is rotated through 90°
- confirm reduction by X-ray.

Posterior

This is uncommon, but may result from a seizure. Posterior dislocations often go unnoticed, so there may be a significant delay between injury and diagnosis. The arm may be held adducted and internally rotated; external rotation and abduction cause pain. Manual reduction is only effective if the injury is of recent onset, otherwise surgical reduction should be performed.

Rotator cuff injury

The rotator cuff is comprised of the supraspinatus, infraspinatus, teres minor and subscapularis muscles, which arise from the scapula and attach onto the humerus. The primary function of the rotator cuff is to stabilize the shoulder joint.

Rotator cuff injuries are commonly due to tendon, rather than muscle, injuries; these include tears and inflammation within the tendon(s), or their associated bursa, leading to impingement between the acromion and the humeral head. Common clinical syndromes include

- painful arc syndrome (pain on abduction between 45° and 160°) suggesting supraspinatus tendonitis or a partial tear
- subacromial impingement syndrome (pain on abduction between 60° and 120°)
- pain on any abduction, suggesting calcification of the rotator cuff.

Management

NSAIDs ± steroid injection are the mainstay of treatment unless a complete tendon tear has occurred, in which case tendon repair should be considered. Shock-wave therapy can also be used for calcific tendonitis.

Rupture of long head of biceps

The patient may report feeling something 'going' or 'popping'. A ball of muscle is usually visible on elbow flexion. Management is with analgesia and surgical reattachment of the tendon to the humerus (biceps tenodesis).

Clavicle fractures

These are often related to a fall on an outstretched hand. Lateral fractures may need internal fixation, but most others can be managed with analgesia and immobilization in a broad sling for 3 weeks.

Spinal column injury

Suspect an associated spinal injury in the following situations: calcaneal fractures, facial injury, sternal dislocation, head injury.

Principles of investigation and management

Investigation of suspected spinal injury usually requires plain X-ray imaging, in at least two planes. CT will provide more detailed bone imaging, but MRI should be performed first if neural damage is suspected. Analgesia and immobilization are appropriate initial management until further assessment of the injury can be made. Thereafter, spinal surgery may be necessary for unstable fractures.

Specific spinal injuries

Cervical

Specific guidance on the assessment and management of suspected cervical spine injury is given in 'Major trauma', p. 254.

Whiplash

Damage to the anterior musculoligamentous components often follows sudden flexion with rebound hyperextension of the neck, e.g. during RTA. Severe muscle spasm follows and there may be an associated vertebral body avulsion fracture. Cervical X-rays should be performed; however, rest, analgesia and soft collar support is usually all that is required.

Thoracic

The thoracic spine is supported by the ribs and therefore it is less susceptible to injury than other areas. However, when thoracic spine injury occurs, it may be associated with injury to the lungs, heart or oesophagus and care should be taken to exclude these.

Lumbar

Wedge compression

Hyperflexion of the spine around the axis of a vertebral body leads to anterior wedging of the vertebral body. These are usually stable fractures, but if the degree of wedging exceeds 20° there may significant instability due to injury to the lamina or pedicles.

Burst fractures

These are associated with axial loading of the spine and may propel fragments of bone into the spinal canal causing damage to the spinal cord. Spinal column instability is common with burst fractures, particularly those which have associated laminar and or pedicle involvement.

Facial injury

Facial bone fractures

These usually follow trauma and are described using the 'Le Fort' classification:

- I: separation of the upper maxilla from the tooth-containing maxilla
- II: subluxation of the middle one-third of the face; the airway is at risk
- III: involves the space between the supra-orbital margins; may be associated with a CSF leak causing CSF rhinorrhoea.

It is important to ensure the patient's airway is not threatened by inhaled teeth. After assessment, facial fractures should be referred to maxillofacial surgery for consideration of reduction or internal fixation depending on the injury.

Mandibular dislocation and fracture

Mandibular fractures may be identified using mandibular X-rays or orthopantomography (OPG) and should be suspected when there is jaw malocclusion or a mobile fragment. Mandibular fractures should be discussed with the maxillofacial surgeons for consideration of ORIF.

Where there is evidence of dislocation, it should be reduced by a competent individual. Sedate the patient and with the thumbs pressing downward on the back teeth the chin can be lifted up with the fingers of both hands.

Head injury

Clinical assessment

Assess ABC, neurological function and conscious level using the Glasgow Coma Scale (see 'Clinical scores', p. 9, and the 'Unconscious patient', p. 217). Check for evidence of other injuries and antegrade and/or retrograde amnesia. Send samples for FBC, U&E, ECG, ABG and consider blood alcohol and drug levels. Clean and explore any wounds (see 'Wound assessment and suturing', p. 272).

Criteria for admission

Some patients should be admitted for neurological observation and may require CT head scanning.

Admission and urgent CT

- GCS <13 at any time since the injury or a GCS <14, 2h after the injury
- a new focal neurological defect
- open or depressed skull fracture or basal skull fracture (suggested by 'panda' eyes, otorrhoea, rhinorrhoea)
- post-event seizure.

Admission for simple observation ± non-urgent CT

- more than one episode of vomiting or any loss of consciousness
- age >65 or history of coagulopathy
- involvement in a serious accident or amnesia (more concerning if this extends for >30 min before the injury).

Where none of these criteria are met, patients can be discharged with a head injury information leaflet, provided they have somebody to look after them at home.

Neurological observation

Patients who are admitted should have standard observations plus regular monitoring of GCS, pupillary size and symmetry. If signs of raised intracranial pressure develop (rising BP, slowing pulse, respiratory failure, dilated pupils, extensor posture), arrange an urgent CT and discuss the use of 20% mannitol with a senior (5 mL/kg IV over 15 min). Patients with evidence of a brain haematoma/subdural collection should be discussed with the regional neurosurgical unit.

Nerve injury

The likelihood of recovery is dependent on the severity of the original nerve damage. Nerve injury can be classified as follows:

- neuropraxia: pressure-associated temporary loss of conduction
- axonotmesis: damage to the nerve but not of the endoneural tube
- neurotmesis: division of the nerve.

Specific types of nerve injury

Brachial plexus injury

Erb–Duchenne

There is involvement of C5/6: the arm hangs at the side, the forearm is pronated, the wrist flexed and there is loss of sensation over deltoid, lateral forearm and hand.

Klumpke

There is involvement of C8/T1: claw hand, loss of sensation over ulnar side of arm. It may be associated with a sympathetic trunk lesion causing Horner's syndrome.

Median nerve injury

The median nerve supplies most of the muscles of the volar forearm, the thenar muscles and two lumbricals. It supplies sensory innervation for the thumb, index, middle and half of the ring finger.

Injuries to the median nerve may result in severe disability. Injury at the wrist tends to cause loss of thumb opposition and abduction. High injuries lead to loss of wrist flexion, ulnar deviation, loss of thumb opposition, abduction and flexion and may also result in loss of finger flexion. Test the patient's ability to oppose and abduct the thumb. To test abduction, with the patient's palm upwards, check whether they can keep their thumb pointing upwards, as you apply pressure in the direction of the fingers.

Ulnar nerve injury

Ulnar nerve injury usually occurs following trauma to the elbow. Injury results in loss of sensation to the little finger and half of the ring finger. Adduction and abduction of the fingers may be impaired (especially in high injuries) and the resulting paralysis gives the classical presentation with 'claw hand'.

Radial nerve injury

Usually results from injury to the humerus or elbow, or from local compression of the radial nerve as it travels around the humeral shaft, e.g. 'Saturday night palsy', which occurs after falling asleep with the arm over a chair.

Injury to the nerve results in loss of extension of the wrist, fingers and thumb. There is wrist drop and poor grip strength. Sensation is impaired over the dorsum of the forearm and posterior aspect of the first interdigital cleft.

Management of nerve injury

Minor nerve injures (neuropraxia) will usually resolve spontaneously. If recovery is likely to be prolonged, a splint or support should be used to maintain the affected limb in an anatomical position. Neural dysfunction due to compression by adjacent structures should be relieved surgically. Urgent surgical repair may be necessary for neurotmesis and specialist help should be sought.

ACUTE LEG PAIN

Leg pain is a common reason for presentation to A&E, GP surgeries and a variety of hospital specialties. There may be a history of trauma or injury or associated features on examination including leg swelling, skin changes, limb deformity or weakness. The causes of acute leg pain can be classified into trauma, infection and vascular problems.

Trauma

Trauma may result in a variety of insults to the skin, soft tissues and bones of the leg. For detailed guidance see 'Major trauma', p. 254, and 'Fractures and minor trauma', p. 259.

Infection

Cellulitis

Common symptoms include unilateral or bilateral leg swelling, erythema and a sensation of warmth in the leg(s). These may be accompanied by fever and systemic upset. Cellulitis usually develops insidiously, in contrast to deep venous thrombosis, which may be more acute. There may a history of trauma or a skin break. Chronic leg ulceration, venous stasis and interdigital fungal infection are also risk factors. Lymphadenopathy ± lymphangitis may be present.

Check FBC, U&E, LFT, CRP and blood cultures. Any skin blisters should be aspirated and the material sent for culture. ECG and CXR should be requested in patients over 40, and those in whom there are other reasons to do so, e.g. evidence of sepsis syndrome. The extent of any erythema should be marked with a pen: this allows objective assessment of any change in the size of the affected area over time.

Treatment involves leg elevation, IV antibiotics and DVT prophylaxis (see 'Common prescribing', p. 109). Follow your local protocol when choosing antibiotics; however a commonly used regime is intravenous flucloxacillin (1.2 g 6-hourly) and benzylpenicillin (1.2–2.4 g 6-hourly). When converting to oral treatment, use flucloxacillin and penicillin V.

Necrotizing soft tissue infection

Necrotizing fasciitis

This is a severe, rapidly progressive condition associated with destruction of all skin layers and often accompanied by sepsis and multi-organ failure. It usually develops at sites of trauma, injection or following surgery and is more common in diabetic or immunocompromised patients. Acute erythema with central anaesthesia rapidly evolves into gangrenous ulceration. Necrotizing fasciitis is classified according to the causative organism:

- type I: caused by Enterobacteriaceae and anaerobes
- type II: caused by *Streptococcus pyogenes* group A.

If the diagnosis is suspected clinically check FBC, U&E, LFT, CRP, Coag, blood cultures and Ca^{2+} (hypocalcaemia can occur secondary to fat necrosis). Ensure blood is sent for a group and save. Urgent surgical debridement of the limb is essential, so do not delay in referring to orthopaedics or plastic surgery, depending on local policy.

Look for evidence of sepsis syndrome and shock (see 'Shock', p. 250). Fluid resuscitation should be early and aggressive if there is evidence of either. Start high flow oxygen and broad-spectrum intravenous antibiotics, e.g. benzylpenicillin (2.4 g 4-hourly), clindamycin (600 mg 6-hourly) and ciprofloxacin (400 mg 12-hourly). Mortality can be up to 80% and amputation may be necessary in up to 50% of patients.

Clostridium infections

Clostridia may colonize wounds, but do not always cause spreading infection. However, *Clostridium perfringens, tetani* and *botulinum* can cause anaerobic cellulitis and gas formation in the wound. The latter two organisms are more common in IV drug abusers.

'Gas gangrene' develops when the infection invades healthy surrounding tissue, usually following deeply penetrating wounds. It is associated with severe pain and skin tenderness and progresses rapidly. Gas bubbles may be felt under the skin. Systemic sepsis, shock and multi-organ failure can result.

Urgent investigations should include routine blood samples, CK, fibrin and blood cultures. An ECG and CXR should be performed. If there is evidence of shock, fluid resuscitation should be aggressive (see p. 251). Antibiotic treatment should be started immediately, using a similar regime to that suggested above for necrotizing fasciitis, but with the addition of IV metronidazole (500 mg 6-hourly). Surgical debridement is required. Some centres advocate hyperbaric oxygen. Pain can be severe and should be managed appropriately (see 'Common prescribing', p. 107).

Septic arthritis and osteomyelitis

See 'Rheumatology', p. 283.

Vascular problems

Deep venous thrombosis

History and examination

DVT is notoriously difficult to diagnose clinically; however, the patient may complain of a painful, swollen leg which may be red and feel hot. Other factors from the history that suggest a diagnosis of DVT include a relatively sudden onset and the presence of risk factors (see PTE in 'Breathlessness', p. 152).

Investigations

Many units have specific investigation protocols and you should follow these, where provided. An assessment of the probability of the patient having a DVT and their risks in regard to anticoagulation must be conducted before any blood tests are ordered. Routine bloods should be checked, including platelets, U&E, LFT and Coag, which will be useful if subsequent treatment with anticoagulation is to be considered.

D-dimers are now available in most units for investigation of suspected DVT. These are fibrin degradation products and are elevated in any fibrinolytic state, e.g. thrombosis, sepsis, malignancy, pregnancy. D-dimers must always be interpreted in combination with a pre-test probability score (see 'Breathlessness', p. 153) and an understanding of the specific assay used. In patients with a low or intermediate pre-test probability of DVT, a negative VIDAS D-dimer result reliably excludes a DVT and no further imaging is required. Other assays, e.g. SimpliRED, are less sensitive and can only exclude DVT in patients with a low pre-test probability. DVT cannot be excluded in patients with a positive D-dimer or those with a high pre-test probability (in whom a D-dimer should not be checked); therefore further tests are required. In most centres this will involve venous Doppler ultrasound examination. A positive D-dimer is extremely non-specific and should never be used as the sole indication for further investigation.

If the Doppler is negative in patients with a high clinical suspicion, a repeat scan should be requested in 3–7 days. Patients with suspected DVT should also have an ECG and CXR, if only as a baseline comparison, should symptoms of possible pulmonary thromboembolism develop later. Young patients and those with a recurring presentation of DVT should be considered for more detailed investigation of possible thrombophilic states (see 'Coagulation disorders', p. 282). However, such investigation is unlikely to change the need for long-term anticoagulation in recurrent disease.

Treatment

Elevate the leg. LMWH and warfarin should be used as per the treatment of pulmonary thromboembolism (see 'Breathlessness', p. 154). See p. 109 for warfarin doses and duration of therapy.

Acute arterial ischaemia

Patients present with an acutely painful, weak limb. Peripheral pulses will be reduced compared with the other side and there will be reduced capillary refill. Pallor and mottling may develop. Reduced sensation is a late sign. Risk factors for arterial ischaemia include:

- local thrombosis, e.g. recent trauma, pre-existing peripheral vascular disease (especially if complicated by dehydration)
- arterial graft
- malignancy
- potential embolic sources, e.g. AF, MI, prosthetic valve, aortic aneurysm.

Investigation should focus on identifying any embolic source, defining the severity of any potential sequelae, e.g. sepsis, and preparing the patient for surgery, if appropriate. Check FBC, U&E, Coag ± thrombophilia screen, G+S and request an ECG and CXR. Consider echocardiography if examination findings, ECG or CXR suggest cardiac pathology. Doppler ultrasound of the affected limb and urgent review by a vascular surgeon should be requested. Interim treatment with IV heparin should be considered (see p. 109).

WOUNDS AND BURNS

Wounds

Assessment

Enquire about the origin of the wound, any animal contact, glass injury and any associated symptoms that might suggest other injuries. Document the patient's tetanus status, if they know it (Table 9.7).

Clinical examination should start with ABCDE (see 'Major trauma', p. 254). Look for evidence of shock (see 'Shock and fluid balance', p. 250). Document the size, site and nature of wound, e.g. abrasion, puncture, incision (sharp edges but can be deep), laceration (rough edges and more superficial). Comment in your notes whether the wound is full-thickness, as suggested by exposure of subcutaneous fat.

Check for a distal neurovascular deficit by palpating the peripheral pulses and assessing capillary refill time, distal sensation and muscle power. If these are abnormal, seek senior help. If you suspect glass or metal fragments in the wound, X-ray the area.

Wounds sustained during an accident or assault may result in legal action and you may be required to explain your findings in court. Therefore, ensure that your notes are clear and legible and state only what you know to be the case. Whatever the patient has told you is simply alleged by them unless you can personally substantiate it.

Cleaning and deeper inspection

Clean the superficial wound area with water or saline. Use local anaesthetic, if deeper cleaning, scrubbing of abrasions, or exploration to identify foreign bodies or assess the involvement of deeper structures is required.

Management

Wound closure techniques are described in 'Suturing', p. 63. Guidance on tetanus prophylaxis is provided in Table 9.7. The following wounds are defined as high risk: heavy soil or manure contamination, wounds >6h old, puncture wounds including cat bites and wounds in areas of poor circulation.

A 5-day course of antibiotics, e.g. amoxicillin (500mg 8-hourly) and flucloxacillin (500mg 6-hourly) should be prescribed if the wound communicates directly with bone or appears infected. Patients with bites should be given antibiotics, e.g. co-amoxiclav (625mg 8-hourly). Patients with valvular heart disease should receive antibiotic prophylaxis as per the BNF.

Table 9.7 Tetanus prophylaxis in patients with wounds

Prior tetanus status	Clean low-risk wound	High-risk wound
Full course or booster <10 years ago	No prophylaxis needed	If contaminated by manure, give human anti-tetanus immunoglobulin (HATI) 250–500 units IM
Partial course or booster ≥10 years ago	Give tetanus booster: 0.5 mL IM tetanus toxoid	Give both tetanus booster and HATI
Not immunized or unknown status	Start tetanus course	Start tetanus course and give HATI

Burns

Most burns are minor and can be treated as an outpatient. However, major burns are associated with a significant risk of death, due to the risk of inhalational lung injury, hypovolaemic shock and secondary infection. Burns should be classified according to their cause, depth and extent.

Cause

Burns may result from thermal (including contact with a heat source, naked flame or scald), electrical, chemical, radiation or friction injury. Electrical and chemical burns, in particular, may cause considerable damage to underlying tissue.

Depth

Burn depth was previously classified as 1st, 2nd or 3rd degree, but should now be described using the following classification:

- superficial: epidermis only, red with no blisters
- partial thickness: affects upper dermis with blanching redness and some blisters
- deep dermal: very painful, non-blanching, sometimes mottled and blistering
- full thickness: numb, firm, white, brown or black with vessel thrombosis.

Extent

This should be expressed as the percentage of the patient's total body surface area (TBSA) involved. The extent of a burn correlates directly with in-hospital mortality and can be determined using Wallace's rule of nine, where each whole arm = 9%, the head = 9%, each side of the trunk and each whole leg = 18% and the perineum = 1%. Lund–Browder charts are more accurate and can be used in both adults and children as they take into account the person's age and the different proportions of the head and limbs in growing children.

Immediate assessment and investigations

Clinical assessment should start with ABC and consideration of the patient's need for analgesia. Airway oedema and signs of inhalational lung injury may not develop immediately and regular monitoring is required. Findings suggestive of inhalational injury include stridor, breathlessness, singed nose hair and eyebrows, facial or neck burns and carbon deposits or inflammatory change in the oropharynx.

Carbon monoxide (CO) poisoning should be actively excluded: remember that oxygen saturations will be inaccurate. Perform an ABG and check the carboxyhaemoglobin level (<20% is rarely associated with symptoms). Where appropriate, start high flow oxygen (this expedites dissociation of CO from haemoglobin).

Look for evidence of poor perfusion, hypovolaemia and shock (see p. 250). Any patient with widespread or large burns (affecting >20% of their body surface area) is likely to need intravascular volume support. Insert at least 2 wide-bore cannulae and start an IV infusion of crystalloids, ideally Hartmann's solution. The approximate volume required in the first 24 h can be calculated as = 4 mL × weight (kg) × %TBSA involved; give half of this volume in the first 8 h and the rest over the next 16 h, titrated against heart rate, blood pressure and urine output.

Where possible, check the voltage of the source of an electrical burn. Look for entry and exit wounds, perform an ECG and take samples for serum troponin and urinary myoglobin. With chemical burns, obtain as much detail as possible about the causative agent and take care not to contaminate yourself with it.

All patients should have co-morbidities documented, as these are likely to influence their outcome. Samples should be taken for FBC, U&E, LFT, Coag and cross-matching. A CXR should also be performed as a baseline and to look for evidence of the development of ARDS.

Burns management

Initial measures

After ABC has been addressed, analgesia should be given and any non-adherent clothing removed. Garments that are stuck down should be left and removed during formal debridement. Brush away any dry chemical powder and lavage affected areas with large amounts of cold water.

Referral and admission

Patients with burns affecting the face, hands or genitalia should be discussed early with the local plastic surgery team. Those with widespread or large burns should be discussed with the nearest regional burns unit.

Indications for admission to hospital

- evidence of inhalational, chemical or electrical injury
- burn size >15% TBSA at any age, or >10% in the very old or young
- full thickness burns
- burns involving a delicate area, e.g. hands, face, feet, perineum
- other injuries or illnesses contributing to the burn or hindering its recovery.

General wound management

Specialist advice should be sought. In general, the affected areas should be cleaned with chlorhexidine. A non-adherent dressing such as silver sulfadiazine paraffin gauze or Jelonet® should then be applied. Hands can be enclosed in plastic bags containing silver sulfadiazine. Tetanus toxoid should be given and the dressings changed on alternate days, with particular attention paid to evidence of developing infection. Circumferential burns may require a longitudinal incision over the length of the burn to avoid compromising distal circulation and nerve function.

SECTION 3

Specialties and cancers

10 Specialty acute presentations

HAEMATOLOGICAL

Presentation

Symptoms attributable to a blood disorder are non-specific and wide-ranging. Anaemia may be associated with fatigue, breathlessness and worsening of existing cardiovascular diseases resulting in angina, claudication, syncope or palpitations. Spontaneous bleeding or haemarthrosis may indicate a coagulopathy or thrombocytopenia. Infection may reflect an underlying white blood cell dyscrasia. In addition, systemic symptoms such as weight loss, sweats and a fever are associated with a variety of blood disorders (see 'Leukaemia and lymphoma', pp. 370 & 373). Therefore, the diagnosis of these conditions requires a high index of suspicion and is often based on blood test abnormalities. Clinical signs may be subtle or absent and are not limited to one system. Abnormalities may include:

- eyes: conjunctival pallor, yellow sclera indicating jaundice, fundal haemorrhage
- mouth: angular stomatitis, telangiectasia, smooth tongue, mucosa petechiae, tonsillar enlargement, gum hypertrophy
- hands: koilonychia, telangiectasia
- cardiorespiratory: tachycardia or signs of heart failure
- neck and axilla: nodal enlargement and, if present, site, tenderness, mobility, character (soft, rubbery)
- abdomen: splenomegaly, hepatomegaly, nodes, ascites
- joints and feet: limited movement or swelling, impaired peripheral circulation
- urine: for blood or urobilinogen.

Red blood cell disorders

These are classified based on the mean corpuscular volume (MCV) of the red cell population. Microcytic anaemias are characterized by low MCV (<76 fL); macrocytic anaemias are characterized by a high MCV (>100 fL). Remember that the MCV is an average and if there is a bimodal distribution of red cell volumes (e.g. a microcytic anaemia due to chronic bleeding in combination with a reticulocytosis due to a more acute haemorrhage) the MCV can be misleading. If in doubt, ask haematology to examine a blood film.

Microcytic and normocytic anaemias

Causes include:

- iron deficiency: this is most common and is associated with red cell hypochromia
- bleeding or haemolysis: may be associated with a reticulocytosis
- thalassaemia: target cells with basophilic stippling on the blood film and haemolysis; see below
- sideroblastic anaemia: dimorphic cells on the blood film
- anaemia of chronic disease: this may result from malignancy, chronic infection or inflammation; it may also result in normochromic, normocytic anaemia.

Iron deficiency

Gastrointestinal loss, menstrual blood loss and pregnancy are the most common causes. Malabsorption (e.g. due to hypochlorhydria or coeliac disease) should also be considered. Serum ferritin is a helpful indicator of low iron stores; however it can also be low in hypothyroidism and may be elevated as part of the acute phase response. In such situations, a transferrin or total iron binding capacity should be checked.

Further investigation should focus on the suspected aetiology, e.g. endoscopy for gastrointestinal blood loss, serum antigliadin antibodies or TTG ± duodenal biopsy for coeliac disease, or stool examination for parasites.

Transfusion is rarely required, but should be considered where the anaemia exacerbates other diseases, e.g. IHD. Oral ferrous sulphate (200 mg 8-hourly) for 3–6 months is usually sufficient if a cause can be identified and treated. Otherwise indefinite replacement may be required. Ferrous gluconate (300 mg 12-hourly PO) can be used if patients are intolerant of ferrous sulphate.

Thalassaemia

This group of inherited conditions is characterized by underproduction of the globin chains within the haemoglobin molecule. There are several genetic abnormalities which affect the production of α and β chains, resulting in α and β thalassaemia, respectively. Homozygotes for these mutations develop thalassaemia major, while heterozygotes develop thalassaemia minor (also known as thalassaemia trait).

β-Thalassaemia is the most common and is found predominantly in Mediterranean populations. In the minor variety, there is only mild hypochromic anaemia with punctuate basophilia and target cells. However, the major form results in an inability to make HbA and severe hypochromic anaemia from the first few months of life, with erythroblastosis and raised levels of fetal haemoglobin (HbF). Allogeneic bone marrow transplantation is an effective treatment, if a donor can be found. Otherwise, repeated transfusion (with desferrioxamine to reduce iron overload), bone marrow support with folic acid 5 mg daily, and splenectomy are alternatives. Screening of a potentially affected fetus should be considered.

α-Thalassaemia is most common in South-East Asian communities. α-Thalassaemia major can cause hydrops fetalis and fetal death. Patients with less severe forms of the disease have a higher survival rate, but often need support similar to that for β-thalassaemia.

Macrocytic anaemias

Causes include:

- vitamin B_{12} deficiency
- folate deficiency
- alcohol
- hypothyroidism
- artefact, commonly caused by reticulocytosis, e.g. in haemolysis or active bleeding.

Vitamin B_{12} deficiency

Causes include hypochlorhydria, e.g. following gastric surgery, pancreatic insufficiency, coeliac and Crohn's diseases, dietary deficiency, e.g. vegetarians and pernicious anaemia.

Neurological sequelae, due to demyelination, can result from significant B_{12} deficiency and can occur in the absence of anaemia. Symptoms include paraesthesiae, numbness and, if left untreated, ataxia and subacute combined degeneration of the cord.

Pernicious anaemia

This results from autoantibody-mediated atrophy of the parietal cells of the gastric mucosa. These cells are responsible for the production of intrinsic factor (IF), which is necessary for B_{12} absorption in the small intestine. PA may be associated with other autoimmune diseases. Anti-parietal cell antibodies are sensitive, but non-specific markers of PA; the presence of intrinsic factor antibodies is pathognomonic.

Schilling's test can be used to distinguish pernicious anaemia from other causes of B_{12} deficiency: This involves co-administration of 1 mg of oral and intramuscular radio-labelled vitamin B_{12}. The IM injection saturates body stores of B_{12} and encourages renal excretion of the oral dose. A 24-h urine collection is then performed. Normal patients will excrete around 10% of the oral dose; excretion of <5% is considered abnormal. To differentiate between PA and other causes of B_{12} malabsorption, B_{12} dosing is repeated, this time with addition of oral intrinsic factor. PA is indicated by normalization of B_{12} excretion on the second urine collection; a second abnormal result indicates a malabsorptive problem in the distal small intestine, e.g. coeliac or Crohn's disease.

Treatment of PA involves administration of hydroxocobalamin (1000 µg IM in 5 doses over 2–3 days, followed by the same dose every 3 months indefinitely).

Folate deficiency

Causes include poor dietary intake (leafy vegetables, cereals, seeds), drugs that interfere with folate metabolism (e.g. methotrexate, phenytoin), malabsorption (e.g. due to coeliac disease), pregnancy and haemolysis.

Treatment is folic acid (5 mg PO daily for 3 weeks, then 5 mg weekly). B_{12} levels must be checked before treatment is started. If these are not available, it is safer to assume and treat concomitant B_{12} deficiency to avoid precipitating B_{12}-associated neuropathy.

Haemolytic anaemias

In health, a red cell circulates for 90–120 days before it is destroyed within the reticuloendothelial system. Accelerated red cell lysis leads to haemolytic anaemia; patients may present with typical symptoms of anaemia and jaundice is common, due a rise in unconjugated bilirubin. There are many causes of haemolytic anaemia, broadly grouped into hereditary and acquired conditions.

Hereditary haemolytic anaemias

These are not immune mediated; therefore the direct Coomb's test will be negative. They are subclassified into:

- red cell membrane defects, e.g. hereditary spherocytosis and hereditary elliptocytosis
- enzyme deficiencies, e.g. glucose-6-phosphate dehydrogenase (G6PD), pyruvate kinase or pyrimidine 5'-nucleotidase
- haemoglobinopathies, e.g. sickle cell disease (see below) and thalassaemia (see above).

Hereditary spherocytosis

Commonly found in northern Europeans and Japanese and usually inherited in an autosomal dominant fashion. Defective production of cytoskeletal proteins results in large, spherical red cells which are visible on a blood film. These spherocytes are fragile, prone to haemolysis and are filtered by the spleen, resulting in anaemia. Patients may be asymptomatic or present with anaemia or complications related to haemolysis, e.g. pigment gallstones. The osmotic fragility test is positive.

Severe anaemia may result from infection (an aplastic crisis may be seen with parvovirus infection) or folate deficiency, e.g. during pregnancy. Management involves life-long folic acid prophylaxis (5 mg once weekly) ± splenectomy. Any transfusions must be given slowly. Families should be screened.

Hereditary elliptocytosis

May be autosomal dominant or recessive and is less common than hereditary spherocytosis in the UK. It usually causes an asymptomatic abnormality on the blood film. Occasionally results in neonatal haemolysis or a chronic compensated haemolytic state (managed as per hereditary spherocytosis).

G6PD deficiency

An X-linked recessive condition, this confers a malarial protective advantage to female heterozygotes, but is more severe when it affects Caucasians and Orientals. Infection and a range of drugs can precipitate haemolysis, as can ingestion of a form of broad bean (this is known as favism). Occasionally neonatal haemolysis can occur. Features include non-spherocytic intravascular haemolysis with 'bite' and blister cells on the blood film.

Pyruvate kinase deficiency

This is inherited as an autosomal recessive trait with varying degrees of anaemia. Characteristic 'prickle cells' like holly leaves are seen on the blood film.

Sickle cell disease

This results from a single glutamic acid to valine substitution at position 6 of the β-globin polypeptide chain. An autosomal recessive disease, it results in a preponderance of HbS and the fully expressed sickle cell phenotype only in homozygotes. Heterozygotes produce a mixture of HbA and HbS (termed AS), and express a far less severe, and often asymptomatic, phenotype described as sickle 'trait'. Sickle trait confers resistance to falciparum malaria, hence the mutation has perpetuated in sub-Saharan Africa, which has the highest incidence of the condition.

Sickle cell anaemia produces abnormally shaped red cells that become stuck in small vessels. Because of its role as a filtration system for the bloodstream this leads to multi-infarct splenic injury and autosplenectomy, often by the end of childhood. Other serious complications include parvovirus B19 infection, which can lead to severe aplastic anaemia, and sickling crises, which may be precipitated by hypoxia, infection, hypothermia or dehydration. Examples of these include:

- bone vaso-occlusive crisis: affects small vessels in bones (often hands and feet in children, and long bones, ribs and vertebrae in adults); presents with acute severe bone pain ± fever or tachycardia
- sickle chest syndrome: commonest cause of death in adult sickle disease; ventilatory failure due to fat emboli following bone marrow infarction
- sequestration crisis: end-organ venous thrombotic occlusion with acute painful enlargement; often affects spleen or liver.

Patients require protection against infection with encapsulated organisms. They should receive regular pneumococcal vaccination, daily penicillin V prophylaxis and vaccination against *Haemophilus* and hepatitis B should be considered. Hydroxycarbamide may be beneficial and daily folic acid supplements should be given. A crisis will require analgesia, oxygen, fluids and antibiotic cover. In severe cases, exchange transfusion may be considered.

Acquired haemolytic anaemias

Acquired haemolytic anaemias are classified into immune-mediated causes (direct Coombs' test is positive) and non-immune-mediated causes (direct Coombs' test is negative).

- immune-mediated acquired haemolytic anaemias include autoimmune conditions (see below), allo-immune conditions, e.g. haemolytic disease of the newborn (see 'Obstetric', p. 318), and drug-induced haemolytic anaemia, most commonly due to methyldopa and high-dose penicillin
- non-immune-mediated acquired haemolytic anaemias may be due to the direct action of drugs on red blood cells (e.g. dapsone, sulfasalazine, arsenic); trauma (e.g. mechanical heart valves); infections (e.g. malaria, *Clostridium perfringens*); or microangiopathic haemolysis (e.g. in haemolytic uraemic syndrome, disseminated intravascular coagulation, thrombotic thrombocytopenic purpura and HELLP syndrome).

Autoimmune haemolytic anaemia

Red cell antibodies can be 'warm agglutinins', binding best at 37°C, or 'cold agglutinins', binding best at 4°C.

Warm agglutinin disease accounts for 80% of cases and is usually due to IgG antibodies. It is associated with haematological malignancy, other solid tumours, connective tissue disease, drugs (e.g. penicillin, quinine), inflammatory bowel disease and HIV infection. Haemolysis with spherocytes is seen on a blood film and the direct Coombs' test is positive.

Management involves treatment of the underlying cause and oral steroids (1 mg/kg prednisolone). Splenectomy or immunosuppression may be necessary in refractory disease.

Cold agglutinin disease is usually due to complement-binding IgM antibodies. It is associated with low-grade B-cell lymphoma and infection, e.g. mycoplasma, glandular fever. Treatment includes keeping the extremities warm and oral steroids.

Polycythaemia

Polycythaemia can be relative (due to a reduction in circulating plasma volume) or genuine, due to increased red cell mass. Genuine polycythaemia may be:

- primary: due to the myeloproliferative disorder, polycythaemia rubra vera (PRV)
- secondary: to chronic hypoxia or increased erythropoietin secretion (most commonly from renal tumours).

Polycythaemia may present with pruritus (which is often worse after a hot bath), gout, angina and arterial thromboses. Treatment is of the underlying cause in secondary polycythaemia, although venesection may be required temporarily to reduce the risk of thrombotic complications. PRV is treated by venesection of approximately 500 mL blood every 7 days until the haematocrit is <0.45. Aspirin is used to limit the risk of thrombosis. Interferon or hydroxycarbamide is used as a myelosuppressant.

White blood cell disorders

Neutropenia

This is defined as a neutrophil count $<1.5\times10^9$/L. Causes include cytotoxic drug therapy, infection, connective tissue disease, alcohol or bone marrow infiltration. Infection in neutropenic patients is poorly tolerated and can result in shock and rapid deterioration. Patients with neutropenic sepsis should be reviewed urgently and admitted for observation and treatment (see 'Neutropenic sepsis', p. 246).

Neutrophilia

Causes include bacterial infection, inflammation, infarction, trauma including surgery, malignancy, myeloproliferative disorders, exercise, pregnancy and steroid use. Treatment should be directed to the underlying cause.

Lymphopenia

Defined by a lymphocyte count $<1\times10^9/L$. Associations include connective tissue disease, sarcoid, renal disease, lymphoma, drugs and severe combined immunodeficiency syndrome. Lymphopenia results in defective cell-mediated immunity and infection with viruses, fungi or TB.

Lymphocytosis

Due to infection, e.g. viral or whooping cough, or lymphoproliferative disease.

Eosinophilia

Due to allergic disorders, parasitic infection, drug hypersensitivity, connective tissue and skin diseases and malignancy.

Platelet disorders

Thrombocytopenia

May present with purpura, spontaneous bruising or haemorrhage. A bone marrow examination may be helpful to determine the cause, which will be due to either:

- reduced marrow production: marrow infiltration by tumour, leukaemia or myeloma; chronic alcohol excess; vitamin B_{12} deficiency; drugs (e.g. thiazides); idiopathic
- excessive platelet consumption: DIC (see below), idiopathic thrombocytopenic purpura (see below), viral infection, e.g. EBV, bacterial infection, thrombotic thrombocytopenic purpura; splenomegaly; liver and connective tissue diseases.

Idiopathic thrombocytopenic purpura

In children, ITP is often preceded by a viral infection, but in adults it is more commonly associated with connective tissue disease. Females are affected more often than men. Autoantibodies to platelet glycoprotein result in premature platelet consumption. This results in increased production of platelet precursors in the bone marrow (megakaryocytes).

In children, spontaneous bleeding and purpura are often self-limiting but steroids may be necessary. Severe cases require platelet transfusion and IV immunoglobulin. In adults, steroids are often less effective and IV IgG may be needed. Splenectomy is used for relapsing cases.

Thrombocytosis

This can be reactive (infection, chronic inflammation, malignancy, haemolytic anaemia or haemorrhage, trauma and tissue damage), due to myeloproliferation or primary megakaryocyte proliferation. Complications include stroke and other vascular events, or bleeding due to platelet dysfunction.

Pancytopenia

This term describes the combination of anaemia, leucopenia and thrombocytopenia and may be due to:

- defective cell production due to bone marrow infiltration (e.g. by solid tumours, lymphoma, myeloproliferative disorders); hereditary or acquired aplasia, e.g. drug related or viral
- excess cell destruction (hypersplenism) is seen in myelofibrosis, portal hypertension and some infections, e.g. malaria.

Bone marrow aspiration and trephine biopsy may be necessary if the diagnosis is not clinically apparent.

Coagulation disorders

These are broadly divided into hereditary and acquired conditions.

Hereditary

Haemophilia

Haemophilia A

This is an X-linked inherited deficiency of factor VIII. Symptoms develop around 6 months of age and include spontaneous bleeding into joints and muscles and an increased bleeding tendency after trauma.

Factor VIII concentrate infusion is required for bleeding episodes and prior to surgery, and should be followed by a course of tranexamic acid. With repeated transfusion some patients may develop antibodies to factor VIII, rendering it ineffective. Activated clotting factors VIIa or FEIBA (factor VIII inhibitor bypassing activity) should be used instead.

Patients transfused before 1985 were exposed to an increased risk of transfusion-transmissible infections for which screening was not undertaken before this date. Thus, there is an increased incidence of hepatitis A, B, C, and HIV in haemophiliacs of this generation. Concerns persist regarding prion-related infections.

Haemophilia B

Also referred to as 'Christmas disease', this results from a reduction of factor IX and manifests much as haemophilia A, but is less common. Treatment is with factor IX concentrate.

Other clotting cascade deficiencies

Anti-thrombin deficiency

This is a protein that inactivates certain clotting factors. Deficiency produces a prothrombotic tendency. The condition is exacerbated by heparin.

Protein C+S deficiency

Protein C and S affect the inactivation of clotting cascade factors V and VIII. An inherited deficiency of either leads to a prothrombotic tendency.

Von Willebrand disease

Although common, this is usually mild. It is inherited as an autosomal dominant disorder (chromosome 12), but individual expression can vary significantly. A protein deficiency occurs linked to the carriage of factor VIII and also the adherence of platelets to damaged tissue. Bruising, epistaxis and excess bleeding following trauma or surgery can result. Testing shows a low factor VIII level and a prolonged bleeding time. Desmopressin can temporarily raise the level of the protein involved. Severe episodes require transfusion of factor VIII concentrate.

Acquired

DIC

Endothelial damage from infections (e.g. Gram-negative or streptococcal), tumours or obstetric complications can trigger tissue factor expression, activation of the clotting cascade through the extrinsic pathway, and consumption of platelets, clotting factors and fibrinogen by intravascular coagulation. Blood tests show thrombocytopenia, a prolonged PT, APPT and a low fibrinogen. Treatment is that of the underlying cause and in particular of any associated infection, dehydration, acidosis or hypoxia. Platelet transfusion ± fresh frozen plasma may be necessary.

General

Liver disease and warfarin over-anticoagulation can lead to abnormal clotting with excess bleeding. See 'Warfarin', p. 110.

RHEUMATOLOGICAL

Rheumatological symptoms are a common reason for attendance at GP surgeries, A&E and a variety of hospital specialties. The most common acute presentations involve joint pain or stiffness and their causes, in adults and children, are detailed below.

Acute monoarthritis

The priority is to establish the diagnosis and commence appropriate therapy. The most important disorder to consider is septic arthritis; others include crystal arthritis, haemarthrosis, reactive arthritis or inflammatory monoarthritis. A careful history is important: ask about previous similar episodes, recent illnesses, medication, family history and a history of bleeding disorders or anticoagulation.

Clinical features

In septic arthritis, the history is usually short and is of pain in the affected joint for days rather than weeks. If examination reveals a hot swollen tender joint with restriction of movement, then urgent investigation is required.

Investigation

In a native joint, synovial fluid should be aspirated and the samples sent for polarizing microscopy, Gram-stain and culture before starting antibiotics; some microbiologists prefer the sample to be sent to the laboratory in blood culture bottles. If a prosthetic joint is affected, always refer to an orthopaedic surgeon.

Blood cultures should also be obtained and other relevant investigations include FBC, ESR, CRP and renal function. Plain radiology would not be expected to show any changes in an acute septic arthritis, but may point to an alternative diagnosis, e.g. chondrocalcinosis suggesting pseudogout. Ultrasound has a role in assisting joint aspiration in joints that are not easily accessible, such as the hip. In osteomyelitis, plain radiography may show bone destruction, but MRI is the best imaging modality. Deep bone biopsy may also be necessary.

Management

If septic arthritis is suspected IV empirical antibiotics should be commenced and the choice refined following investigation results. If the diagnosis is confirmed these should be continued for up to 2 weeks IV, followed by around 4 weeks of oral therapy. Flucloxacillin (2 g 6-hourly) ± gentamicin would be a normal first-choice regime. In the case of penicillin allergy, use either clindamycin (450–600 mg 6-hourly) or a 3rd generation cephalosporin, instead. However, alternative drugs may be necessary if there is a high risk of Gram-negative infection (2nd or 3rd generation cephalosporin, e.g. cefuroxime 1.5 g 8-hourly) or MRSA (vancomycin plus 2nd or 3rd generation cephalosporin).

In addition, a septic joint should be drained to dryness as soon as possible. Local protocols will determine whether this is by closed needle or by arthroscopy. Hip infection should involve early specialist advice from orthopaedics.

Osteomyelitis can be managed with similar antibiotics to that for septic arthritis (including fusidic acid), but a longer duration of IV treatment may be necessary. Surgical input is often required for drainage, debridement and bone stabilization and all cases should be managed in consultation with orthopaedics.

New-onset inflammatory polyarthritis

The most important diagnosis to consider is rheumatoid arthritis (RA). This is because early diagnosis and prompt treatment of RA has been shown to improve outcome. However, there are no satisfactory diagnostic criteria for early RA and traditional diagnostic criteria do not apply (these employ features such as nodule formation and radiological erosion which are only present in established disease). Reflecting this difficulty, the term 'undifferentiated inflammatory polyarthritis' is often used to describe patients with an early inflammatory arthritis in whom a specific diagnosis cannot yet be made.

Clinical assessment

History

The following features are important discriminators and should be elicited from the history:

- duration of symptoms
- associated features, e.g. morning stiffness
- family history of RA or other arthritis
- personal or family history of associated conditions, e.g. psoriasis or inflammatory bowel disease
- any recent history of sexually transmitted or diarrhoeal illness; uveitis or conjunctivitis; rash or fever; symptoms associated with a connective tissue disorder such as dry eyes, oral ulceration, photosensitive or other skin rash or Raynaud's phenomenon.

The history may also include features suggestive of an alternative diagnosis. A history of limb girdle stiffness in a patient over the age of 50 may suggest polymyalgia rheumatica, whereas a very acute monoarthritis in a patient on diuretics may suggest gout. Also consider the possibility of rarer presentations, e.g. lymphoma, myeloma, sarcoid and vasculitis.

Examination

The pattern of joint involvement is an important factor. RA, for example, is charac teristically symmetrical, whereas psoriatic arthritis and other seronegative arthritides are frequently asymmetrical. RA is a polyarthritis with almost universal involvement of the hands or feet. A large-joint oligoarthritis or monoarthritis is uncommon in RA, but may occur in spondyloarthritis, reactive arthritis or gout. Predominant spinal involvement may suggest ankylosing spondylitis or another of the spondyloarthropathies. It is also helpful to record whether there is arthralgia alone or definite synovitis, e.g. a positive metacarpal or metatarsal squeeze test.

Investigation

While history and examination are the most important methods of determining if there is inflammatory arthritis, some investigations are helpful. These will usually be carried out in specialist centres and should not delay referral; see below.

- IgM rheumatoid factor is associated with poor prognosis (especially in high titre) and may be helpful in confirming the diagnosis
- antibodies to cyclic citrullinated peptides (anti-CCP antibodies) have a high specificity for RA, are a reliable marker of persistent disease and, if available, are useful markers in early or undifferentiated arthritis
- ESR and CRP can be of value
- serological assays for organisms that cause a reactive arthropathy, where relevant
- plain radiology is seldom helpful in establishing a diagnosis in early disease
- ultrasound and MRI are more sensitive at detecting synovitis, but are best organized from the rheumatology clinic, where they will be used to direct management.

Management

Specialist input

All patients with a new inflammatory arthropathy should be referred promptly to a rheumatologist. The purpose of this early referral is to allow recognition of persistent inflammatory arthritis and to start treatment with effective disease-modifying therapy at the earliest opportunity. Some centres have specific 'early arthritis' clinics or local protocols to ensure that such patients are seen promptly.

Management of established rheumatoid arthritis

There is still controversy about how best to use disease-modifying anti-rheumatic drugs (DMARDs). Sequential monotherapy, 'step-up' and 'step-down' regimens are all still widely used. The British Society for Rheumatology website is a good source of up-to-date treatment guidelines.

The role of biological drugs is a rapidly changing field. At present in the UK, the use of anti-TNF drugs (infliximab, etanercept and adalimumab) is restricted to those who have failed conventional DMARD therapy. However, there is recent evidence to support their use in early disease and recommendations may change in the future as a result. Newer biological agents which have recently been licensed include rituximab, which is an anti-B cell antibody, and abatacept, which blocks T-cell co-stimulation. Other biological drugs are likely to become available in the future. While it is not possible to discuss individual treatment strategies in detail here, there are some general practice points which apply in the outpatient clinic.

Familiarize yourself with departmental policies regarding assessment and drug monitoring. Most rheumatology departments will have agreed shared-care policies with local GPs showing what monitoring is being carried out, by whom and how often. Many patients will also have a patient-held record of results.

There are now many well validated assessment tools that are being incorporated into routine clinical practice and used to guide changes in treatment. If a disease activity score (DAS) or other measure is usually recorded, find out what this means and what action should be taken.

Use the whole team, e.g. involvement of the specialist nurse, podiatrist, orthotist, physiotherapist and occupational therapist may be appropriate for a patient with foot pain and poor mobility.

Review drug therapy and discuss this with your consultant. In patients with active disease, escalate drug doses and consider combination or biological therapy. If the disease is well controlled consider reducing or stopping NSAIDs or steroids. Ask if the department has a protocol for stepping down DMARD therapy for patients in remission. Also consider intra-articular steroid for active joints. Ask for advice: rheumatology is a complex branch of medicine and expert input is valuable.

Low back pain

Low back pain is common with a lifetime prevalence of up to 70%. The important aspects of managing chronic low back pain include correctly diagnosing those patients with a specific cause for their pain, achieving pain relief and preventing disability.

About 90% of patients with low back pain will have 'non-specific low back pain'. In the remaining 10% underlying causes can be found. These include vertebral fracture, ankylosing spondylitis, infection or malignancy. Features that suggest an underlying cause have been described as 'red flags' and include:

- onset <20 or >55 years
- non-mechanical or thoracic pain
- previous history of carcinoma, steroids or HIV
- feeling unwell, weight loss or widespread neurological symptoms
- structural spinal deformity.

Investigation

Imaging is generally only helpful in 'red flag' patients and is not generally recommended for non-specific back pain. MRI may be useful where there are radicular symptoms, e.g. prominent unilateral leg pain, numbness and paraesthesia, leg pain induced by straight leg raising.

Management

In acute low back pain, non-steroidal anti-inflammatory drugs and early mobilization are of value. Most acute low back pain will resolve within 1–2 weeks. Predictive factors for chronicity include a large number of personal, psychosocial and occupational factors. The most important of these include obesity, depression (especially when associated with somatization) and job dissatisfaction.

In patients with chronic low back pain, treatments employed include supervised exercise therapy with encouragement to remain active, analgesics, acupuncture, 'back schools' and cognitive behavioural therapy. In those with manual occupations, liaison with the employer to facilitate an early return to work on lighter duties may be appropriate.

Acute joint pain in children

Arthritis in children may present in different ways to adults. Musculoskeletal symptoms are common in childhood and only a small proportion of these will represent juvenile arthritis. Many children do not complain of joint pain and the clinical signs can be subtle. Some children will present with a limp or arm dysfunction. Restriction of range of movement at a joint is an important clinical sign. A subset of children will present with prominent systemic upset and constitutional features such as fever, lethargy, weight loss or irritability. It is important to ask about associated features, such as eye symptoms and rash.

Presentations

On the basis of the number of joints affected in the first 6 months of disease, juvenile idiopathic arthritis is classified into six groups.

Oligoarthritis

This typically occurs in girls under 5 years of age. These children have a high frequency of anti-nuclear antibodies and chronic anterior uveitis which may be silent. For the majority the prognosis is good, although a significant minority have persistent disease.

Psoriatic arthritis

Psoriatic arthritis can affect boys or girls and the diagnosis requires a personal or family history of psoriasis. In some patients, the arthritis may precede the psoriasis.

Enthesitis

Enthesitis (inflammation at the insertion or either tendon or ligament) related arthritis most frequently affects older boys and shares some features with ankylosing spondylitis in adults. These children may present with a lower limb oligoarthritis often associated with enthesitis at the plantar fascia or Achilles insertion. There may be a family history of ankylosing spondylitis or inflammatory bowel disease.

Polyarthritis

This is less common in children than in adults. A proportion of children with multiple joint involvement will have a symmetrical polyarthritis, associated with a positive rheumatoid factor, and a disease which clinically resembles rheumatoid arthritis in the adult. In younger children the disease is usually seronegative. Prognosis in polyarticular disease is poorer than in oligoarticular disease and persists, in a significant proportion, into adult life.

Systemic arthritis

The diagnosis is challenging because the majority of symptoms are extra-articular and may include very non-specific features such as fever, rash, weight loss and lymphadenopathy. In these patients it is important to exclude other diagnoses. About one third develop a severe polyarthritis.

Other

Patients who fit no category or more than one category.

Limb girdle stiffness

Shoulder soft tissue injury (see 'Shoulder injuries', p. 266) and inflammatory arthritides may be responsible for limb girdle stiffness. However, an important condition to consider is polymyalgia rheumatica (PMR). Where PMR is present, a significant number of patients will also have giant cell arteritis (GCA) which is important to recognize because it can cause blindness.

Polymyalgia rheumatica

Presentation

This inflammatory disorder affects females more than males (3:1) and is diagnosed when three or more of the following criteria are present: age >65, ESR >40 mm/h, bilateral upper arm tenderness, morning stiffness of >1 h, onset of illness <2 weeks, depression and/or weight loss. The diagnosis is confirmed by a rapid clinical response to corticosteroids.

Polymyalgia rheumatica can present acutely with pain and stiffness or have an insidious onset where systemic symptoms predominate. A low-grade fever may be present.

Investigation and diagnosis

Blood tests commonly reveal a raised ESR; there may also be an elevated CRP, a normochromic, normocytic anaemia and a raised alkaline phosphatase. As the presentation of PMR may overlap with that of other conditions (myeloma, rheumatoid arthritis, connective tissue disease, myositis, fibromyalgia, osteomalacia), it is worth considering these in the investigation and including: protein electrophoresis, rheumatoid factor, autoantibodies, CK, calcium and phosphate.

Management

Treatment is with prednisolone (15 mg PO daily; reduced after 4 weeks to 10 mg daily). A dramatic response should be seen within 72 h. The daily dose is then reduced by 1 mg every 4–6 weeks over 6–12 months until it reaches 5 mg. Thereafter, the dose can usually be reduced by 1 mg every 3–4 months over 2 years. NSAIDs can also be used to help pain as the dose is reduced.

Relapses are common and respond to a temporary increase in the steroid dose before a slower further titrated reduction. If continued high doses are needed, or if corticosteroids cannot be withdrawn after 2 years, steroid-sparing agents, such as methotrexate or azathioprine, should be considered.

Giant cell arteritis

Presentation

This inflammatory process usually affects females more than males (4:1) and those aged 70 or over. It is rare in the under 50s. It often affects the temporal artery and can cause headache, jaw claudication (suggested by pain on chewing), blurring of vision, scalp tenderness over the temporal artery and, if untreated, blindness. It can also be associated with systemic symptoms similar to those described in PMR and there is significant overlap between the two conditions; 50% of patients with giant cell arteritis will also have PMR and about 10% of those with PMR will have GCA. GCA may affect large arteries elsewhere and may result in aortic aneurysms or large artery thrombosis, e.g. CVA.

Investigation and diagnosis

Diagnosis is on the basis of clinical findings, a raised ESR and a temporal artery biopsy. However, a negative biopsy cannot exclude the diagnosis and arrangements for biopsy should not delay treatment.

Management

There is an immediate threat to the patient's vision. Therefore, patients with GCA should be treated with high doses of steroids initially, e.g. prednisolone 40–50 mg daily with a slow reduction towards a 10 mg daily dose, over 6 weeks. Thereafter, doses should reduce by 1 mg/month, but a maintenance dose will be needed for at least a year. Relapses are managed with further dose increases and should prompt the consideration of steroid-sparing agents.

All patients requiring corticosteroids at over 7.5 mg/day for more than 3 months should have bone protection prescribed, e.g. bisphosphonates ± in women, hormone replacement therapy. Bone density should be measured by dual-energy X-ray densitometry (DEXA), ideally at the start of treatment. Likewise, gastric protection, e.g. omeprazole, should be considered.

Skin, muscle and systemic symptoms

Systemic symptoms may be caused by the inflammatory arthritides or their treatment. However, it is important to consider the possibility of other pathologies that may cause similar symptoms.

Systemic lupus erythematosus

Epidemiology and aetiology

Systemic lupus erythematosus (SLE) is the commonest of the multisystem connective tissue diseases (CTD). It affects 3/10 000 Caucasians and is more common in Afro-Caribbean races (20/10 000). About 90% of affected individuals are women. SLE results from the production of anti-nuclear antibodies; at least 50 different antigen targets have so far been identified.

Presentation

SLE may present with any number of a wide range of clinical features. Of these, arthritis associated with Raynaud's phenomenon is the most common. Mucocutaneous features include the classical butterfly facial rash (Fig. 10.1), discoid lupus and livedo reticularis (a feature of anti-phospholipid syndrome).

A variety of joint symptoms may occur, including a small joint synovitis similar to RA. However, joint deformities are rare. There is an increased risk of venous thromboembolism and miscarriage due to production of anti-phospholipid antibodies (anti-phospholipid syndrome). Renal involvement (lupus nephritis) is heralded by haematuria, proteinuria and worsening renal impairment.

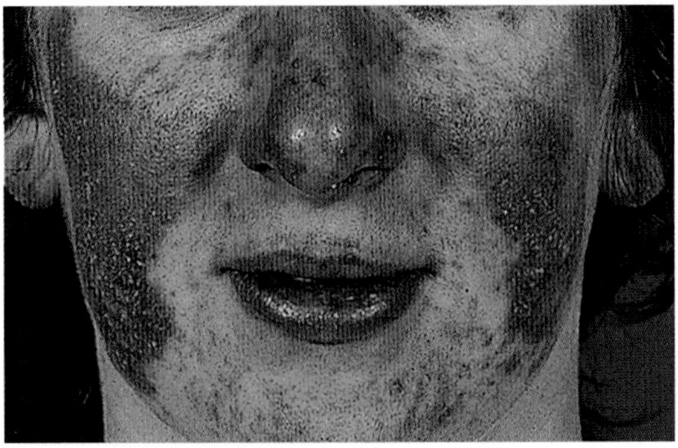

Figure 10.1 Butterfly facial rash typical of SLE.

Table 10.1 Most common features of SLE

Feature	Characteristics
Malar (butterfly) rash	Fixed erythema, typical distribution, spares nasolabial folds
Discoid rash	Erythematous raised patches; adherent keratotic scar and follicular plugging
Photosensitivity	Rash in response to sunlight
Oral ulcers	Often painless
Arthritis	Involving two or more peripheral joints; non-erosive
Serositis	Pleuritis (effusion, rub or convincing story) or pericarditis (effusion, rub or ECG changes)
Renal	Persistent proteinuria >0.5 g/24 h or cellular casts on microscopy
Neurological	Seizures or psychosis in the absence of another cause
Haematological	Haemolytic anaemia or leucopenia/lymphopenia/ thrombocytopenia, on two occasions, in the absence of another cause
Immunological	Anti-dsDNA in abnormal titre or antibodies to Sm antigen or positive anti-phospholipid antibodies
ANA disorder	Abnormal titre of ANA by immunofluorescence

Diagnosis and investigation

Diagnosis requires recognition of typical symptoms and signs and demonstration of circulating anti-nuclear antibodies (ANA). Patients who are ANA-negative are unlikely to have SLE unless they are anti-Ro positive. Although antibodies to double-stranded DNA (anti-dsDNA) are classically associated with SLE, these are present in only 30–50% of patients. The revised American Rheumatism Association criteria for the diagnosis of SLE require at least four of the 11 most common features of SLE for diagnosis (Table 10.1).

Management

All patients should avoid excessive sunlight and UV exposure and the use of high-factor sun blocks is essential. Patients with mild disease may only require intermittent analgesic or NSAIDs for joint symptoms. Oral hydroxychloroquine (200–400 mg daily) is often effective in controlling skin or more troublesome joint disease. Short courses of oral prednisolone (e.g. 40–60 mg daily) may be required for flairs of synovitis, pleuropericarditis or skin disease. The dose should be weaned oncecontrol is achieved and steroid-sparing agents may be useful, e.g. azathioprine, methotrexate. Life-threatening disease, such as cerebral, renal or pulmonary vasculitis, often requires pulsed IV methylprednisolone (0.5–1 g daily) and/or cyclophosphamide (0.375–1g/m^2 every 2–4 weeks). Patients with anti-phospholipid syndrome should receive life-long anticoagulation with warfarin after a first venous thromboembolic event.

Prognosis

The 5-year survival rate exceeds 90%. However, mortality in those who have had the disease for many years is higher, due to an increased incidence of cardiovascular disease, possibly reflecting long-term steroid use. Therefore, the lowest effective steroid dose should always be used. Poor prognostic features include development of lupus nephritis, pulmonary fibrosis (may be associated with 'shrinking lung syndrome') and pulmonary hypertension.

Systemic sclerosis

Epidemiology and aetiology

Systemic sclerosis (previously termed 'scleroderma') is most common in the fourth and fifth decades and affects 1–2/10000 people. It is four times more common in women. The classical hallmark of systemic sclerosis is sclerodactyly and Raynaud's phenomenon ± digital ischaemia. The cause is unknown and, unlike SLE, there are no consistent racial or genetic associations.

Presentation

Raynaud's phenomenon is often the earliest clinical feature, usually followed by skin disease.

Skin disease is characterized by shiny, taut fingers with erythema and tortuous dilatation of capillary loops in the nail-fold bed. Classical facial features include thinning of the lips and radial furrowing around the mouth. Patients with skin involvement limited to distal sites (below knee and elbow, but excluding the face) are said to have limited cutaneous systemic sclerosis (LCSS). Those with more extensive skin disease are described as having diffuse cutaneous systemic sclerosis (DCSS). A proportion of patients with LCSS have the CREST phenotype (calcinosis, Raynaud's phenomenon, oesophageal involvement, sclerodactyly and telangiectasia) (Fig. 10.2).

Arthralgia is common, but functional limitation of the hands is due to skin thickening rather than joint disease. Myositis may lead to muscle pain and weakness. Erosive joint disease is uncommon. Gastrointestinal involvement may include severe oesophagitis, dysphagia and recurrent upper GI bleeding from antral vascular ectasia ('water melon stomach') in up to 20% of patients.

Pulmonary and renal complications are a major cause of morbidity and mortality. Fibrosing alveolitis is more common in diffuse disease; pulmonary hypertension is more common in limited disease and CREST syndrome. Hypertensive renal crisis is heralded by malignant hypertension and acute renal failure; it is more common in diffuse disease and may be fatal.

Diagnosis and investigation

The diagnosis is mainly a clinical one. The majority of patients will be ANA-positive; additional anti-topoisomerase-1 and anti-centromere antibodies will be present in 30% of patients with DCSS and 60% patients with LCSS, respectively. Antibodies to Scl-70 are found particularly in pulmonary fibrosis associated with systemic sclerosis.

Management

Patients should be taught simple measures to avoid peripheral cold exposure. No treatment has been shown to be effective in controlling skin disease; however, prompt high-dose antibiotic treatment of local infection is essential. Calcium

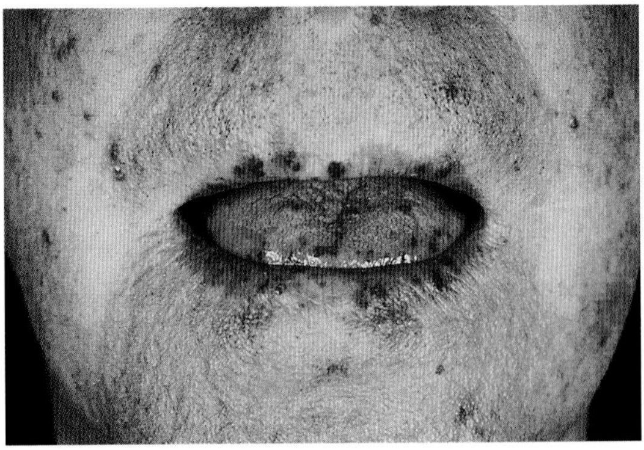

Figure 10.2 Typical facial appearance in CREST syndrome.

channel antagonists (e.g. nifedipine) may be effective for Raynaud's phenomenon. Severe digital ischaemic disease should be treated with regular infusions of intravenous epoprostenol. Steroids can be helpful in myositis and ACE inhibitors should be used to treat hypertensive renal crises (even in the presence of renal impairment). Pulmonary hypertension should be treated with anticoagulation and IV epoprostenol or oral bosentan/sildenafil, depending on disease severity.

Prognosis

The 5-year survival rate is approximately 70%. Poor prognostic features include advanced age at diagnosis, diffuse disease, a high ESR, proteinuria, a low transfer factor or other evidence of pulmonary hypertension.

Polymyositis and dermatomyositis

Epidemiology and aetiology

Polymyositis and dermatomyositis are the commonest forms of the idiopathic inflammatory myopathies. Their aetiology is unknown and genetic associations vary amongst different racial groups. Despite this, there is no significant geographical variation in disease incidence, which is approximately 2–10 per million/year.

Presentation

Both conditions are characterized by muscle weakness and pain. Polymyositis usually presents with progressive symmetrical proximal muscle weakness, e.g. the patient will complain of difficulty rising from a chair, or brushing their hair. The onset is usually over weeks to months, but may be more rapid. Pharyngeal or respiratory muscle involvement is an ominous sign. Interstitial lung disease may develop and is particularly associated with the presence of anti-Jo antibodies.

Dermatomyositis presents with identical muscle features, but additional skin signs. These may include:

- Gottron's papules: scaly erythematosus or violaceous plaques over the extensor surfaces of the finger joints
- heliotrope rash: violaceous discoloration of the eyelids, usually associated with peri-orbital oedema (Fig. 10.3)
- shawl-distribution rash: violaceous eruptions over the shoulders, upper back and upper chest.

Both conditions may be associated with systemic features including fever, weight loss and fatigue and there is an increased risk of malignancy (risk increased by 30% in polymyositis and by 300% in dermatomyositis).

Diagnosis and investigation

Proximal myopathy without neuropathy is highly suggestive, especially if associated with systemic features. CK is often elevated, but a normal CK does not exclude the disease. However, it is a useful means of monitoring disease activity in the longer

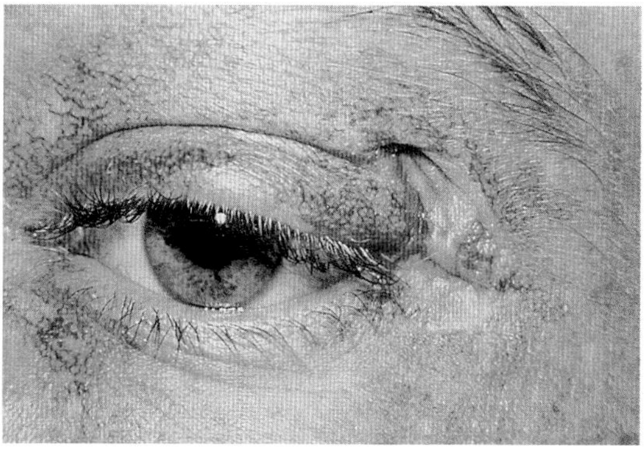

Figure 10.3 Heliotrope rash typical of dermatomyositis.

term. Electromyography will confirm myopathy and the absence of neuropathy. Muscle biopsy is required to confirm the diagnosis and will show fibre necrosis and regeneration associated with an inflammatory cell infiltrate. MRI can be used to identify an appropriate area of muscle for biopsy. If underlying malignancy is suspected (based on symptoms or excessive weight loss), screening CT or breast mammography should be considered.

Management

High-dose oral prednisolone (40–60 mg daily) is usually required to achieve control. This can be tapered by 25% per month to a maintenance dose of 5–7.5 mg/day. Patients with pharyngeal or respiratory muscle involvement may require initial treatment with IV methylprednisolone (1 g daily for 3 days). Azathioprine or methotrexate can be used as second-line or steroid-sparing agents. Ciclosporin, cyclophosphamide, tacrolimus and IV immunoglobulin are reserved for refractory disease, in which setting a steroid-induced myopathy should be excluded and consideration given to the need for re-biopsy.

Mixed connective tissue disease

This an overlap syndrome which may include clinical features commonly found in SLE, systemic sclerosis and dermato/polymyositis. Raynaud's phenomenon is commonly present, in addition to synovitis and oedema of the hands and fingers and muscle pain and weakness. Anti-ribonucleoprotein (anti-RNP) antibodies are often present. Treatment is similar to that of the more specific connective tissue diseases.

DERMATOLOGICAL

The skin is the largest organ of the body and performs several vital functions. It is a barrier to physical agents, ultraviolet light and microorganisms, helps regulate body temperature and prevents loss of body fluids. In addition, it is involved in sensory and autonomic functions, immune surveillance and is essential for vitamin D hydroxylation.

Skin disorders are common and, for patients admitted acutely, it helps to be able to distinguish conditions that require supportive management from those that demand acute investigation or specialist input. In addition, skin changes may act as markers of systemic disease or internal malignancy, a selection of which is listed below:

- coeliac disease: dermatitis herpetiformis
- diabetes: necrobiosis lipoidica, disseminated granuloma annulare, xanthelasma, xanthoma
- thyroid disease: pretibial myxoedema, xerosis
- inflammatory bowel disease: pyoderma gangrenosum
- malignancy: acanthosis nigricans, dermatomyositis, ichthyosis, pruritus.

Assessment

This requires a full history and examination of all the skin with good lighting. Ask about family history, recent medication and contact with possible allergens, such as leather, latex, cosmetics or jewellery. Examine the distribution (e.g. flexor, extensor, palmar, glove or dermatomal), symmetry and morphology of any skin problem and look for evidence of photo-exposure. Record a description of the condition using the mnemonic: 'Skin Specialists Often Suggest Suncream' (SSOSS):

- Site on body
- Size (measure with tape measure)
- Outline (clear demarcation or indistinguishable from, e.g., surrounding erythema)
- Shape (linear or round)
- Surface (flat, raised, excoriated, scaly).

Table 10.2 Basic skin terminology

Terminology	Description
Macule	Localized flat area of colour or textural change
Papule	Solid elevation, usually <0.5 cm
Nodule	Solid elevation, usually >0.5 cm
Patch	Localized flat area of colour or textural change, usually >1 cm in diameter
Plaque	Raised plateau-like elevation of skin, usually >2 cm in diameter
Vesicle	Clear fluid-filled elevation, usually <0.5 cm
Blister/bulla	Large fluid-filled elevation, usually >0.5 cm (tense or flaccid)
Pustule	Pus-filled elevation, of variable size; may be infected or sterile
Excoriation	Scratch
Purpura	Bruised discoloration due to leakage of red blood cells
Telangiectasia	Collection of abnormally visible dilated blood vessels
Lichenification	Thickened skin with prominent markings

The terminology that is used to describe common lesions is unique to dermatology, and you should be familiar with the most basic terms (Table 10.2).

Common inflammatory rashes

Psoriasis

Psoriasis is a chronic, inflammatory disease affecting 1–3% of the population (Figs 10.4 and 10.5 overleaf). There is a genetic predisposition, but other factors may also precipitate psoriasis as listed in Table 10.3. There are various clinical phenotypes:

- classic chronic psoriasis: presents as well-defined red plaques with silvery scale, usually on extensor surfaces and scalp
- guttate psoriasis: a more acute eruption (tiny 'raindrop' lesions) on torso and limbs that commonly follows a streptococcal throat infection
- flexural psoriasis: glazed red plaques (with little scale) that often affect the axillae, genitalia, gluteal cleft, sub-mammary area and umbilicus
- pustular psoriasis: may be localized, affecting palms and soles with yellow sterile pustules which become brown on healing, or as a more generalized form; see 'Skin failure and emergency dermatology', p. 306
- scalp and nail disease: nail pitting, ridging and separation of the distal edge of the nail from the nail bed (onycholysis) are common problems
- joint involvement: psoriatic arthropathy is common and seen in up to 5% of cases and may pre-date skin disease.

Treatment

Patients should be reassured that the disease is not contagious and is treatable, but should be aware that most subtypes will relapse. Topical therapy is the safest approach, with emollients providing relief from itch and scale. A number of topical agents can be used, including vitamin D analogues, coal tar preparations, steroids, dithranol, keratolytics and retinoids. Depending on disease severity or the psychological impact of the disease, phototherapy with either narrow-band ultraviolet B (UVB) or ultraviolet A with psoralen photosensitizer (PUVA), or systemic therapy may be needed. If atypical, or poorly responsive to treatment, consider a biopsy to exclude conditions such as cutaneous lymphoma or secondary syphilis.

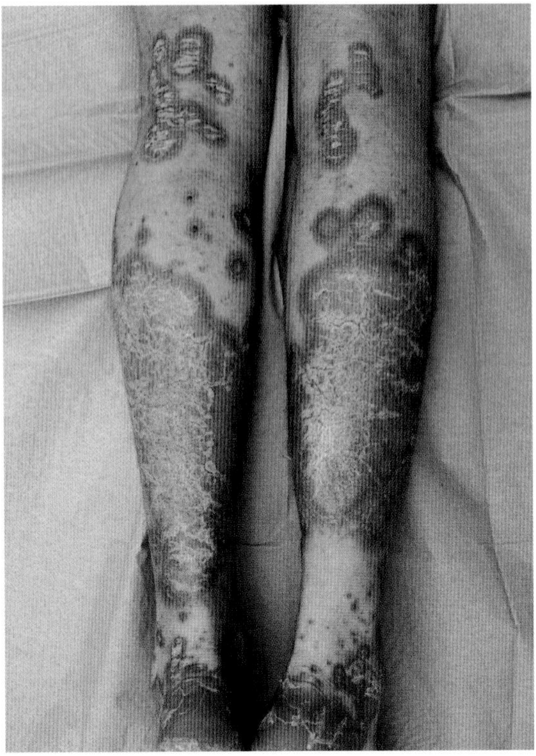

Figure 10.4 Chronic plaque psoriasis.

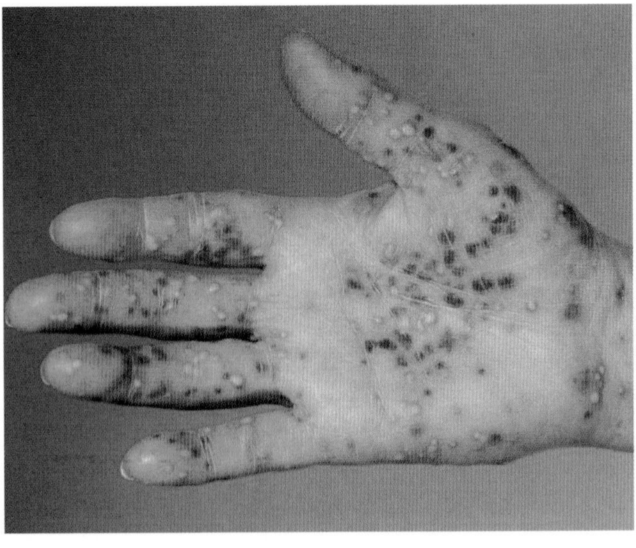

Figure 10.5 Pustular psoriasis showing pustules of variable size and healing pustules which fade with brown pigmentation.

Table 10.3 Precipitating factors in psoriasis

Precipitating factors	Details
Infection	Streptococcal sore throat (triggers guttate psoriasis)
Drugs	β-blockers, lithium, antimalarials may exacerbate or trigger
Sunlight	May exacerbate in a minority of patients (10%)
Genetics	Association with HLA Cw6, B13, B17
Trauma (Koebner phenomenon)	Psoriasis may be triggered at a site of injury, e.g. scratch marks giving rise to a linear pattern
Stress	Difficult to assess, but a history of significant stress is often obtained

Eczema

Eczema is a non-infectious itchy inflammatory condition, often also referred to as dermatitis (Figs 10.6, 10.7, overleaf). Eczema can be classified based its distribution, morphology and aetiology (Table 10.4, p. 297). It may also be described according to the duration of symptoms:

- acute eczema: the cause is usually exogenous and presentation is with redness, papules, oedema, pain, vesicles and, sometimes, large blisters
- chronic eczema: occurs with scaling, fissuring and thickening (lichenification).

With all types of eczema, there may be a superimposed irritant or allergic component. Irritant contact dermatitis may be due to a variety of abrasive and chemical substances, and barrier protection such as gloves is essential.

Allergic contact dermatitis may be identified by history (e.g. reactions to cheap earrings suggests nickel allergy); by examination looking at the distribution of the eruption (e.g. under watchstrap buckle, suggesting nickel allergy); or by patch testing looking for a type IV hypersensitivity reaction. The latter should be considered in anyone with eczema unresponsive to treatment, and with all patients with hand dermatitis.

Treatment

This should include copious emollients, soap substitutes, avoidance of irritants and excessive dust or animal dander, use of protective gloves and cotton clothing. Keeping nails cut short prevents excessive skin damage. In children with atopic eczema, bandaging and wet wraps are a useful adjunct, and sedating antihistamines may provide some benefit from itch.

Specific treatments include topical steroids, topical immunomodulators such as tacrolimus or pimecrolimus (Elidel®), tar bandages, topical or systemic antibiotics, phototherapy and immunosuppressants.

Lichen planus

This is less common than psoriasis and eczema and presents with extremely pruritic (itchy) polygonal purple papules (Fig. 10.8, p. 297). They often appear in a symmetrical pattern involving wrists, forearms, acral sites and lower legs. In mucosal and genital areas, Wickham's striae (a lacy white network) and ulceration may be more prominent than papules. Generalized spread may occur and, if nails or scalp are affected, scarring may result.

Treatment

Although self-limiting, symptomatic treatment with potent or super-potent topical steroids is usually necessary. In more resistant cases, systemic steroids or phototherapy can be used.

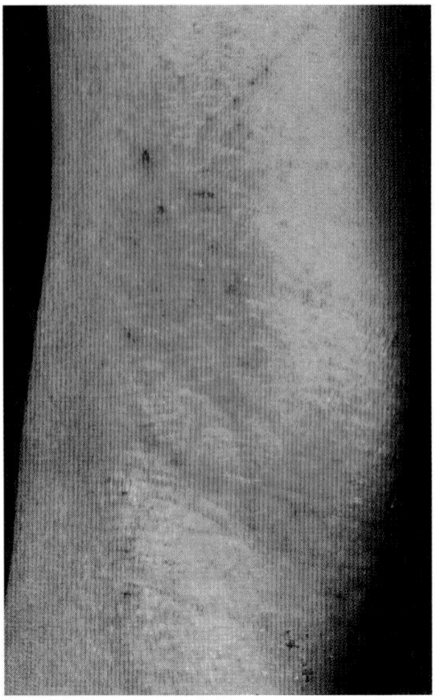

Figure 10.6 Flexural atopic eczema.

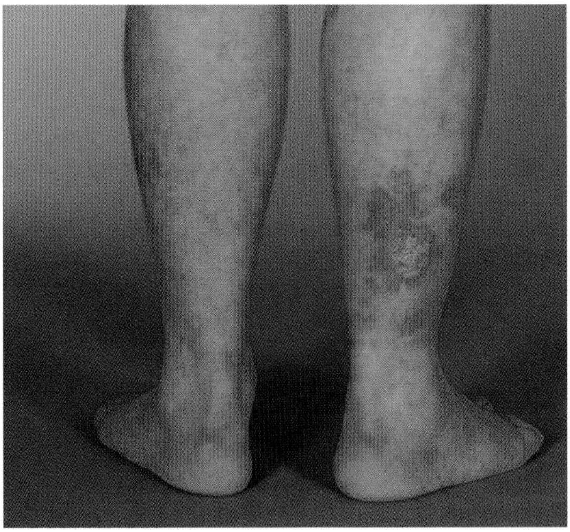

Figure 10.7 Venous eczema, with evidence of haemosiderin pigmentation and superficial varicosities.

Table 10.4 Description of common eczema subtypes

Type	Appearance
Atopic	An inherited disease present in up to 15% of infants, although 75% would have cleared before adulthood; in babies, facial involvement is common; in the older child, the pattern changes to flexural disease (antecubital and popliteal fossae); positive family history of atopy (asthma, hayfever, allergic conjunctivitis) is seen in the majority; adults may develop recurrent disease later in life
Seborrhoeic	Affects the central area of the face and eyebrows, V of chest
Discoid	Scaly itchy circular patches, usually on limbs and torso; often mistaken for 'ringworm'
Pompholyx	Small vesicles on palms and soles; very itchy
Venous	Affects the lower limbs, usually bilaterally, and is linked to venous insufficiency; other features include haemosiderin deposition, lipodermatosclerosis (red tight skin), and ulceration. Frequently misdiagnosed as bilateral cellulites
Asteatotic	Dry, fissured ('crazy pavement') appearance of skin, usually lower legs, particularly in the elderly
Lichen simplex	Heaped up areas of chronic lichenified eczema; common on shins, nape of neck, or readily accessible sites

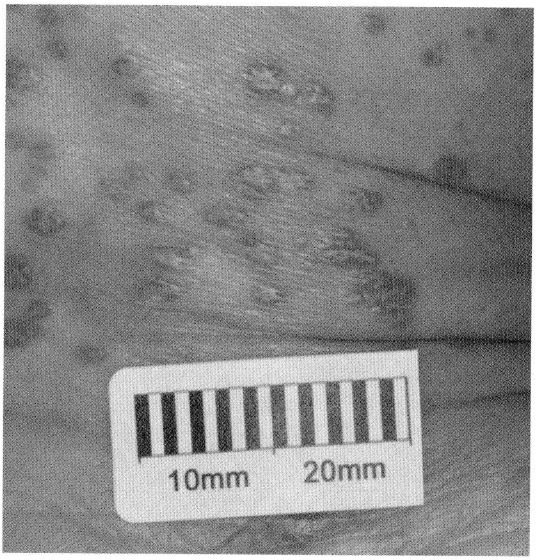

Figure 10.8 Flat-topped polygonal purple papules of lichen planus.

Skin tumours

Skin tumours usually present as an incidental finding to the non-dermatologist. It is important that you are able recognize the features of malignant skin disease (Table 10.5 and Figs 10.9–10.15).

Table 10.5 Common skin tumours

Diagnosis	Description	Treatment
Benign lesions		
Seborrhoeic wart (Fig. 10.9)	Common, often multiple and pigmented with a stuck-on appearance; predilection for face and torso	Reassurance
Skin tags	Polypoid, flesh-coloured, usually multiple; commonest in axillae, groin, around neck	Reassurance
Dermatofibroma	Firm papule or nodule, usually solitary in the legs; sometimes pigmented and/or scaly; dimples when surrounding skin is compressed	Reassurance
Pyogenic granuloma (Fig. 10.10)	Red/purple rapidly growing nodule, which bleeds readily; may occur at site of previous injury and is common on fingers; important differential is amelanotic melanoma	Surgical removal for histological assessment
Chondrodermatitis nodularis helicis	Painful papule on the helix/antihelix of the ear; often mistaken for a basal cell carcinoma but due to inflammation of cartilage	Pressure alleviation, surgery, cryotherapy or topical/intralesional steroids
Pre-malignant lesions		
Actinic keratosis (Fig. 10.11)	Scaly keratotic, occasionally red; either single lesion or diffuse change due to excessive ultraviolet exposure; may treat with immunomodulators, e.g. imiquimod, 5-fluorouracil cream	Cryotherapy, photodynamic therapy, immunomodulators, diclofenac 3% gel, surgery
Bowen's disease (intra-epidermal squamous cell carcinoma) (Fig. 10.12)	Pink scaly plaque, usually solitary and slow growing; usually seen on the lower legs of older females	Observation; treatments as for actinic keratosis
Keratoacanthoma (Fig. 10.13)	Rapidly growing nodule, with thick keratin plug; usually regresses spontaneously within 6 weeks of appearance; may mimic a squamous cell carcinoma	Surgical removal for histological assessment
Malignant lesions		
Basal cell carcinoma (Fig. 10.14)	Skin-coloured papule with overlying telangiectasia, pearly appearance and/or rolled edge; slow growing, with risk of local invasion, but rarely metastasizes; four clinical variants	Surgery, cryotherapy, imiquimod, (PDT), radiotherapy
Squamous cell carcinoma (Fig. 10.15)	Fleshy papule, arising de novo or from a pre-existing actinic keratosis; may progress rapidly to a dome-shaped nodule, or an ill-defined ulcer	Surgery, radiotherapy
Malignant melanoma	Macule, patch or nodule, with variable pigmentation, and occasionally loss of pigment either in parts (regression) or completely (amelanotic melanoma); four clinical variants	Surgery, palliative chemotherapy (for advanced disease), regular follow-up

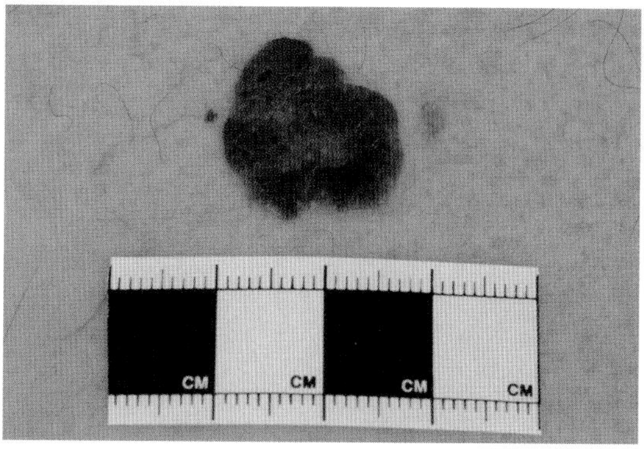

Figure 10.9 Pigmented seborrhoeic wart. Note the stuck-on appearance, with small inclusions (pseudohorn cysts).

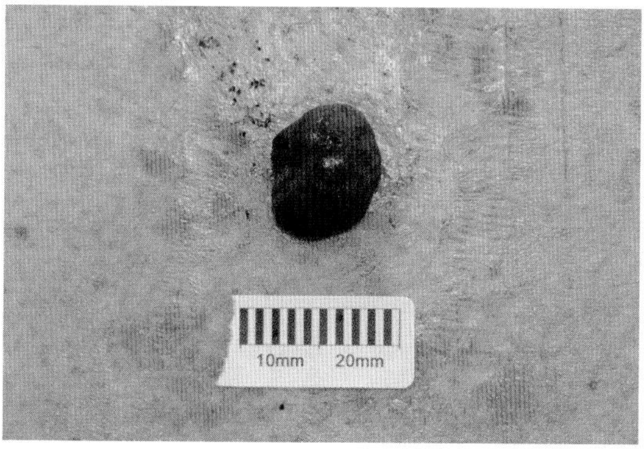

Figure 10.10 Pyogenic granuloma.

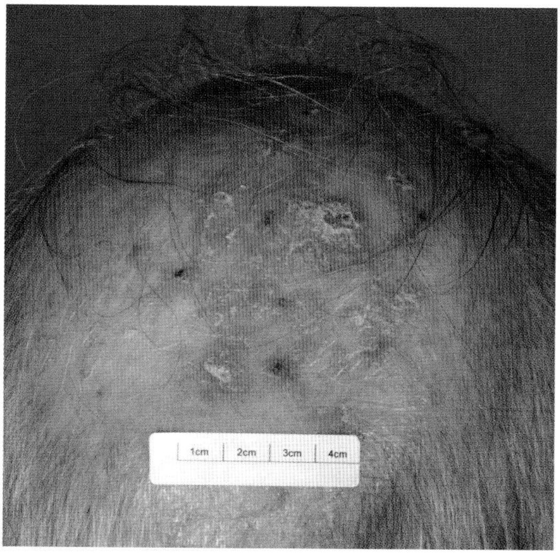

Figure 10.11 Actinic keratoses.

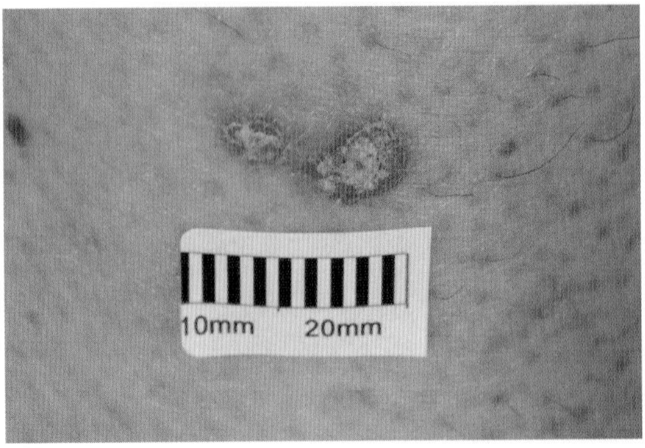

Figure 10.12 Bowen's disease (intra-epithelial squamous cell carcinoma).

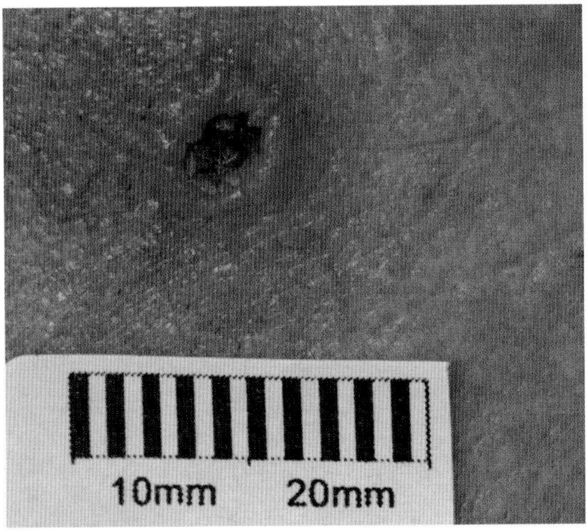

Figure 10.13 Keratoacanthoma showing crateriform periphery and central keratotic area.

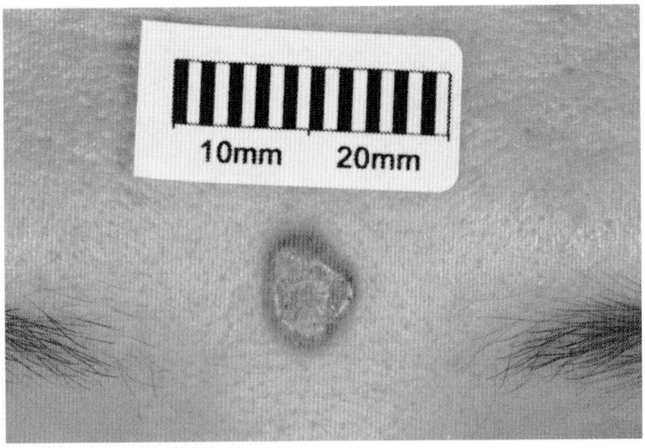

Figure 10.14 Basal cell carcinoma.

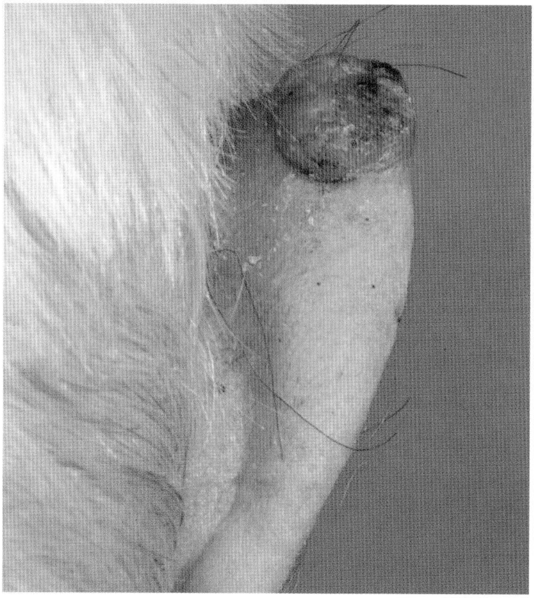

Figure 10.15 Squamous cell carcinoma; commonly occurs on the ear of males.

Assessment of possible malignant lesions

The following features are suspicious of malignant disease:

- A: Asymmetry
- B: irregular Border
- C: variation in Colour and pigmentation
- D: changes in size or Diameter.

Itching, bleeding, oozing and crusting are less sinister features. The risk of malignant change in most melanocytic naevi is small, with the exception of large congenital naevi and dysplastic (markedly irregular) naevi.

Melanoma identification

There are various types of melanoma, which you should be able to recognize:

- superficial spreading malignant melanoma (Fig. 10.16a): this is the most common; it predominantly affects the legs and females more than males
- lentigo maligna melanoma (Fig. 10.16b): this most commonly affects the face; if entirely intra-epidermal it is described as lentigo maligna; excision is curative, although it is prone to local recurrence
- nodular malignant melanoma (Fig. 10.16c): the trunk is most commonly affected and males more often than females; tends to grow rapidly and prognosis depends on the depth of the tumour
- acral lentiginous malignant melanoma (Fig. 10.16d,e): most commonly affects the palms, soles and nail beds (subungual); it is often diagnosed late with poorer prognosis.

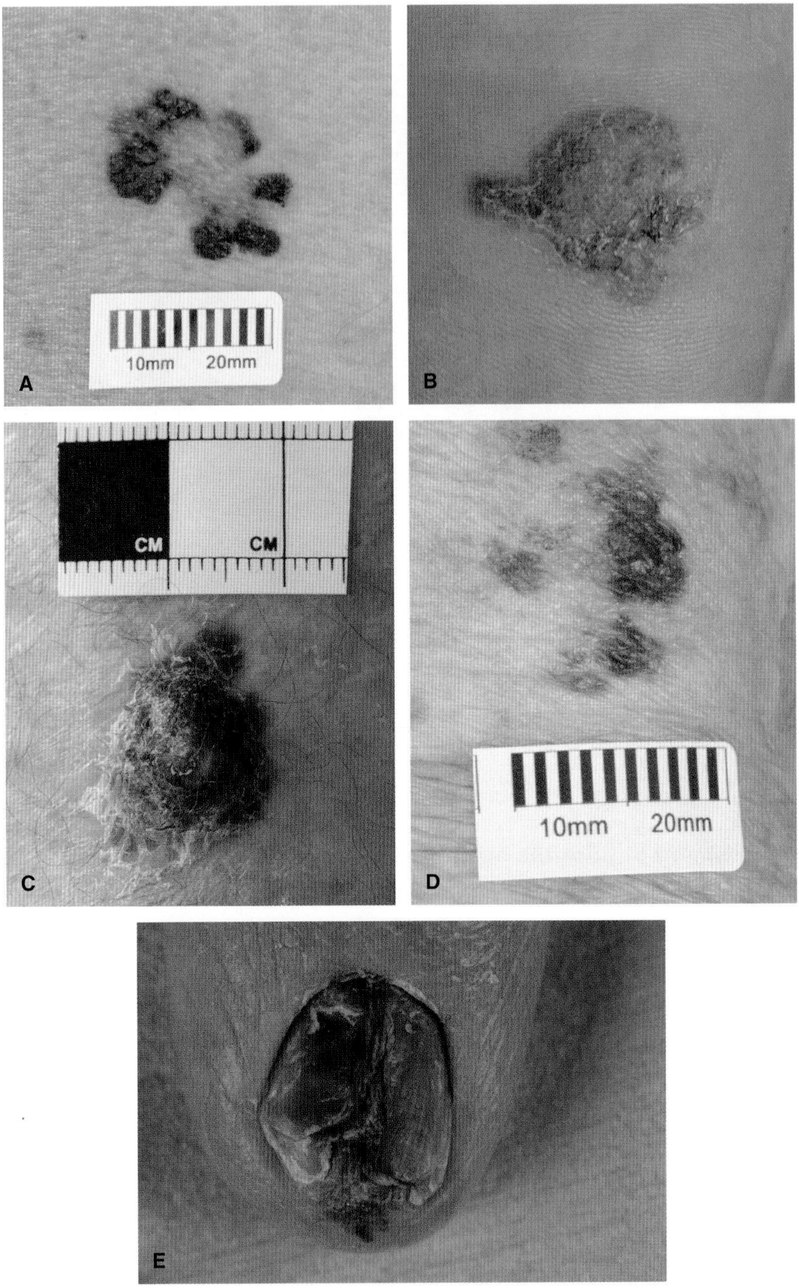

Figure 10.16 (A) Superficial spreading malignant melanoma, showing areas of loss of pigment (regression) centrally. (B) Acral lentiginous melanoma on the sole. (C) Nodular melanoma. (D) Lentigo maligna melanoma, with diffuse pigmentary change. (E) Subungual melanoma (acral).

Common and important problems

Blistering

Blistering may be generalized or localized (Figs 10.17 below, 10.18 overleaf).

Generalized

- bullous pemphigoid: presents with tense blisters that may occur anywhere, but usually spare mucosae; may be preceded by an itchy red eruption, occasionally with urticoid lesions; requires active treatment, usually with systemic steroids
- pemphigus vulgaris: flaccid blisters can occur on both skin and mucosal sites but this is rare in the UK Caucasian population; other pemphigus variants may produce a more warty scaly appearance; potentially life threatening if not treated aggressively
- dermatitis herpetiformis: itchy vesicular eruption, usually on extensor surfaces such as elbows, knees, buttocks; it responds to a gluten-free diet (and dapsone); all patients have a gluten-sensitive enteropathy (coeliac disease) although many are asymptomatic
- chronic bullous disease of childhood and linear IgA disease: rare, but should be considered in a child with a non-healing vesicular eruption; in adults, it has a similar presentation to bullous pemphigoid.

Localized

- porphyria: tense blisters on photo-exposed sites (dorsa hands, face), fragile skin, scarring, milial cysts, hyperpigmentation and hypertrichosis
- epidermolysis bullosa: a group of inherited blistering disorders in children with several subtypes, some of which can be fatal; blisters are triggered by trauma, usually on extremities and mucosal sites, and often lead to scarring
- infectious causes: bacterial and viral infections often produce vesicles/blisters (see 'Skin infections', p. 305)

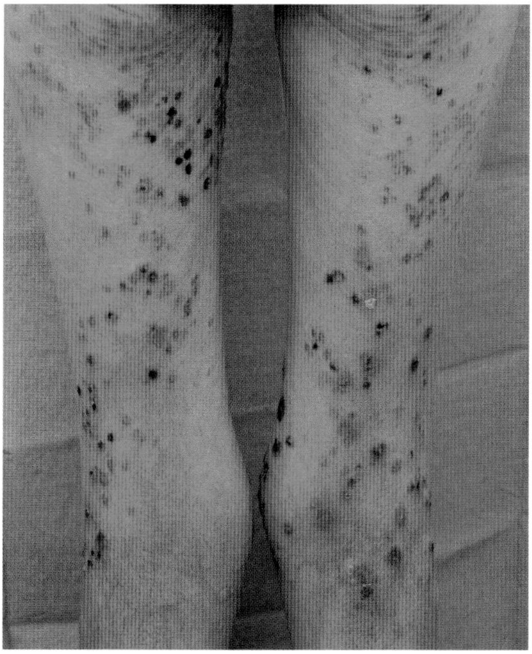

Figure 10.17 Bullous pemphigoid. Most of the lesions are excoriated, but there are a couple of intact tense blisters near the left knee.

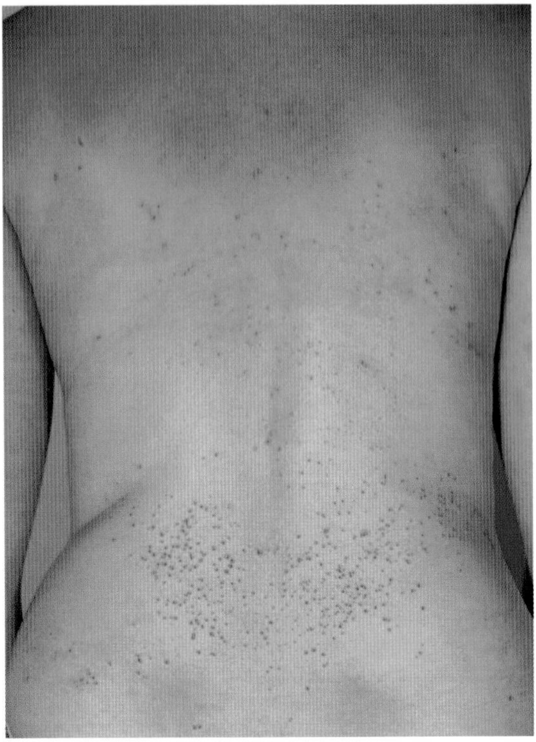

Figure 10.18 Typical distribution of dermatitis herpetiformis. Intact vesicles are seldom seen due to excoriation.

- cutaneous vasculitis: palpable purpura, generally on the legs, but may extend to buttocks, arms and abdomen; may blister and ulcerate; potentially serious if due to systemic disease.

The red face

Patients with a red face are usually very embarrassed about their appearance, and will often demand urgent treatment. Problems may be acute or chronic:

- acne: comedones (blackheads and whiteheads), pustules, papules and nodules
- rosacea: pustules, papules, telangiectasia (broken visible blood vessels), a history of excessive flushing, grittiness of the eyes
- seborrhoeic dermatitis: scaling and redness around the nose, mouth, eyebrows and V of chest
- allergic contact dermatitis: contact with an allergic trigger, e.g. nail varnish, plant pollen, perfumes, hair dye, cosmetics
- connective tissue disease: stigmata of connective tissue disease, e.g. Raynaud's, nail-fold telangiectasia or heliotrope rash (purple rash on the eyelids)
- infection: systemically unwell with pyrexia, e.g. erysipelas, cellulitis, 'slapped cheek' or fifth disease
- systemic: joint disease or heart murmur, e.g. mitral stenosis.

Hair loss (alopecia)

A systematic approach is important in the assessment of hair loss. Look for evidence of scarring, note the distribution (patchy or diffuse) and examine the underlying scalp. Scarring alopecia presents with a shiny scalp with loss of follicular openings or alteration of texture, and should be referred urgently. Types of hair loss are described in Table 10.6.

Table 10.6 Patterns of hair loss and common causes

	Patchy	Diffuse
Non-scarring	Alopecia areata: circular patches of hair loss with normal looking scalp	Androgenetic alopecia: bitemporal and vertex in males, crown of scalp in females (now called female pattern hair loss)
	Severe psoriasis or eczema: scaly scalp Fungal infection: boggy or scaly scalp	Telogen effluvium: excessive shedding Thyroid disease Connective tissue disease
Scarring	Discoid lupus erythematosus: scaly plaques, with atrophy, erythema and follicular plugging Lichen planus: perifollicular erythema	Pseudopelade Folliculitis decalvans

Skin infections

Skin infections are usually managed in primary care. You should be able to recognize the following common infections.

Bacterial

- impetigo: vesicles with yellow crusting, usually due to staphylococcus or streptococcus; spreads rapidly, and can be highly infectious
- staphylococcal 'scalded skin' syndrome: large sheets of red skin which shed to leave denuded areas; usually affects young children
- cellulitis: infection of subcutaneous tissue, usually with streptococci; unilateral leg involvement is common; where there is bilateral redness of the legs, suspect venous insufficiency.

Viral

- warts: infection due to papillomavirus; treatments include reassurance, paring, keratolytics and cryotherapy
- molluscum contagiosum: pearly umbilicated flesh-coloured papules, usually in clusters, due to a pox virus; treatments are poorly tolerated in younger children, but include cryotherapy, surgery or expression of contents
- herpes simplex: primary infection may produce a herpetic whitlow (painful cluster of vesicles/pustules on the finger) or acute gingivostomatitis
- chickenpox (varicella zoster): crops of vesicles, on an erythematous base, in a predominantly truncal distribution
- herpes zoster: tense blisters, often haemorrhagic, with associated tingling and pain, in a dermatomal, unilateral distribution; caused by recrudescence of varicella zoster virus.

Fungal

- dermatophyte infections (ringworm): affects isolated toenails, with crumbly discoloured nails; skin involvement is less common, manifesting as an itchy scaly rash with well-defined edges and central clearing (Fig. 10.19); it may go undiagnosed for long periods, especially if topical steroids are used (tinea incognito)
- pityriasis versicolor: velvety brown macules with subtle scale affecting truncal areas; due to a commensal yeast, it can be difficult to eradicate.

Infestation

- scabies: severely itchy rash affecting wrists, palms and soles and flexures, but often non-specific elsewhere; nodules on the penis are diagnostic; ask about contacts with similar symptoms and look for burrows, reactive eczema, numerous excoriations and pustules on the acral surfaces.

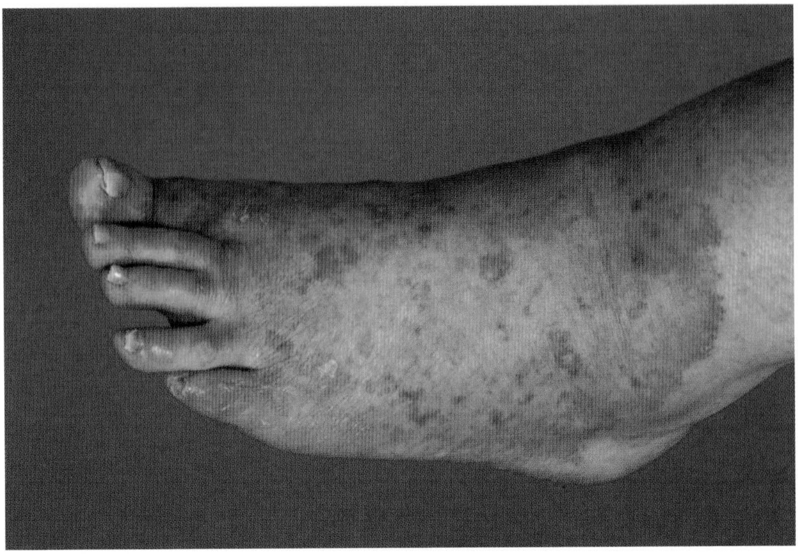

Figure 10.19 Dystrophic toenails due to fungus, with spreading infection on dorsum of foot (tinea pedis). Note the well-demarcated edge.

Skin failure and emergency dermatology

Although uncommon, it is important to know how to manage dermatological emergencies when they present. If extensively inflamed, skin failure may occur, with resultant disruption of many of its vital functions (see p. 292). General measures include admission (ideally to a ward with skilled dermatology nurses), monitoring of vital signs, fluid balance and nutritional input, while observing for signs of complications such as cutaneous and respiratory infection, hypothermia and multisystem failure. Treatment with bland topical emollients and good skin care, often with a specialized mattress, is essential.

Angioedema and urticaria

This is the most common of the emergencies, and often presents acutely to A&E.

- urticaria: transient, generally very itchy (pruritic) wheals or hives
- wheals: pink papules or plaques which are readily identifiable and fade within 24 h of onset
- angioedema: a more oedematous area that commonly affects lips and eyelids.

In acute urticaria, the eruption may be extensive, sudden ± associated with angioedema. Provoking factors such as foods can sometimes be elicited on history, and routine blood tests are not usually necessary. However, most urticarias will last for over 6 weeks, with no obvious trigger (chronic idiopathic).

Treatment

Short- and long-acting antihistamines are given, occasionally intravenously. Admission is not essential. Systemic steroids are sometimes given for an acute severe eruption. Adrenaline (epinephrine) is not usually required. If there is no response to adequate treatment, check FBC, LFT, TFT, ANA and urinalysis to exclude systemic disease. If an allergy to foodstuffs is considered to be the trigger, allergen-specific serum IgE may be measured.

Other variants

- physical urticarias: triggered by cold, heat, sun, pressure and water; antihistamines are recommended with, where possible, avoidance of triggers
- urticarial vasculitis: rare and characterized by urticated areas which last longer than 24 h and usually fade leaving a bruise-like appearance; investigations should include an autoantibody screen
- hereditary angioedema: a very rare and potentially fatal autosomal dominant condition that usually presents in childhood; 10% due to new mutations; angioedema causes respiratory or abdominal symptoms; if suspected, check C_1 esterase inhibitor levels.

Erythroderma

This is said to be present if at least 90% of the body surface is affected by redness (erythema), with or without scaling (dry flaky skin). Onset may be rapid (within a few days) or more gradual over a period of weeks. The patient may be unwell, with shivers, malaise, and even pyrexia. Oedema and reactive (dermatopathic) enlargement of lymph nodes are common. Causes include eczema, psoriasis, cutaneous lymphoma/Sézary syndrome, drug reaction and pityriasis rubra pilaris.

Treatment

Topical steroids, systemic steroids and other immunosuppressants are used depending on the aetiology and the response to general measures.

Toxic epidermal necrolysis and Stevens–Johnson syndrome

Toxic epidermal necrolysis

Toxic epidermal necrolysis (TEN) is a condition that still has high mortality, despite advances in medicine. It is usually the result of an idiosyncratic reaction to a drug. The most commonly implicated drugs are anticonvulsants, antibacterial sulphonamides, non-steroidal anti-inflammatory drugs, allopurinol and antimalarials.

The skin becomes red and necrotic, and complete shedding of the epidermal layer ensues, with >30% body surface involvement (Fig. 10.20). Mucosal involvement is usual and may result in scarring.

All drugs should be stopped, if possible. The use of systemic agents such as steroids, immunoglobulins and other immunosuppressants is somewhat controversial, but, if used, need to be given in the early phases of the disease.

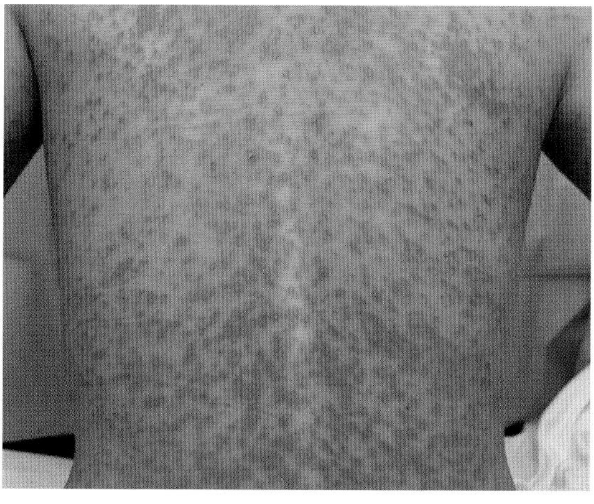

Figure 10.20 Stevens–Johnson syndrome.

Stevens–Johnson syndrome

Stevens–Johnson syndrome (SJS) is thought to be a milder reaction to drugs. Both SJS and TEN are now thought to represent a spectrum of the same disease, with SJS affecting <10% body surface area, and an overlap SJS/TEN syndrome if involvement is 10–30%.

Erythema multiforme

This presents with classic target-like macules, papules and blisters. It is more commonly due to infections, particularly herpes simplex, and the clinical picture is less severe.

Eczema herpeticum

This should be suspected if the patient is systemically unwell, with a background history of atopic eczema. Infection, due to herpes simplex, causes an extensive eruption of vesicles, which later become pustular or ulcerated, usually on the head and neck area. Secondary impetiginization may cause crusting of lesions.

Treatment

Although potentially fatal, due to involvement of internal organs, it is readily treatable with antiviral agents, usually given intravenously.

Generalized pustular psoriasis

This is a rare but serious form of psoriasis, where sheets of sterile pustules develop on an erythematous base. The onset is often sudden, with rapid progression, and an acutely unwell patient. Skin swabs and blood cultures should be taken to exclude infection.

Treatment

Treatment includes topical vitamin D analogues or systemic therapy (methotrexate or ciclosporin).

EAR, NOSE AND THROAT

A variety of ENT conditions present acutely. They can be very painful so gentle examination is important, especially in children.

Ear

Pain (otalgia)

Otitis externa

This usually presents with itch, pain and discharge and is usually caused by minor trauma to the ear canal, e.g. with a cotton bud. There may be watery discharge, an inflamed external auditory canal, cellulitis and debris preventing a view of the tympanic membrane.

Remove the debris with gentle syringing or suction clearance, and take a swab for culture and sensitivity. In mild cases, use local antibiotic and steroid preparations, e.g. neomycin dexamethasone spray or gentamicin hydrocortisone drops. In severe cases, admit and treat with intravenous antibiotics.

Otitis media

This often presents with pain, dullness of hearing and preceding upper respiratory tract infection. Initially, there may be a bulging red tympanic membrane, but later the tympanic membrane perforates with purulent discharge. The onset of facial weakness in a patient with a history of chronic otitis media or the finding of a perforation and/or cholesteatoma is an acute ENT emergency and requires advice from senior medical staff.

Send a sample of the discharge for culture and sensitivity. Prescribe systemic broad-spectrum antibiotics ± decongestants, e.g. xylometazoline nose drops locally or pseudoephedrine systemically. If mastoiditis develops (fullness and tenderness in the post aural region), arrange a CT and, if there is no resolution within 24 h, consider surgical intervention.

Referred otalgia

Where there is pain in the ear, but no obvious otological cause, it is usually due to acute referred pain from temporomandibular joint dysfunction, dental caries or abscess.

Sudden hearing loss

This may be conductive or sensorineural in nature.

Conductive

- impacted wax: remove the wax by syringing, if necessary, with a preceding course of ceruminolytic drops, e.g. Cerumol 2 drops 6-hourly
- acute secretory otitis media: may develop as part of an upper respiratory tract infection, due to eustachian tube blockage, and is treated as per otitis media; examination will reveal a dull and retracted tympanic membrane which will have a yellowish appearance and a fluid level or air bubbles may be visible in the middle ear
- local trauma to the ear: may result in perforation with hearing loss and is usually obvious from the history and findings on examination.

Sensorineural hearing loss

Sudden sensorineural hearing loss is usually due to a viral or vascular cause or more rarely an acoustic neuroma. If of recent onset, steroids and an anti-viral agent may be prescribed, along with an anti-platelet preparation such as clopidogrel.

Tinnitus

Tinnitus is noise, usually ringing, that is heard in the ears and for which there is no external source. Some patients also experience hearing loss. Causes include viral infection, wax, vascular events, presbyacusis, acoustic nerve trauma or neuroma, otitis media, Ménière's disease, ototoxic drugs, hypertension, anaemia.

History should specifically enquire about head injury, otorrhoea, otalgia, vertigo, family history of deafness or tinnitus and drugs. After otoscopy and basic hearing tests, a tympanogram should be undertaken and, if a neuroma is suspected, an MRI requested.

Treatment depends on the cause. Betahistine may help in Ménière's disease, and aural masking by white noise generators can provide relief. Cochlear nerve transection can be considered in severe cases, but results in deafness.

Nose

Epistaxis

Nosebleeds are a common reason for emergency attendance to ENT or A&E. These can range from relatively trivial self-limiting episodes to severe life-threatening events, requiring multiple blood transfusions or surgical intervention. The most common site of epistaxis is from a vascular plexus antero-inferiorly on the nasal septum (Little's area).

Treatment

- start with ABC
- simple pressure over the soft tissue of the nose may be enough to stop the bleeding
- if severe, obtain IV access, check FBC, U&E, LFT, Coag and cross-match

- consider causes: stop medication that may exacerbate bleeding, e.g. warfarin, aspirin, clopidogrel, LMWH; exclude underlying systemic disease, e.g. thrombocytopenia, significant hypertension
- identify the bleeding point.

Bleeding point

- inspect the nose using a Thudicum's nasal speculum and a headlight; suction may be needed to remove clot or continuing blood flow
- topical local anaesthesia and decongestion is usually helpful and can be applied for 5 min before examination, e.g. Co-Phenylcaine®
- cautery: if a bleeding point is seen, the area can be cauterized with a silver nitrate stick (95% best)
- packing: if the bleeding continues, or no bleeding point is seen (posterior source), nasal packing is usually required, e.g. Merocel® expanding packs or Vaseline®-impregnated ribbon gauze
- balloon catheters: if bleeding continues, balloon catheters can be inserted to occlude the posterior choanae and are often required bilaterally
- continued bleeding: surgical intervention will be required and can include septoplasty to allow access to the bleeding vessel and packing, or arterial ligation (e.g. ethmoidal, in the troublesome epistaxis which may follow nasal and facial trauma); embolization of the bleeding vessels is another option.

Rhinitis

This can be allergic or vasomotor (where allergens cannot be detected). Allergic rhinitis can be seasonal, e.g. hayfever, or perennial. The history is usually one of sneezing, rhinorrhoea and itch, often with nasal obstruction. Examination may reveal swollen turbinates.

Continuous treatment over several months is usually required and includes nasal corticosteroids or sodium cromoglycate and antihistamines. Occasionally, nasal cautery or turbinate reduction surgery is considered.

Throat

Sore throat

A sore throat is most commonly due to tonsillitis, quinsy or pharyngitis.

Tonsillitis

Symptoms and signs can occur at any age, especially in the younger age group. The aetiology is often initially viral. Where pus is present, secondary bacterial infection has occurred. While it is often streptococcal, consider the possibility of glandular fever or underlying haematological conditions. For example, in leukaemia, there may be large erythematous tonsils with or without cervical lymphadenopathy and systemic signs of infection.

If the infection is mild and the patient is able to swallow, treatment with antibiotics and encouraging fluid intake may be sufficient. If more severe, or the patient is unable to swallow, they should be admitted for intravenous fluids and antibiotics, e.g. benzylpenicillin (1.2 g 6-hourly) and metronidazole (500 mg 8-hourly). Exclude glandular fever by the monospot test before using co-amoxiclav.

Quinsy

Tonsillitis may progress to a peritonsillar abscess (quinsy). The pain is more severe and localized to one side. Examination shows tonsillitis with additional fullness of the peritonsillar area on the affected side. In addition to antibiotic therapy, aspiration is usually required after spraying with topical local anaesthetic (xylocaine 10%). A 10 or 20 mL syringe with a wide-bore needle should be inserted into the most prominent part of the swelling, usually half-way between the upper pole of the tonsil and the base of the uvula. Up to 10 mL of pus (usually 3–4 mL) should be aspirated. This often provides immediate relief, but if the swelling recurs further aspiration may be required. Alternatively, incision and drainage at the same site may be carried out.

Tonsillar haemorrhage post-tonsillectomy

Following a tonsillectomy, haemorrhage may complicate recovery. It may be primary, reactionary or secondary.

Primary bleeding occurs during the course of the operation and should be dealt with at the time. Reactionary bleeding occurs within the first 24h of surgery, most commonly within the first 6h. If small, it may be possible to dislodge the resulting clot by gargles, e.g. hydrogen peroxide. If large, it may have to be removed with Gwynne Evans tonsillar dissector. If a small bleeding point is seen, pressure should be applied with a swab soaked in 1:10000 adrenaline. If this is unsuccessful, or the bleeding point is large, the patient should be taken back to theatre.

Secondary haemorrhage is defined as bleeding after the first 24h, most commonly between 5 and 10 days postoperatively. This occurs because of infected slough separating from the tonsil bed. Examination often reveals no significant bleeding point, but if a clot is present prescribe antibiotics and treat as in reactionary haemorrhage above. Should the bleeding continue or recur, surgery may be required.

Pharyngitis

Pharyngitis usually occurs in patients who have already had a tonsillectomy or their tonsils have already regressed. Examination reveals erythema of the oropharyngeal mucosa including lymphoid tissue of the posterior pharyngeal wall. It is managed similarly to uncomplicated tonsillitis, i.e. antibiotic and supportive therapy as required. Laryngoscopy should be carried out in severe cases to ensure there is no supraglottic extension which may compromise the airway.

Neck swellings

Acute neck swellings are usually infective. As with any swelling, the site, size, tenderness and mobility should be recorded. Examine the entire head and neck looking for evidence of a primary infection. Other causes of neck swelling include thyroid lumps, thyroglossal cysts (typically midline, at the level of the hyoid bone in the younger age group), branchial cysts (lateral swelling at middle one-third of sternomastoid muscle in the older age group), cystic hygromas, carotid body or parotid tumours and dermoid cysts.

Neck space abscesses

If a large infected gland or group of glands coalesce and liquefy, an abscess will result. The patient will be systemically unwell. The commonest abscesses are parapharyngeal and submandibular, secondary to tonsillar/pharyngeal infection and dental sepsis. The patient may have trismus, making examination more difficult. Imaging with CT can be helpful. Treatment with intravenous antibiotics will be required and, if resolution does not occur within 24h, surgical drainage is necessary.

Parotid swelling

This may present as part of a viral illness, classically mumps, or be seen as a retrograde ductal infection secondary to dehydration, debilitation and sepsis. Supportive symptomatic treatment and antibiotics is indicated. The patient may also require nasogastric feeding to reduce saliva production. Parotid tumours can also cause swelling.

Stridor

Stridor is an inspiratory airway noise indicating airway obstruction or narrowing above the level of the main tracheal carina, e.g. in the supraglottic (above the vocal cord) and glottic (vocal cord) areas. It should be differentiated from stertor which is the noise produced by collapse of the pharyngeal airway.

If the patient has rapidly progressive symptoms, suggesting impending upper airway obstruction (most commonly due to acute epiglottitis or an inhaled foreign body), summon anaesthetic help immediately. Do not attempt to inspect the larynx until facilities are available for immediate endotracheal intubation, or cricothyroidotomy if the former proves impossible.

Infection

Upper airway infections are more common in children, e.g. acute epiglottitis (caused by *Haemophilus influenzae* type B) or acute laryngotracheobronchitis. (For the management in children see 'Paediatric', p. 335.)

Treatment

- IV antibiotics if bacterial infection likely
- steroids, e.g. dexamethasone (150 µg/kg PO or IV)
- humidified oxygen
- nebulized adrenaline, e.g. 400 µg/kg using 1 mg/mL solution (maximum dose 5 mg), with repeated doses at 30 min and 2–3 h if required
- temporary endotracheal intubation may be necessary.

Malignancy

An endobronchial tumour or a lymph node mass narrowing the proximal airways can cause stridor. Treat with IV steroids (e.g. dexamethasone 8 mg twice daily) and refer to oncology for urgent local radiotherapy or chemotherapy.

Retained secretions

Secretions are a common cause of stridor in patients with a weak cough, especially those recently discharged from ITU. Chest physiotherapy is essential and regular suction may be required in patients with a tracheostomy.

Pharyngeal narrowing or occlusion

This may be due to vomit, blood, or the tongue following an acute neurological event, drug overdose, trauma, or cardiorespiratory arrest. The threat to the upper airway is often transient and ventilation may improve as conscious level rises. 'Bag and mask' ventilation with subsequent intubation and ventilation may be required until then (see 'Cardiac arrest', p. 11).

Inhaled foreign body

Inhaled foreign bodies are usually fairly small, e.g. peanuts, part of a drinks can ringpull or, in children, part of a toy. When larger items impact in the larynx, immediate intervention is mandatory. In the hospital setting, an anaesthetist and senior ENT help are required urgently. If the foreign body is small enough to penetrate the larynx and be impacted in the trachea or bronchi, then early bronchoscopy will be required to avoid distal lung collapse and permanent lung injury.

Laryngeal oedema

This is classically seen in patients with anaphylaxis, but is also associated with burns and inhalation of noxious gases. Treatment is with steroids, but ventilation may be required.

Oropharyngeal obstruction

Fish bones

The commonest sites for impaction are the tonsils or tongue base. A headlight and tongue depressor should be used to examine and localize the bone and, if necessary, proceed to indirect or flexible laryngoscopy to examine the posterior tongue base and oropharynx. Topical local anaesthetic spray (xylocaine 10%) can be beneficial. The bone can be removed with forceps.

Food bolus

Food, often incompletely chewed meat, can impact in the pharynx or oesophagus. The commonest sites are just beyond the cricopharyngeus or any of the narrower areas of the oesophagus, for example aortic arch level or cardia.

The patient may have retrosternal discomfort and be unable to swallow, either drooling or spitting saliva. If there is no bone present, intramuscular hyoscine butylbromide 20 mg can be administered and the patient given fizzy drinks, to encourage displacement of the bolus. This can be repeated after an interval of 30 min if necessary. If this is unsuccessful, the patient is likely to require endoscopy.

Dental plates

An impacted dental plate will almost certainly require rigid endoscopy for removal. A lateral soft tissue X-ray of neck and a CXR should be taken to exclude perforation of the pharynx/oesophagus.

Facial pain

Acute sinusitis

There may be a history of preceding upper respiratory tract infection with associated nasal discharge. The patient is usually pyrexial and examination may reveal swelling over the affected paranasal sinus/sinuses with tenderness. Rhinoscopy reveals mucopus in the nasal cavity. Treatment consists of decongestants and antibiotic therapy.

Orbital cellulitis

This causes pain, redness, proptosis and limitation of ocular movements. A CT scan is usually required to exclude associated sinusitis or orbital abscess. Admit for intravenous antibiotics and close monitoring of visual function and systemic status. Close liaison with ophthalmology is required.

Foreign bodies

Children commonly present with foreign bodies in the ear or nose. Only experienced staff should attempt to remove a foreign body as, if the first opportunity is wasted, subsequent treatment can be much more difficult.

Removal of a foreign body from the ear is best carried out with syringing or suction if the child is cooperative. If they are uncooperative, a general anaesthetic will be required. If the foreign body is in the nose, the removal is usually best carried out with a curved instrument, e.g. eustachian catheter, to place behind the foreign body and pull it forwards, rather than risk displacing it more posteriorly with instruments such as forceps, given the danger of aspiration. Theatre may be required, particularly if there is a risk of the child aspirating the object. With both ears and nose it is important to examine the other ear or nostril to ensure that no other foreign bodies are present.

Trauma

See 'Facial injury', p. 268.

OPHTHALMIC

Patients with ophthalmic conditions may present acutely to a variety of clinical specialities other than ophthalmology, e.g. medicine and A&E.

Examination

Ophthalmological examination should be combined with neurological assessment including pupillary reactions, ocular movements and examination of visual fields to confrontation.

External examination of the eye itself should include assessment of colour, presence of any exudate, position of eyelids, eversion of the subtarsal plate and clarity of cornea. Further assessment of the cornea and anterior chamber can be made with the ophthalmoscope set on +10 using fluorescein stain to highlight corneal abnormalities. The posterior segment of the eyes should be examined after dilation of pupils with the ophthalmoscope set at 0. This allows the lens, vitreous, optic disc, macula, retinal vessels and retinal periphery to be examined.

Red or sore eyes

Acute angle-closure glaucoma

This is an ophthalmic emergency, which can lead to permanent visual loss. It commonly affects women over the age of 60 and is characterized by acute pain, blurred vision, headache, nausea and vomiting. Signs include generalized redness, cloudy cornea, mid-dilated and poorly reactive or non-reactive pupil and a shallow anterior chamber.

Immediate treatment should be given with intravenous acetazolamide and topical intraocular pressure-lowering agents. Resistant cases require oral glycerol 50% or intravenous hyperosmotic agents (mannitol 20% IV). Definitive treatment requires iridotomy (laser or surgical).

Corneal ulcers and keratitis

These are associated with intense pain, lacrimation, photophobia and secondary disturbance of vision. Patients with contact lens related ulcers or keratitis need urgent assessment.

Bacterial keratitis

Signs include corneal ulceration with infiltration, associated with hypopyon (a fluid level of pus in the anterior chamber) in some cases. The commonest pathogens are staphylococci or streptococci. Corneal scrapes should be sent for culture and sensitivity and topical broad-spectrum antibiotics prescribed.

Adenoviral keratitis

The cornea may show multiple punctuate subepithelial opacities. Use a short course of a weak topical steroid and topical antibiotics.

Herpes simplex keratitis

The typical lesion is a dendritic ulcer, best seen on fluorescein staining. Use topical antiviral treatment (e.g. aciclovir ointment 5 times daily). This should be continued for 3 days following clinical resolution. Involvement of corneal stroma requires additional topical steroids. Oral antiviral therapy is reserved for frequent recurrences.

Acute conjunctivitis

This usually presents with redness, itching and watering of the eyes. It is usually infective or allergic. Topical antibiotics should be prescribed for bacterial conjunctivitis; topical antihistamines ± steroids for allergic and vernal conjunctivitis; topical tetracycline and oral azithromycin for chlamydial conjunctivitis. In the latter setting, a referral should be made to genitourinary medicine.

Blepharitis

This is a chronic inflammatory condition affecting the lid margins with crusting, dry eyes and irritation. Treatment includes regular lid hygiene, lubricants ± topical antibiotics.

Episcleritis

This is a patch or nodule of inflammation of the episcleral tissue underneath the conjunctiva, usually causing mild discomfort. It is usually self-limiting. The majority of cases are idiopathic, but 10% are associated with connective tissue disorders. Topical steroids are used in severe and symptomatic cases.

Scleritis

This may present with boring pain and can be sight-threatening. There is sectorial, dusky red discoloration of the eye, which is tender to touch. Scleritis may be anterior (nodular, diffuse or necrotizing) or posterior. A total of 50% of patients have an associated systemic disorder, e.g. connective tissue disease, Reiter's syndrome, ankylosing spondylitis, inflammatory bowel disorders, herpes zoster, syphilis or TB.

Topical steroids and oral non-steroidal anti-inflammatory agents are used. Systemic steroids and other immunosuppressive agents may be required in sight-threatening disease, particularly in patients with systemic connective tissue disorders.

Corneal abrasion

This usually occurs secondary to trauma and causes a breach of the corneal epithelium resulting in intense pain, lacrimation, photophobia and blurred vision. The abraded area stains green with fluorescein. Treat with topical antibiotic ointment for 5 days and an eye pad for 24 h.

Corneal foreign bodies

These result in irritation, pain and lacrimation. Most are small, superficial and embedded in the anterior cornea. Eversion of the upper eyelid is necessary to exclude subtarsal foreign bodies. High-velocity foreign bodies can penetrate the eye with little evidence of entry site (e.g. grinding injury). In these cases, an X-ray of the orbit may demonstrate metallic intra-ocular/orbital foreign bodies

Most superficial foreign bodies can be removed, under topical anaesthesia, using a sterile needle and slit lamp. This should be followed by topical antibiotics for 5 days.

Lid malposition and eyelash abnormalities

Entropion, ectropion and trichiasis may all cause red, sticky and watery eyes. Occasionally corneal abrasion and ulceration may occur. Treat with topical lubricants ± removal of misdirected lashes with tweezers. Surgical correction is required if the lid malposition is significant.

Herpes zoster ophthalmicus

This occurs following infection of the ophthalmic division of the trigeminal nerve. Patients commonly report prodromal symptoms of pain before the appearance of a vesicular skin rash along the distribution of the nerve. Ocular complications include conjunctivitis, keratitis or iritis.

Treatment with oral aciclovir (800 mg five times daily for 1 week) is most effective if commenced within the first 72 h of onset of the rash. Topical aciclovir use is not known to be effective in zoster keratitis. Topical steroids are the mainstay of treatment for disciform keratitis and iritis. Intravenous aciclovir is indicated in the immunocompromised and in those with retinal necrosis.

Acute anterior uveitis (iritis)

This is characterized by dull pain and photophobia. It is usually unilateral, with redness around the corneoscleral limbus and small irregular pupils stuck down to the anterior surface of the lens (posterior synechiae).

A history of recurrent episodes is common in those who are HLA-B27 positive. Systemic associations include ankylosing spondylitis, Reiter's disease, seronegative arthritis and sarcoidosis. Treat with a cycloplegic and intensive topical steroids, tapered over a 4–6-week period. Severe cases may require periocular or systemic steroids.

Preseptal cellulitis

This is characterized by swelling and erythema of the lids and periorbital region and may be associated with sinusitis, hordeolum (stye) or trauma. The eye is usually unaffected. Adults are treated with oral antibiotics. However, children require admission and intravenous antibiotics because of the risk of progression to orbital cellulitis.

Orbital cellulitis

See 'Ear, nose and throat', p. 308.

Dry eyes

They are usually associated with dysfunction of the lacrimal gland often in conjunction with blepharitis. Sjögren's syndrome (dry eyes and dry mouth) may be primary or secondary (associated with other connective tissue disorders like rheumatoid arthritis, SLE, systemic sclerosis, dermatomyositis or primary biliary cirrhosis). Treatment is with topical lubricants (drops, gels or ointment).

Adnexal and other lid disorders

Hordeolum (stye)

This is an acute suppurative infection (commonly staphylococcal) that presents as a painful, tender lid swelling, centred around a lash follicle at the lid margin. Treat with a warm compress and oral antibiotics. If an abscess develops, removing the involved lash facilitates drainage of pus.

Chalazion (tarsal cyst)

This is a chronic granulomatous and usually painless inflammation of the meibomian glands. It may resolve spontaneously, or become secondarily infected causing pain and tenderness. Treatment involves a warm compress and lid hygiene, with oral antibiotics if there is secondary soft-tissue infection.

Other causes of red or sore eyes

- subconjunctival haemorrhage
- orbital inflammatory syndrome
- active thyroid eye disease
- carotico-cavernous fistula.

Visual loss and disturbance

Many conditions can alter or cause loss of vision. Some are outlined below. A summary of the different types of visual disorder and the conditions that cause these can be found in Tables 10.7 and 10.8.

Table 10.7 Loss of vision

Sudden painless	Sudden painful	Gradual
Retinal vascular occlusion (arterial or venous) Anterior ischaemic optic neuropathy Retinal detachment Vitreous haemorrhage Age-related macular degeneration (wet type) Cerebrovascular accident	Acute angle-closure glaucoma Optic neuritis	Cataract Chronic glaucoma Age-related macular degeneration (dry type) Diabetic maculopathy Toxic/nutritional optic neuropathy Posterior uveitis

Table 10.8 Transient visual disturbance

Flashes and floaters	Transient visual obscuration/loss
Posterior vitreous detachment with or without retinal tear	Transient ischaemic attack
Retinal detachment	Migraine
Vitreous haemorrhage	Giant cell arteritis
Posterior uveitis	Raised intracranial pressure
	Intermittent angle closure glaucoma

Anterior ischaemic optic neuropathy (AION)

If untreated, this may result in bilateral blindness. Infarction of the optic nerve head presents with sudden visual loss, a relative afferent pupillary defect, pale sectoral disc oedema and disc haemorrhages. Patients are usually over 65 years of age. AION can be classified as arteritic (if secondary to giant cell arteritis) or non-arteritic when it may be associated with hypertension, diabetes and hyperlipidaemia. Look for symptoms of giant cell arteritis (temporal headache, jaw claudication, scalp tenderness, myalgia and weight loss). The ESR is significantly elevated in 90% of patients.

Arteritic cases should be treated with high-dose intravenous and oral steroids for 12–18 months, depending on patient symptoms and ESR. In non-arteritic cases treatment is directed at predisposing risk factors.

Retinal detachment

This can be rhegmatogenous (associated with a retinal tear) or non-rhegmatogenous (exudative or tractional). Rhegmatogenous detachment is the commonest type, presenting with symptoms of flashing lights, floaters and field defects. Risk factors are myopia, trauma, complicated cataract surgery, aphakia and vitreoretinal disease. The detached retina has a convex configuration, appearing grey with dark blood vessels. Treatment is with retinal reattachment surgery.

Retinal vascular occlusions

There is usually sudden, unilateral and painless visual loss, which can be complete or partial. The central or branch retinal arteries or veins may be involved. Risk factors include age, systemic hypertension, diabetes, hypercholesterolaemia and smoking.

In central retinal artery occlusion, the retina appears pale and the arteries appear attenuated with a cherry red appearance of the macula. Retinal vein occlusions are characterized by dilated, tortuous veins associated with multiple retinal haemorrhages. Treatment involves detection and treatment of the underlying systemic risk factors.

Diabetic retinopathy

See 'Diabetes mellitus', p. 187.

Age-related macular degeneration (ARMD)

Affects central vision in those aged over 50 years and can be classified as dry or wet. Fundus examination may show macular drusen (discrete yellow spots), retinal pigmentary changes (hyperpigmentation or hypopigmentation), exudates, haemorrhages and neovascular membranes. Laser photocoagulation or intravitreal injections of anti-vascular endothelial growth factor agents may help preserve visual function in a select group of patients with wet ARMD.

Optic neuritis

Inflammation of the optic nerve is usually idiopathic in origin, but may be the first sign of multiple sclerosis. Patients are usually between 18 and 45 years of age. Visual deterioration occurs over a few days and is associated with painful eye movements, colour vision deficit and visual loss. A relative afferent pupillary defect is present. Initially, the optic disc appears normal in retro-bulbar neuritis but is swollen in optic neuritis.

Recovery begins in a few weeks and continues for several months. About 75% of patients regain visual acuity. However, some may be left with subtle colour vision loss and pupil and contrast sensitivity abnormalities. Pulsed steroid therapy is reserved for bilateral cases and uniocular patients.

Ocular trauma

A thorough history is important. An urgent ophthalmic referral should be considered after initial assessment using an ABCDE approach.

Blunt injuries

These account for 80% of ocular injuries. Ocular signs may include corneal abrasions, hyphaemia, iris tears, dislocated lens, retinal detachment and vitreous haemorrhage. A facial X-ray or CT scan may be required to exclude a blow-out fracture or globe rupture.

Penetrating injuries

It is important to ascertain a history of impact with sharp objects or projectile foreign bodies (e.g. hammering metal on metal, injury with broken glass, knives). Eye signs include lid laceration, corneal/scleral laceration, shallow anterior chamber or a distorted pupil.

Chemical injuries

These merit immediate thorough irrigation of the eye after instillation of topical anaesthetic. The nature of the chemical (alkali more damaging than acid) including its physical form (liquid, particulate, gas) is important. Removal of particulate matter with eversion of upper lids is required. The pH of the eye should be checked and irrigation continued until neutral.

Proptosis

The commonest cause is thyroid eye disease and is due to swelling of extraocular muscles and lymphocytic infiltration of orbital tissue. Other causes include orbital cellulites, tumours, haematoma or idiopathic orbital inflammatory syndrome. Protection and care of the cornea may be necessary, including lateral tarsorrhaphy. Severe cases of thyroid eye disease may require systemic steroids.

OBSTETRIC

Although pregnancy is a normal physiological state it can be associated with significant health risks to both mother and baby. Pregnant women routinely present acutely to a variety of specialties, so an understanding of the physiological changes and common problems encountered during pregnancy is essential for all doctors. This section reviews these topics and relates them to the antenatal, term and postnatal periods.

Physiological adaptations to pregnancy

Physiological changes have evolved to protect both mother and baby during pregnancy and delivery. However, their effect on other body systems can precipitate new disease, affect pre-existing conditions and alter the expected response to drugs.

Haematological

- erythropoiesis is dramatically increased and red cell mass increases by around 30%; this can lead to iron, folic acid and, to a lesser extent, vitamin B_{12} deficiency
- plasma volume increases by 50%, leading to haemodilution and 'physiological anaemia' despite the increase in erythropoiesis
- WCC rises, principally due to an increase in polymorphonuclear leucocytes; levels may be as high as 16×10^9/L in the third trimester, rising to 25–30$\times 10^9$/L during labour
- levels of clotting factors increase (particularly fibrinogen and factor VIII, but also factors VII, IX, X and XII to a lesser extent); plasminogen levels are also increased, although the net effect is a procoagulant state; this has evolved to reduce blood loss at the time of delivery, but increases the risk of VTE 10-fold.

Cardiovascular

- the heart is displaced upwards and to the left by the enlarging uterus
- cardiac output increases by approximately 1.5 L/min (around 40%); this is largely due to an increase in stroke volume with a smaller rise in heart rate
- systemic blood pressure (diastolic more than systolic) declines slightly in pregnancy; this is due to the vasodilating effects of progesterone.

Respiratory

- progesterone levels stimulate respiratory drive resulting in a 40% rise in tidal volume and a 65% rise in alveolar ventilation; this leads to physiological hyperventilation, a fall in maternal $PaCO_2$ and rapid clearance of fetal CO_2 across the placenta.

Renal

- GFR increases by 50%, resulting in a fall in serum urea and creatinine levels and impaired tubular reabsorption of glucose; this can lead to glycosuria
- the kidneys increase in size, including dilatation of the renal pelvis and ureters which can lead to urinary stasis and an increased risk of pyelonephritis.

Others

- gut motility is reduced leading to constipation and delayed gastric emptying; relaxation of the oesophageal sphincter may also result in heartburn
- the cervix enlarges and softens and ectropions are common; the vagina hypertrophies and there is an increase in vaginal secretions due to desquamation of cells
- cortisol, ACTH, TSH and MSH are all increased and thyroxine can increase 2–3-fold.

Antenatal care

The aim of antenatal care is to identify and obviate health risks to the mother and baby. Pregnancy is usually confirmed in the community setting with a urinary pregnancy test and the expected date of delivery (EDD) is calculated using Nägele's rule: first day of LMP, then subtract 3 months and add 7 days.

The booking visit

This is usually performed at approximately 12 weeks' gestation. It is the key element in establishing a tailored plan for the antenatal care of each individual pregnancy. A booking history should include menstrual and contraceptive history, previous obstetric history, past medical and surgical history, family history of relevant medical, obstetric or genetic conditions, smoking history and current medications and allergies.

An ultrasound scan should be performed to confirm viability, establish the number of fetuses, and date the pregnancy. Fetal biometry in the first trimester has been shown to be more accurate for dating than Nägele's rule and is now considered the gold standard. Prenatal testing for trisomy 21 may also be offered at this visit (see below).

Midwife-led antenatal clinic follow-up is standard practice for women who are designated low risk at their booking visit and remain so throughout pregnancy. A modified pattern of care will be required for women in moderate and high risk categories, whose care should be consultant-led. Initial investigations at booking include, FBC, Glu, blood group, hepatitis B serology, rubella, syphilis, HIV and an MSSU.

Prenatal testing

There are various approaches to prenatal screening programmes for structural and karyotypic fetal anomalies in the UK. However, the following are increasingly part of standard practice:

- first trimester trisomy 21 screening: combined nuchal and serum biochemical screening; performed at 10–13 weeks' gestation; 85–90% detection rate and 5% false positive rate
- fetal anomaly scan: performed at 20 weeks' gestation; 80% detection of major malformations
- invasive diagnostic prenatal testing: offered to women designated to be at high risk of karyotypic anomalies on the basis of history or screening tests
- chorionic villus sampling: placental biopsy performed from 11 weeks' gestation; 2% miscarriage rate
- amniocentesis: amniotic fluid analysis performed from 15 weeks' gestation; 1% miscarriage rate
- cordocentesis: fetal blood analysis; extracted via umbilical cord usually from 20 weeks; 1–5% risk of fetal loss.

Complications of pregnancy

Nausea and vomiting

About 80% of pregnant women experience nausea and 50% experience vomiting. Mild nausea and vomiting are often relieved by simple dietary measures, e.g. eating frequent small meals high in carbohydrates. Moderate symptoms may be treated by a range of therapies including ginger extract, vitamin B_6, acupressure, and other conventional antiemetics, e.g. cyclizine (50 mg 8-hourly). These symptoms are usually self-limiting, and resolve by the second trimester. However, for a small number of women they can cause serious morbidity.

Hyperemesis gravidarum

Occurs in 1 in 200 pregnancies and is characterized by dehydration, electrolyte disturbance and over 5% weight loss. It is a diagnosis of exclusion after other causes of vomiting have been ruled out, e.g. urinary tract infection, gastritis, cholecystitis. It occurs more frequently in multiple or molar pregnancy.

Management

Admit severe cases for IV fluid rehydration and parenteral antiemetics. Correct any electrolyte imbalance. In refractory cases, consider:

- ranitidine (150 mg 12-hourly) or omeprazole (20 mg daily)
- corticosteroids: hydrocortisone (50 mg intravenously 8-hourly) for 1 day, followed by prednisolone (30 mg/day), reducing weekly to lowest effective dose (usually 15 mg) within 5 weeks
- thiamine (50 mg 8-hourly orally) or Pabrinex® (250 mg IV weekly), particularly in women with multiple admissions or severe weight loss
- enteral and parenteral feeding may be required on rare occasions.

Anaemia

'Physiological anaemia' occurs due to relative haemodilution and does not require specific treatment. Pathological anaemia during pregnancy is defined as a haemoglobin <10g/L and is often due to a relative haematinic deficiency. Serum ferritin, folate and vitamin B_{12} levels should be checked in all women. Consider haemoglobin electrophoresis in relevant risk groups (see below).

Iron deficiency is the commonest cause of anaemia in pregnancy in the UK and is often dietary in origin. Start oral supplements. Parenteral iron is rarely required. Macrocytic anaemias due to folic acid or vitamin B_{12} deficiency should be treated with appropriate supplements. True vitamin B_{12} deficiency in pregnancy is rare but should be treated with IM hydroxycobalamin.

Haemoglobinopathies

Thalassaemia and sickle cell disease are autosomal recessive conditions and prenatal diagnosis is available for both. Screening in the UK is offered after a risk factor assessment during the booking antenatal visit.

- women with minor thalassaemia traits may develop mild to moderate anaemia; however this does not usually pose a significant threat to mother or fetus
- women with major thalassaemia traits may develop severe anaemia requiring repeated blood transfusion; antenatal care should be multidisciplinary with both obstetric and haematology involvement
- women with sickle cell disease have an increased risk of miscarriage, preterm labour and stillbirth; these risks can be minimized by ensuring adequate hydration, avoiding infection and regular blood transfusions to maintain a high proportion of HbA in the maternal bloodstream.

Haemolytic disease of the newborn

This results from the transfer of maternal blood group antibodies across the placenta. These antibodies result in lysis of fetal red cells bearing the relevant antigen, causing fetal anaemia and, in severe cases, hydrops fetalis and death. Rhesus isoimmunization is the commonest cause; others include ABO incompatibility, anti-Kell antibodies and anti-Duffy antibodies.

Regardless of the immunological origin, fetal red cell lysis results. This leads to a rise in unconjugated bilirubin in the fetal bloodstream which, before birth, can be cleared by the placenta. However, following delivery unconjugated bilirubin accumulates, resulting in neural toxicity and kernicterus if untreated. This is characterized by hypertonia, opisthotonia, seizures, sensorineural impairment, cerebral palsy and, ultimately, death.

Anti-D prophylaxis

Anti-D antibodies develop following feto-maternal haemorrhage in a Rhesus D negative woman carrying a Rhesus D positive fetus (83% of the UK population are Rhesus positive). Anti-D prophylaxis should be given according to one of the regimes below (depending on local policy):

- 500 IU anti-D IM administered at 28 weeks and 34 weeks
- 1500 IU anti-D IM administered at 28 weeks.

Antenatal anti-D immunoprophylaxis is also given for a range of potentially sensitizing events in non-Rhesus sensitized Rhesus D negative women including:

- bleeding beyond 12 weeks' gestation
- surgical or medical management of ectopic pregnancy
- surgical or medical management of first trimester miscarriage
- abdominal trauma
- invasive prenatal tests or external cephalic version
- intrauterine death.

Following these events, 250 IU of anti-D should given if the pregnancy is <20 weeks' gestation; 500 IU should be administered when >20 weeks' gestation. After

20 weeks' gestation, a Kleihauer test should also be performed to determine the size of any potential feto-maternal haemorrhage and the dose of anti-D should be adjusted accordingly.

Management of isoimmunized pregnancies

Pregnancies are identified as being at risk on the basis of a history of isoimmunization in a previous pregnancy or as a result of the antenatal blood group surveillance undertaken at booking and in the third trimester.

Until recently, women with significant blood group antibodies had to undergo serial amniocentesis to check for haemolysis and thus fetal anaemia. This has now been superseded by a non-invasive test for fetal anaemia using Doppler assessment of the middle cerebral arteries. Where Doppler screening suggests fetal anaemia, cordocentesis and intrauterine transfusion is undertaken if the gestational age is <34 weeks; elective delivery and neonatal treatment is advocated at or beyond 34 weeks' gestation.

Diabetes in pregnancy

Gestational diabetes

This affects 2–5% of pregnancies in the UK, usually develops in the third trimester and leads to an increased risk of fetal macrosomia, birth injury and possibly an increased risk of perinatal mortality.

Risk factors include a family history of type 2 diabetes, obesity, maternal age >35 years, previous delivery of a macrosomic baby, previous unexplained congenital anomaly (particularly neural tube or cardiac defects) and Asian ethnicity.

Various screening protocols exist; these incorporate urine testing for glycosuria, random blood glucose testing and oral glucose tolerance tests (OGTT). Regardless of the screening protocol, the 75g OGTT remains the gold standard test. Gestational diabetes is present when fasting glucose >5.5mmol/L or 2h glucose is >9.0mmol/L.

Management

The aims of treatment are to normalize glycaemic control and avoid complications. For the majority of women, dietary measures will be sufficient, but a small proportion will require insulin or oral hypoglycaemics. Blood glucose monitoring should be performed at least four times daily.

Women with satisfactory dietary control, without evidence of fetal macrosomia, can usually deliver normally. Those requiring insulin or oral hypoglycaemics should be delivered by 40 weeks' gestation, treatment discontinued and normal diet resumed postnatally. A repeat OGTT should be performed 6 weeks postnatally.

Women with gestational diabetes should be informed that this confers a lifetime risk of developing diabetes of 25–50% and they should be encouraged to modify their lifestyle accordingly.

The effect of the pregnancy on pre-existing diabetes

Pregnancy may lead to a worsening of previous diabetic control, retinopathy and nephropathy. During the first trimester, hypoglycaemia is common and antenatal visits are often fortnightly or weekly until these episodes have resolved and glycaemic control is optimized. During the second trimester, glycaemic control often remains relatively stable, but deteriorates early in the third trimester due to the physiological changes of pregnancy. These include dramatically increased insulin requirements due to a combination of increased gluconeogenesis and insulin resistance.

The outcome for pregnancies with pre-existing type 1 and type 2 diabetes are similar and all patients not controlled on diet alone should be treated with insulin. Insulin does not cross the placenta and is safe for the developing fetus. Some type 2 diabetics may be treated with oral hypoglycaemic agents, but long-term safety data are not available for these drugs in pregnant patients and they are not licensed for this indication.

Women with diabetes contemplating pregnancy should attend a formal pre-pregnancy clinic and optimize control prior to conception, aiming for an HbA_{1c} within the normal range (<6.5%). Following delivery, insulin requirements fall significantly and usually to pre-pregnancy levels, or at least half the dose of insulin taken prior to delivery. Oral hypoglycaemics can be recommenced, but should be avoided if the patient is breast-feeding.

The effect of pre-existing diabetes on the pregnancy

Pre-existing diabetes confers an increased risk of miscarriage, pre-term labour, pre-eclampsia, macrosomia (>50%), shoulder dystocia (8%) and Erb's palsy. Folic acid 5 mg PO daily should be given pre-conceptually to minimize risk of neural tube defects. Ultrasound surveillance should be offered and usually includes:

- first trimester scan to confirm viability
- second trimester fetal anomaly scan including echocardiography
- monthly growth scans from 28 weeks' gestation
- fetal surveillance by regular cardiotocography may also be employed from 34–36 weeks' gestation.

Unfortunately, current monitoring techniques are poor predictors of fetal outcome. It is still unclear why some babies die, although an acute metabolic cause is likely. Due to the limitations of current fetal surveillance, delivery is often planned at 38–39 weeks. If macrosomia is suspected, delivery by elective caesarean section is recommended.

Abdominal pain in pregnancy

Pregnant women are susceptible to the same diseases that cause abdominal pain as non-pregnant women. However, the presentation of these conditions may be altered because abdominal viscera are often displaced by the gravid uterus. Consider the following causes:

- upper abdominal pain: costochondritis, cholecystitis, cholangitis, hepatitis, severe pre-eclampsia, appendicitis; peptic ulcer disease is rare in pregnancy
- flanks: pyelonephritis, appendicitis (right flank only), musculoskeletal, ovarian cyst accident
- central abdomen: abruptio placentae, labour, fibroid degeneration
- lower abdomen: symphysis pubis diastasis, lower UTI, ectopic pregnancy (Table 10.9), ovarian cyst accident; pelvic inflammatory disease is rare due to alterations in cervical mucus.

If a surgical cause for abdominal pain seems likely, remember that laparotomy in the first trimester carries a risk of miscarriage approaching 10%. This falls to 1–2% in the second and third trimesters.

Table 10.9 Criteria for management of ectopic pregnancy

Clinical findings	Ultrasound findings	β-HCG	Management
Haemodynamically stable; no significant pain	Empty uterus No adnexal mass No free fluid	<2000 IU	Conservative
	Empty uterus or pseudosac Adnexal mass <4 cm No free fluid	<5000 IU	Medical: methotrexate (50 mg/m^2 IM)
Often asymptomatic; may have abdominal pain	Empty uterus or pseudosac ± Adnexal mass >4 cm ± Free fluid	Any level	Surgical

Urinary tract infection

The risk of lower urinary tract infection (UTI) does not increase in pregnancy. However, the risk of a UTI developing into pyelonephritis is increased (to around 20%) due to ureteric dilation and relative urinary stasis. Therefore all bacteriuria, even if asymptomatic, should be treated. Where possible, this should be based on culture and sensitivity results, but the following is a guide:

- asymptomatic: 3 days of amoxicillin 500 mg 8-hourly, or cefalexin 500 mg 8-hourly
- symptomatic: 7 days of amoxicillin 500 mg 8-hourly, or cefalexin 500 mg 8-hourly.

Fibroids

A small minority of fibroids grow during pregnancy and undergo 'red degeneration'. This occurs when fibroid growth outstrips its blood supply causing central necrosis and severe pain. This should be managed conservatively with analgesics. Rarely, pedunculated fibroids may undergo torsion, necessitating surgery.

Ovarian cysts

Serous cysts and dermoid tumours are the commonest ovarian tumours found in pregnancy. Although benign, they can undergo torsion or haemorrhage and cause acute abdominal pain. Laparotomy and ovarian cystectomy or oophorectomy is often recommended for large tumours, but is best deferred until the second trimester.

Asymptomatic, small cysts found incidentally at booking ultrasound do not require treatment or follow-up. Complex cysts, or cysts measuring over 5 cm, should be followed up by repeat ultrasound scan at 13–14 weeks' gestation.

Hypertension, pre-eclampsia, eclampsia

These are often referred to as the hypertensive disorders of pregnancy. They are serious disorders that are associated with an increase in maternal and fetal morbidity and mortality. Since they often remain asymptomatic until severe complications develop, antenatal screening is essential.

Hypertension

This is defined as a blood pressure above 140/90 mmHg. It may predate conception or be pregnancy-induced (gestational) and may occur with or without proteinuria. Proteinuria is defined as >0.3 g urinary protein loss in 24 h or proteinuria of '++' or more, on two separate occasions at least 4 h apart.

Management

The aim of antihypertensive treatment is to reduce the risk of a maternal cerebrovascular accident. This is particularly associated with a systolic BP >170 mmHg or a diastolic BP >110 mmHg. Treatment should not be overly aggressive as uteroplacental perfusion may be compromised. Generally, a target systolic BP of 140–150 mmHg and diastolic BP of 90–100 mmHg is sufficient. Women with pre-existing renal disease should be treated more aggressively; aim for a BP <130/80 mmHg. Atenolol is associated with intrauterine growth restriction and its use should be discouraged. ACE inhibitors are contraindicated in pregnancy as their use has been associated with skull defects, fetal renal failure and intrauterine death.

Pre-eclampsia

This is defined as gestational hypertension with proteinuria. Pre-eclampsia complicates approximately 5–6% of UK pregnancies. It is an immune-mediated disease triggered by the fetoplacental unit, affecting a variety of maternal end organs including kidney, liver and brain. It is also associated with reduced uteroplacental perfusion leading to intrauterine fetal growth restriction.

Severe pre-eclampsia

Severe pre-eclampsia is relatively rare (5/1000) and is defined as a systolic BP >170 mmHg and/or a diastolic BP >110 mmHg, plus proteinuria over 1 g/L. This definition is extended to women with less severe hypertension and proteinuria, but two or more of the following clinical features:

- severe headache
- visual disturbance
- severe epigastric pain and/or vomiting
- clonus or papilloedema
- hepatic tenderness, ALT or AST >70 IU/L or PLT $<100\times10^9$/L.

Management of pre-eclampsia

The key elements are maternal and fetal surveillance, drug treatment when necessary and planned delivery. Asymptomatic women, with mild to moderate disease (BP <170/110 mmHg and proteinuria <1 g/24 h), can be managed as outpatients. Twice-weekly monitoring at a maternity day-care unit should be performed including assessment of BP, urinary protein estimation, FBC, U&E, urate, LFT and cardiotocography. Ultrasound assessment of fetal growth and umbilical artery Doppler may also be required.

Inpatient management is required for women with severe pre-eclampsia and should also be considered for women with early-onset (<32 weeks) mild to moderate disease due to the greater potential for rapid disease progression. Consider the following:

- intravenous antihypertensives, e.g. labetalol (50 mg IV bolus followed by IV infusion of 40 mg/h; max 160 mg/h) or hydralazine (5 mg bolus followed by IV infusion of 10 mg/h); contraindicated in SLE, severe tachycardia, high-output cardiac failure and porphyria
- oral antihypertensives: methyldopa (250 mg PO two or three times daily; max 3 g/day) or labetalol (200 mg PO 8-hourly; max 2.4 g/day) or nifedipine (10–20 mg PO twice daily)
- IV magnesium sulphate: this is an effective means of preventing progression to eclampsia; see below for dosage.

Eclampsia

Eclampsia is rare and affects 5/10 000 pregnancies. It is defined as one or more convulsions superimposed upon pre-eclampsia.

Treatment and stabilization of the mother is essential before any intervention in the interests of the fetus is contemplated. Magnesium sulphate should be given as a 4 g IV bolus over 5–20 min, followed by a 1 g/h IV infusion for 24 h after the last seizure. Frequent maternal monitoring is required whilst on the infusion, e.g. BP, heart rate, pulse oximetry, respiratory rate, deep tendon reflexes. Once stabilized, fetal assessment should be performed and delivery expedited.

Bleeding in pregnancy

Bleeding in pregnancy is relatively common, but creates enormous anxiety. For the majority, a normal pregnancy outcome can be anticipated, but management should be tailored to both gestational age at referral and diagnosis.

First trimester bleeding

This is rarely life threatening and can originate from anywhere in the genital tract. It may be painless or painful. A speculum or vaginal examination is not required when assessing a single episode of minor bleeding, but should be performed if bleeding is heavy or recurrent. This allows inspection of the cervix for clot, dilatation and removal, if necessary, of any products of conception (POC).

General management

- mild bleeding: less than or the same as that of a normal period; manage as outpatient, refer to EPAS (Early Pregnancy Assessment Service)
- moderate bleeding: more than a normal period, but haemodynamically stable; perform speculum, arrange ultrasound as inpatient or via EPAS outpatient service
- severe bleeding: more than a normal period and haemodynamically unstable; admit, resuscitate (see 'Shock', p. 250), consider ergometrine (0.5 mg IM) and early surgical intervention.

Products of conception

POC or clot distending the cervical canal may cause cervical shock through vagal stimulation, bradycardia and hypotension. Management is based on fluid resuscitation and removal of POC using a speculum and sponge forceps. This should be performed where the patient is being assessed, does not require anaesthesia and is usually immediately effective. Further treatment should be guided by senior advice and relates to the size of the retained POC.

Mid-trimester bleeding

This is relatively infrequent. It is often benign, but may signal miscarriage or preterm labour, particularly if associated with a mucoid discharge suggestive of 'show'. Under these circumstances a speculum examination should be performed to assess cervical dilatation and to exclude local causes.

Third trimester bleeding (antepartum haemorrhage)

Although often attributable to causes in the lower genital tract, assessment should exclude potentially life-threatening placenta praevia and abruptio placentae. There is a risk of postpartum haemorrhage for both abruptio placentae and placenta praevia and prophylactic measures should be employed.

Placenta praevia

This refers to a placenta lying within the lower uterine segment (LUS) after 24 weeks' gestation. The incidence varies with gestation, but occurs in approximately 2–3% of term pregnancies. Classically, bleeding is painless, the uterus is soft and the presenting part high.

- type I (minor): extends into LUS but does not reach cervical os
- type II (minor): extends to internal cervical os but not across it
- type III (major): extends partially across cervix at full dilatation
- type IV (major): extends fully across cervical os at full dilatation.

Vaginal delivery may be possible with type I praevia, but caesarean section is indicated for types II–IV. The timing of delivery is related to presentation. If there are no symptoms or there is minimal bleeding, aim for delivery at 37–38 weeks' gestation. Otherwise, delivery is indicated where there are signs of maternal or fetal compromise; consider steroids if gestation <36 weeks.

Abruptio placentae

This describes separation of a normally sited placenta after the 20th week of pregnancy, before the birth of the baby. Appropriate resuscitation should be undertaken and consideration given to early delivery; this decision will be influenced by both disease severity and gestational age.

Thromboembolic disease in pregnancy

Pregnancy is a procoagulant state and, with an increasingly sedentary lifestyle and prevalence of obesity among mothers, venous and pulmonary thromboembolism (VTE) has become the leading cause of maternal death in the UK in recent years.

VTE is 10 times more common in pregnant than in non-pregnant women of the same age. Symptoms, signs and investigation of DVT and PTE are as per

'Acute leg pain', p. 270 and 'Breathlessness', p. 139 respectively. Although levels of D-dimers increase physiologically during pregnancy, a negative result has the same exclusion value as in a non-pregnant woman. Current evidence suggests that CTPA and V/Q scanning can both be used without significant risk to the fetus. However, radiation dose to the pregnant breast is increased with CTPA.

Management

Pregnant women with massive PTE (defined by hypotension or RV dilatation) should be treated as described in 'Breathlessness', p. 139. In all other situations, LMWH is the treatment of choice. Although tinzaparin is the first drug of choice for treatment of PTE in other patients, in pregnancy there are limited safety data for this drug as compared to enoxaparin.

Enoxaparin is given twice daily and the dose is adjusted to booking weight (not weight at the time of event): <50 kg, 40 mg; 50–69 kg, 60 mg; 70–89 kg, 80 mg; >90 kg, 100 mg. Warfarin is teratogenic and is contraindicated in pregnancy. For more information, see 'Anticoagulation', p. 110.

LMWH can be changed to an IV infusion of unfractionated heparin once the mother goes into labour. For a planned delivery, LMWH should be discontinued 24 h prior to induction of labour or planned caesarean section. This is important to remember as regional anaesthesia, e.g. an epidural, is contraindicated for 12 h following prophylactic LMWH, for 24 h following treatment dose LMWH and for 6 h after IV heparin.

Duration of therapy

LMWH should be continued throughout the pregnancy, for at least 6 weeks postnatally and until at least 3 months of treatment has been given in total. Following delivery, women should be offered a choice of maintaining LMWH or converting to warfarin, as both drugs are safe if they plan to breast-feed. Warfarin should not be commenced until the third postnatal day.

Inferior vena caval filters

A temporary caval filter should be considered for women who develop iliac vein thrombosis in the perinatal period or women with recurrent PTE despite adequate anticoagulation.

Labour

Labour is characterized by 'show', regular uterine contractions and progressive effacement and dilatation of the cervix. Prolonged labour has been arbitrarily defined as labour lasting >24 h in a primigravida and >16 h in a multigravida.

Definitions

First stage

This commences with the onset of labour and ends when the cervix is fully dilated. It is subdivided into the latent and active phases and is also characterized by descent of the fetal head.

- latent: variable length; commences from the onset of regular contractions and ends when the cervix is effaced and 3 cm dilated
- active: normal progression through this phase is defined by at least 0.5 cm of cervical dilatation per hour.

Second stage

This stage commences at full dilatation and ends with delivery of the baby. It has a propulsive and expulsive stage. It is considered prolonged if over 2 h in a primigravida and over 1 h in a multigravida.

Third stage

Starts with the delivery of the baby and ends with delivery of the placenta.

Normal labour

- descent: the head enters the pelvic inlet in an occipitotransverse position and descends through the maternal pelvis
- flexion: the head flexes as it descends and meets the pelvic floor muscles leading to a smaller diameter of presentation and thus easier passage through the birth canal
- internal rotation: the head rotates as it hits the pelvic floor to an occipitoanterior position
- extension: the flexed head descends to the vulva and the base of the occiput comes into contact with the base of the inferior rami of the pubis and the head extends until it is delivered
- restitution: the head rotates to the natural position relative to the shoulders
- external rotation: the shoulders rotate into the anteroposterior diameter of the pelvis when they reach the pelvic floor
- delivery of the shoulders: lateral flexion of the trunk posteriorly to deliver the anterior shoulder followed by lateral flexion of the trunk anteriorly to deliver the posterior shoulder is followed by rapid expulsion of rest of baby.

Abnormal labour

There are many conditions which predispose to abnormal labour:

- inefficient uterine contraction: predominantly occurs in primigravid labours and is treated with oxytocin
- relative cephalopelvic disproportion: common, particularly in primigravidae, and often associated with a deflexed occipitoposterior position
- true cephalopelvic disproportion: rare, <5% cases; causes include fetal macrosomia, contracted pelvis
- malpresentation: brow presentation (1 in 1500), face presentation (1 in 600), compound presentation, shoulder presentation, breech presentation
- others: obstructing pelvic tumours, large fibroids disrupting normal propagation of contractions.

Pre-term labour

Pre-term birth is defined as delivery before 37 completed weeks' gestation and complicates 5–8% pregnancies in the UK. It remains one of the leading causes of perinatal mortality and morbidity. Risk factors include multiple pregnancy, previous pre-term birth, antepartum haemorrhage, cervical incompetence, smoking, teenage pregnancy, BMI <18, low socioeconomic class, drug abuse, bacterial vaginosis and asymptomatic bacteruria.

In women presenting with regular uterine activity, accurate prediction of subsequent pre-term labour remains difficult. Fetal fibronectin testing may prove useful in this setting, being 97% negatively predictive for birth within 14 days.

Treatment

The risks to the mother and fetus of delivering prematurely need to be weighed against the risks of trying to prolong the pregnancy. Treatment options include steroids, tocolytics and antibiotics:

Steroids

Steroid use encourages fetal lung maturation and reduces the risk of intraventricular haemorrhage, necrotizing enterocolitis and neonatal death, e.g. betamethasone (12 mg IM × 2 doses 24 h apart) administered from 24–36 completed weeks' gestation.

Tocolytics

Tocolytics prolong pregnancy in the short term; however, there is no evidence that this improves neonatal morbidity or mortality. Therefore, they cannot be recommended routinely. However, they do have a role in prolonging the pregnancy for 48 h, to allow sufficient time for steroids to have an effect or for in utero transfer. They should not be used after this period.

Commonly used tocolytics in the UK include atosiban, nifedipine, ritodrine and indometacin. Atosiban IV is recommended as first-line therapy due to its preferential side-effect profile.

Antibiotics

Infection remains one of the leading causes of pre-term birth. Antibiotic therapy prolongs pregnancy and improves fetal outcome if the mother's membranes have ruptured. If not, they should not be given. A common regime is erythromycin (250 mg 6-hourly) for 10 days.

Fetal monitoring

Electronic fetal monitoring (EFM) was initially introduced in the 1970s in the belief that it would improve the detection of fetal hypoxia, thereby reducing cerebral palsy and perinatal mortality. Subsequent evidence has not proven this and most obstetric units in the UK now adopt a policy of intermittent auscultation rather than EFM of the fetal heart in labour for low-risk women. EFM by cardiotocography (CTG) is reserved for women designated to be at high risk of developing intrapartum fetal hypoxia, e.g. pre-eclampsia, diabetes, intra-uterine growth restriction, antepartum haemorrhage, multiple pregnancy, breech presentation.

Intermittent auscultation

Intermittent auscultation (IA) of the fetal heart involves an assessment of heart rate, rhythm (regular or irregular), accelerations or decelerations and should be commenced at the onset of active labour. The auscultation may be via hand-held Pinard or Doptone, which allows greater mobility.

IA should be performed immediately after a contraction for at least 1 full minute, at 15 min intervals in the first stage of labour and 5 min intervals during the active second stage of labour. If any abnormalities are detected, electronic fetal monitoring should be instituted.

Cardiotocography

The cardiotocograph (CTG) provides a continuous linear trace recording of the fetal heart beat and uterine contractions. The frequency is recorded via an external transducer: a normal contraction pattern ≤5 contractions in 10 min. An intrauterine pressure catheter is the only means of assessing the strength of contractions and this is not routinely used. A frequency of >5 contractions in 10 min is associated with uterine hyperstimulation and may lead to fetal hypoxaemia.

Fetal heart rate monitoring definitions

- baseline rate: normal 110–160 b.p.m., tachycardia >160 b.p.m.; bradycardia <110 b.p.m.
- variability: normal 5 b.p.m., reduced <5 b.p.m.; increased >25 b.p.m. (often termed saltatory)
- accelerations: a rise in the baseline rate of 15 b.p.m. sustained for at least 15 s
- decelerations: a fall in the baseline rate which may be subtle or marked.

A CTG with normal fetal heart rate, normal variability and the presence of at least two accelerations in 20 min is termed 'reactive' and implies adequate fetal oxygenation. A non-reactive CTG may be indicative of fetal sleep, be secondary to drugs (particularly opiates) or may be due to fetal hypoxaemia.

Variability is the single greatest determinant of fetal hypoxaemia when compared with the other factors above. Normal variability is reassuring. Reduced variability, particularly if prolonged (>90 min), is associated with an increased risk of fetal hypoxaemia.

Decelerations are common in labour particularly in the second stage and are often benign. However, if severe (a fall in baseline rate ≥60 b.p.m. sustained for 60 s), or accompanied by other adverse features such as fetal tachycardia, fetal bradycardia and, in particular, reduced variability, fetal hypoxaemia is likely. Certain specific patterns of deceleration are seen: cord compression, often variable in shape and timing in relation to uterine contractions; uteroplacental insufficiency, usually occurs late in timing in relation to uterine contractions.

Fetal blood sampling

This technique of measuring pH via fetal scalp sampling is seen as complementary to FHR monitoring and when used in conjunction with CTG may reduce caesarean section rates.

- pH >7.25: normal
- pH 7.20–7.25: borderline, repeat 30 min
- pH <7.20: abnormal – deliver.

Neonatal assessment

The Apgar score is used to assess the newborn infant and the response following an episode of resuscitation (Table 10.10). It comprises an assessment of five components: heart rate, respiratory effort, muscle tone, reflex irritability and colour. A 5 min Apgar score of 7–10 is normal. A score of 4–6 is intermediate but the risk of adverse neurological outcome increases when the score is ≤3 at 10, 15 and 20 min.

The score is best interpreted when applied to full-term infants as lack of maturity in pre-term infants will affect their normal tone and reflex irritability. Moreover, the score, as it should be applied to a spontaneously breathing infant at birth, cannot be applied in the same way to an infant requiring resuscitation at birth. Nevertheless, an Apgar score at 0 at 10 min of age is a significant indicator that further resuscitative intervention is unlikely to be successful and the change in score between 1 and 5 min is a good indicator of the response to resuscitation.

Table 10.10 The Apgar score

Variable	Score		
	0	1	2
Colour	Blue or pale	Acrocyanotic	Completely pink
Heart rate (b.p.m.)	Absent	<100	>100
Reflex irritability	None	Grimace	Active withdrawal
Tone	Limp	Some flexion	Active motion
Respiration	Absent	Weak cry/hypoventilation	Good crying

Postpartum complications

Postpartum haemorrhage

This is defined as blood loss in excess of 500 mL (minor) or 1000 mL (major) following delivery. Assessment should follow Advanced Life Support in Obstetrics guidelines which involve consideration of the four Ts:

- Tone: atonic uterus (70%)
- Tissue: retained placental tissue
- Trauma: perineal, vaginal, cervical or uterine tears
- Thrombin: inherited or iatrogenic coagulopathy.

Management

Resuscitate if shocked (see 'Shock p. 250). Urgent transfusion will be required. Cross-match 4 units and liaise with haematology if FFP or cryoprecipitate is required (see 'Blood products', p. 122). Consult with senior colleagues and consider the following:

- Syntocinon (5 IU IV, then 40 IU over 4 h), ergometrine (0.25–0.5 mg IV), carboprost (Hemabate®) (0.25 mg IM repeated every 15 min for up to 8 doses), misoprostol (800 μg PV) or misoprostol (1000 μg PR)
- rub up a contraction: place a hand on uterine fundus and press firmly with a rotating motion
- bi-manual uterine compression
- ensure placenta is complete and uterus is empty
- suture visible tears and look for others, e.g. cervical tears
- book theatre for examination under anaesthetic
- consider need for additional procedures including insertion of Rusch balloon catheter, B-Lynch suture, uterine artery embolization and hysterectomy.

Retained placenta

This affects 2% of pregnancies, may be partial or complete and is associated with PPH. Treatment involves manual removal under anaesthesia (usually regional) with antibiotic cover to reduce the risk of endometritis.

Postpartum sepsis

Can affect 1–8% of deliveries and accounts for 0.6/100 000 maternal deaths. Endometritis and caesarean section wound infection are the commonest causes in the UK. Other causes include perineal wound infection, urinary tract infection, mastitis, chest infection (particularly following general anaesthesia), and rarely peritonitis and necrotizing fascitis. Postpartum sepsis has been increasing in recent years, perhaps related to increasing maternal obesity and increasing caesarean section rates.

GYNAECOLOGICAL

Although most commonly encountered by trainees working in specialist units, gynaecological problems may present acutely to other specialties including general practice, surgery and A&E. A working knowledge of the most common presentations is therefore desirable.

Menstrual disorders

Heavy menstrual bleeding

Menorrhagia describes recurrent heavy periods with blood loss in excess of 80 mL. However, this term has been superseded in recent years by the more useful definition 'heavy menstrual bleeding (HMB)'. This is defined as excessive menstrual blood loss which interferes with a woman's physical, social, emotional and/or quality of life. HMB is usually of benign origin, but has significant costs in terms of healthcare resources in both primary and secondary care.

Examination should look for signs of abdominal masses including fibroids and, in women over 45 with persistent intermenstrual bleeding, assessment should include transvaginal ultrasound ± biopsy of the endometrium.

The principal aim of treatment is to improve quality of life. If pharmacological treatment is proposed, the choice of agent used should reflect the woman's own wishes, including any preference for hormonal versus non-hormonal methods, and their need for contraception or the maintenance of fertility. A levonorgestrel releasing intrauterine system is first-line treatment, but this is expensive and is associated with some side-effects, e.g. breast tenderness, headache and irregular bleeding. Combined oral contraceptives, NSAIDs and tranexamic acid are second-line agents with oral progestogen norethisterone, injectable progestogen or gonadotrophin releasing hormone analogues used in other cases. Where fibroids are found, other treatment may be necessary.

Post-menopausal bleeding (PMB)

This is defined as vaginal bleeding occurring over 12 months after amenorrhoea in a woman of the age where the menopause can be expected. It accounts for 5% of all referrals to gynaecology departments in the UK. Outpatient assessment should be on an urgent basis, reflecting the underlying risk of malignancy. In the UK, PMB is often assessed at 'one stop' clinics where pelvic examination, cervical smear, transvaginal ultrasound, endometrial sampling and hysteroscopy can all be performed as required. Treatment is dependent on the diagnosis reached during this assessment:

- secondary to HRT use: treatment modification
- vaginal atrophy: topical oestrogens, or systemic oestrogens and progestogens if non-hysterectomized
- endometrial hyperplasia: progestogens or total abdominal hysterectomy (TAH) and bilateral salpingo-oophorectomy (BSO)
- endometrial carcinoma: see p. 364.
- cervical carcinoma: see p. 363.
- ovarian carcinoma: see p. 361.

Gynaecological cancers should be managed either in cancer referral centres or by clinicians with a special interest and surgical expertise in gynaecological cancer with liaison via regional managed clinical gynaecological cancer networks.

Abdominal/pelvic masses

Abdominal and or pelvic masses may be detected in women presenting with a variety of gynaecological symptoms including abdominal pain, dysmenorrhoea and menstrual disturbance. Alternatively, they may be incidental findings in women having examinations or investigations for other reasons. The majority of gynaecological masses arise in the ovary and uterus but masses may also be found in the fallopian tube, cervix, vagina and vulva.

Ovarian cysts

Although ovarian cysts are extremely common, the majority are functional and benign. They can be classified as:

- functional cysts
- surface epithelial: 75% of benign and 90–95% of malignant tumours
- sex-cord stromal: 5–10% of tumours
- germ cell: 15–20% of tumours.

Incidence increases with age and peaks between the ages of 40 and 49 years. Malignant cysts tend to be commoner at the extremes of age, i.e. in childhood or after 50 years. Ovarian cysts and tumours can be classified as follows:

The risk malignancy index (RMI) should be used to determine likelihood of malignancy, particularly if complex cysts are seen or the woman is postmenopausal. The RMI index recommended by the Royal College of Obstetricians and Gynaecologists is summarized in Table 10.11. Where the RMI is <25, a conservative approach may be appropriate. Alternatively, laparoscopic cystectomy or oophorectomy may be performed if the index of suspicion is high. If RMI is >25, referral via a managed clinical network is appropriate.

Table 10.11 Risk malignancy index for ovarian tumours

Characteristics		RMI score
Ultrasound features (U)		
Multilocular cyst; solid areas; bilateral lesion;	None	0
evidence of metastases; presence of ascites	Two or more abnormalities	3
Menopausal status (M)		
Pre-menopausal		1
Post-menopausal		3
CA125 (U/mL)		Level

RMI score = U × M × CA125 level
Low risk, RMI <25; moderate risk, RMI = 25–250; high risk, RMI >250

Fibroids

Fibroids are benign tumours derived from the smooth muscle of the myometrium and are found in 20% women over the age of 35 years. They are extremely common in Afro-Caribbean women, and are variable in size and location. They are mostly asymptomatic, but can cause heavy menstrual bleeding leading to anaemia and abdominal pain secondary to degeneration or torsion. They usually regress after the menopause. Treatment is aimed at alleviating symptoms and includes analgesia, myomectomy, uterine artery embolization and hysterectomy.

Abdominal pain in gynaecology

Pelvic and lower abdominal pain are common. A careful history and examination should help to differentiate between gynaecological and non-gynaecological causes. Treatment is tailored to diagnosis and, although often effective in the acute setting, can be extremely challenging in the longer term.

Physiological pain

Ovulatory

Usually mid-cycle lasting 2–3 days. Treat with simple analgesics and/or combined oral contraceptive pill.

Dysmenorrhoea

Treat with simple analgesics and or combined oral contraceptive pill.

Acute pain

Ruptured ectopic pregnancy

Ectopic pregnancy is defined as any pregnancy that occurs outside the uterus. The majority develop in the fallopian tubes; the remainder occur in the abdomen, ovary or cervix. Rupture can lead to shock and carries a significant mortality risk.

Presentation

Presentation is highly variable: symptoms may include lower abdominal pain with vaginal blood loss. Peritonitis and shock suggest tubal rupture. Examination may reveal mild pelvic tenderness or a rigid abdomen in keeping with peritonitis. It is very unusual to feel a pelvic mass as an ectopic pregnancy is normally too small and soft to be palpable.

Investigation

Routine blood tests and a cross-match sample should be sent. A pregnancy test is usually positive. Transvaginal ultrasound can be useful in determining the presence of a viable intrauterine pregnancy. Haemoglobin is often reduced in proportion to the amount of blood lost.

Management

Intravenous fluid resuscitation is necessary if the patient is haemodynamically compromised. Appropriate analgesia should be provided and early obstetric referral made. Surgical intervention should not be delayed.

Ruptured ovarian cyst and ovarian torsion

Ovarian cysts are often discovered incidentally on routine ultrasound examination; their management is described on p. 332. Occasionally, they may be complicated by rupture or torsion (both are more common on the right side; torsion is more likely to occur in females under 30 years of age).

Presentation and investigation

Acute onset of abdominal pain suggests cyst rupture, but ovarian torsion or ectopic pregnancy need to be actively excluded. Examination findings can vary greatly from lower abdominal tenderness to overt peritonitis and septic shock. Pelvic examination may reveal a pelvic mass or adnexal tenderness.

The WBC may be normal or mildly elevated. Haemoglobin may be decreased if there is associated haemorrhage. Blood, urine and cervical cultures should be performed in all patients. All females of child-bearing age should have a pregnancy test. Imaging studies such as abdominal ultrasound or CT scanning may be useful in haemodynamically stable patients.

Management

All patients who are haemodynamically unstable need rapid and adequate fluid resuscitation. Analgesia should be titrated to patients' needs. Early referral to surgery or gynaecology is mandatory.

Chronic pain

Pelvic inflammatory disease (PID)

This is a disease of the female upper genital tract and describes inflammation of the uterus, fallopian tubes and adjacent pelvic structures. It is caused by organisms ascending from the vagina (particularly *Neisseria gonorrhoea* and *Chlamydia trachomatis*). It can occur at any age; sexually active females below the age of 25 years are most commonly affected.

Presentation

Symptoms and signs depend on the organism and the severity of the infection, e.g. patients with gonococcal PID tend to present acutely with severe abdominal pain, nausea and vomiting and fever. Most patients present with bilateral lower abdominal pain accompanied by vaginal discharge or irregular vaginal bleeding. Alternatively, women may present with the sequelae of chronic infection, e.g. ectopic pregnancy, infertility or chronic pelvic pain.

Examination may reveal lower abdominal tenderness with voluntary guarding; in severe cases there may be peritonitis. Pelvic examination should be performed in all females with suspected PID.

Investigation

The WBC and CRP may be elevated, but are normal in 50% of cases. All patients should have a urinalysis and a pregnancy test performed. Imaging (initially in the form of pelvic ultrasound) is merited in all patients in whom there is diagnostic doubt or if complications are suspected, e.g. tubo-ovarian abscess. Consider testing for other sexually transmitted diseases if chlamydia or gonorrhoea is cultured.

Management

All patients with PID require antibiotics and treatment should not be delayed. Consult your local antibiotic prescribing protocols, but options include norfloxacin (400 mg 12-hourly), metronidazole (400 mg 8-hourly), ampicillin (500 mg 6-hourly) and oxycycline (200 mg daily). Antibiotics should be given IV to patients who are systemically unwell. Gynaecological assessment should be sought as soon as possible. Tracing and treatment of sexual contacts is required.

Endometriosis

This is defined as the presence of endometrial tissue outside the uterus, resulting in a chronic inflammatory reaction. The most commonly affected sites are the pelvic organs and peritoneum, although the bowel and other distant sites may be affected. Pain is usually cyclical causing severe dysmenorrhoea. Associated symptoms include deep dyspareunia, fatigue and infertility. Pelvic examination is often normal; however, in advanced disease a fixed retroverted uterus, thickened tender uterosacral ligaments or enlarged ovaries may be found. Laparoscopy is the gold standard for diagnosis. A number of treatment options are available and are summarized below:

- naproxen (250 mg 8-hourly)
- hormonal: continuous combined oral contraceptive pill; danazol (200 mg 8-hourly); gestrinone (2.5 mg twice weekly) or medroxyprogesterone acetate (10 mg 8-hourly); gonadotrophin releasing hormone analogues; levonorgestrel intrauterine system
- surgical: laparoscopic ablation of endometriotic lesions, laparoscopic cystectomy, TAH ± BSO; total abdominal hysterectomy ± BSO; usually effective providing all endometriotic lesions are removed; concurrent BSO improves symptomatic relief and reduces need for repeat surgery.

Other causes of pain

Other gynaecological causes of pain include pelvic congestion syndrome, fibroids (see above), pregnancy or congenital haematometra or haematocolpos.

PAEDIATRIC

ABC

Regardless of cause, the assessment and treatment of the acutely sick child should follow the APLS/EPLS guidelines.

Airway

Ensure that the child has a clear airway and is able to maintain it. If no, open the airway with a head tilt/chin lift (see 'Airway management', p. 12); call for help from anaesthetic (ICU) and senior colleagues.

Breathing

Check that the child is breathing and observe for spontaneous respiration; if present, give oxygen and continue with assessment; if not, apply an appropriately sized mask and provide bag and mask ventilation with high flow oxygen; again call senior colleagues as soon as possible.

Circulation

Check the pulse. If absent, begin cardiac compressions (15:2); refer to APLS guidelines. If present, assess skin colour, perfusion, heart rate, blood pressure, level of consciousness. If compromised, gain intravenous or intraosseous access (if able and trained to do so) and give 20 ml/kg normal saline by bolus; repeat if necessary. See also 'Shock', p. 342.

General assessment

Observation

When assessing a sick child, some of the most important information will be gained by careful observation:

- Is the child behaving normally for its age?
- How are they responding to their surroundings?

- Are they interested (they should be) or at least appear wary?
- Is the child awake, asleep, drowsy (should they be)?
- Do they smile or interact with you?
- Do infants (approx. 1 year old) recognize strangers and seek comfort from carers?
- Can the irritable child be distracted with a toy (this may be reassuring)?
- Is the child moving normally?

History

With very young children, the available history will come from the parents or carer (although you must remember to involve the patient if they are developmentally able to do so). It is often better to ask the parent or carer about responses to the symptom you might expect rather than the symptom itself, e.g. instead of asking 'Do they have a sore throat?', ask whether the child is dribbling, refusing food, irritable or distressed.

Enquire about past medical and birth history, stage of development and vaccination history (Tables 10.12, 10.13).

Table 10.12 Developmental milestones

Smiles	6–8 weeks
Reaches out for toys	3–4 months
Sits securely unsupported (straight back)	6–8 months
Picks up small object, either rake or pincer	8–9 months
Beginning to chew food with 'lumps'	8–9 months
Walks	12–18 months
Kicks ball, joins two words together	2 years
Climbs stairs, alternate feet per step	3.5 years

Table 10.13 UK vaccination schedule

Age	Vaccine
2 months	Combined: Diphtheria, Tetanus, Pertussis, Polio, *Haemophilus influenzae* type B Pneumococcal
3 months	Combined: Diphtheria, Tetanus, Pertussis, Polio, *Haemophilus influenzae* type B Meningococcal type C
4 months	Combined: Diphtheria, Tetanus, Pertussis, Polio, *Haemophilus influenzae* type B Meningococcal type C Pneumococcal
12 months	Combined: *Haemophilus influenzae* type B, Meningococcal type C
13–15 months	Combined: Measles, Mumps, Rubella (MMR) Pneumococcal
3–4 years	Combined: Diphtheria, Tetanus, Pertussis, Polio
13–18 years	Combined: Tetanus, Pertussis, Polio

Examination

Once you are satisfied with ABC, further assessment for specific causes can take place.

Child-friendly approach

Examine the child on the parent's lap or, if older, on a bed with a parent close by. As above, observation is of crucial importance, particularly in young children. Older children can be examined using a more adult-type approach. The parts of the examination that require minimum cooperation should be performed first; e.g. observation of the chest and auscultation of chest and heart before moving the child for abdominal examination. Uncomfortable procedures, such as examining the ears, should be left to last.

Basics

Check pulse, blood pressure, respiratory rate and temperature (Table 10.14), in addition to more general observations, such as their colour, skin temperature and perfusion. Examine the fontanelle: the average time for fontanelle(s) to close is 18 months, but some can close normally as early as 9 months. If the fontanelle is present, assess whether it is full, sunken or bulging; see Table 10.15 for signs and levels of dehydration.

Table 10.14 Normal values of heart rate and respiratory rate in children

Age	Resting heart rate (b.p.m.)	Respiratory rate (b.p.m.)
Neonate and infant	100–160	40–60
1–5 years	80–120	25–40
6–12 years	60–110	12–24

Table 10.15 Signs, level of dehydration and likely fluid deficit

Level of dehydration	Signs	Fluid deficit (%)
Mild	Dry mucous membranes; complaining of thirst	<5
Moderate	As mild plus tachycardia, sunken eyes and/or fontanelle, loss of skin turgor	5–10
Severe	As moderate plus 'shocked', cool periphery, poor perfusion, altered conscious level	>10

Chest

Observe the child's breathing rate and pattern; look for evidence of chronic chest disease or respiratory distress (e.g. tachypnoea), intercostal or subcostal indrawing, tracheal tug, use of accessory muscles, nasal flaring or expiratory grunt. Nasal discharge is suggestive of a viral URTI. Listen for stridor, wheeze, or cough: the very common paediatric conditions of croup and bronchiolitis have very typical coughs (see p. 339).

Skin

Examine the skin for rashes (and check whether any rash blanches on pressure). Note any signs of inflammation: swelling, bruises or other abnormal marks. Remember to undress the child and take the nappy off if present (often best left until the end of the examination).

Systems

Formal examination techniques and method of systems examination in children vary according to age, and focus on likely pathologies. This is especially so for cardiovascular disease, where congenital rather than acquired diseases (as in adult medicine) predominate.

Common acute presentations

Stridor

The commonest cause of stridor is laryngotracheobronchitis (croup), although in infants congenital causes should also be considered, e.g. laryngomalacia. Following the introduction of haemophilus immunization, epiglottitis is now rare. However, true vaccine failures do occur, and bacterial tracheitis can present in a very similar way; with a stridulous, apparently septic child, with or without drooling. Stridor, due to foreign body inhalation, is of very sudden onset, with no prodrome and either an appropriate history or occurring in an unsupervised child (see 'Ear, nose and throat', p. 308).

Croup

Usually occurs in children aged 1–3 years; it is rare before 6 months and after 5 years. It is viral in aetiology, most commonly due to parainfluenza.

Presentation and assessment

Children usually have a 1–3 day history of URTI symptoms prior to the development of stridor, hoarseness and a characteristic 'barking' cough. Typically, they are miserable with a low-grade fever but do not appear septic or systemically unwell, unlike those with epiglottitis. Try to keep the child settled on the parent's lap with minimal intervention, as they get much worse when upset. Look for signs of respiratory distress (see above). Think about the possibility of impending respiratory failure in a child who becomes sleepy or drowsy with shallow or slowing respiration. Do not examine the throat as it adds little information and can result in sudden airway obstruction, especially in epiglottitis.

Treatment

Airway management is the priority; supportive measures will be adequate in most and intubation is not usually necessary. This will depend on the degree of respiratory distress and level of oxygen saturation:

- severe: marked intercostal recession, tracheal tug, respiratory rate above 40/min or slow with minimal chest wall movement, respiratory failure; intubation may be required, get senior help
- mild/moderate: moderate intercostal recession, tracheal tug, respiratory rate 30–40/min; give oral dexamethasone (150 μg/kg) or prednisolone (1–2 mg/kg) plus humidified oxygen as required
- minimal: little or no intercostal recession, respiratory rate near normal; supportive therapy only.

Children with moderate to severe croup not responding to steroids should be given nebulized adrenaline solution 1:1000 (1 mg/mL), 400 μg/kg (max 5 mg) repeated if necessary after 30 min. Close monitoring thereafter is essential because the effects only last 2–3 h. Rebound can and does occur so consideration should be given to intubation, if necessary.

Cough

Many respiratory problems in children and young people present with cough, often with typical characteristics:

- croup: barking cough
- bronchiolitis: moist cough

- asthma: dry cough ± wheeze
- whooping cough: whoop of sudden inspiration following a spasmodic bout of coughing often associated with cyanosis or facial redness.

Pneumonia and chest infection

Presentation and assessment

Pneumonia and chest infections should be suspected in children with a cough not suggestive of the above diagnoses. Infection may be caused by viruses, atypical organisms such as *Mycoplasma pneumoniae* or bacteria. Clinical features are often similar, with prodromal URTI symptoms followed by breathlessness and cough.

Examine for respiratory distress and focal chest signs such as discrepant air entry, crepitations, wheeze and, in the older child, dullness to percussion. A CXR is justified for those with focal signs and significant respiratory distress. If systemically unwell, investigation should include FBC, inflammatory markers and blood cultures. Throat swabs, ASO or mycoplasma titres may be appropriate.

Treatment

Most children will have a viral infection and should be managed supportively with supplemental oxygen as required, antipyretics (paracetamol or ibuprofen) and fluids (oral, nasogastric or intravenous) as needed. Bacterial pneumonia is relatively uncommon, but if the child is acutely unwell or septic, has radiological collapse or consolidation and/or raised inflammatory markers, antibiotics should be considered.

If community-acquired bacterial infection is suspected, oral amoxicillin should be used (or a macrolide if allergy exists or atypical infection is suspected). Flucloxacillin can be added if *Staph. aureus* is suspected (measles, influenza or cystic fibrosis). Children with severe infection should receive a third-generation cephalosporin intravenously, plus a macrolide if atypical infection is possible.

Wheeze and breathlessness

Wheeze is very common in children whether accompanied by breathlessness or not. The common causes depend on the age of the child. In infants, bronchiolitis is the most common cause, while in older children, asthma is more common. Rarer causes include aspiration, and infective causes such as pneumonia, foreign body inhalation or external compression.

Bronchiolitis

Presentation and assessment

Bronchiolitis is a very common respiratory disease, occurring, most commonly, in infants aged 3–6 months. It presents with poor feeding, cough (paroxysmal, moist and wheezy), irritability, and fever, often preceded by prodromal URTI symptoms with sneezing and runny nose. In those <3 months, it can present with apnoea in the absence of any initial respiratory symptoms.

Bronchiolitis is caused, in 75% cases, by the respiratory syncytial virus (RSV), with peak prevalence in winter. In many infants, the disease is mild, lasting 3–7 days, and can be managed at home. However, hospital admission is required in a significant minority, particularly those with pre-existing medical problems, such as prematurity, cardiac or respiratory conditions.

Examine for basic observations and also for hyperinflation. Auscultation may reveal inspiratory crepitations and expiratory wheeze.

Appropriate investigations include nasopharyngeal aspirate to aid infection control and reduce unnecessary antibiotic treatment. CXR and ABGs are not helpful in mild disease and should only be performed in children with respiratory distress.

Treatment

This is entirely supportive; monitoring of oxygen saturation in those with respiratory distress is advised. Feeding may be a problem due to the increased work of breathing; nasogastric feeding is indicated in this situation and some children will require intravenous fluids. Usually, antibiotics are not required. There is insufficient evidence to justify the use of antivirals, β_2 agonists, anticholinergics, nebulized epinephrine or corticosteroids.

Asthma

Presentation and assessment

Asthma is one of the commonest reasons for admission to hospital in children and young people. In pre-school children, cough may be the only feature of chronic asthma. In infancy and early childhood, viral infection is the commonest trigger for acute exacerbations. Older, school-aged children may have more marked atopic features and/or chronic symptoms, such as exercise-induced cough and wheeze.

The assessment of children with asthma should be according to the British Thoracic Society and SIGN guidelines available on the relevant websites and casualty wall charts. Generally, the assessment is similar to that for adults (see 'Breathlessness', p. 141). However, in children, criteria for moderate and severe asthma are as per Table 10.16.

Table 10.16 Asthma severity

Age	Moderate	Severe
<2 years	SpO_2 ≥92%; audible wheeze; using accessory muscles; still feeding	SpO_2 <92%; cyanosis; respiratory distress; too breathless to feed
2–5 years	SpO_2 ≥92%; no features of severe asthma	SpO_2 ≥92%; heart rate >130/min; respiratory rate >50/min; use of accessory muscles; too breathless to talk or eat
>5 years	SpO_2 ≥92%; PEF ≥50% best or predicted; no features of severe asthma	SpO_2 ≥92%; PEF <50% best or predicted; heart rate >120/min; respiratory rate >30/min; use of accessory muscles

It is worth noting that routine chest X-rays in children should be avoided unless there are other clinical indicators that merit this, e.g. severe asthma or signs of a pneumothorax. Blood gas analysis in children with asthma should be reserved for those patients with a severe exacerbation not responding to treatment.

Treatment

The treatment of children with severe asthma is much as per that for adults (see 'Breathlessness', p. 139). However, note that drug doses vary: hydrocortisone 4 mg/kg IV (where indicated); prednisolone is given in soluble form and in children the oral dose is 10 mg daily for those under 2 years of age; 20 mg daily for those aged 2–5; and 30–40 mg daily for those over 5 years of age. Nebulized salbutamol is usually given in doses of 2.5 mg and where ipratropium is being used the dose is only 0.25 mg. Those with mild to moderate asthma should be treated as follows:

- salbutamol inhaler 2–4 puffs (giving 1 puff every 30 s) via a spacer and mask; repeat every 2 min until stable, increasing the number of puffs given by 2 at every repetition, up to a maximum of 10; repeat again 2–4-hourly
- consider oral prednisolone: dose according to age, as above
- if repeat salbutamol is required within 1 h, treat as severe (see above).

Once acute symptoms are settling think about whether treatment of chronic asthma is needed or changes to their existing treatment are appropriate. Details of the treatment of chronic asthma are given in the BNF for Children, based on British Thoracic Society and SIGN guidelines.

Septicaemia and shock

Septicaemia is one of the commonest causes of shock in acute paediatrics. Others include hypovolaemia as a result of vomiting and diarrhoea and rarer causes such as anaphylactic shock.

Presentation and assessment

A child who is developing shock will have many of the features of the acutely sick child with observations outside quoted normal ranges (see Table 10.14, p. 337). In addition, specific features include decreased skin perfusion: a delay in capillary refill (>2–3 s) and cool, mottled, pale skin. Altered consciousness indicates inadequate perfusion of the brain.

Initial features may be subtle, such as inattention, agitation or irritability. Decreased urine output occurs. Hypotension is usually a late sign and can indicate imminent cardiorespiratory arrest. Also, there may be signs or symptoms attributable to underlying causes of the infection such as pneumonia, urinary tract infection or meningitis.

Immediate general management

Immediate treatment should be given, following BLS and APLS guidelines as discussed briefly above. Shock should be treated with intravenous normal saline, initially 20 mL/kg bolus. Further fluids and early inotropic support should be given, as guided by senior colleagues, or in discussion with your local PICU (see also 'Shock and fluid balance', p. 250).

Meningococcal infection

Meningococcal infection is caused by *Neisseria meningitidis* of 3 subgroups (A, B, and C). Routine immunization now occurs to serotype C, although infection with type B is the most common. The clinical illness can include septicaemia and/or meningitis and is often preceded by a relatively short history of non-specific illness and fever. Unfortunately, the child can progress to meningococcal septicaemia within a matter of hours. Immediate recognition and treatment is required.

Meningococcal septicaemia

On examination, the child will usually have the features of shock, along with the classical non-blanching petechial rash, which may progress to purpuric lesions with skin necrosis. Investigations should include FBC, U&E, LFT, Coag, blood cultures, inflammatory markers and ABG.

Treat initially for shock (as above) and give ceftriaxone (80 mg/kg IV). For an estimate of weight in children aged 1–10 use: weight (kg) = (age in years + 4) × 2.

If the condition is suspected when working in primary care, intravenous or intramuscular penicillin (1.2 g for adults and children over 10 years; 600 mg for a child of 1–9 years; 300 mg for a child under 1 year) should be given prior to immediate transfer to hospital.

Meningococcal meningitis

Although commonly caused by *N. meningitidis*, meningitis can also be caused by pneumonococcus and haemophilus. The latter is now uncommon following the introduction of routine haemophilus vaccination. Before the age of 3 months, group *B* streptococcus and *Listeria* predominate.

Patients frequently have symptoms of URTI or mild febrile illness for 1–3 days prior to developing meningitis. Features are again those of the acutely sick child. However, the young infant in particular may have non-specific features such as poor feeding, irritability or persistent crying. In addition to features of shock, look for evidence of meningism such as neck stiffness, Kernig's and Brudzinski's signs. Infants may have a tense, full fontanelle but neck stiffness is a late sign. They may have an altered conscious level and seizures can occur, either focal or generalized.

Investigations are similar to those for septicaemia above. The diagnosis is confirmed by lumbar puncture; however, this should only be done after discussion with a senior colleague and when there are no contraindications, e.g. abnormal conscious level, focal neurology, features of raised intracranial pressure, abnormal coagulation, and severe uncorrected shock.

Treatment is as for septicaemia. Older children should receive ceftriaxone 80 mg/kg IV. In addition, infants under the age of 3 months should be given ampicillin ± gentamicin or similar, according to your local guideline.

Seizures

Febrile convulsions are common in children and are usually associated with a fever above 39°C. They are rare before the age of 9 months and generally do not occur after the age of 5 years.

Presentation and assessment

Typically, seizures in children are generalized, tonic-clonic in nature, short-lasting and self-terminating. However, they may be prolonged and febrile convulsions are the commonest cause of status epilepticus in children. Despite the most likely cause of a convulsion being fever, other causes must be considered including meningitis, encephalitis, hypoglycaemia, other metabolic abnormality, or underlying structural brain abnormality.

Check the BM. Further investigations should be guided toward excluding meningitis and/or identifying a focus of infection, e.g. UTI, URTI, chest infection. If metabolic disease is suspected, discuss with senior colleagues.

Treatment

Treatment is required where convulsions do not self-terminate after 5–10 min: lorazepam (100 μg/kg IV; max 4 mg). If IV access is not available, buccal or nasal midazolam or rectal diazepam should be used (see BNFC). Treat any fever with paracetamol (15 mg/kg, 6-hourly) ± ibuprofen (5 mg/kg, 8-hourly).

Vomiting and diarrhoea

Presentation and assessment

Vomiting and diarrhoea are non-specific features of many diseases presenting in infants and children, e.g. meningitis, UTI, chest infection or URTI. In the absence of specific features of these illnesses, the child may have infective gastroenteritis, most commonly caused by viral infection (rotavirus). Bacterial gastroenteritis can also occur and should be suspected if blood is present in the stool.

Look for evidence of dehydration and shock (see Table 10.15). Abdominal examination typically reveals a soft, diffuse and mildly tender abdomen with no masses palpable. The presence of other features, either in the abdomen or elsewhere, should immediately raise the possibility of another cause, which in the abdomen includes intussusception, intestinal obstruction and appendicitis. Investigation should include stool samples for identification of viruses and bacterial causes. U&E are appropriate if significant dehydration is present.

Treatment

This should be according to local guidelines and is based on the degree of dehydration:

- mild: water, juice (with sugar) or rehydration solution 5 mL every 5 min; if tolerated progress back to normal fluids
- moderate: oral rehydration fluids (deficit + maintenance) 5 mL every 5 min, increasing volume when tolerated
- severe: IV rehydration after fluid resuscitation as per 'Shock', p. 251, e.g. 0.45% saline + 5% dextrose over 48 h (maintenance + deficit); if sodium is abnormal consult local guidelines or senior colleague.

Abdominal pain

Presentation

Abdominal pain in children is common; infants will cry intermittently and draw their legs up, whereas older children can indicate the area of pain. Abdominal pain may be accompanied by vomiting or diarrhoea. Bilious vomiting and peritonism are late signs in children.

Specific diagnoses to consider in acute abdominal pain include mesenteric adenitis, appendicitis, obstruction, intussusception, gastritis and gastroenteritis. Conditions which cause chronic abdominal pain such as constipation, food intolerance, coeliac disease and colic can present acutely; similarly disease processes outside the abdomen can cause abdominal pain, such as Henoch–Schönlein purpura, pneumonia or diabetic ketoacidosis.

Assessment and treatment

History should include specific enquiry for features suggesting obstruction such as bile-stained vomiting, distended abdomen, presence of blood in any vomit (common in Mallory–Weiss tears, but oesophageal varices do occur in children). Younger children with intussusception initially have abdominal pain with clear vomit or foodstuffs, but go on to develop bilious vomit and later will pass blood-stained 'redcurrant jelly' stools. The presentation of appendicitis is similar to that in adults; see p. 165.

Examination should look for distension, guarding and or rebound tenderness, masses and organomegaly, as well as the presence or absence of bowel sounds.

The management indicated will depend on the underlying cause. Therefore, any child with acute abdominal pain should be discussed at an early stage with a paediatrician and/or a surgeon.

Neonatal jaundice

Jaundice is normal in a term infant who is <2 weeks old. However, if this persists, a pathological cause should be considered. The most important distinction to make is between unconjugated hyperbilirubinaemia as seen in physiological or breast milk jaundice and conjugated hyperbilirubinaemia of biliary atresia or hepatitis.

History should include questions about stool colour (pale stools may indicate biliary obstruction/atresia), feeding pattern, presence of vomiting or the possibility of congenital infection. Investigations vary and local protocols should be consulted, but commonly will include:

- urine for urinalysis, culture and test for galactosaemia
- FBC, blood film, reticulocyte count, blood group and Coombs' test for possible haemolysis
- TFT to exclude hypothyroidism
- congenital infection screen: blood and urine for *Toxoplasma*, rubella and CMV
- others, e.g. tests for cystic fibrosis and α_1-antitrypsin deficiency.

Management should be directed at the underlying cause, but often includes coloured light phototherapy. This reduces serum bilirubin levels and the incidence of serious complications such as chronic bilirubin encephalopathy (kernicterus).

SURGICAL LUMPS

Clinical assessment

When presented with a lump, it is important to take a short history regarding the duration, rate of growth and symptoms associated with the lump, e.g. pain, fever, weight loss, etc. Often, patients will tell you that the lump was only noticed recently despite it being relatively large. This can be for a number of reasons. It may only recently have become painful, the patient may have lost weight making it more obvious or they may have been trying to ignore it subconsciously. After a brief history, examine the lump remembering the eight 'Ss' summarized in Table 10.17.

Table 10.17 The 8 Ss of assessing lumps

Skin	Any changes in the colour or temperature of the skin?
Size	Get an accurate idea of the size using a ruler if necessary
Site	What surrounding structures might the lump be related to?
Surface	Feel for the consistency of the lump and define its margins
Sore	Tenderness suggests an inflammatory aetiology or rapid growth
Stuck	Is the lump fixed to the skin/muscle or surrounding structures?
Sounds	Listen for bruits or bowel sounds
Special	Reducibility, fluctuance, transillumination, other lymph nodes, contralateral side

Common skin lumps

Ganglion

A ganglion is a collection of gelatinous fluid surrounding joints or tendon sheaths. They are caused by the degeneration of fibrous tissue and are usually painless, although they can interfere with tendon function. They are spherical, tense and fixed and are most common around the wrist and foot. They can be left to resolve spontaneously (50% within 5 years), aspirated (around 80% recur) or excised (around 20% recur).

Lipoma

These are formed by the benign growth of fat in the subcutaneous tissues. They can occur anywhere, although they are more common in the upper limbs and upper body, and can be multiple. They are soft, lobulated and freely mobile beneath normal skin. They can also occur in muscles (tensing the muscle makes the lump disappear). They can be removed for cosmetic reasons although reassurance is often all that is necessary. Very large or painful swellings should be removed as they may suggest liposarcoma, although these are rare.

Lymph nodes

Lymphadenopathy is most commonly caused by infection or malignancy. Infective causes include glandular fever, tuberculosis and a variety of common bacteria and viruses. Malignant lymphadenopathy may be primary (see 'Lymphoma', p. 373) or reflect spread from a distant or local tumour.

Clinical assessment

History

Painful lymphadenopathy is usually associated with acute enlargement, most commonly due to infection. Painless, fixed, large nodes or nodes that are matted together strongly suggest malignancy.

Examination

The most common sites are the axilla, groins and neck, and all groups should be palpated. Nodes that feel rubbery, particularly those <1 cm in diameter, are unlikely to be malignant. Examine the region drained by the lymph node group to look for any causative pathology and remember that supraclavicular lymphadenopathy can be caused by lung or upper GI tumours.

Investigation

Consider appropriate blood tests and microbiological samples, as directed by the clinical picture. ENT examination, CXR or GI investigations may also be appropriate, depending on the lymph node group involved.

Ultrasound can be used to characterize lymph node structure (typically abnormal in malignant disease) and direct a biopsy. A tissue diagnosis often requires fine needle aspiration or excision biopsy, which is preferable if lymphoma is suspected.

Moles, melanomas, basal cell carcinomas, seborrhoeic warts

See 'Dermatology', p. 292.

Sebaceous cysts

These arise from sebaceous glands commonly related to hair follicles. They usually occur on the scalp, face, ears, back and scrotum. They are not found on the palms or soles of feet. They are smooth, spherical, tense and attached to the skin. Around half will have a related punctum through which a cheesy material may discharge. Patients notice them when they catch on clothing or become infected. Treatment involves excision, usually under local anaesthetic. Recurrence is common if the entire cyst wall is not removed.

Skin tags

These are pedunculated papillomas or benign overgrowths of skin. They can occur anywhere, forming skin-coloured, warty growths usually on a narrow stalk. Treatment is by simple excision under local anaesthetic.

Hernias

Presentation and assessment

Patients may report discomfort in the groin and an intermittent lump which disappears when they lie down.

Typically the swelling can be reduced into the abdomen. Small hernias are often best examined with the patient standing. Ask the patient to identify the area of concern and attempt to reduce it. Position yourself such that you can place your hand where their hand has been (i.e. usually standing behind them). Once reduced, asking the patient to cough makes the lump either palpable or visible (cough impulse). Small hernias can be difficult to diagnose, so listen carefully to the history.

Strangulation

It is important that strangulation is recognized and managed quickly. Strangulated hernias are irreducible (incarcerated), extremely painful and tender to touch. The skin overlying the hernia may become red, indicating ischaemia of the contents of the hernia and necessitating swift surgical intervention. There may also be features of small bowel obstruction present with abdominal distension, obstructive bowel sounds and vomiting (see 'Acute abdominal pain', p. 165). The risk of strangulation is greater with a femoral hernia than an inguinal hernia and these should be repaired urgently; see below.

Types of hernia and management

Inguinal hernias

Inguinal hernias arise just above the inguinal ligament and may extend into the scrotum. They can be divided into indirect hernias which pass through the internal inguinal ring with the cord structures, or direct hernias which protrude into the inguinal canal through a weakness in the fascia of the anterior abdominal wall. Clinically differentiation between the two types is unreliable and of little relevance since their treatment is the same.

Elective hernias can be repaired by either open or laparoscopic approaches, usually using a mesh repair. Local anaesthetic repair is possible for patients unfit for general anaesthesia.

Femoral hernias

Femoral hernias are less common than inguinal hernias and are more common in women than in men (usually over the age of 50). They arise below and lateral to the pubic tubercle (the opposite of inguinal hernias), although they can bulge up over the inguinal ligament. They are more tense and difficult to reduce than inguinal hernias because the femoral ring is less compliant. This also makes them more at risk of incarceration and so all femoral hernias should be repaired on an urgent basis. Femoral hernias are commonly missed, so always keep the diagnosis in mind when seeing a patient with small bowel obstruction.

Epigastric hernia

An epigastric hernia occurs through a defect in the linea alba anywhere between the umbilicus and the xiphisternum. They are often tense with no cough impulse and can be mistaken for a lipoma. The key to the diagnosis is their position. Patients also complain of pain which can be worse at the time of eating.

Epigastric hernias can be confused with divarication of the recti which is a separation of the rectus muscles seen in children but occasionally persisting into adulthood. It can also occur during pregnancy.

Incisional hernias

The diagnosis of an incisional hernia should be straightforward. They occur at the site of a previous surgical wound and are more common following a wound infection. They are also associated with obesity, steroid use and other factors which suggest impaired healing. Incisional hernias often have a wide neck making strangulation less likely. There is a significant recurrence rate after repair of incisional hernia, so it is important to explain the risk to benefit ratio before surgery is considered.

Umbilical hernias

The most common hernia is a paraumbilical hernia which arises immediately beside the umbilical cicatrix causing the pit to take on a crescentic shape. A true umbilical hernia coming through the centre of the umbilicus is much rarer. They are more common in obesity and should display the features of other hernias, i.e. reducibility and cough impulse. The defect is often small which makes incarceration more likely and, therefore, repair should be advised.

Non-hernia groin lumps

Ectopic testis

An ectopic testicle occurs when there is failure of decent into the scrotum from the embryonic position in the abdomen. Occasionally the testicle can be mobilized into the scrotum in early life but if discovered late it should be removed as there is a 20–40-fold increased risk of testicular malignancy.

Femoral artery aneurysm

This is usually associated with an expansile pulsation in the groin (if you place fingers on either side, they should be pushed apart as well as upward). If found, you should check the opposite side and check other limb pulses. Femoral aneurysms are often bilateral and are associated with an increased incidence of popliteal aneurysms.

Lymph node

See above.

Saphena varix

A saphena varix is caused by swelling of the long saphenous vein over an incompetent sapheno-femoral junction. The swelling is compressible, disappears when the patient lies down and is often associated with obvious varicose veins.

Scrotal lumps

Epididymal cyst

These cystic swellings contain fluid and are related to the epididymis which can be felt separate from the testis. Ultrasound can again be helpful and small cysts are usually painless with reassurance being the only necessary treatment.

Epididymo-orchitis

Epididymo-orchitis is most commonly due to sexually transmitted infections in men under 35 or a urinary tract infection in those over 35. Symptoms include unilateral testicular pain, urethritis or urethral discharge. There may be tenderness of the affected side as well as palpable swelling in the epididymis. The main differential diagnosis is testicular torsion which will often cause more severe pain of sudden onset. Occasionally scrotal exploration will be required to differentiate between the two as testicular salvage requires prompt diagnosis. The diagnosis of epididymo-orchitis requires urine samples for culture and sensitivity. Antibiotic treatment should be started empirically, in addition to analgesia, bed rest and scrotal support.

Hydrocele

A hydrocele is caused by a collection of fluid in the sac surrounding the testicle. This can be primary (no known cause) or secondary to infection, trauma or a testicular tumour. True scrotal swellings can be diagnosed by being able to get above the swelling (as opposed to an inguino-scrotal hernia). A hydrocele will not be separate from the testis and will transilluminate because it is full of fluid. In children, it is related to a patent processus vaginalis which can be tied off, leading to resolution. In adults, it can be treated by surgical drainage and stitching the sac inside out. Scrotal ultrasonography is required preoperatively to exclude a testicular tumour.

Testicular tumour

Any lump related to the testicle should be treated as a tumour until proven otherwise. They are usually painless with a feeling of 'heaviness'. A history of trauma will often be given, but do not let this falsely reassure you. Refer urgently to urology, check β-HCG, α-FP and arrange an ultrasound. Exploration is the definitive investigation. Treatment of testicular cancer is discussed in 'Cancer', p. 369.

Perianal lumps

Abscesses

Abscesses can develop anywhere. In the perianal region the commonest cause is infection in the anal glands. An abscess presents with redness of the skin and is acutely tender to touch. The swelling may be tense or display fluctuance. Incision and drainage is the initial treatment although a fistula should be suspected if the abscess is recurrent.

Haemorrhoids

Haemorrhoids are vascular cushions present in all adults that probably contribute to continence. They can bleed (1st degree) and/or prolapse (2nd degree) and can become thrombosed and permanently prolapsed (3rd degree).

Inspection will reveal purple/red swellings covered by mucosa typically at 3, 7 and 11 o'clock positions. Treatment of symptomatic haemorrhoids includes dietary advice and laxatives for constipation, rubber band ligation or haemorrhoidectomy. Extensively thrombosed and ulcerated haemorrhoids can be mistaken for rectal prolapse or anal carcinoma.

Perianal haematomas

These present as a small, purple, acutely tender, pea-sized lump in the perianal region following an episode of straining. It is caused by a ruptured capillary forming a haematoma. It will resolve spontaneously after a few days or the haematoma can be evacuated under local anaesthetic with rapid relief.

Skin tags

Perianal skin tags are often related to haemorrhoids and may itch or bleed. However, they are frequently asymptomatic requiring no treatment.

Head and neck lumps

See 'Ear, nose and throat', p. 308.

Breast lumps

All patients with new breast lumps should be referred to the breast clinic for 'triple assessment' involving clinical examination, radiological (mammogram or ultrasound) and pathological assessment (FNA or core biopsy). The presentation, detailed assessment and management of breast cancer is discussed in 'Cancer', p. 353.

Clinical examination

Before you examine a breast lump, make the patient comfortable, usually sitting at 45°, and always have a chaperone with you. Inspection for skin changes or any change in the contour of the breast should be performed with the patient's arms by their side and then with hands behind their head. Palpation should cover the four quadrants of the breast and the area behind the nipple. The axilla should also be examined; bring the patient's arm down toward their side to allow access to the apex.

Cancers and palliative care

11

PERFORMANCE STATUS AND QUALITY OF LIFE

Performance status

Performance status is a means of stratifying the functional ability of patients with malignant disease. Drawing on the multiple factors that contribute towards a clinician's overall judgement of a patient, it has been found to be a good predictor of mortality and fitness for therapy. However, it is still largely subjective and can be difficult to interpret in patients with habitually sedentary lifestyles. The two main performance status scales used are the World Health Organization/Eastern Cooperative Oncology Group (WHO/ECOG) and Karnofsky (KPS) scales. Table 11.1 illustrates the WHO/ECOG scale.

Quality of life

Quality of life (QoL) is a multidimensional characteristic of an individual's existence. It encompasses their capacity for physical functioning, their experience of disease and treatment-related symptoms, and their social and psychological well-being. Several tools have been developed to assess quality of life with varying levels of complexity and specificity for specific tumours, e.g. Functional Living Index Cancer (FLIC); European Organisation for Research and Treatment of Cancer Quality of Life Questionnaire (EORTC-QLQ).

In contrast to performance status, quality of life measurements are usually patient self-assessments rather than clinician-performed assessments. Where a cancer cannot be cured it is especially important to evaluate treatments in terms of their impact on overall QoL, rather than whether or not they simply improve control of a specific symptom. Indeed, such treatments can sometimes

Table 11.1 WHO/ECOG performance status scale	
Score	**Status**
0	Normal activity, fully active without restriction
1	Restriction of strenuous activity, can do light work
2	Ambulatory and capable of self-care, but unable to carry out any work activities: up and about >50% of waking hours
3	Capable of limited self-care, confined to bed/chair >50% of waking hours
4	Completely disabled, cannot undertake any self-care, totally confined to bed or chair

reduce QoL, through the development of side-effects or complications. Likewise, it should be remembered that the impact on QoL of any cancer intervention is very patient-dependent.

LUNG CANCER

Epidemiology and aetiology

In the UK, lung cancer is the second most common cause of cancer in men and the third most common cause of cancer in women. Unfortunately, mortality rates have changed little over the past 10 years and lung cancer is now the commonest cause of cancer-related death.

Tobacco smoking is the principal risk factor for the development of lung cancer, and is thought to contribute to 90% of cases. Other risk factors include a family history in a 1st-degree relative, previous chest radiotherapy, cannabis smoking (more carcinogenic than tobacco) and exposure to asbestos, silica (if in the presence of silicosis), polycyclic hydrocarbons, radon and nitrogen oxides. Genetic abnormalities have also been associated with lung cancer, e.g. chromosome 3p21 deletion, mutation of the *p53* gene and altered expression of oncogenes such as c-*erb*-B2 and N-*myc*.

Screening

Symptoms of lung cancer often develop late, and patients commonly present with incurable, metastatic disease. Although lung cancer screening seems logical, the results of recent studies have been disappointing. Plain CXR screening has been shown to be insensitive, while CT is limited by low specificity and a high incidence of false positive pulmonary nodules. Various bio-markers have shown promise, but none has been shown to be sufficiently predictive.

Presentation

Common presentations include a new (or changed) cough, haemoptysis, dyspnoea, chest pain, wheeze, a slow to resolve or non-resolving chest infection, fatigue, weight loss and anorexia. Early symptoms may easily be confused with an exacerbation of chronic lung disease, e.g. COPD, mandating a high index of suspicion, careful examination of the CXR and follow-up to ensure complete resolution of symptoms and radiological changes.

Advanced disease is suggested by arm or facial swelling due to superior vena caval obstruction; hoarseness due to tumour involvement of the recurrent laryngeal nerve; cardiac arrhythmias due to pericardial involvement; fits or limb weakness due to cranial metastases; or bone pain due to metastases or pathological fractures.

A variety of clinical findings may be present, e.g. finger clubbing, lymphadenopathy, wheeze, stridor, lung consolidation or collapse, pleural effusion, signs of organ or bony metastases, anaemia, paraneoplastic neurological syndromes, Horner's syndrome.

Investigation, pathology and staging

Investigation

Investigation priorities are three-fold: obtain a tissue diagnosis, stage the disease accurately and assess the patient's cardiorespiratory fitness and potential operability (see also 'Performance status', p. 349). The majority of patients with lung cancer will have significant smoking-related co-morbidity.

Initial investigations should include CXR, FBC, U&E, LFT, Ca, LDH, oxygen saturation and spirometry (see p. 89). If the CXR is concerning or clinical suspicion persists, these should be followed by urgent CT scanning of chest, liver and adrenals. Isotope bone and CT brain scanning are not performed routinely, but undertaken where there is clinical suspicion of metastatic disease.

Since the majority of lung cancers arise centrally from main or segmental bronchi, a histological diagnosis can be obtained by flexible bronchoscopy. Peripheral lesions (about 20% of cases) should be biopsied percutaneously, under CT guidance. This approach carries a significant risk of pneumothorax and, therefore, adequate lung function is essential (FEV_1 >1 L). Alternative approaches to tissue diagnosis in difficult cases include:

- fine needle aspiration or biopsy of palpable cervical nodes
- transbronchial lung biopsy: under fluoroscopic guidance where FEV_1 >1 L
- transbronchial needle aspiration of mediastinal lymph nodes (TBNA), with or without endobronchial ultrasound (EBUS) guidance
- surgical mediastinoscopy, mediastinotomy, or open lung biopsy
- biopsy of liver metastases.

Pathology

Lung cancer is classified into two main pathological groupings: small cell lung cancer (SCLC) and non-small cell lung cancer (NSCLC). SCLC metastasizes early and is rapidly progressive. NSCLC is further divided into squamous, adenocarcinoma, large cell and undifferentiated NSCLC.

Squamous tumours are more common in older men, often account for cavitating lesions, are slower growing, often appear centrally, but are also usually responsible for Pancoast's syndrome (Horner's syndrome and brachial plexus symptoms secondary to an apical tumour). Adenocarcinomas are found peripherally more often than some other types, more commonly affect women and have a greater potential to metastasize early.

Less common forms of lung cancer include broncho-alveolar carcinoma (probably a variant of NSCLC) and the carcinoid tumours. The latter are often polypoid and benign; however, they have a similar neuroendocrine origin to SCLC and some may show malignant features. Carcinoid syndrome is suggested by flushing, diarrhoea and cough. Primary pleural cancers are usually due to adenocarcinoma or asbestos-associated mesothelioma (thickened lobulated pleura on CT).

Staging

Small cell lung cancer (SCLC)

Staging for SCLC is relatively simple:

- limited disease: contained within one hemi-thorax, including pleural effusion, ipsilateral mediastinal nodes and ipsilateral supraclavicular nodes
- extensive disease: any disease beyond this.

Table 11.2 Staging of NSCLC

Stage	TNM	Description	5-year survival (%)
Ia	T1 N0 M0	Tumour <3 cm and surrounded by normal lung/pleura	75
Ib	T2 N0 M0	Tumour >3 cm or involves a main bronchus (>2 cm away from the carina), the visceral pleura or associated with localized collapse of the adjacent lung	55
IIa	T1 N1 M0	T1 tumour with peribronchial or ipsilateral hilar nodes	50
IIb	T2 N1 M0 T3 N0 M0	T2 tumour with peribronchial or ipsilateral hilar nodes Tumour involves either the chest wall, mediastinal pleura, diaphragm, pericardium or major bronchi within 2 cm of carina or they are associated with collapse of the entire lung distal the lesion; no nodal involvement	40
IIIa	T3 N1 M0 T1–3 N2 M0	T3 tumour with peribronchial or ipsilateral hilar nodes T1–3 tumour with ipsilateral mediastinal or subcarinal nodes	10–35
IIIb	Any T4 N3 disease	Tumour involves the oesophagus, trachea/carina, great vessels or heart, or is associated with a malignant effusion or satellite nodules in the same lobe Involves contralateral hilar or mediastinal and ipsilateral supraclavicular nodes	<5
IV	Any M1	Metastases, including satellite lesions in a separate lobe	<5

Additional markers of an adverse prognosis in SCLC include a low sodium, raised LDH, weight loss and poor performance status.

Non-small cell lung cancer (NSCLC)

The Mountain classification, based on the TNM system, is used. Increasing stage is associated with decreasing 5-year survival (Table 11.2). Patients with stage I and II disease have potentially resectable disease and should be discussed with, or referred to, a cardiothoracic surgeon. Performance status, cardiopulmonary function and the presence of significant weight loss will determine whether the patient is operable.

Survival and management

Lung cancer has one of the worst rates of survival of all cancers: 5-year survival is approximately 7% and many patients die within a few months of diagnosis. Prognosis depends on the type and stage of disease.

Small cell lung cancer treatment

SCLC should be treated with combination chemotherapy, incorporating a platinum-based agent. In limited disease, this is given with curative intent over four cycles. However, the dose and duration of treatment may be limited by performance status and co-morbidity. Only a small proportion of patients will achieve disease remission and, of those, late relapse with cranial metastases is common. Therefore, patients who do achieve an apparently complete response to therapy should be offered consolidative chest radiotherapy and prophylactic cranial radiotherapy to reduce the incidence of relapse.

Non-small cell lung cancer treatment

Surgery

Five-year survival rates of 55–75% can be achieved when the tumour is resectable (stage I or II) and the patient is operable (adequate cardiorespiratory reserve, good performance status, limited co-morbidity). Some centres will also offer surgery to patients with stage IIIa disease after down-staging chemotherapy. Unfortunately, most patients present with irresectable disease (stage IIIb or V) or have other co-morbidities that preclude safe surgical intervention.

Radical radiotherapy

Patients with stage I or II disease, not suitable for surgery due to co-morbidity, should be offered radical radiotherapy. This offers a survival advantage, assuming they have sufficient lung reserve and the total tumour volume (including any lymphadenopathy) can be confined within a sufficiently small radiotherapy field.

Chemotherapy

Platinum-based chemotherapy should be offered to patients with advanced NSCLC (stage IIIb or IV) in whom it can improve symptoms, QoL and survival (usually by a number of months rather than years). Chemotherapy may also be offered to patients with stage IIIb disease in some centres, in an attempt to down-stage the disease and facilitate surgical resection.

Palliative treatment

When active anti-cancer measures are not feasible, due to poor performance status or significant co-morbidity, or as an adjunct to chemotherapy, palliative (low-dose) radiotherapy may improve symptoms such as pain (e.g. from bone metastases), cough and haemoptysis. Patients with brain metastases should be treated with high-dose steroids (e.g. dexamethasone 8 mg PO 12-hourly) and offered cranial radiotherapy if they have a favourable response.

Recent lung collapse due to an obstructing central tumour can sometimes be palliated with endobronchial laser therapy and stenting. Superior vena caval obstruction (SVCO) is a medical emergency requiring urgent radiotherapy. Stenting is sometimes used beforehand to maintain patency until the radiotherapy effect is established. The effect of steroids in SVCO remains debatable.

Associated COPD, anaemia or pleural effusion should be treated. General measures for the management of breathlessness in advanced malignancy are described in 'Palliative care', p. 376.

BREAST CANCER

Epidemiology and aetiology

Breast cancer is the most common cancer in the UK with over 44 000 new cases per year and a life-time risk of the disease in women of 1 in 9. It predominantly affects women over the age of 50 and there is an increased incidence in those with a family history, early menarche and late menopause, nulliparity, a later age of initial child-bearing, use of the oral contraceptive pill or HRT and exposure to chest radiation. There is also an association with alcohol consumption, dietary fat intake, obesity, height and higher social class. Lower incidence is associated with multiple pregnancies, breast-feeding and regular physical exercise.

Certain defective genes are known to be strongly associated with breast cancer, e.g. *BRCA* (BReast CAncer) *1* and *2*. In addition, there are a variety of other genetic factors involved, e.g. over-expression of the epidermal growth factors; amplification of the *myc* oncogene.

Screening

In the UK, women between 50–70 years of age are invited every 3 years for screening by two-view mammography. Those over 70 years of age are not routinely invited, but may request continuing surveillance if they wish.

Presentation

Patients may present through the national screening programme or with local symptoms such as a lump or pain in the breast, discharge from the nipple or skin changes such as tethering or ulceration. Symptoms such as axillary swelling, breathlessness or bony pain are concerning and should prompt exclusion of nodal and metastatic disease (present in about 20% of patients).

Investigation, pathology and staging

Investigation

Patients should be seen in a multidisciplinary breast clinic. This allows clinical assessment by a specialist surgeon, review of relevant breast imaging (ultrasound, mammography) and early tissue sampling, by either aspiration or core biopsy. MRI may be used in some centres or in patients with breast implants, in whom ultrasound is less accurate. Routine haematological and biochemical tests should be checked in all patients. A chest X-ray, liver ultrasound or isotope bone scan should be performed if metastatic disease is suspected.

Pathology

Most breast carcinomas are adenocarcinomas; these are subdivided into in-situ carcinomas, invasive lobular cancers and the more common invasive ductal forms. Other, rarer forms of breast cancer include medullary, mucinous and inflammatory tumours, e.g. peau d'orange carcinomas and Paget's disease of the nipple.

Tumours are graded pathologically into high, intermediate and low grade based on the level of cell differentiation. Oestrogen, progesterone and human epidermal growth factor (HER2) receptor status should also be assessed and used to identify patients for hormone therapy; see below.

Staging

The disease is staged pathologically and requires axilliary node sampling in all but non-invasive cases (stage 0). Staging allows grouping of tumours into early (stage I), locally advanced (stages II and III) and metastatic (stage IV) disease.

- stage 0: non-invasive cancer, i.e. lobular or ductal carcinoma in situ
- stage I: invasive tumours up to 2 cm without further spread
- stage II: invasive tumour 2–5 cm and/or limited axillary node involvement
- stage IIIa: invasive tumour >5 cm or axillary nodes that are clumped together or to surrounding tissue
- stage IIIb: invasive tumour of any size involving skin, chest wall or internal mammary glands, including inflammatory breast carcinoma
- stage IV: metastatic spread.

Survival and management

Combined treatment involving surgery, chemoradiotherapy and hormone treatments achieve 5-year survival rates of around 80% with an estimated 20-year survival rate of about 65%.

Surgery

Surgical resection should be offered to patients with early or locally advanced disease. The operation that is indicated depends on the stage of the disease:

- stage 0: lumpectomy or mastectomy
- stage I: breast-conserving surgery (with counselling of the risk of further surgery if resection margins are not clear) or modified radical mastectomy
- stage II and III: radical mastectomy; patients with large cancers should be considered for neo-adjuvant chemotherapy.

All patients with invasive disease require axillary surgery and should be considered for postoperative radiotherapy. Patients under 70 years of age with early breast cancer should also be considered for adjuvant chemotherapy.

Hormone therapy

All pre-menopausal women with oestrogen receptor positive disease or unknown oestrogen sensitivity and all post-menopausal women should be considered for hormone therapy in the form of tamoxifen. In post-menopausal women this should be changed to an aromatase inhibitor after 2–3 years and such drugs should be first-line hormonal treatment in post-menopausal women with advanced disease.

Chemotherapy

Patients with advanced disease can be considered for chemotherapy, particularly taxane-based. The monoclonal antibody treatment trastuzumab (Herceptin®) may improve survival in those with advanced disease and HER2 positive status, when given in combination with chemotherapy. In pre-menopausal women with advanced disease, the combination of tamoxifen with ovarian ablation can also be used. Bisphosphonates may be helpful for those with bone pain and megestrol acetate may help control hot flushes.

COLORECTAL CANCER

Epidemiology and aetiology

Colorectal cancer is the second most common cancer in the UK, accounting for over 16 000 deaths per year and 10% of all cancer-related deaths. Risk factors include:

- age >50
- a diet rich in red meat and saturated animal fats and deficient in dietary fibre, fresh fruit and vegetables, calcium and folic acid
- colorectal adenomas or longstanding inflammatory bowel disease
- acromegaly
- previous uterosigmoidostomy or radiotherapy
- obesity and a sedentary lifestyle
- smoking and alcohol use
- genetic factors, e.g. germline mutations in DNA repair genes result in hereditary non-polyposis colon cancer (HNPCC) and inactivation of certain tumour suppressor genes, including *APC*, K-*ras* and *p53*, causes familial adenomatous polyposis (FAP).

Environmental risk factors probably account for 80% of sporadic cases. Genetic factors are particularly important in patients with hereditary cancer syndromes.

Presentation

This varies and is particularly dependent on the site of the primary tumour. Left-sided lesions, in the descending colon, commonly present with fresh rectal bleeding and early bowel obstruction. Right-sided tumours, particularly those in the caecum, are more likely to result in symptoms of anaemia (from occult GI blood loss), altered bowel habit and obstruction (which is a late feature). Anorectal tumours commonly cause early bleeding, mucous discharge and tenesmus (a sensation of incomplete bowel emptying). Other general features include colicky lower abdominal pain, weight loss and fatigue. A small proportion of patients present with complications of obstruction and perforation, including acute peritonitis, local abscess or fistula formation.

Clinical examination may be normal, or there may be evidence of anaemia, iron deficiency, recent weight loss or a palpable abdominal mass. Craggy hepatomegaly suggests metastatic disease. Low rectal tumours may be palpable on PR examination which should be performed in all patients in whom the diagnosis is suspected.

Screening

The NHS Bowel Cancer Screening Programme has recently been introduced. Previous randomized controlled trials have shown that faecal occult blood (FOB) testing every 1–2 years, followed by colonoscopy if necessary, can detect early-stage colorectal cancers and reduces mortality by 16%. The UK screening programme offers FOB testing to all patients aged 60–69. Patients are sent FOB testing kits and instructions for their use and are asked to post them back to a central laboratory. Those with positive results are referred for further assessment ± colonoscopy, if indicated.

Investigation, pathology and staging

Investigation

All patients should have routine haematological and biochemical tests, including Coag. Colonoscopy is the investigation of choice, as rigid sigmoidoscopy will detect less than one-third of all colorectal cancers. Colonoscopy also allows tissue sampling for histological confirmation, screening for synchronous lesions and removal of adenomatous polyps. Barium enema is an alternative in very frail patients, but it is less sensitive and non-specific.

Cross-sectional imaging is essential for staging. CT scanning is sufficient in most cases and will demonstrate intra-abdominal nodes and liver metastases if present. However, pelvic MRI or endoanal ultrasound is necessary to stage rectal cancers accurately. Serum carcinoembryonic antigen (CEA) is elevated in some patients at diagnosis, but is not sensitive enough to be used as a screening test. However, where it is high at diagnosis, it can be used to assess treatment response. It is also used to detect early recurrence during follow-up.

Pathology

Approximately 95% of tumours are adenocarcinomas and most result from malignant transformation of an adenomatous polyp; 65% occur in the rectosigmoid; 15% occur in the caecum and ascending colon. Synchronous tumours are found in 2–5% of patients. Colorectal cancers are usually polypoid or circumferential and they spread by invading outwards through the bowel wall; see 'Staging', below.

Staging

Disease stage at diagnosis, using Dukes' classification, is the principal determinant of survival:

- A: tumour confined within the bowel wall
- B: tumour extending through the bowel wall, but not associated with spread to draining lymph nodes or distant metastases
- C: any tumour associated with spread to draining lymph nodes
- D: any tumour associated with distant metastasis.

Survival and management

The 5-year survival rate in patients with Dukes' A, B, C and D disease is >90%, 65%, 30–35% and <5%, respectively.

Surgical resection is potentially curative and should be performed by a specialist colorectal surgeon. The operation required will depend on the site and size of the primary tumour. All resections involve removal of the tumour surrounded by an adequate resection margin and including all draining lymph nodes. A primary anastomosis of the bowel will be performed, if possible, but all patients should be counselled regarding the risk of being left with a stoma. Patients who present acutely with bowel obstruction or peritonitis will usually require a stoma, at least in the short term. However, a secondary anastomosis can often be performed once the acute illness has resolved. Rectal cancers are particularly prone to early recurrence, even after removal of all visible disease. This risk can be reduced and survival improved by the use of total mesorectal excision.

Patients with pathologically staged Dukes' A disease do not require adjuvant therapy after surgery. Those with Dukes' B disease and inadequate resection margins should be offered adjuvant radiotherapy to reduce the chance of local recurrence. Adjuvant chemotherapy with 5-FU improves survival by 4–13% in patients with Dukes' C disease.

Fit patients with Dukes' D disease will sometimes be offered surgery to palliate obstruction, pain or bleeding. However, palliative chemotherapy with 5-FU (and irinotecan as second-line) is the more conventional treatment offered and may provide a survival benefit. Other palliative measures include pelvic radiotherapy, endoscopic laser therapy and stenting for rectal symptoms.

OESOPHAGEAL CANCER

Epidemiology and aetiology

In the UK, oesophageal cancer accounts for about 7000 deaths every year. A number of common risks have also been identified. These include excessive alcohol consumption, smoking, obesity and a poor diet. The following factors are associated with an increased risk:

- age (most patients are >60), male sex (twice as common as females) and a family history
- tobacco smoking and heavy alcohol use, especially if taken together
- gastro-oesophageal reflux disease and its consequence, Barrett's oesophagus (adenocarcinoma)
- obesity, although this may reflect the increased incidence of reflux disease
- dietary nitrosamines, e.g. salted and smoked meats
- previous mediastinal radiotherapy
- coeliac disease (squamous cell carcinoma)
- Plummer–Vinson syndrome (anaemia and oesophageal webbing), tylosis and Howel–Evans syndrome.

Risk reduction has been seen with aspirin or other NSAID use and consumption of fruit and green and yellow vegetables.

Presentation

Symptoms are uncommon in early disease. However, as the tumour enlarges, the patient may present with dysphagia, which may be associated with pain (odynophagia), burning retrosternal discomfort, weight loss, nausea and vomiting, regurgitation of food or haematemesis. Aspiration pneumonia can result from altered oesophageal motility and vomiting. Metastatic disease can lead to presentation with jaundice or respiratory symptoms.

Obvious clinical signs may be absent in many cases, but look for lymphadenopathy, evidence of weight loss and nutritional deficiency and carefully examine the abdomen. Compressive effects in the mediastinum may result in superior vena cava obstruction.

Investigation, pathology and staging

Investigation

Initial investigations should include routine haematological and biochemical blood tests, including LFTs and Coag, and a CXR. Upper GI endoscopy should be performed at an early stage. This allows direct visualization of the tumour and biopsy for histological confirmation and classification. A barium swallow may show an obstructing lesion in the oesophagus, but will need to be followed by endoscopy, unless the patient is extremely frail.

CT scanning of the chest, abdomen and pelvis is routinely performed for staging purposes; see 'Staging', below. This allows identification of metastatic disease and suspicious lymph node masses. Because CT tends to under-stage the disease, endoscopic ultrasound (EUS) is now routinely performed in many centres before treatment decisions are made. Positron emission tomography (PET) is an alternative means of identifying metabolically active lymph node (or other) masses if plain CT imaging and EUS are indeterminate.

Pathology

Most tumours are either adenocarcinomas or squamous cell carcinomas. Small cell carcinomas are uncommon and behave similarly to those originating in lung. Adenocarcinomas most commonly occur distally and are closely associated with reflux disease and Barrett's oesophagus. Squamous cell carcinomas are more common proximally.

Staging

This is based on the TNM stage of the disease and is classified as follows:

- stage I: disease confined to the lamina propria or submucosa (T1 N0 M0)
- stage IIa: disease extends into the muscularis propria (T2 N0 M0) or adventitia (T3 N0 M0), but without nodal or metastatic spread
- stage IIb: T1 or T2 tumour with regional lymph node involvement (T1 or T2 N1 M0)
- stage III: T3 tumour with local lymph node involvement (T3 N1 M0) or any T4 tumour, indicated by local invasion into tissues around the oesophagus, but without distant metastases (T4, any N, M0)
- stage IV; distant metastases, e.g. lung or liver (any T or N plus M1).

Survival and management

Overall 5-year survival is only 6–9%. If the disease in confined to the oesophagus (stage I and IIa disease), oesophagectomy is the treatment of choice, assuming the patient is fit enough. Unfortunately, 5-year survival is disappointing even in these patients (around 30%), but can be improved by the addition of neo-adjuvant chemotherapy with cisplatin or 5-flurouracil (5-FU).

Approximately 70% of patients present with metastatic or locally advanced disease, but palliative treatments may still be worthwhile. These include oesophageal stenting, laser ablation and photodynamic therapy. Palliative radiotherapy can reduce tumour size and improve swallowing, particularly in patients with squamous cell carcinoma, which tends to be radiosensitive.

STOMACH CANCER

Epidemiology and aetiology

The incidence of stomach cancer varies greatly across the world. It is particularly common in Japan, Korea and China, where it is responsible for 11% of all male deaths. In the UK, stomach cancer accounts for about 6000 deaths every year. Risk factors include:

- age >50 and male sex
- *H. pylori*, which leads to chronic atrophic gastritis
- obesity, smoking and alcohol
- a diet rich in nitrosamines, e.g. salted and smoked meats, and deficient in fresh fruit and vegetables
- pernicious anaemia, adenomatous gastric polyps and previous partial gastrectomy
- genetic factors, including mutations in E-cadherin (associated with hereditary diffuse gastric cancer) and *APC* (associated with familial polyposis coli, stomach cancer and other malignancies).

Presentation

The majority of patients present with advanced disease. Common symptoms include weight loss (60%) and dyspepsia (50%). Anorexia and nausea occur in approximately one-third. Presentation with acute GI bleeding or anaemia is less common. Occasionally, early stomach cancers may be found on endoscopy performed for dyspepsia alone.

Clinical examination is often normal, but may reveal signs of anaemia, evidence of weight loss, an epigastric mass or palpable supraclavicular lymphadenopathy (Troisier's sign). Metastatic disease is suggested by jaundice, hepatomegaly or ascites.

Investigation, pathology and staging

Investigation

No sufficiently accurate screening test exists and symptoms are often vague. Therefore, upper GI endoscopy is mandatory in patients with 'alarm' features (weight loss, anaemia, vomiting, haematemesis, malaena, dysphagia or a palpable mass). This allows multiple biopsies and brush cytology to be taken from any visible abnormalities. Endoscopic ultrasound can be used to define the extent of tumour spread through the stomach wall. CT scanning is required for staging. If the disease appears resectable this should be followed by laparoscopy to exclude peritoneal seeding.

Pathology

Some of 50% of tumours develop in the antrum, 20–30% in the body, and 20% in the cardia. Of these, 95% are adenocarcinomas and can be further classified into 'intestinal' and 'diffuse' types. The former is associated with chronic atrophic gastritis and a better prognosis. The latter is often poorly differentiated. Linitis plastica is an uncommon infiltrating, scirrhous cancer which results in a 'leather bottle stomach'.

Staging

This is based on the extent to which the tumour has invaded through the three layers of the stomach wall (mucosa, muscle layer and serosa), the number of local lymph nodes affected and the presence of metastatic disease.

- stage Ia: tumour confined to the mucosa with no abnormal lymph nodes
- stage Ib: tumour confined to the mucosa, but associated with 1–6 local lymph nodes or tumour that extends directly into the muscle layer
- stage II: tumour confined to the mucosa, but associated with 7–15 local lymph nodes; tumour that extends directly into the muscle layer and is associated with 1–6 local lymph nodes, or tumour that has spread directly into the serosa, but without any associated lymphadenopathy
- stage IIIa: tumour that has spread to the muscle layer and is associated with 7–15 local lymph nodes; serosal tumour associated with 1–6 local lymph nodes, or tumour that is invading adjacent structures in the abdomen, but is not associated with any lymphadenopathy
- stage IIIb: serosal tumour associated with 7–15 local lymph nodes
- stage IV: tumour invading adjacent structures and associated with at least one abnormal lymph node; any tumour associated with more than 15 abnormal lymph nodes, or tumour associated with distant metastases.

Survival and management

Overall 5-year survival is <30%, although this improves to 50–60% in patients with early disease who are fit enough for surgery. The operation performed will depend upon the disease stage and the site of the primary tumour. Total gastrectomy and lymphadenectomy will usually be required and proximal tumours involving the oesophagogastric junction may require an additional distal oesophagectomy. A partial gastrectomy may be sufficient for small, distal tumours. There is no evidence that chemotherapy (neo-adjuvant or adjuvant), or postoperative radiotherapy improve survival.

Irresectable, locally advanced disease can be treated with palliative combination chemotherapy, incorporating 5-FU. Endoscopic laser ablation may be used to palliate bleeding or dysphagia. Stenting may improve swallowing in patients with tumours of the cardia.

PANCREATIC CANCER

Epidemiology and aetiology

In the UK, pancreatic cancer accounts for about 7000 deaths every year. It is twice as common in men and is associated with smoking, excessive alcohol consumption, obesity, chronic pancreatitis and increasing age. Around 5–10% of patients have a genetic predisposition, e.g. MEN, hereditary non-polyposis coli or hereditary pancreatitis.

Presentation

The disease classically presents with obstructive jaundice (pale stools/steatorrhoea, dark urine, often associated with severe itch), weight loss and/or epigastric pain radiating to the back. Less common presentations include diarrhoea, vomiting from duodenal obstruction, acute pancreatitis or diabetes mellitus.

Examination may reveal signs of significant weight loss, excoriation marks, an epigastric mass or hepatomegaly. A palpable but non-tender gallbladder in a jaundiced patient is highly suggestive of distal biliary obstruction due to a pancreatic tumour (Courvoisier's sign).

Investigation, pathology and staging

Investigation

LFTs are likely to show an obstructive pattern with a high bilirubin. Routine indices, including a random blood glucose and Coag, should also be checked. Dual-phase, contrast-enhanced spiral CT will show the vast majority of tumours and is essential for staging. Laparoscopy allows histological confirmation and identification of smaller metastases and spread into local vessels. In patients not fit for surgery, ultrasonography, CT-guided biopsy or endoscopic ultrasound-guided FNA can be used to obtain a tissue diagnosis. ERCP is not usually used for diagnosis because of its low sensitivity and the risk that it will precipitate acute pancreatitis. However, ERCP does allow stent placement to relieve obstructive jaundice. CA19-9 is a useful tumour marker measured in some centres.

Pathology

A total of 90% of pancreatic cancers are adenocarcinomas; 70% arise in the head of the pancreas. The disease metastasizes early and the vast majority of patients have metastatic disease at presentation.

Staging

Only 15–20% of patients present with resectable stage I disease. Since there is no mortality benefit from what is extensive abdominal surgery in the remaining 80%, accurate staging is essential.

- stage I: tumour confined to the pancreas without lymph node involvement (stage Ia: tumour <2 cm; stage Ib: tumour >2 cm)
- stage II: tumour extending beyond the pancreas, into the duodenum, bile duct, portal or superior mesenteric vein, but not involving the coeliac axis or superior mesenteric artery (stage IIa); any stage I tumour that is associated with regional lymph node spread (stage IIb)
- stage III: any tumour involving the coeliac axis or superior mesenteric artery irrespective of lymph node status
- stage IV: tumour associated with distant metastasis.

Survival and management

Overall 5-year survival is approximately 3% and median survival is 4–6 months. This is increased to 12–19 months in patients with stage I disease who undergo complete resection and have a 5-year survival rate of 15–20%. 'Complete resection' involves a pancreaticoduodenectomy (Whipple's procedure). There is some evidence of improved survival with adjuvant 5-FU ± gemcitabine, but pancreatic cancer is inherently resistant to most chemotherapy regimes.

For the majority of patients, treatment is focused on palliative measures. Pain can be controlled using opiate analgesia ± coeliac plexus neurolysis, by percutaneous or endoscopic ultrasound-guided alcohol injection. Jaundice and itch can be relieved by choledochojejunostomy, in patients who are fit enough for surgery, or ERCP in others.

OVARIAN CANCER

Epidemiology and aetiology

Ovarian cancer is the commonest gynaecological cancer in the UK, affecting approximately 1 in 70 women and resulting in around 4500 deaths per year. The cause of ovarian cancer is unknown. Increased risk is associated with nulliparity. Conversely, factors that limit the number of ovulations, such as the combined oral contraceptive pill and breast-feeding, are protective. Up to 10% of ovarian cancers are hereditary and associated with a family history of ovarian or breast cancer. The lifetime risk of ovarian cancer among *BRCA* (BReast CAncer) *1* or *2* gene carriers may be up to 7 times that of non-carriers.

Screening

Screening for ovarian cancer, using a combination of clinical examination, pelvic ultrasound and serum CA125 measurement, may be offered to patients with a strong family history of ovarian cancer and/or breast cancer. However, the efficacy (and potential morbidity associated with intervention following a false positive result) is not known and this practice should not be regarded as 'evidence-based'.

Presentation

The survival rate of ovarian cancer is poor due to the majority of patients presenting late with advanced disease. Symptoms are often non-specific and vague and are frequently associated with metastatic disease. Typical symptoms include abdominal distension or bloating, weight gain or loss, anorexia and malaise. Patients may also present with symptoms relating to an ovarian cyst. The risk malignancy index should be applied to determine likelihood of ovarian cancer (see 'Abdominal/pelvic masses', p. 332).

Breathlessness may be related to pleural effusion. Urinary symptoms or DVT may result from local pressure effects. Abnormal vaginal bleeding (usually postmenopausal) is a less common presentation.

A fixed, hard, irregular pelvic mass may be felt on abdominal, vaginal and rectal examination and there may be associated supraclavicular, axillary or inguinal lymphadenopathy.

Investigation, pathology and staging

Investigation

Routine blood tests, serum CA125, chest X-ray and abdominal ultrasound should be followed by CT or MRI of the abdomen and pelvis. Where there is doubt as to the source of the primary, endoscopy of the upper and lower gastrointestinal tract and barium contrast studies may be useful. In younger patients AFP and β-HCG should be measured, as germ cell tumours are the commonest gynaecological malignancy in the first two decades of life.

Pathology

The pathological classification of ovarian tumours and the risk assessment of likely malignancy in ovarian growths are outlined on p. 332.

Staging

Staging is by laparotomy and involves assessment of anatomical spread:

- stage I: disease confined to one or both ovaries (Ic includes the presence of surface disease/ruptured ovarian capsule or malignant ascites/positive peritoneal washings)
- stage II: involvement of one or both ovaries with pelvic structures involved
- stage III: stage I/II with peritoneal implants outside the pelvis or with positive retroperitoneal lymph nodes
- stage IV: involves distant metastases (including liver parenchyma/positive pleural fluid cytology).

Survival and management

Ovarian cancer commonly presents with advanced disease and, as such, curative surgical resection is rarely possible. Tumour debulking is commonly performed, followed by adjuvant combination chemotherapy with paclitaxel and a platinum-based agent. This therapy is associated with a high incidence of side-effects and the overall 5-year survival rate remains poor at 41%. Survival correlates not only to the stage of disease and tumour grade, but also the patient's age at presentation. Recurrent disease may be treated with second-line chemotherapy, secondary cytoreductive surgery or palliative surgery, most frequently indicated for bowel obstruction.

CERVICAL CANCER

Epidemiology and aetiology

Cervical cancer causes about 1300 deaths in the UK per year. The major risk factor for the development of cervical cancer is human papilloma virus (HPV) infection. This far outweighs other known risk factors such as smoking, an early age of onset of sexual activity, increasing number of sexual partners and low socio-economic group. HPV 16 is the most commonly encountered viral subtype.

Screening

In the UK, the NHS Cervical Screening Programme (NHSCSP) was introduced in 1988. Women aged 20–64 (20–60 in Scotland) are screened by a cervical smear test every 3–5 years. The programme has had a dramatic effect, halving the mortality of cervical cancer from the time of its introduction. Patients with mild dyskaryosis should be invited for a repeat smear in 6 months. Those with moderate or severe dyskaryosis, or persistent abnormalities should be referred for colposcopy to exclude invasive cervical carcinoma or its precursor, cervical intraepithelial neoplasia (CIN), which in the vast majority of cases can be treated colposcopically.

Presentation

Cervical cancer is usually asymptomatic in the early stages: invasive and pre-invasive disease may be identified through screening. Early symptoms include post-coital bleeding, inter-menstrual bleeding or offensive vaginal discharge. Advanced disease may present with back pain, dysuria, haematuria, rectal bleeding or lower limb lymphoedema.

Investigation, pathology and staging

Women with abnormal cervical cytology on smear testing should undergo colposcopy, which involves visual assessment of the cervix and allows for the biopsy of suspicious areas under direct vision. Of the cervical malignancies, 85% are squamous or adenosquamous carcinomas, which are associated with a more favourable prognosis than the less common adenocarcinoma. Staging is based on clinical examination, cystoscopy and chest X-ray.

- Stage 0: pre-invasive disease – cervical intraepithelial neoplasia (CIN)
- stage I: tumour confined to the cervix
- stage II: tumour extending into, but not beyond, the upper two-thirds of the vagina or parametrium
- stage III: tumour extending into the lower one-third of the vagina or involving the pelvic sidewall
- stage IV: locally invasive disease involving the bladder or rectum or metastatic disease outside the pelvis.

Survival and management

In patients with micro-invasive stage disease (which is often asymptomatic and discovered through cervical screening), cone biopsy or diathermy excision may be all that is required. For all other stages of disease, surgical resection by radical hysterectomy with pelvic lymphadenectomy is indicated. In some cases of small volume disease, in women wishing to conserve their fertility, trachelectomy (radical excision of the cervix) and pelvic lymphadenectomy may be considered appropriate.

Adjuvant pelvic radiotherapy is used in patients with positive pelvic lymph nodes, or where disease is found at the specimen excision margins. Radical radiotherapy is used for patients unfit for surgery, or those with advanced disease deemed unsuitable for surgery. Further surgery (such as pelvic exenteration), radiotherapy and chemotherapy may all be used as palliative therapies, or in the treatment of recurrent disease.

In women who receive treatment, 5-year survival for microinvasive stage I disease approaches 100%, falling to 70–85% for small volume stage I and II tumours, 50–70% for large volume stages I and II tumours, 30–50% for stage III, and 5–15% for stage IV disease.

ENDOMETRIAL CANCER

Epidemiology and aetiology

The number of deaths per year is similar to that of cervical cancer in the UK (1200/year). High levels and, in particular, high postmenopausal levels of oestrogens are a recognized risk factor for endometrial cancer. Causes include obesity (due to peripheral conversion of oestrogens to androgens in adipose tissue), oestrogen therapy unopposed by progestogens, tamoxifen therapy, late menopause and polycystic ovarian syndrome (PCOS). Genetic factors also appear important and there is an established linked to hereditary non-polyposis colorectal cancer (HNPCC).

Screening

Screening is not useful for endometrial cancer, where early investigation of symptoms, usually vaginal bleeding, is the most appropriate approach.

Presentation

Endometrial cancer usually presents with vaginal bleeding in post-menopausal women. Up to 10% of women with post-menopausal bleeding (PMB) will have an underlying endometrial cancer, with the risk increasing with age.

Investigation, pathology and staging

Investigation

Transvaginal ultrasound scanning (TVS) is the preferred first-line investigation of PMB. If the endometrial thickness is ≤3 mm the probability of malignancy is reduced from 10% to 0.6–0.8%. Endometrial tissue sampling can usually be easily performed as an outpatient examination and allows for reliable histological assessment. Hysteroscopic examination with endometrial curettage should be performed where PMB is associated with tamoxifen use, or where TVS is suspicious of malignant disease (easily treated benign pathology such as endometrial polyps or submucous fibroids). This is increasingly performed as an outpatient procedure without the requirement of a general anaesthetic.

Pathology

A total of 95% of endometrial cancers are adenocarcinomas arising from the endometrium. Other subtypes, such as papillary serous adenocarcinomas and clear cell carcinomas, are more aggressive and are associated with up to 50% of all relapses.

Staging

The staging of endometrial cancer is based on surgical and subsequent pathological findings, although MRI may be used preoperatively to assess myometrial invasion and the presence of nodal disease. Renal tract ultrasound or IVU should be performed if there is a clinical suspicion of ureteric or bladder involvement.

- stage I: tumour confined to corpus
- stage II: tumour confined to corpus and cervix
- stage III: tumour spread beyond corpus but not outside pelvis; may include pelvic or para-aortic lymph nodes
- stage IV: bladder or rectal involvement or distant metastases.

Survival and management

The majority of endometrial cancers present at an early stage: this is reflected in an overall 5-year survival rate of 75%. Curative surgical resection is usually possible by total abdominal hysterectomy and bilateral salpingo-oophorectomy. Adjuvant radiotherapy may be offered to patients based on the stage and grade of disease. Progestogen therapy is not recommended for women who have undergone surgery for early-stage disease, as it does not improve overall survival; it may, however, have a role in those unfit for surgery, or with advanced disease. The role of chemotherapy is limited to palliation for women with advanced or recurrent disease.

PROSTATE CANCER

Epidemiology and aetiology

In British men, prostate cancer is the commonest form of malignancy and the second most common cause of cancer-related death. The majority of cases are diagnosed in patients over the age of 70. The risk of developing prostate cancer is increased in those with a family history affecting a 1st-degree relative, especially if the relative was diagnosed before the age of 60. This may be related to inheritance of a recessive or X-linked gene, although this has yet to be identified. The risk is also increased in men of white African or black Caribbean origin and patients with a high dietary fat intake. A lycopene-rich diet (e.g. tomatoes) may be protective and diabetes mellitus is also associated with a lower risk of the disease, possibly because of lower testosterone levels.

Screening

Population screening for prostate cancer is not routine. In part, this reflects the limitations of the blood test most commonly used to identify disease, prostate specific antigen (PSA). About two-thirds of those with raised levels will not have prostate cancer and 20% of those with the disease do not have raised levels. There is also considerable inter-laboratory variation in testing and biological variation related to age and other factors. Other bio-markers are being evaluated, but, as yet, none has proven sufficiently reliable.

Presentation

Prostatic enlargement can cause urinary symptoms with urinary retention or reduction of flow, frequency, incontinence or dysuria. However, these are not ubiquitous and the patient may present with bony metastases, e.g. back pain, sclerotic lesions, sciatica secondary to vertebral collapse. Marrow infiltration may also cause recurrent anaemia and fatigue.

Clinically, a firm nodular immobile mass may be felt on rectal examination and there may also be supraclavicular lymphadenopathy or hepatomegaly.

Investigation, pathology and staging

Investigation

Check PSA, but be aware that it may be falsely elevated after digital examination of the prostate and should never be considered diagnostic of prostate cancer in isolation. A trans-rectal ultrasound-guided biopsy (TRUS) is required for histological confirmation. CT is used to assess local and distant spread. A raised alkaline phosphatase suggests bone metastases and should prompt further assessment with radio-isotope bone scan, CT or MRI.

Pathology

Prostate cancer is an adenocarcinoma which usually arises in the posterior lobe of the prostate and spreads through local structures such as the rectum.

Staging

Prostate cancer is staged anatomically and pathologically.

Anatomical staging

This follows the TNM classification. The most important distinction to make is between tumours that are confined to, or have spread beyond, the prostate gland.

- early disease includes T1 and T2 tumours which remain confined within the prostatic capsule
- locally advanced disease describes T3 and T4 tumours which have invaded beyond the capsule; these may, or may not, be associated with nodal spread or distant metastases.

Pathological staging

The Gleason system scores the microscopic appearance of the cancer from 2 to 10, with higher scores being associated with less well differentiated tumours and a poorer prognosis. The score is most reliable when used to assess large prostatectomy samples following surgery.

Gleason scoring of the smaller biopsies obtained via TRUS are less reliable, particularly those with lower scores. However, useful early prognostic information can be gained when the Gleason score of a TRUS biopsy sample is 6 (well differentiated), 7 (moderately differentiated) or 8 (poorly differentiated).

Survival and management

The 5-year survival rate is approximately 70%. Patients with early disease, a low PSA and low Gleason score can be curatively managed by either radical prostatectomy or radical radiotherapy, assuming they are fit. Both prostatectomy and radical radiotherapy are associated with complications, including incontinence, impotence, urethral stricture and urethral fistula. Patients who proceed to prostatectomy and are found to have more advanced disease than was expected benefit from anti-androgens or, occasionally, bilateral orchidectomy.

In patients over 70 years, observation, serial PSA measurement and repeat biopsy is sometimes justified on the basis of the slow disease progression expected, the paucity of symptoms that usually result from the condition and the likelihood of death from other co-morbidity.

Those with locally advanced disease are managed with radiotherapy, preceded by anti-androgens, e.g. cyproterone acetate. Long-term treatment is given by depot injection of LHRH analogues, e.g. goserelin. Serial PSA monitoring may predict the development of metastatic disease before symptoms develop.

In those with metastatic disease, temporary disease control can be achieved by hormone treatment followed by chemotherapy (e.g. docetaxel) in fitter patients. Bone pain from metastases may respond to bisphosphonates (e.g. zoledronic acid), which also reduce the risk of fracture and vertebral collapse, but do not alter survival.

BLADDER CANCER

Epidemiology and aetiology

Bladder cancer accounts for just under 5000 deaths per year in the UK. It is more common in smokers and in those exposed to aniline dyes and polycyclic hydrocarbons.

Presentation

Bladder cancer usually presents with painless haematuria. Other symptoms may include dysuria, frequency or incomplete voiding.

Investigation, pathology and staging

Investigation

The key diagnostic test is cystoscopy. Urine cytology is highly specific but relatively insensitive. Urinary markers, such as bladder tumour associated antigen and nuclear matrix protein, are more sensitive but lack sufficient specificity to replace cystoscopy. An IVU or CT urogram is used to assess the renal outflow tract and staging of the tumour is by a combination of US, CT or MRI ± isotope bone scanning.

Pathology

Transitional cell tumours are the most common type of bladder cancer (90%). Others include squamous carcinoma (5%) and adenocarcinoma (2%).

Staging

Staging is based on the extent of tumour involvement of the bladder wall (Tis = in situ; Ta = epithelial; T1 = lamina propria; T2 = superficial muscle, T3 = deep muscle ± perivesical fat; T4 = prostate or adjacent muscle) and differentiation of the tumour.

Survival and management

About 80% of bladder cancers are confined to the detrusor muscle at diagnosis. After local treatment (see below), 70% of these will recur within 2 years; however, they are unlikely to invade the deeper muscle layers. For this reason, bladder cancers were previously referred to as 'bladder warts'. Survival is much better than for some other cancer types and approximately 80–90% of patients with superficial tumours will be alive after 5 years. However, in those with disease invading muscle, the 5-year survival rate is <50%.

Superficial tumours

Many transitional cell cancers can be treated locally at the time of cystoscopy but close follow-up with regular cystoscopy is necessary. Bacille Calmette-Guérin (BCG) immunotherapy should be offered to patients with early superficial tumours and those with carcinoma in situ on biopsy. In the latter, it may reduce the rate of progression to invasive carcinoma, although this is still seen in 50% and regular follow-up by cystoscopy is necessary.

Advanced disease

Bladder resection and/or radiotherapy should be considered. Recurrence after surgery alone is approximately 15% and after radiotherapy alone can be up to 50%. However, this must be offset against the operative mortality risk of cystectomy (5%). Neo-adjuvant radiotherapy has no benefit, but adjuvant chemotherapy may have a role. Palliative radiotherapy is used in those with metastatic disease.

RENAL CANCER

Epidemiology and aetiology

Approximately 7000 new cases of renal cancer occur each year in the UK. The disease is more common in males (2:1) and in those over 50. Known risk factors include smoking, a family history of kidney or thyroid cancer, obesity and exposure to asbestos or cadmium. There is an increased incidence in von Hippel–Lindau syndrome. Wilm's nephroblastoma is an uncommon form of renal cancer that presents in childhood.

Presentation

Renal cancers most commonly present with haematuria, flank pain and/or a loin mass. A significant proportion are discovered incidentally on abdominal imaging organized for another reason. Less common clinical features include PUO, hypertension, polycythaemia (erythropoietin production) and hypercalcaemia (PTH-like hormone production). About 30% of patients present with metastatic disease, which may be widespread and often includes cannonball lung lesions.

Investigation, pathology and staging

Investigation

Routine blood tests, including FBC, ESR, U&E, LFT and Ca^{2+}, should be checked in all patients. Contrast-enhanced CT scanning allows differentiation between cystic and solid lesions and provides essential staging information regarding lymph node, renal vein and IVC involvement. Ultrasound can be useful in assessing possible cystic masses if CT is indeterminate. IVU is not used routinely because of its low sensitivity and specificity.

Renal arteriography was previously used routinely to determine the involvement of vascular structures prior to surgery. This has now been largely superseded by MR angiography or inferior venacavography. Radio-isotope bone scanning should be performed if bony metastases are suspected clinically.

Most renal cancers are deemed surgical or non-surgical based on imaging alone and a histological diagnosis may not be made until after resection. If a tissue diagnosis is felt necessary preoperatively or in patients not fit for surgery, a percutaneous biopsy may be attempted using US or CT guidance.

Pathology

Renal carcinomas can be classified into clear cell (80–90%), papillary (10–15%) and chromophobe (4–5%) and graded using the Fuhrman nuclear grading system. They may extend into the renal vein and inferior vena cava.

Staging

Anatomical staging is based on radiological appearances:

- stage I: tumour confined to the capsule of the kidney
- stage II: tumour invading into the perinephric fat but not Gerota's fascia
- stage III: tumour that has spread into the renal vein or inferior vena cava (IIIa), regional lymph nodes (IIIb) or both (IIIc)
- stage IV: tumour invading adjacent structures or distant organs.

Survival and management

Renal cancers discovered incidentally usually have a better prognosis. Overall, 5-year survival is around 50% but this is largely dependent on stage. The 5-year survival rates in stage I, II, III and IV disease are 94%, 79%, 12–25% and <20%, respectively.

Radical nephrectomy should be offered to all patients with disease confined to the kidney, who are fit enough. This involves removal of the perinephric fat, regional lymph nodes and any involved vascular structures. Palliative nephrectomy with adjuvant immunotherapy (with interferon or interleukin-2) improves survival and symptoms in fit patients with metastatic disease.

Radiotherapy should be offered as the primary treatment modality in patients who are not fit enough for surgery.

Renal cancers are generally poorly responsive to chemotherapy. Therefore, immunotherapy (e.g. interferon and IL-2, above) and biological agents have been developed and trialled with some success. New oral multi-targeted tyrosine kinase inhibitors, e.g. sunitinib and sorafenib, may be useful in metastatic disease.

The lungs are the commonest site of metastasis (cannonball), but these lesions can also be resected. Patients with bony metastases should be offered palliative radiotherapy.

TESTICULAR CANCER

Epidemiology and aetiology

About 2000 new cases of testicular cancer occur in the UK each year. Approximately 1 in 500 men aged 15–50 will develop the disease. It is more common in affluent social classes and Caucasians. Risk factors include a positive family history and fertility disorders, orchitis and a history of undescended testes.

Presentation

Patients most commonly present with a painless testicular swelling. This may described as 'a heaviness' and there may be a history of minor trauma, which should not dissuade you from the diagnosis. Less common modes of presentation include gynaecomastia (β-HCG production) or symptoms of metastatic disease, e.g. seminomas commonly spread to para-aortic nodes and cause back pain; teratomas are more likely to spread haematogenously, resulting in lung, liver, bone or brain metastases.

Investigation, pathology and staging

Investigation

Ultrasound should be used to define the nature of any testicular swelling. This should be followed by chest and abdominal CT if there is no evidence of a non-malignant cause, e.g. hydrocele, epididymitis. Tumour markers can be useful in staging and measuring response to treatment: β-HCG is produced by trophoblastic elements in seminomas and teratomas; α-FP is not found in seminomas but produced by yolksac elements.

Histological diagnosis is made at orchidectomy; see below. Preoperative tissue sampling is not advised because of a risk of malignant seeding if the mass is malignant.

Pathology

Testicular cancers can be classified into seminomas (40%) and teratomas (50%). Lymphomas are the most common form in men >50 years of age, but are rare below this age.

Staging

Staging uses CT, CXR and tumour markers to assess spread.

- stage 1: limited to the testicle (stage 1M: tumour marker rises after surgery)
- stage 2: spread to abdominal nodes; subclassification by largest lymph node size (a <2cm, b 2–5cm, c >5cm)
- stage 3: extra-abdominal nodes
- stage 4: extra-lymphatic metastasis (L1 = 3 lung metastases; L2 = 3 pulmonary nodules; L3 = 3 lung metastases greater than 1 or 2cm; H+ = liver metastases).

Survival and management

The 5-year survival rate exceeds 95% in patients with stage I disease. Therefore, early detection by regular self-examination is of paramount importance. Treatment is by radical inguinal orchidectomy (testicular conservation may be possible in those with tumours under 2cm). Indications for adjuvant therapy will depend on the histology of the orchidectomy sample.

Patients with stage I–IIb seminomas should receive infradiaphragmatic lymph node radiotherapy. In patients with large volume disease, combination chemotherapy may be more effective than radiotherapy alone. Those with stage 2c or greater are offered chemotherapy. Teratomas are not radiosensitive and patients with stage 2 disease or above are offered combination chemotherapy.

A subset of patients are predisposed to invasive carcinoma, e.g. maldescent, atrophy or age <30, and a biopsy of the contralateral testicle may reveal intratubular germ-cell neoplasia. Additional irradiation is required to reduce the risk of progression to invasive disease and sperm storage should be offered prior to therapy.

LEUKAEMIA

Epidemiology and aetiology

There are approximately 7000 new cases of leukaemia per year in the UK and 4300 deaths. Acute leukaemia is less common than chronic leukaemia and lymphoblastic forms predominate. Of these, acute lymphoblastic leukaemia (ALL) is commonest among children while chronic lymphoblastic leukaemia (CLL) is most common amongst males over the age of 50.

Specific chromosomal mutations are associated with the leukaemias. The Philadelphia chromosome results from a translocation between chromosomes 9 and 22. The chimeric gene (*bcr–abl*) is produced and codes for a 210kDa protein with tyrosine kinase activity that results in increased cell division and inhibited DNA repair.

A total of 95% of patients with chronic myeloid leukaemia (CML) have the Philadelphia chromosome. The Philadelphia chromosome may be present in ALL (25–30% of adults; 2–10% of children) and rarely in acute myeloid leukaemia (AML).

Presentation

Presentation varies according to the type of disease. Acute leukaemias are characterized by the accumulation of immature precursors in the bone marrow. This leads to bone marrow failure with resultant anaemia, recurrent and severe infection and/or signs of thrombocytopenia, e.g. petechial rashes, excessive bruising, mucosal bleeding.

Chronic forms may also present with bone marrow failure, but are often detected incidentally after a routine blood test reveals a raised WBC. Other symptoms, which predominate in chronic forms of the disease, but may also affect those with acute leukaemia, include:

- fever, lethargy, night sweats and other flu-like symptoms
- weakness, fatigue, dizziness, nausea or diarrhoea
- hepatomegaly and splenomegaly
- bone or joint pain.

Investigation and pathology

Investigation

Initial investigations should include FBC (with differential WBC), Coag, ESR, U&E, LFT, LDH and calcium. The white cell count is often increased, but may be normal or low. Anaemia and thrombocytopenia suggest extensive bone marrow involvement. Check folate, B_{12} and ferritin, reticulocyte count and a direct Coombs' test. A baseline ECG should be performed along with a CXR (to identify intrathoracic lymphadenopathy).

Further investigation by bone marrow aspiration and trephine will allow microscopic evaluation of bone marrow cells and structure. Specific cells may be seen within the bone marrow of patients with leukaemia. In AML, Auer rods are seen in the cytoplasm of blast cells and are diagnostic.

In addition, blood or bone marrow samples should be sent for cytogenetics and immunophenotyping. This permits further categorization of the cancer and can be used to determine appropriate therapy. Investigations that contribute to staging include LP, CT and MRI. If cardiotoxic chemotherapeutic agents are being considered, echocardiography may be necessary to assess baseline cardiac function.

Pathology

Leukaemias are classified based on the cell line involved:

- lymphocytes: lymphoblastic (also known as lymphocytic) leukaemia
- myelocytes (precursor granulocytic white cells): myeloid (also known as myelogenous) leukaemia.

Further classification is dependent on the cell type, size and level of maturity and differs for each form of leukaemia.

Survival and management

The prognosis of patients with leukaemia, and the need for treatment, varies greatly and is dependent on the type of disease they have. The acute leukaemias tend to be more aggressive, although they are also more sensitive to therapy and cure may be possible.

Acute leukaemia

The potentially curative chemotherapeutic regimes available result in significant bone marrow suppression and side-effects. Patients require hospitalization, isolation and, where appropriate, antibiotic/antifungal prophylaxis and blood product transfusion (red cell concentrate and platelets). In some cases, treatment with granulocyte colony stimulating factor (G-CSF) allows more rapid recovery from neutropenia and a shorter hospital stay.

'Induction' chemotherapy aims to achieve 'complete remission'. However, achieving this simply means that no disease can be detected with the available assessment methods. With no further treatment, most patients would eventually relapse.

Acute lymphoblastic leukaemia

- induction chemotherapy: the agents used will depend on local protocol or relevant clinical trials; there may be accompanying steroids, allopurinol and folinic acid
- consolidation therapy: 4–8 months in children; 1–3 months in adults
- CNS prophylaxis: children with T-cell leukaemia, high WBC or CSF leukaemic cells; either cranial irradiation supplemented by intrathecal (IT) methotrexate, high-dose systemic methotrexate or IT chemotherapy
- maintenance therapy or progression to bone marrow transplant depends on the type of ALL and the age of the patient.

The 5-year survival rate is 85% in children and 40% in adults. Prognosis is poorer in patients with certain cytogenetic abnormalities, e.g. the Philadelphia chromosome (see above), abnormalities on the short arm of chromosome 11, and those with a high WBC count (>100 000/mm^3).

Acute myeloid leukaemia

Many different chemotherapeutic plans are available for the treatment of AML. Treatment begins with induction chemotherapy and appropriate supportive therapy. In contrast to ALL, about 15% of patients have resistant disease and further induction therapy may be required with alternative chemotherapeutic agents.

Post-remission therapy is individualized according to the patient's prognostic factors and their general health:

- low-risk patients (e.g. low-risk tumour cytogenetics) only require an additional course of consolidation chemotherapy; 5-year survival 76%
- intermediate-risk patients (e.g. those with normal cytogenetics): further treatment is tailored to the patient and ranges from single additional course consolidation chemotherapy to bone marrow transplantation; 5-year survival 48%
- high-risk patients (e.g. high-risk cytogenetics or underlying MDS): allogenic stem cell transplantation is recommended if the patient is likely to tolerate the transplant and an appropriate donor can be found; 5-year survival 21%.

Despite aggressive therapy, only 20–30% of patients enjoy long-term disease-free survival. Relapsed AML treatment includes stem cell transplant and novel therapies including monoclonal antibody-linked cytotoxic agents. Prognosis for relapsed AML is poor.

Chronic leukaemia

Chronic myeloid leukaemia

Young patients may be considered for allogeneic bone marrow transplantation, although the transplant-related mortality is high. Tyrosine kinase inhibitors such as imatinib (Gleevec®) specifically target the activated fusion protein with tyrosine kinase activity coded for by the Philadelphia chromosome (see above).

Prognosis for those receiving specific tyrosine kinase inhibitors is good, with reports of over 80% 5-year survival.

Chronic lymphoblastic leukaemia

CLL is largely incurable; however, it tends to progress slowly in most cases and, therefore, many patients will not require therapy. In these patients, a 'watch and wait' approach is adopted and 5-year survival is 75%.

Older patients with more advanced disease may benefit from chemotherapy, as do young patients who are experiencing symptoms. Other treatment options include radiotherapy, splenectomy and, in young patients, bone marrow transplantation. Specific indications for treatment include:

- anaemia or thrombocytopenia
- progression to a later stage of disease
- painful splenomegaly or lymphadenopathy
- lymphocyte doubling time of <12 months.

LYMPHOMA

Epidemiology and aetiology

Lymphoma is more prevalent and results in a greater number of deaths than leukaemia. Non-Hodgkin's lymphoma (NHL) accounts for approximately 10 000 cases/year in the UK and 4500 deaths. The incidence of NHL is highest in patients aged over 50. In contrast, Hodgkin's disease (HD) is less common (approx. 1500 cases and 300 deaths/year) and tends to affect younger patients (aged between 15 and 40).

Presentation

Patients with HD and NHL often present with lymphadenopathy. They may also describe fatigue, itch (due to eosinophilia) or systemic 'B' symptoms, such as night sweats, weight loss and fever. If there is bone marrow involvement, there may be evidence of anaemia, recurrent infection or thrombocytopenia.

In HD, cervical and supraclavicular nodes are most commonly involved (80–90%) and about one-third of patients describe systemic symptoms. Rarely, they also describe lymph node pain after alcohol consumption. On examination, 30% will have splenomegaly; hepatomegaly may occur, but is less common.

Patients with NHL may also present with lymphadenopathy, although it is less likely to be confined to a single area. Intrathoracic or intra-abdominal lymphadenopathy may result in symptoms such as shortness of breath, chest pain, cough, abdominal pain or leg oedema.

Investigation, pathology and staging

Investigation

Initial investigations should include blood tests for FBC (with differential WBC), Coag, ESR, U&E, LFT, LDH and calcium, and a CXR (to identify intrathoracic lymphadenopathy).

Lymph node biopsy is essential for histological diagnosis. In many cases, this can be taken from a palpable node under local anaesthetic. However, mediastinoscopy, laparoscopy or CT-guided biopsy may be necessary.

A CT scan of the neck, chest, abdomen and pelvis is required for staging MRI and PET scanning may also be useful. Since some of the chemotherapeutic agents are cardiotoxic, a baseline echocardiogram should be performed. If CNS involvement is suspected clinically, an LP should be performed.

Bone marrow sampling should be performed in all patients with NHL and those with HD in whom marrow infiltration is suspected clinically. Other investigations that should be performed in suspected NHL include:

- immunophenotyping of surface antigens: distinguishes T or B cell lineage
- immunoglobulins: some lymphomas are associated with IgG or IgM paraproteins

- uric acid measurement: high levels are associated with an increased risk of tumour lysis syndrome when treatment is started; see below
- HIV testing: should be considered if appropriate risk factors are present (see 'HIV testing', p. 414).

Pathology

Several classification systems exist for lymphoma. They may be classified by grade and range from aggressive (high-grade) tumours to indolent (low-grade) tumours. In addition, they may be classified by cell type and size, as well as whether they are diffuse or follicular. The most commonly used classification system is the WHO classification that separates lymphoma into HD (characterized by Reed–Sternberg cells) and NHL which includes a variety of subclassifications, e.g. mature B cell neoplasms, mature T cell and natural killer (NK) cell neoplasms, immunodeficiency-associated lymphoproliferative disorders.

Staging

The staging of both HD and NHL is based on the Ann Arbor classification system which considers the number of lymph node regions involved and their relative positions:

- stage I: a single lymph node region (I), or a single extralymphatic site (Ie)
- stage II: two or more node regions on the same side of the diaphragm (II), or one lymph node region and a contiguous extralymphatic site (IIe)
- stage III: two or more node regions on opposite sides of the diaphragm, which may include the spleen (IIIs) and/or limited contiguous extralymphatic organs (IIIe) or sites (IIIes)
- stage IV: disseminated involvement of one or more extralymphatic organs.

Further classification is made by the absence (A) or presence (B) of systemic symptoms (see p. 374).

Survival and management

Hodgkin's disease

Treatment options depend on disease stage. Early disease may be treated with radiotherapy alone although the choice depends on the age, sex, disease bulk and histological subtype. The dose to normal tissues can be limited and fertility is usually preserved. Over 90% of patients with stage IA are cured by radiotherapy alone. Females who receive breast irradiation during treatment are at an increased risk of breast cancer.

Treatment options in more advanced disease include combination chemotherapy with or without radiotherapy. Common combination chemotherapy regimes include ABVD (adriamycin® (doxorubicin), bleomycin, vinblastine and dacarbazine) and ChIVPP (chlorambucil, vinblastine, procarbazine, prednisolone). 70% of patients who require chemotherapy are cured, although the 15% of patients who do not respond to initial chemotherapy have a poor prognosis.

Non-Hodgkin's lymphoma

Treatment will depend on the stage of disease, the histological type of disease, whether it is indolent or aggressive, as well as the age and general health of the patient. Initial treatment for the majority of patients will be chemotherapy. CHOP is the commonest combination therapy used and stands for cyclophosphamide, hydroxydaunorubicin (doxorubicin), Oncovin® (vincristine) and prednisolone. Doxorubicin is cardiotoxic and, therefore, patients with cardiovascular disease are given modified combination treatment referred to as COP or CVP. Where the histological type is B cell in origin, rituximab (a monoclonal antibody) is added to the therapy (R-CHOP).

Although combination therapy is often well tolerated, side-effects include nausea and vomiting, haemorrhagic cystitis and alopecia. Neutropenia is common by the second week of treatment and prophylactic antibiotics and antifungals should be prescribed along with suitable mouth care.

The rapid breakdown of cells can lead to tumour lysis syndrome, which can result in hyperkalaemia, hyperphosphataemia, hyperuricaemia, hypocalaemia and acute renal failure. Patients are prescribed allopurinol PO or IV, depending on the risk (according to tumour type and chemotherapeutic agents) and appropriate fluid hydration.

Localized disease may be amenable to treatment with radiotherapy. In particular, where there is evidence of CNS involvement, cranial radiotherapy is given along with intrathecal chemotherapy. Haematopoietic stem cell transplantation or bone marrow transplantation may be considered in patients with disease recurrence.

Prognosis depends on the stage and type of disease. Indolent disease is generally not curable, but is typically slowly progressive and responds temporarily to therapy. Aggressive NHLs are potentially curable with combination chemotherapy. Diffuse large B cell lymphoma is the most common type of lymphoma that is considered curable: if there is complete remission for 3 years, the patient is considered cured.

MYELOMA

Epidemiology and aetiology

There are 3800 new cases of multiple myeloma and 2400 deaths per year, with the majority occurring in patients over the age of 50.

Presentation

Patients classically present with bone pain secondary to fractures, vertebral collapse, or hypercalcaemia with or without evidence of bone marrow failure. In addition, they may have evidence of renal failure secondary to paraprotein deposition, hypercalcaemia, infection, NSAID use, amyloidosis or dehydration. Hyperviscosity syndrome may manifest as a retinal bleed, bruising, heart failure or cerebral ischaemia.

Investigation, pathology and staging

Investigation

To make a diagnosis, two of the following criteria must be met:

- malignant plasma cells in the bone marrow
- serum/urinary paraprotein band
- skeletal lesions.

Initial investigations should include blood tests for FBC, Coag, ESR, U&E, LFT, LDH, calcium and albumin. A skeletal survey should be performed (CXR, skull and long bone X-rays) to look for lytic lesions. In addition, X-rays of painful bony areas should be performed to look for evidence of fractures.

Blood and urine should be sent for electrophoresis, in particular Bence Jones proteinuria (see below). If a paraprotein is identified, immunoelectrophoresis can determine the type and amount of paraprotein. The degree of immune paresis can be determined by measuring plasma immunoglobulins.

Bone marrow aspiration and trephine are used to assess the degree of infiltration. If there is evidence of spinal pathology, an MRI spine should be performed. In addition, serum β_2-microglobulin estimation may provide useful prognostic information.

Pathology

Monoclonal proliferation of plasma cells results in a paraprotein band that is seen on protein electrophoresis. In some cases, only light chains are produced; where they are excreted in the urine, this is referred to as Bence Jones proteinuria.

The majority of the plasma cells exist in the bone marrow. In addition to producing immunoglobulin, they also secrete cytokines which stimulate osteoclast activity and result in net bone absorption and hypercalcaemia. If the proliferation of the plasma cells in the marrow is significant, bone marrow failure can result.

Survival and management

In the majority of patients, the aim of treatment is disease control rather than cure. However, in patients under 55 years who have a sibling donor, allogeneic bone marrow transplantation may be curative. Where patients are asymptomatic, treatment may not be required.

Initial treatment

This will depend on the mode of presentation and symptoms or complications:

- renal impairment: see 'Renal impairment', p. 213; however allopurinol may help to prevent urate nephropathy
- hypercalcaemia: see 'Electrolytes', p. 206; bisphosphonates delay any other skeletal events and are helpful in the treatment of hypercalcaemia and should be given long term
- bone pain: appropriate analgesia should be given (see 'Common prescribing', p. 107); avoid NSAIDs in renal failure
- fractures: reduction and immobilization should be attempted (see 'Minor trauma and fractures', p. 259) although they usually require open reduction and internal fixation.

Further therapy

The majority of patients receive chemotherapy regimes, e.g. melphalan and prednisolone. Frail elderly patients receive it orally while younger patients (<65) receive melphalan intravenously at high doses. Treatment continues until falling paraprotein levels reach a plateau. If the paraprotein level later rises (relapse) most patients will respond to further treatment with melphalan.

Radiotherapy can be used to treat localized bone pain unresponsive to analgesia and is also indicated in emergency treatment of spinal cord compression due to extradural plasmacytomas.

Autologous stem cell transplants should be considered in all patients aged <65 years, although this has limited impact on survival. Where treatment fails to control disease, second and third line treatments in the form of thalidomide and bortezomib (a proteasome inhibitor) may be considered.

PALLIATIVE CARE

Palliative care physicians use drug therapy as part of a comprehensive management plan addressing the physical, psychological, social and spiritual needs of the patient. Careful clinical assessment is essential and great care should be taken to identify mechanisms that may be contributing to symptoms: fear, depression, loneliness can all be expressed as physical complaints. Terminally ill patients often have specific problems with medications. For example, oral therapies may be difficult to tolerate because of anorexia, nausea, a dry mouth or difficulty swallowing. It is important to review the cardex regularly and discontinue non-essential medications.

Most hospital units have local palliative care guidelines containing useful advice on prescribing and other issues; these should be consulted where available.

Pain relief

When choosing appropriate analgesia, it is important to determine the source, type, severity and frequency of pain. The pain control ladder should be used to guide analgesic escalation (Fig. 11.1).

Morphine and dose titration

When deciding on the initial dose of morphine, consider the size, age and organ function of the patient, e.g. an elderly patient may only require 5 mg morphine 4-hourly initially. Always start with a short-acting opiate, e.g. Sevredol® 10 mg. Titrate the dose upwards by 30% each day, remembering to increase breakthrough analgesia in proportion as you do so, until pain is controlled or side-effects develop. Once an adequate 4-hourly dose has been established, change to a slow-release morphine product, e.g. MST®. To calculate the necessary 12-hourly dose, divide the total Sevredol® used in 24 h by 2. Ensure that the breakthrough dose (of a short-acting opiate such as Sevredol®) equals one-sixth of the total daily dose of the long-acting agent.

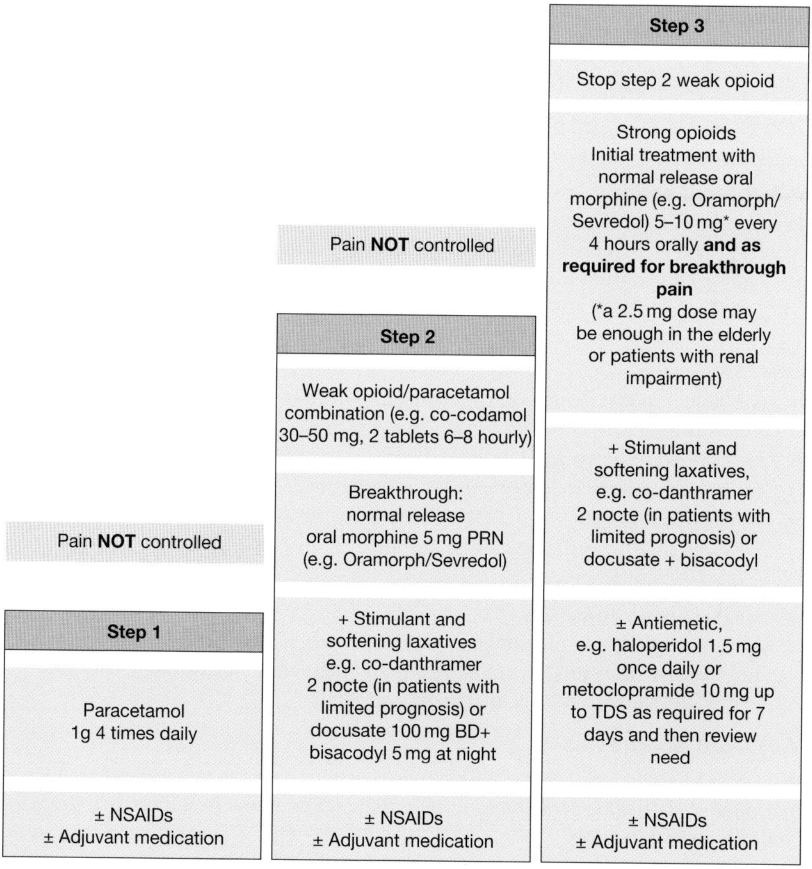

Figure 11.1 The pain control ladder.

Table 11.3 Potency of opioid analgesics

Analgesic	Route	Potency[a]	Example
Codeine	Oral	1/10	Morphine 6 mg = codeine 60 mg
Dihydrocodeine	Oral	1/10	Morphine 6 mg = dihydrocodeine 60 mg
Tramadol	Oral	1/5	Morphine 10 mg = tramadol 50 mg
Oxycodone	Oral	2	Morphine 20 mg = oxycodone 10 mg
Diamorphine	SC	3	Morphine 3 mg = diamorphine 1 mg
Morphine	SC	2	Morphine 20 mg oral = 10 mg SC
Oxycodone	SC	4	Morphine 20 mg = oxycodone 5 mg SC
Morphine	IM	2	Morphine 20 mg oral = 10 mg IM
Morphine	IV	3	Morphine 30 mg oral = 10 mg IV
Fentanyl	Transdermal		Morphine 90–120 mg daily = 25 μg transdermal fentanyl

[a] Potency compared with oral morphine.

Opiate requirements will change over time, so it is important regularly to review the effect of the dose.

Opioid toxicity

Opioid toxicity is suggested by drowsiness and confusion, altered visual fields, vivid dreams, hallucinations, pin-point pupils and myoclonus. If pain is controlled, reduce the dose of morphine by one-third and ensure that the patient is well hydrated (IV or SC fluid may be required). Where there is poor pain control, ensure good hydration and use adjuvant therapies or alternative opioids.

Alternative opioids

It is worth remembering that these are no more effective than oral morphine, although their different side-effect profiles can offer advantages. As with traditional opiates, breakthrough analgesia should always be prescribed. Opiates vary in their potency and a change in dosage will be required when converting from one form to another (Table 11.3).

Oxycodone

- available in normal and controlled-release oral preparations and parenteral preparations
- does not have active metabolites: useful if renal function is unstable
- less hallucinations, itch, drowsiness and confusion.

Transdermal fentanyl

- used in patients with stable pain, this is a second line treatment and should only be commenced under guidance from seniors or the palliative care team
- patch changed every 72 h
- lag time of 6–12 h until pain control effective; therefore if converting from oral slow-release morphine the patient should be given their normal (final) oral dose at the same time that the patch is applied.

Adjuvant analgesics

Non-opioid analgesics target specific pain mechanisms (e.g. inflammation, neuropathy) and should be considered in all patients. Situations in which they are particularly useful include:

- bone pain: NSAIDs, e.g. diclofenac (50 mg 8-hourly) often co-prescribed with a PPI such as lansoprazole (30 mg daily)

- neuropathic pain: amitriptyline (10–25 mg at night); anticonvulsants, e.g. sodium valproate (100–200 mg twice daily), carbamazepine (100–200 mg twice daily), gabapentin (100–300 mg at night); or steroid, e.g. dexamethasone (8–16 mg daily in divided doses)
- liver capsule pain: steroids, e.g. dexamethasone (4–6 mg daily); or NSAID (as above)
- non-pharmacological agents also offer pain relief: radiotherapy; transcutaneous electrical nerve stimulation (TENS).

Syringe drivers

If the patient becomes unable to tolerate oral medications, the total daily dose of opioid should be given subcutaneously via a syringe driver over 24 h (for conversion ratios between agents see Table 11.3). Where available, diamorphine is preferable to morphine given its greater tissue solubility.

The administration route of other medicines, such as antiemetics or anxiolytics, may also need to be changed and some can be added to the syringe pump solution. Metoclopramide and cyclizine should not be used together since they may cause precipitation. Water can be used as a diluent in most syringe drivers except those containing levomepromazine, when saline should be used.

Gastrointestinal symptoms

Constipation

Opioids reduce gut motility, so effective laxative treatment should be prescribed including a peristaltic stimulant. As the dose of morphine increases it is likely that the laxative dose will also need to increase.

- co-danthramer (1–2 tablets daily), which is a stool softener combined with a peristaltic stimulant
- dual prescription of an osmotic laxative like lactulose (10 mL twice daily) and a peristaltic stimulant such as senna (2 tablets at night).

Nausea and vomiting

Nausea and vomiting can occur for a variety of reasons and it is important to establish the most likely cause before deciding on therapy:

- opioids commonly cause nausea at the start of treatment: treat with metoclopramide (10 mg 8-hourly) or haloperidol 1.5 mg daily (treatment may only be required for the first days)
- hypercalcaemia: treat the hypercalcaemia (see 'Electrolytes', p. 206) and treat nausea with haloperidol (1.5 mg daily)
- renal failure: treat the underlying cause and use haloperidol 1.5 mg daily
- mechanical bowel obstruction: cyclizine (50 mg 8-hourly)
- raised intracranial pressure: cyclizine (50 mg 8-hourly).

Anorexia

Patients with cancer often develop anorexia and associated cachexia. The patient's senses of smell and taste can be altered and often there is a preference for sweet and salty food and a dislike or metallic taste with red meat. To maintain sufficient calorific intake, they should be encouraged to experiment with different foods. Using smaller, more regular portions and avoiding the smell of food preparation can also help. Options for pharmacological treatment include prednisolone (20 mg/day) or megestrol acetate (160 mg daily titrated to 160 mg 8-hourly). Treatment should be tried for 2 weeks and, if it is not effective, discontinued. If continuing with prednisolone, use a maintenance dose of 10 mg daily.

Dry mouth, candidiasis and ulcers

These are common complaints in this group of patients. It is important to stress the importance of good mouth care, with daily assessment and tooth brushing after each meal and before bedtime. Soft white paraffin can be applied to dry or broken lips. Other specific measures include:

- dry mouth: chlorhexidine (0.2%) mouthwash 3–4 times daily for 1 min
- candidiasis: chlorhexidine (0.2%) mouthwash twice daily for 1 min plus fluconazole (50–100 mg daily for 7–14 days)
- angular cheilitis: miconazole gel topically 4 times daily
- ulcers: identify cause and use chlorhexidine (0.2%) mouthwash to prevent infections
- herpetic lip ulcers: aciclovir 5% cream 5 times daily for 5 days
- herpetic mouth ulcers: aciclovir tablets or suspension (200 mg 5 times daily for 5 days)
- malignant ulcers or staphylococcal mucositis: flucloxacillin (250–500 mg 6-hourly)
- anaerobic lesions: metronidazole (400 mg 8-hourly).

Respiratory symptoms

Dyspnoea

In patients with terminal disease, breathlessness is common and is often multifactorial. Priorities in the assessment and management of dyspnoea in this setting include:

- identify and treat, where possible, the cause, e.g. pleural effusion, lymphangitis or anaemia
- optimize the treatment of co-morbid conditions, e.g. asthma or COPD
- opioids are often helpful because of their central action to reduce respiratory drive (e.g. Oromorph® 5–10 mg)
- benzodiazepines can be effective in low doses (e.g. diazepam 1–2 mg 8-hourly)
- oxygen should be provided for all patients to use as required
- continuous oxygen therapy should be prescribed for hypoxic patients although it may need to be controlled in those with concomitant type 2 respiratory failure.

Cough

The cause of the cough should be identified and specific treatment considered:

- cancer related: airway obstruction, pulmonary infiltration, fistula formation, mucus production
- treatment related: post-radiotherapy fibrosis, chemotherapy, ACE inhibitors, β-blockers
- others: infection, COPD, bronchiectasis, aspiration, effusion, pulmonary oedema.

Symptomatic management of cough includes:

- simple linctus (5 mL 6–8-hourly)
- codeine linctus (15 mg in 5 mL: 5–10 mL 6–8-hourly)
- oral morphine solution (2.5–5 mg 6–8-hourly) titrated accordingly with cover for constipation.

Secretions

Towards the end of life, respiratory secretions can become troublesome and require treatment. When suctioning and positioning fail to produce adequate benefit and symptoms are causing distress to the patient or family, pharmacological therapy can be initiated, e.g. hyoscine hydrobromide (400 μg SC titrated upwards to 600–2400 μg daily).

Other symptoms

Agitation

This may be due to pain, opiate toxicity, a blocked catheter, constipation, infection or new medications. Only when these causes have been excluded or treated should pharmacological treatment (benzodiazepines or haloperidol) be considered.

Depression

All patients should be assessed for the presence or risk of depression. There are no universally accepted diagnostic criteria for depression in palliative care, but it is important that patients with low mood are assessed to establish the duration and persistence of their symptoms. Where persistent low mood is highlighted, they should be offered psychological support and assessed for active suicidal ideation.

Not all patients will be keen on pharmacological therapy, but where they are, it is worth considering whether the patient suffers from neuropathic pain: if so, choose an antidepressant that will be active against this, e.g. amitriptyline (75 mg at night; 25 mg in elderly or frail patients). Neither paroxetine nor fluoxetine is appropriate for use in palliative care. Alternative antidepressants include sertraline (50 mg daily), citalopram (20 mg daily) or lofepramine (70 mg at night).

Fatigue

Fatigue is a common problem in cancer patients and has multiple contributory causes. Where reversible causes exist, they should be treated, e.g. treatment of anaemia, medication review, dietetic advice and appetite stimulants in anorexia (see above). Consideration needs to be given to addressing physical, emotional and practical needs and help should be tailored to maximize independence and maintain self-esteem.

Hiccups

There are many causes of hiccups which may or may not be related to the patient's current condition. Most causes are gastrointestinal although hiccups can occur secondary to medication. Treatment options should be directed at the cause where identified, but pharmacological approaches include chlorpromazine (25–50 mg 3–4 times daily) and haloperidol (1.5 mg 3 times daily).

Itch

Itch can be a significant problem for some patients and has many causes. Look for evidence of:

- unusually dry skin: avoid heat, hot baths or drying agents (e.g. calamine) and moisturize regularly with an emollient like aqueous cream
- unusually wet skin: use barrier cream in skin folds after washing and aim to reduce sweating
- change in skin colour: consider iron deficiency anaemia, jaundice, poor venous drainage, ischaemia or local tumour
- skin damage: infection, pressure damage or skin disorders
- other causes: opiate use.

Where local measures fail to control itch, systemic drug therapy can be tried. Antihistamines (e.g. chlorphenamine 4 mg 4–6-hourly), chlorpromazine, cimetidine, phenobarbital and rifampicin may be helpful. Where jaundice is the cause of the itch, consider cholestyramine (4–8 g daily).

Sweating

Excessive sweating occurs in about 16% of patients with advanced cancer. While treatment of reversible causes should always be considered first, other pharmacological treatment can give symptomatic relief.

Associated with fever

- paracetamol (1 g 4–6-hourly)
- NSAID: ibuprofen, diclofenac or naproxen at normal doses.

Not associated with fever

- NSAID: high-dose naproxen (e.g. 250–500 mg twice daily)
- cimetidine (400–800 mg at night)
- antimuscarinics: amitriptyline (10–50 mg at night), levomepromazine (unlicensed: 3–6 mg at night)
- thalidomide and thioridazine may be given under specialist advice.

Associated with androgen depletion

- megestrol (40 mg daily: response after 2–4 weeks): titrated at monthly intervals.

Liverpool Care Pathway

An integrated and structured approach to the care of terminally ill patients is essential, irrespective of whether they are in a hospice or a mainstream clinical ward. A standardized 'palliative care' approach can be extended to patients in non-specialist (and specialist) centres through the use of protocols and integrated care pathways, such as the Liverpool Care Pathway. These documents assist clinical teams in the identification of the patient who is dying, the review and management of symptom control, and the choice of necessary ongoing medications and those that can be discontinued. In addition, they support the recording of appropriate clinical assessments and communication between professionals.

On the ward 12

TIME AND 'TAKE' MANAGEMENT

General time management

Managing time effectively will allow you to complete your work with the minimal amount of stress instead of 'fire-fighting' all day. Working late every day does not mean that you are more committed than your colleagues and evolving time management skills is important to a career in medicine:

- know what the job is, what you are expected to achieve and by when
- expect the 'unexpected'
- have regular systems in place that allow you to see at a glance what has been done and what you still have to do
- prioritize urgent work over less urgent and know the difference
- re-evaluate and adjust your priorities and worklists as you go through each day
- delegate appropriately
- know when you are 'slowing down'; take breaks and know when to ask for help.

Organizing yourself

- use a notebook, at least A5 in size and preferably including a 'page-a-day' diary
- at the front, make a list of all the patients in your care that you can keep adding to or deleting as the days pass: include patient identifier numbers, dates of birth, working diagnosis and allergies
- for each day, write down the list of jobs you are given for each patient; indicate alongside those which have been completed and those for which you have seen results
- carry a list of blood and other request forms, referral forms and discharge prescriptions in the back of the book.

A daily routine

At the start of the day

- identify and familiarize yourself with any overnight admissions
- check if any of the patients on the ward were unwell overnight and were seen by the overnight team; review them yourself before the ward round

- find out if any new tasks have been allocated to you as a result of overnight activity; add them to your worklist for the day
- review results from the tests you ordered yesterday or the day before.

During the day

- try to get things done as soon as they are requested, e.g. fill out blood forms on the ward round
- fill out requests for tests that involve other departments, e.g. radiology, as early as possible, since other people need to organize their work too
- predict discharges: even if some drugs might change on the ward round it is worth having the rest of the discharge form prepared
- make sure that you are not doing tasks that should be done by others; learn to say 'no' if you are given inappropriate tasks
- take your breaks: you will be much more efficient
- leave jobs that do not require much energy until the end of the day
- if you are struggling, ask for help and, if you have time to spare, offer it.

At the end of the day

- check your list for any requests not actioned or results not back: make a note in your diary reminding you to do, or check, these tomorrow or on the appropriate day
- check that all routine tasks for the evening and night-shift have been completed before you leave, e.g. fluid, warfarin or insulin prescriptions
- prepare any outstanding blood forms that need to be ready first thing for phlebotomy the next day
- if you know you will not get something done before you finish, say so and pass it on to the overnight team
- review any ill patients and decide if they will need further review overnight
- make time for an effective handover (see 'Verbal communication', p. 385).

The 'take'/'on-call'

If you are organized in your regular work, your performance during 'take' or 'on-call' duties will reflect this. On a receiving shift you can expect that:

- the volume of work may be greater
- the patients may be sicker, mandating more urgent action
- the work will be more unpredictable
- you will be part of a team, required to respond to the triage assessment made by others and acting timeously to requests from all members
- you will have more staff to help you and you should delegate where appropriate
- the work will rarely stop and you will need to make more effort to plan breaks that 'fit in', including taking food with you to avoid going hungry in case there is no time to visit the shop; work with the others in the team to plan when you will each take time out.

Working at night

The majority of hospitals now employ 'hospital at night' teams to provide out of hours care. These teams are comprised of a number of doctors from different hospital specialties, who between them have the full range of skills and competences required to deliver safe clinical care overnight. Most teams also incorporate senior nursing staff who have been trained to assess patients and perform basic procedures, including cannulation. Such senior nurses will often be the first port of call for ward-based nursing staff if they need a cannula inserted or a patient reviewed. If required, a medical member of the team will then be called.

The 'hospital at night' team also softens traditional boundaries between specialties and, irrespective of their 'base', the whole team is expected to work together. Doctors working in specialties that are traditionally quiet overnight will be expected to assist their colleagues working in busier areas, e.g. medical units, A&E. Senior trainees from one specialty may also be called to assist junior trainees in another with procedures.

The hospital at night system works best if there is a formal handover from day to night staff. This allows sick patients on the wards and other potential problems to be highlighted (see 'Handover', below). Remember the 'golden rules' of working out of hours:

- when you see patients, WRITE IN THE NOTES
- if you do not know what to do or are concerned, CALL SOMEONE.

VERBAL COMMUNICATION

Good communication is essential between colleagues and with patients and their families.

Communicating with colleagues

Handover

In hospital practice, good handover between day and night shift teams is crucial. It provides the only opportunity to inform night staff about sick patients and may well be their only link to events occurring during the day. Handovers aim to convey important information from one party to another in a way that can be easily understood and actioned. This includes information about:

- unwell patients or others who need review or discharge
- patients who have the potential to become unwell
- pending investigations that need to be reviewed
- other jobs that need to be completed.

Before the handover meeting, it helps to prepare a list of the information you want to communicate and to distinguish urgent cases or tasks from routine ones. In many hospitals the formal evening handover is a regimented affair involving several hospital departments. Pay attention and make notes: you might be asked to see the patients discussed later.

Telephone

Telephone communication has to be conducted without the benefit of non-verbal cues. This makes it difficult to know how well your message is being understood at the other end. To make the most of such communication:

- be clear: speak audibly and slowly
- be structured: see ISBAR below
- be organized: have relevant information to hand, e.g. recent investigation results; if making a referral or phoning a senior colleague, you may also wish to jot down the key points you want to make under the ISBAR headings; see below.

ISBAR

The person at the other end of the phone needs to hear information in a form they can follow, allowing them to build a picture they can visualize. This is particularly true if they have just woken up: give them a minute to waken up properly to avoid having to repeat the story. One way of structuring these calls uses a technique based around the mnemonic ISBAR:

- **I**dentify: identify yourself, the person you are speaking to and the patient
- **S**ituation: summarize the key problem and why you are calling; if it's urgent, say so!
- **B**ackground: give a structured synopsis of the story; only provide the relevant information
- **A**ssessment: say what you think is going on; stating the obvious is helpful
- **R**equest: outline what you want them to do.

Communication with patients and families

You will need to talk to patients and families on a regular basis about investigations, diagnosis and treatment. Good communication involves patients and/or carers in a two-way discussion, rather than being simply a process of imparting information. It is often as much about listening to what is said and observing non-verbal cues as it is about talking.

Whom to communicate with

You have a duty of confidentiality to adult patients. Before you communicate with any family member or representative about them, you need to seek their consent. Families do not always understand this and may expect you to pass information over the phone when they call the ward, to answer questions when you meet them in the corridor or to be advised of results before the patient. They may also express a wish for you not to tell the patient something or insist on coming with a patient into a clinic consultation room.

However, the patient may not like or trust a particular family member, or they may wish to tell the family selected information in their own way and at their own pace. Any adult who is mentally capable, even if they are elderly or dependent on others, has the right to choose with whom they will share the information and when they will do it.

In the case of inpatients, it can help to clarify the lines of communication at the outset. Identify their main contact or next of kin. Clarify whether any information should be held back from the contact pending discussion with the patient. When dealing with outpatients, check with the patient before they come into the consultation room if they wish their relatives to accompany them.

How to communicate

Communicating well comes with practice; the following principles are a guide:

Environment

- try to create a comfortable environment which is quiet
- ensure privacy and prevent interruptions, e.g. give your bleep to somebody else
- avoid having a desk between you and the patient/family; it will act as a barrier
- sit at the same eye level as the patient: do not stand over them.

Background and agenda

- explain who you are
- if you are talking to a relative of the patient, verify who they are and what relationship they have with the patient
- clearly introduce what the meeting is for and what you hope to cover in it, e.g. 'I have the results of your test: I'd like to go through the results and then talk about some of the treatment options'
- find out what they know already: 'can you tell me what you have been told so far'
- establish if there is anything else they want you to address.

Main conversation

- avoid medical jargon
- try to keep to the structure you outlined at the start
- if you have a lot to say, try to break it up into manageable sections to avoid overwhelming the patient/family
- be aware of your body language: adopt an open position, i.e. avoiding crossed arms/legs
- regularly check whether they have any questions
- answer any questions honestly.

Closure

- ask if they have any remaining questions or concerns
- summarize what you think are the main points from the discussion.

Breaking bad news

This task is best performed in a controlled environment by experienced clinicians. However, all doctors may be required to do so in an emergency situation. If you are not prepared, it will be stressful for you and for the patient/family.

Preparation

Know the case and the proposed medical plan. Consider what questions the patient/family are likely to ask. Ideally, inform the patient that their results should be available on a certain day, at a certain time and check if they would like to be told them, and also if they would like any family members to be with them at the time.

Know what you want to say ahead of time, but be prepared to adjust this depending on the response to the initial outline of information you give.

Environment

Take a minute to review the room that you will meet in (see 'How to communicate', p. 386). Remember that patients or family may get upset or become aggressive: position yourself with a clear exit (see 'Aggression and violence', p. 420).

Take a member of nursing staff with you. Ideally, it should be one who knows the patient and their family. Let them know beforehand what you are going to say and see if they have any comments.

The 'bad news' discussion

Several suggested formats exist for this type of discussion. Whichever approach you adopt, it must be individualized to the patient/family and reflect what information they want to know, their personality and cultural background:

Prepare the patient

Announce that the information you are about to give them is concerning. Wait to check if they wish you to proceed.

Share the information

Outline what you know about the patient's illness, e.g. their diagnosis or other test results.

Pause

Once the diagnosis has been given, it is usual to pause to allow the patient time to absorb the implications of the news. This is particularly appropriate if the diagnosis is cancer or another life-threatening/debilitating illness. Once you feel comfortable that the patient is ready to move on, address any additional pieces of information relevant to subsequent treatment decisions, e.g. whether the cancer has advanced or not.

Discuss options

Outline what you think the options are for the next steps. This may involve a suggested plan for further investigations or referral for potentially curative treatment. Even if you can only offer palliative therapy try to emphasize what can be done for the patient, however small.

Listen to what they think and agree a plan

Use questions regularly to explore what the patient understands and what they wish to consider in terms of treatment. Use the answers to shape the discussion about the plan of action. You must always be honest with the patient and their family and must always be wary of raising false hopes, ensuring any questions they ask are answered directly and honestly. Once you have a plan, ensure that the patient is in agreement with it.

Offer support

Consider what other means of emotional and practical support can be offered, especially where no active disease-modifying treatment is available, e.g. Macmillan support and financial entitlements.

Reflect and summarize

Encourage the patient to reflect on what they have heard; clarify if they have any remaining concerns or queries and then summarize what you have discussed. This helps to ensure that they take away the most important parts of the consultation.

Enquiries about prognosis

Patients or families may ask how long someone has got to live. This is a difficult question to answer, not least because prognosis is a difficult thing to predict accurately. Therefore:

- ensure that the patient appreciates the vagaries of such a prediction
- only answer the question if you have factual information on which to base your response (e.g. some knowledge of the likely outcome of their disease)
- use broad expressions like 'months rather than years' instead of giving absolute lengths of time, e.g. '6 months'; if a specific time is given, some patients will count this down to the last day and then seem surprised that they are still alive
- if the question is asked by someone other than the patient, and the patient is present, first check they wish to discuss this
- consider asking the question back, i.e. 'How long are you expecting?' to gauge the detail they wish.

Handling emotions

Patients and family members will, unsurprisingly, display a variety of emotions when bad news is broken. You must be able to make an assessment of their emotional state.

Anger is a common response to bad news and it may be related to many factors. It is important to recognize anger where it appears and have some understanding of how to handle it:

- acknowledge the anger: 'I can see how angry you are about your father's death'
- legitimize the anger: 'It must be hard for you that he became unwell so quickly'
- encourage expression: 'Can you tell me how you are feeling just now'.

In response to bad news, patients will usually progress through the 5 stages of grief, although they may not start with the first or progress in a stepwise fashion:

- denial: 'it can't be happening'
- anger: 'why me? it's not fair'
- bargaining: 'just let me live long enough to ...'
- depression: 'I can't go on like this'
- acceptance: 'okay, this is happening'.

WRITTEN COMMUNICATION

Case-notes

You will spend a large proportion of your time writing in patients' notes. For any interaction between you and the patient, or their family, the notes are the only enduring record of what happened or what was said. They will inform those who share in the care of your patient and will also be crucial to any defence of your actions in court. Therefore, write legibly and document the date and time of every entry. Also sign and print your name and add a contact number. Examples of when to make entries in the notes include:

- whenever you attend a patient, e.g. ward round, urgent review, procedure
- to comment on results you have seen
- whenever you make a significant change to prescribed medication
- after gaining consent, be it verbal or written (see 'Consent', p. 406)
- when certifying a death, when you should include details of what was documented (see 'Death Certification', p. 400).

Discharge documentation

You will be responsible for creating discharge documentation for patients under your care. These documents are extremely important because they summarize the key problems and events that took place during a patient's admission. Your colleagues will use them to understand what happened and to guide further action during the patient's visits to general practice, outpatient departments or in the event of readmission. It is likely that you will be required to produce both interim discharge documents and formal discharge letters.

Interim discharge documents

The purpose of an interim discharge summary is to record a diagnosis and briefly summarize the admission, discharge medication and follow-up plans. It is completed before discharge and is a vital tool for early communication with the GP. Where possible, it is useful to complete the interim discharge ahead of the actual discharge day. This is especially true for a weekend discharge when pharmacy departments often have restricted opening hours and your colleagues will have plenty of other things to do.

It is easy to focus only on the prescription section of the document. However, it is also extremely important that the correct diagnosis is entered. 'Musculoskeletal chest pain' or 'Troponin-negative ACS' is more helpful than 'Chest pain: MI screen negative'. Likewise, any early action required of the GP should be clearly indicated, e.g. 'repeat U&E within 1 week'.

Remember to list all the medication that a patient is taking on discharge; inaccurate lists can result in patients being restarted on tablets that had been intentionally stopped during admission, or having other medication stopped accidentally.

Some documents will have a separate section for you to record any medications discontinued during an admission; where this exists, it is important to complete it. Where it does not, you will need to include this information elsewhere on the form.

Discharge letters

Diagnosis

It is essential that the diagnoses which prompted admission are documented accurately. Local and national statistics depend upon this information for accurate population disease monitoring and health service planning. In most cases, there will be a list of diagnoses rather than a single diagnosis: the principal diagnosis that was the focus of the admission should be listed first. Remember that it is valid to include obesity and smoking status in the diagnosis list.

Although the main body of the letter will vary widely depending on style, it is worth noting that it is an exercise in communication and not one of prose. Long and tortuous sentences describing the mode of admission are not necessary; nor are long lists of particular blood results. You may find it helpful to follow a structured letter with the following headings:

History

Briefly describe the mode of admission. Concisely describe the history of presenting complaint, followed by a review of relevant past medical history to set the scene for the rest of the letter.

Examination

Highlight the relevant positive and negative findings. There is absolutely no need to describe in detail all the neurological findings for a patient who has presented with a CVA. However, it is helpful to document features that could affect the aetiology or management of a condition, e.g. that she 'had a murmur consistent with aortic stenosis and a right carotid bruit'.

Investigations

It is useful to the reader to have all the results from investigations in one section of the letter, even though they may have occurred throughout the course of a long admission. Again, prose is not required and it is rarely necessary to quote specific blood results, e.g. 'FBC normal. Electrolytes normal'.

Management and progress

In this section of the letter, describe what happened during the admission. Outline any treatments that were started, or procedures that took place, and include any complications that occurred. Summarize events as succinctly as possible, e.g. for a patient with an exacerbation of COPD: 'They were commenced on nebulized bronchodilators, oral antibiotics and steroids. They made an uncomplicated recovery and were discharged home on a reducing dose of oral steroid.'

Follow-up

Outline whether hospital follow-up or specific social services have been arranged. Ensure any clinic appointments are booked, or that you leave a message for the secretary to organize them. Remember that writing the discharge letter is a good opportunity to review and document the results of all the investigations that were performed. State if any are still pending and double check that they have been ordered.

Medication

It is always useful to list the medication prescribed on discharge, especially when there have been changes to treatment. Where relevant, it is important to highlight medication that was discontinued in a separate section.

Other letters

Referral letters

There are often times when patients need to be reviewed by other healthcare professionals as inpatients. The most common method for organizing such a review is by writing a letter. These should be typed and printed where possible. In certain hospitals, letter templates may be available, and in others web-based proformas will enable standardized referrals. Whatever the form of the letter, a copy should be made and filed within the correspondence section of the notes.

Some departments will require referrals to be made on proformas specific to their own specialty, e.g. a geriatrics referral form may have an area for documenting the patient's mini-mental score or whether they can mobilize independently.

If proforma or template is not required, use the following to construct a referral letter:

- patient demographics, including hospital number or other unique identifier
- patient location and supervising consultant
- date of referral and date of admission
- brief history of admission, leading into a sentence about why the review is required
- relevant past medical history and examination findings
- relevant investigations
- relevant drug history
- current plans for therapy
- final summary of the case including what the recipient is being asked to do, e.g. provide an opinion, consider taking over care; be clear about the level of urgency of response needed.

Remember that, while you do need to tell a story, it should be concise and only include the information that is pertinent to the referral. Always sign and date the letter. Consider delivering it yourself since using the hospital mail may result in a delay.

Clinic letters

Once you have reviewed a patient in the clinic, you will need to write to the GP summarizing the consultation. Your letter will also act as a record in the case-notes. However, remember to make notes within the file itself as your letter tape can be lost or erased in error and you may find it hard to remember one case from another. While some outpatient departments will provide a tape and dictaphone, others will not and you will have to get both from the department secretaries, before you go to the clinic. A sample outline for a clinic letter would be as follows:

Problem list

Each current and significant past diagnosis, especially those that are relevant to this particular consultation. Include relevant operations or major treatments, e.g. radiotherapy, and give dates of these.

Medications list

List each of the current medications and consider grouping into 'medications where change is recommended' and 'ongoing medication'.

History

If this is a 'new' case, remember to thank the GP for the referral of this 'x'-aged man or woman. Outline the questions posed in the GP letter and the key points taken from their history. Then, for both 'return' and 'new' patients, state whom, if anybody, accompanied the patient. Move on to describe the history of the presenting complaint, anything relevant from past medical and social history and then systemic enquiry.

Examination

Summarize the relevant positive and negative findings and include any formal scores applicable to the specialty, e.g. performance status.

Investigations

Cover the results of any investigations undertaken on the day and then those that were ordered, or for which results are outstanding.

Verbal communication

Record any particular concerns the patient had, using their words, where possible. Record any specific advice you gave, e.g. risks you outlined before taking consent, side-effects of new treatments, prognosis.

Plan

Summarize what you think the main issues are and what you suggest is done about them. Remember, it is not usually your role to actually change any medication, but rather to suggest the alternative management to the GP.

Follow-up

Note the planned date of any next appointment or intervention.

BEFORE, DURING AND AFTER THEATRE

Preparation for theatre

The preparation of patients for theatre is often the responsibility of the junior doctor. However, most surgical units will have a written preoperative protocol which has been agreed between the surgeons and anaesthetists. You should familiarize yourself with this and any other local policies, including those regarding the ordering of blood products.

The aim of preoperative assessment is to ensure the patient is in the best possible condition for surgery. This requires a thorough history and examination and targeted investigation. In some units, patients attending for elective surgery will have already been assessed at an outpatient preoperative clinic, where a proforma may have been completed and any relevant tests performed in advance.

History and examination

A brief history of the relevant surgical condition is essential. Any recent change in this should be highlighted. Document any other relevant conditions; cardiorespiratory disease is particularly important and may influence the choice and type of anaesthesia offered.

Ask about any previous surgery or anaesthetics, especially including any adverse reactions. Check smoking and alcohol histories. Allergies should be explored and drug history documented: certain medications may interact with anaesthetic drugs; patients on oral steroids may need a temporarily increased dose; drugs like warfarin, aspirin, clopidogrel or combined oral contraceptives may need to be discontinued before an operation.

The main focus of the examination should be on the condition requiring surgery and the cardiorespiratory system. Oxygen saturation on air, respiratory rate, pulse and blood pressure should be documented. Other systems should be examined as appropriate to the clinical situation, e.g. breasts, peripheral arterial system, joints. If appropriate, the site of the operation should be marked with a permanent marker.

Investigations

Investigation policies vary between units, but may include the following tests in the situations listed:

- FBC: females; history of prior or anticipated blood loss; history of possible infection, pre-existing cardiorespiratory disease
- U&E: patients on diuretics or ACE inhibitors; prior hypertension; renal disease; cardiac disease or diabetes; age over 60; history of altered fluid balance, e.g. vomiting
- LFT: previous biliary or liver disease; recent abdominal pain; recent introduction of new drug; history of alcoholism
- clotting: patients on anticoagulants; previous history of liver disease or bleeding
- sickle-cell: Afro-Caribbeans who do not know their status
- cross-match or group and save: follow local blood transfusion policy

- ECG: patients over 50; smokers; history of cardiovascular disease, hypertension, renal disease or diabetes; patients on diuretics or any other drug that may affect the QT interval
- CXR: patients over 60; those with cardiorespiratory disease, new respiratory symptoms or signs
- urine β-HCG: women of child-bearing age.

Further cardiorespiratory assessment may be required prior to major procedures, e.g. blood gases, spirometry or echocardiography.

Prescriptions and prophylaxis

A drug cardex should be completed showing current medication, including any to be withheld prior to surgery (see above). Check your unit's policy with regard to the routine prescription of additional 'as required' medication, e.g. paracetamol.

Remember to assess DVT risk and prescribe LMWH accordingly. If the patient is to have an epidural as part of their procedure, anticoagulants may need to be discontinued (see 'Anticoagulation', p. 109). Immobilized patients should wear anti-embolic stockings unless there is a contraindication, e.g. peripheral vascular disease.

Antibiotic prophylaxis is required for patients with certain conditions, e.g. valvular heart disease, or certain procedures. Check local policy; there is also guidance in the BNF. Some units will use aperients, e.g. Picolax®, to prepare the large bowel prior to instrumentation or surgery.

Consent

This should be completed by the person carrying out the procedure or at the very least someone with a full knowledge of it, the possible complications and alternative treatments (see 'Consent', p. 406).

In theatre

When attending theatre, it is important that you are aware of the basic principles of patient care and your own personal conduct. It is good practice when attending an operation to have introduced yourself to the patient beforehand and familiarized yourself with their case.

General preparation

Blues or greens should be worn and are usually changed between lists. However, they may have to be changed more frequently if they become soiled or after cases involving MRSA infection. A hat and appropriate footwear should be worn before entering any clean area and jewellery should be removed. Hats should be removed before leaving the theatre suite, as should the blues worn in theatre.

Before entering the theatre itself, ensure that your identification is clearly visible. Introduce yourself to a member of theatre staff, who will advise you on the room layout and scrubbing protocol; see below. Ensure that you have eaten and drunk enough before you go to theatre. You may have to stand for a long time without much rest.

Patient and site identification

Each operating theatre will have a protocol for making sure that the correct procedure is carried out on the correct patient and on the correct side. It is good practice for the clinician to see the patient again once they have reached the theatre area, both to reassure them and also as a final check of identification and operating site.

Scrubbing up and the sterile field

For guidance on creating and working in a sterile field, including use of gowns and gloves, see 'The sterile field', p. 19.

Scrubbing with an antibacterial solution reduces the concentration of micro-organisms on the hands (it does not render them sterile). If you have not scrubbed up before, ask one of the nursing staff to show you how. In high-risk operations such as a caesarean section or an HIV case you will need two pairs of gloves.

The first scrub should last around 5 min and brushes should be used on nails only. Scrubbing cleans the hands and arms from the fingers out, much as a wound would be cleaned from the inside out without returning to the centre. Work soap thoroughly around and between the fingers, then over the rest of the hands, around wrists and up towards the elbow, always washing upwards, never back down towards the hands. Always keep your hands above your elbows.

Subsequent scrubs (between cases) should last around 3 min. Rinse from fingers to elbows, again keeping your hands ABOVE your elbows and dry from fingers to elbows with a separate sterile towel for each arm. If you are asked to adjust or hold anything, make sure it has a sterile cover. If you are worried that you may have touched something non-sterile do not be afraid to say. If you are observing, but not scrubbed, keep a good distance between yourself and the sterile area.

Positioning and monitoring of the patient

It is important that theatre noise is kept to a minimum for the comfort of the patient and also to aid good communication. Proper positioning of the patient is vital, not only to allow access for the surgeon and anaesthetist, but also to avoid pressure which can cause tissue and nerve damage.

Monitoring equipment will be applied to the patient to watch for cardiorespiratory instability and will depend on the extent of the procedure. Warming blankets may be applied since thermoregulation is impaired by anaesthesia.

Instrument and swab counts should be carried out both before, during and after the procedure to ensure that none is left in the patient's wound. Any specimens that are taken should be clearly labelled with the patient's details and site of origin. If you are in charge of these, ensure that they reach the laboratory and are not left lying about.

Postoperative care

In the immediate recovery phase, patients are cared for close to the theatre area in case of life-threatening complications, such as haemorrhage. They are monitored to ensure that they are ventilating sufficiently without assistance and that they can protect their own airway. Cardiovascular status is also assessed until they are stable to transfer to the ward. The care of patients on the ward is the responsibility of the entire multidisciplinary surgical team.

General assessment and documentation

- assess pain and mobilization
- check the patient can eat and drink, pass urine, flatus and faeces
- enquire about any nausea or vomiting; check basic physical observations, e.g. pulse, BP, respiratory rate, oxygen saturation, temperature, urine output; check any drain for signs of site infection or dislodgement and for drainage output volume and consistency
- examine chest, abdomen, legs and wound site regularly
- begin each ward round entry in the case-notes with a heading stating how many days have now elapsed following theatre.

Management

- analgesia: good analgesia is essential for deep ventilation and mobilization; it should be planned, include background and breakthrough analgesia and should be re-assessed regularly for adequacy

- fluid balance and haemoglobin: involves an assessment of maintenance requirements, including U&E and Hb, and replacement or correction of any ongoing losses (see 'Prescribing fluid', p. 122)
- nutrition: early enteral nutrition is safe after most surgery and tolerated by the majority of patients; if fasting is going to be prolonged, then parenteral nutrition should be commenced
- antibiotic prophylaxis: single-dose prophylaxis is as effective as multi-dose regimes; prolonged antibiotic therapy is reserved for treating active infection
- thromboembolic prophylaxis: stocking use and LMWH should continue until patients are mobilizing freely (see 'LMWH', p. 110)
- wound care: wounds should be reviewed regularly for signs of infection
- ambulation: early mobilization is important to avoid postoperative complications, but requires good analgesia and physiotherapy involvement.

Complications

Complications can be divided into early and late and their timing is often useful in determining the diagnosis. The following is a brief outline of some of the more common complications.

Early

Partial lung collapse or consolidation

Basal atelectasis/collapse is caused by impaired ventilation and failure to clear secretions. This is a common cause of mild pyrexia immediately postoperatively. The use of humidified oxygen and deep breathing exercises may avoid infection.

Aspiration

Aspiration of gastric contents is most common in patients with an altered conscious level at either induction or recovery from anaesthesia. Significant aspiration leads to bronchospasm and hypoxia with moist crackles and reduced air entry. Antibiotics, suction of the bronchial tree or assisted ventilation may be required.

DVT/PTE

DVTs can be clinically silent or cause pain, swelling and oedema of the lower limb (see 'Deep venous thrombosis', p. 271). The presentation and management of PTE is described in 'Pulmonary thromboembolism', p. 152.

Haemorrhage

This may be obvious after superficial surgery and respond to pressure or placement of a haemostatic suture. After abdominal or thoracic surgery, haemorrhage may be concealed and, unless the possibility is considered, the diagnosis can be late (see 'Shock', p. 250).

Renal failure

If renal function is deteriorating, ensure adequate fluid resuscitation, stop any nephrotoxic drugs, e.g. NSAIDs, and exclude urinary tract obstruction. Invasive monitoring (CVP) may be required and specialist renal advice sought if renal function continues to deteriorate (see 'Acute renal failure', p. 209).

Wound infection

This results in a red or swollen wound that discharges pus or serous fluid. Swabs should be taken and empirical antibiotics commenced, until sensitivities are available.

Wound dehiscence

This affects the superficial layers of skin and subcutaneous fat. It will usually close by secondary intention if dressed appropriately. Complete dehiscence of the abdominal wall is a surgical emergency and is often heralded by a serosanguineous discharge followed by small bowel protruding from the wound. The wound should be covered in sterile saline-soaked swabs and the patient returned to theatre for surgical repair (see also 'Wound closure and dressings', p. 61).

Abscess formation

This will usually lead to a swinging pyrexia and elevated inflammatory markers. A small pleural effusion may be evident if the abscess is just below the diaphragm. Drainage is the most important treatment and may be possible percutaneously after localization.

Paralytic ileus

This may occur after abdominal surgery and causes abdominal bloating and colic. It is usually self-limiting (48–72 h).

Anastomotic leakage

This is commonest after oesophageal or rectal surgery and is one of the most serious postoperative complications. It can lead to generalized peritonitis, abscess or fistula formation. In a deteriorating patient, anastomotic breakdown should be one of the first complications to exclude. This will usually require contrast studies or a CT scan.

Late

Adhesions

Fibrous adhesions form between loops of bowel and can cause obstruction or infarction. They can present in the days following surgery or after many years and are a significant surgical problem, for which there is no clear prophylactic treatment.

Incisional hernia

See 'Surgical lumps', p. 343.

Discharge

General measures in relation to self-care and support should be considered (see 'Discharge documentation', p. 389). In the case of patients following surgery, you should also check the patient can mobilize, eat and drink and has a supply of adequate analgesia and antibiotics, if appropriate. You should also ensure that they know:

- when and where any sutures are to be removed
- when, or if, any follow-up is planned
- when any medication withheld before surgery can be recommenced
- when they can shower, drive, return to work or fly
- what to do in the event of a complication.

Legal and ethical practice 13

THE DOCTOR–PATIENT RELATIONSHIP

According to the UK General Medical Council (GMC), the doctor–patient relationship should 'be based on openness, trust and good communication' and allow the doctor to 'work in partnership with the patient to address their individual needs'. The GMC also advises doctors that, in their relationships with their patients, they are expected to:

- be polite, considerate and honest
- treat patients with dignity
- treat each patient as an individual
- respect patients' privacy and right to confidentiality
- support patients in caring for themselves to improve and maintain their health
- encourage patients who have knowledge about their condition to use this when they are making decisions about their care.

Although these principles of care should be reflected in all doctor–patient relationships, different forms of relationship will evolve depending on the level of trust and willingness expressed by the patient and the level of openness and the communication structure employed by the clinician.

Types of relationship

One current theory describes four forms of relationship with differing levels of patient or doctor control:

- paternalistic: a typical doctor-centred style, often using closed questions to elicit yes or no answers; this style concentrates on the doctor's decisions around diagnosis and treatment rather than the patient's view or experience of their illness
- consumeristic: the patient takes the active role and the doctor accedes to the patient's request for something, e.g. a second opinion

- default: this is essentially an impasse between the doctor and the patient's expectation of the relationship; it usually occurs when the doctor offers the patient a patient-centred approach, involving them in decision-making, but the patient prefers to choose a passive role 'whatever you think best, doctor'
- mutualistic: both patient and doctor jointly exchange information and agree a plan, using an open questioning style.

Patient expectation

Patient expectation influences the role they adopt in the relationship. Older patients often expect a paternalistic approach and can be confused by the more modern mutual sharing of 'power'. If the option to share the decision-making process appears to be rejected, it may be necessary for the doctor to assume control. However, this can be difficult or stressful for doctors trained to practise mutuality, especially where the discussion involves life-threatening decisions. It is worth considering a mental outline of both types of conversation before you see the patient.

It is important not to assume that the patient wishes you to be paternalistic in all areas of their care. They may wish you to decide on whether a referral to another discipline should be made, but may still wish to choose what kind of painkiller to have. It is worth making repeated attempts to engage them in management decisions throughout the consultation. Patient involvement in clinical decision-making has also been shown to improve treatment compliance and reduce the need for repeated consultations with other clinicians.

Potential difficulties

Compliance

It is the responsibility of the doctor to enable the patient to understand their diagnosis and treatment options. However, patients have a choice to take your advice or to leave it. Rejection of the advice given/failure to take medication prescribed can strain the doctor–patient relationship, with doctors feeling that the patient has not fulfilled 'their side of the bargain'. However, the overly righteous doctor risks losing what trust they have been given by the patient. It may be better to accept gracefully patient non-compliance with some aspects of advice or treatment, if it means they continue to attend for advice at all.

Time

Time, or the lack of it, can lead to some doctors feeling pressurized and irritable with patients who take a long time to get to the point or get undressed, those who have a self-inflicted problem, or those with a relatively minor illness. However, it is not the patient's fault that time is short and all patients deserve the same high level of personal courtesy.

Defining boundaries

The doctor–patient relationship is an unusual invasion of personal privacy permissible only by the definition of unspoken boundaries between the two parties. It is important to:

- strike a balance between showing compassion for a patient and allowing personal friendship; where you feel a patient has developed an unhelpful personal attachment to you, it can be worth discussing this with colleagues and arranging a transfer of patient care; meantime you have a duty to maintain patient care
- not enter into romantic or personal relationships with existing, or even prior, patients

- take special care where consultations are not witnessed, e.g. on home visits, not to be too familiar in approach and not to undertake personal examinations at home if these can wait
- be cautious about accepting gifts of significant value from patients
- avoid seeing patients within the context of your home or personal social environment.

The doctor–patient relationship can be a challenging responsibility, but is also a tremendously rewarding privilege.

APPROPRIATE RESUSCITATION AND DNAR

All clinicians have a responsibility to ensure that the treatments they offer are in the best interests of the patient and have a reasonable chance of success. This is particularly true when considering cardiopulmonary resuscitation, since it is invasive, often traumatic and >80% of patients will die at the time of arrest or before discharge from hospital. CPR is often a difficult topic to raise with patients or their families. However, prospective consideration of the appropriateness of resuscitation is essential in the management of all patients at risk of a cardiac arrest. Decisions to withhold resuscitation should, where appropriate, be discussed with the patient and family and be documented.

Advance care planning

Since the majority of patients are not expected to arrest, advance care planning regarding CPR is not necessary or appropriate in this group. If they arrest, resuscitation should be attempted unless they have expressed a contrary wish.

In other patients, there may be clear risk factors for cardiac arrest, including advanced malignancy, recent MI, unstable coronary disease, severe sepsis or respiratory failure. In such patients, the issue of CPR should be considered early, and a decision made, before a crisis arises. Whether this should be discussed with the patient or their family is considered below.

Making a decision not to resuscitate

A 'Do Not Attempt Resuscitation order' (DNAR) can be made by any junior doctor who has full GMC registration, although local protocols may vary and it is advisable to seek senior advice. In all cases, the responsible senior doctor (usually the consultant) should be informed about the decision as soon as possible. A DNAR order may be appropriate in the following circumstances:

- where the patient's condition is such that effective CPR is unlikely to be successful
- where successful CPR is likely to be followed by a length and quality of life that is not in the patient's best interests
- where CPR is not in accordance with the known or expressed sustained wishes of patient who is mentally competent
- where CPR is not in accordance with a valid and applicable advanced life directive, e.g. anticipatory refusal or living will.

Discussion

In critically ill patients, as in all circumstances, it is important to maintain a dialogue with the patient and their family, as well as with nursing and other medical staff. This allows a consensus view on the likely outcome of any resuscitation attempt to be formed by all those involved, including, where appropriate, the patient.

The requirement to discuss a DNAR decision with a patient directly depends on the reason for making the decision. In the case of a terminally ill patient in whom resuscitation would be inappropriate and likely futile, discussion of such a decision may not be necessary. However, many patients in this situation will want to discuss issues in respect of dying and most will appreciate the opportunity to decide how they will die.

Where decisions are to be made that relate to perceived quality of life following resuscitation, discussion is mandatory with the patient (or their nominated representative if they are not competent). The most senior doctor available should undertake such a discussion and, where practical, the responsible senior doctor should be informed beforehand.

If you are involved, it is important to consider the stress that such discussions are likely to create and to approach the topic with sensitivity and honesty. You may need to discuss the specifics of a patient's condition or treatment and should prepare for this ahead (see also 'Verbal communication', p. 385).

Documentation

When the decision has been made, it must be documented appropriately. Refer to your local protocol. Where DNAR forms exist, they should be completed in full, signed and placed in the notes. If no form exists, document clearly in the notes by writing 'Do Not Attempt Resuscitation' rather than 'not for 2222' or 'DNR'. Include the date and time that the decision was made, with whom it was discussed and when the decision should be reviewed.

Review

Decisions regarding whether or not to commence resuscitation should be reviewed by a senior member of the medical team on a regular basis, as per local protocol. This review should take account of any changes in the patient's condition and whether this has any bearing on the previous decision.

DEATH CERTIFICATION

Death certification enables families to register the death of their loved ones and provides a permanent legal record of the event. The family must produce a death certificate to arrange disposal of the body and settle the estate of the deceased. In addition, the causes of death recorded on death certificates are recorded centrally and used to monitor disease patterns in the general population. For all three reasons, the accuracy of what is entered on the certificate is very important.

How to establish a death

Any suitably qualified individual, e.g. registered nurse, can verify that a death has occurred. It is worth noting that there is no legal definition of death in the UK; however, you should examine the body and then write in the notes.

Examine the body

Several Asian religions object to contact with the body: you should wear disposable gloves and keep the body covered with a plain white sheet. Jewish patients should not be touched until 20 min after death:

- check for spontaneous movement, including respiratory effort
- check for reaction to voice and pain (sternal rub or supraorbital nerve)
- palpate at least two major pulses for 1 min
- inspect the eyes looking for dryness, fixed dilated pupils, absence of corneal reflexes and clouding of the cornea

- auscultate the heart and lungs for 1 min each
- remember to note if a pacemaker is present.

Write in the case-notes

- the date and time of death (the time the patient actually died, even if this is according to other staff, rather than your own observations)
- when you were contacted and the date and time of certification, if this is different
- a description of what you did to establish death
- what you wrote on the certificate (see below)
- whether a pacemaker was present
- whether the family know if the deceased wished cremation or not
- whether you have informed the GP or Coroner/Fiscal of the death.

Writing the certificate

Legal certification of the death can only be performed by a doctor who has provided care during the last illness and who saw the patient within 14 days preceding their death (28 days in Northern Ireland), or after death.

In hospital, many doctors can be involved in the final illness, but the proper certification of death is ultimately the responsibility of the consultant in charge. If you are called to see a patient briefly when on-call and they later die, it is wise to leave the certification of death to the 'parent' team who are likely to know them better. Sometimes, the death occurs in situations that require the doctor to report it to the Procurator Fiscal in Scotland, or Coroner in England and Wales, rather than proceed to issue a certificate (see below).

- check that you have the right information; consider whether you are the correct person to certify the death
- obtain the death certificate book (usually one held on each ward)
- if necessary, discuss case with Coroner (Fiscal) before certifying (see below)
- if the case is being referred for a post-mortem examination, a provisional certificate may be issued, but you should indicate that further information from autopsy may be available
- ensure every section of the certificate is complete, including the duration of illnesses
- use black ink and write clearly and neatly, preferably in block capitals
- the 'place of death' refers to the ward, hospital and city of death
- your 'residence' should be given as your work, not your personal address
- your 'qualifications' are your medical degree
- consider the final cause of death (cause Ia); the sequence leading to this (causes I b, c, d, in reverse order of contribution); any other conditions that did not result in cause I, but did contribute in some way to the death (cause II); see also below
- remember to include non-disease states that resulted in the death, e.g. chronic smoking in lung cancer, chronic alcohol consumption in variceal bleeding
- avoid using modes of death, e.g. any organ 'failure', arrest or exhaustion
- write all conditions in full: never use symbols or abbreviations, e.g. TIA
- unacceptable completion will result in refusal of the certificate by the Registrar with distressing delay for the family and notification of your senior colleagues.

Causes of death

When describing the cause of death it is worth noting that organ 'failure', especially without explanation of how it developed, is not an acceptable cause of death. It is wise to give as much detail as possible as to the nature and extent of disease. Abbreviations such as 'COPD' should be avoided and the terms given in full.

In addition, pneumonia and myocardial infarction have been very common diagnoses on death certificates, without always being the real cause of death. Many patients have chest signs and symptoms at death and many patients die suddenly. Therefore, to avoid further questioning by the Registrar, you are best to add as much detail as possible of the final condition and any further evidence in the remainder of the certificate to substantiate these diagnoses.

Discussion with family

As the certifying doctor, you will usually be asked to give the certificate to the family and talk to them about the death. It is worth taking a senior nurse with you.

Family members may be angry at you, other colleagues, the hospital, themselves, other relatives or the GP. It is wise to show that you understand how upset they feel, but not to comment on the actions of other people, especially members of medical or nursing staff. They may also have questions that relate to the death or what to do next:

- what caused the death: if there is any doubt about this, if you do not know the case well, or if any medical mishap was involved, check with a senior what you should say
- when did they die and who was with them: they will need reassurance that it was peaceful, or that the patient was unaware of what was happening
- advice on what to do next: many hospitals have information leaflets you can give families about where and when to register the death and how to contact an undertaker; some families also benefit from the support available from the hospital chaplaincy.

In some cases, it is necessary to contact the Fiscal or Coroner before the certificate can be issued (often the next day). You will need to explain your legal obligation to do this and that any decisions about disposal of the body need to wait until after this.

In other cases, a post-mortem may be considered. It is now recommended that any consent to post-mortem should be taken by a senior member of staff, but you may need to give the family the relevant information leaflet prior to this discussion; see below. It is worth noting that some faiths find post-mortem examinations unacceptable and you should be sensitive to this.

If the patient is to be cremated, additional paperwork will be necessary (see below), so you will need to establish if a cremation is intended. Many Asian faiths prefer cremation, while burial is preferred by some Christian faiths. You should approach this sensitively.

Reporting deaths to the Procurator Fiscal or Coroner

When to report

Legally, the Registrar (the government-appointed individual who checks the validity and acceptability of papers such as death certificates) has the responsibility to report deaths that occur in certain situations to the Fiscal or Coroner. However, when the doctor is aware that such reporting would be necessary, it is usual practice for them to report directly to the Fiscal or Coroner to avoid unnecessary delay. Local practices may vary slightly, but doctors should usually consult the Fiscal or Coroner when:

- no doctor has seen the patient during their last illness and within 14 days before death, or after death
- the patient's identity or usual residence is unknown
- the cause of death is unknown
- the death was sudden and unexpected (deaths within 24 h of hospital admission are included here, where the evidence for cause of death may be lacking, in which case the patient's GP may be asked to certify)

- the death was suspicious, violent (including suicide) or unnatural, e.g. due to an accident, drowning or fire
- the death was due to food poisoning or infectious disease
- the death was due to alcohol or drugs
- the death was due to neglect (by self or others)
- the death was due to industrial disease or occurred at work
- the death occurred in or shortly after release from prison or police custody
- the death occurred following an abortion or attempted abortion
- the deceased is a newborn child
- the deceased is a foster child or a child in the care of a local authority or on a local 'at risk' register (some areas of the UK recommend reporting in the case of any child under the age of 18)
- the death might be due to a case of sudden infant death
- the death might relate to recent surgery or anaesthetic (including procedures such as endoscopy)
- the death might relate to a medical mishap (include cases where the family are clearly unhappy with the care given and may make a formal complaint or seek legal action).

Before phoning the Fiscal or Coroner you should discuss the case with the consultant responsible. This allows them to agree that it is appropriate for them to be contacted, that you are the correct person to phone them (you need to know their case well), whether as a team you are prepared to issue a certificate and what it will say.

What you will be asked

- your details, including qualifications (with dates) and how you knew the patient
- the patient's details, including their address and next of kin
- the GP's details, including address and telephone number, if possible
- why the patient was admitted to the hospital and whether it was an emergency or arranged admission
- in the case of an emergency admission, whether the patient had been attending a GP and whether a diagnosis already been made; whether the patient had any previous medical history (either GP or hospital)
- how ill the patient was on admission; what the clinical findings were and what treatment or management occurred
- whether a surgical (including diagnostic) procedure was carried out; whether it was under general or local anaesthetic; if it was technically successful; what was found; what happened after the operation and if it was an expected/recognized complication
- whether you are prepared to issue a death certificate; if yes, what the certificate will say (discuss this with the consultant before you phone).

Post-mortem examinations

There are two types of post-mortem: a hospital post-mortem that requires consent from the next of kin and a Fiscal or Coroner post-mortem that is carried out by law, in the case of a suspicious or sudden and unexplained death, and does not require consent from a relative.

Formal guidelines now cover the process of seeking consent for, and the undertaking of, a hospital post-mortem. A senior doctor should gain consent from relatives and information should be given about the extent of the examination, any planned retention of organs or removal of samples and how such organs and samples would be disposed of. In addition, where appropriate, relatives' views on the use of any material for teaching should be established. It is likely that your hospital will have a local policy, information sheets and a consent form specific to hospital post-mortems.

Cremation papers

Information about who should complete these and what to record is as described above under 'Writing the certificate', p. 401. However, it is worth noting that the person completing Part I should have attended the patient before the death and seen them after death. In addition, where possible, they should also have certified the death, and be available to discuss the case with the doctor completing Part II. There is a statutory fee for such papers, which is usually paid by the undertaker and sent to you at the address you use on the form.

CAPACITY, CONSENT AND COMPETENCE

The term 'capacity' refers to a person's ability to do something. This includes the ability to make decisions regarding medical treatment and is distinct from 'consent' which is a voluntary agreement made by someone who is both informed and competent.

Capacity is a legal concept and ultimately whether or not a person has capacity can only be decided upon in a court of law. In practice, however, healthcare professionals can make decisions regarding capacity without reference to the courts. The term 'competence' is not a technical legal term, but is effectively synonymous with capacity in routine practice.

Consent is often thought to apply only to clinical procedures or operations. However, it should be sought in regard to all contact with patients, including physical examinations, admission to hospital and the sharing of information in medical reports.

Legal context

You are advised to make yourself aware of current best practice statements in your country of work and to keep your understanding of these updated. There may be specific documents that you will be required to use, because of either local protocol or national legislation. Remember that legislation may vary across the UK. Use your regional websites and, if you have any doubt, check with a senior.

Capacity

Principles of capacity

The guidance under 'Legal context', above should be noted. However, in general the following principles of capacity apply:

- there is a presumption of capacity and, hence, incapacity needs to be demonstrated
- there is no objective test for capacity
- improved communication can enhance capacity
- greater mental capacity is needed to make complex or serious decisions
- capacity can fluctuate and may do so in states like delirium
- patients with capacity have the legal right to make decisions contrary to medical opinion
- capacity is decision-specific and its assessment must relate to a particular decision at a particular time, not a range of decisions over a period of time
- decisions made for patients with incapacity must be in their best interests and should not conflict with any known previous wishes expressed by the patient.

Tests of capacity

There is no objective or 'standard' test of capacity and, while cognitive assessment can be informative, it should not be used in isolation as a test for capacity. Generally, for a patient to be considered as having capacity, they need to be able to understand and retain the information relevant to the decision, to use or weigh that information and to communicate their response through whatever means possible. In assessing capacity it is also important to consider that the degree of capacity required for a decision is partly a function of the complexity of the decision: consenting to undergo coronary artery bypass grafting requires more capacity than consenting to have a flexible cystoscopy under local anaesthetic. Equally, while a lack of capacity can result from mental illness, impaired ability to communicate or learning disability, the presence of these states does not define incapacity.

Lack of capacity

In Scotland, where an adult lacks capacity, the Adults with Incapacity (Scotland) Act 2000 requires that the medical profession, rather than immediate family, decides whether an intervention is in the patient's best interest. Two senior clinicians are required to complete an 'incapacity' consent form. It is still preferable to make the family aware of the reasons surrounding a decision and to seek from them any prior views expressed by the patient regarding treatment options.

In England and Wales, where a patient lacks capacity, the Mental Capacity Act 2005 designates the 'decision-maker' as the person usually responsible for the day-to-day care of the patient; this can be a doctor, nurse or social worker. However, any 'advance statement' made by the patient must be considered and either the patient's designated representative, usual carers, a formal deputy appointed by the Court of Protection, or attorney appointed under Lasting Power of Attorney should be consulted. If no such person is available, an 'independent mental capacity advocate' may be invited to be involved in a decision with serious medical impact (unless otherwise covered by the provisions of the Mental Health Act), or where long-term care is proposed. It is also important to consider how long the patient is expected to regain the degree of capacity required and whether the decision should wait until then.

Capacity and consent in emergencies

Where the patient's life is threatened and they have incapacity and there is no legally entitled surrogate to make the decision, the doctor should act in the best interests of the patient. Such incapacity may simply result from the patient being rendered unconscious, but, whatever the cause, any decisions that are made should not conflict with any known previously expressed wishes of the patient.

Capacity and consent in children

A child under 16 years old may have the capacity to give consent, or deny permission, for a medical procedure or treatment. However, they must be deemed competent to do so, and be judged to understand fully the issues involved by the medical staff caring for them (this is known as 'Gillick' competence). The child should be considered the first person from whom consent is gained, but parents or carers must be fully informed, prior to being asked for permission. If permission is denied you should seek advice of senior colleagues in the first instance. Where the child is not competent to give or withhold consent, a person with parental responsibility may act on their behalf. Where a child, deemed competent, refuses an intervention, English Law allows a person with parental responsibility or the court to authorize an intervention where it is deemed to be in the child's best interest – Scottish law does not allow this.

Consent

Principles of consent

There are four key principles for appropriately gaining consent.

Capacity

The patient must have sufficient capacity to give consent in regard to the particular situation for which consent is sought (see above).

Information

When consent is being obtained, the information that is provided should be honest, be enough and be given with respect to patient's dignity, privacy and confidentiality. It should be supplied in a format the patient can understand, be specific to their circumstances and should:

- describe the benefits, significant risks and options, including that of no intervention
- cover whether the proposed intervention is experimental
- describe the involvement of doctors in training and students
- give the name of the doctor who is in overall charge of the intervention
- remind patients of their right to change their mind.

Freedom of choice

Consent must be given voluntarily before any intervention and without pressure, deceit or undue influence.

Ongoing process

The moment of consent is not a single irrevocable time point. A patient is entitled to change their mind, request additional time and information or withdraw their consent at any time, despite giving consent initially. It is important to review whether a patient still gives their consent to an intervention shortly before it takes place, especially if several weeks or months have elapsed since consent was originally obtained.

Types of consent

Implied consent

A patient undresses to be examined, or holds out an arm for a blood test.

Verbal

Verbal consent is sufficient for minimally invasive interventions associated with low risk, for example a rectal examination or an ultrasound. It is important to document in the notes that verbally expressed consent was obtained.

Written

Written consent is advisable for any intervention that carries a significant risk. Consent forms should be completed using full words, not abbreviations, and should be legible. They should not be altered once signed and the time between obtaining consent and the procedure should be <3 months. Examples where written consent should be obtained:

- a procedure or operation involving any sedation or anaesthetic
- the insertion of any tube or needle through the skin, with the exception of taking blood and inserting peripheral lines
- some legal statutes require written consent for specific interventions such as fertility treatments.

Obtaining consent

Significant risk

Patients do not need to be told about every risk attached to an intervention, but information about significant risk should be shared. The significance of a risk depends on how often it may occur in a series of patients and also how severe it would be, should it occur. A risk that is expected to occur in 1:100 patients undergoing a specific intervention is regarded as significant, but equally a risk of death or severe disablement in 1:10 000 cases after another intervention is still highly significant.

Who obtains consent

It is usually preferable for the individual who will be carrying out the intervention to explain to the patient what is involved and obtain their consent. However, it is possible for you to seek consent on behalf of colleagues, provided that you:

- are suitably trained and qualified
- have sufficient knowledge of the proposed intervention and the risks involved
- act in accordance with current national guidance.

Irregular discharge

Patients who are physically and mentally capable can decide to leave the hospital, even if it is not in their best medical interest. However, when patients decide to leave against medical advice, this decision and their awareness of the risk(s) incurred should be documented using an 'irregular discharge' form.

It is easy to feel that a patient is being unreasonable in this situation, but it is their choice and you should respect it. Explain the concerns you have about their health and why you feel it is best that they stay in hospital. Do not enter into an argument or protracted discussion. Once you have stated your case, if they still choose to go, allow them to sign the form and leave.

It is not normal to make any transport arrangements for such patients and most clinicians would also not offer any discharge medication, tests or follow-up after such a discharge.

CHILD PROTECTION

All doctors have a responsibility for the protection of children. This involves the timely recognition of abuse or neglect, and the subsequent referral of the child or family to the appropriate individual or agency.

All health authorities, trusts and hospitals have their own child protection procedures, documentation and designated officers. It is essential that you familiarize yourself with this information in your induction period. Exact terminology and legal practice vary between countries, but the following provides an introduction to child protection.

Examination, consent and confidentiality

When examination of a potentially abused child is required, consent, preferably written, should be obtained by a senior doctor (see 'Capacity and consent in children', p. 405). The managing consultant should be involved early in any such case.

All children should be examined in the presence of a chaperone (not just the parent or carer) and the chaperone's details should be documented in the notes, along with those of anyone else who was present. This is not only for the protection of the child, but also of the health professional involved. Ideally, it may also help reduce the child's anxiety.

Doctors are obliged to share all necessary information with other statutory agencies (police and social services). The GMC confirms that in cases of suspected abuse, 'you must give information promptly to an appropriate, responsible person or agency, when you believe it is in the best interests' of the child or young person to do so.

Types of child abuse

'Child abuse is any act of commission or omission, which results in harm to the child'

(RCPCH 2006 – Child Protection Companion).

There are four types of child abuse: physical, emotional, neglect and sexual. Abuse or neglect can occur within the family, community, school/residential unit, or health unit.

Physical abuse

Where children have been subjected to physical abuse, the history that they present with often fails to make sense, is inconsistent or changes. It may not explain the injury, or fit with the child's stage of development, e.g. a baby <3 months old apparently rolling off a bed or sofa. The events may not have been witnessed, the carer's response to the injury may have been unusual or inappropriate, or presentation to health services delayed. Children presenting with physical abuse often have a history of multiple attendances to A&E, primary care or both. Check the Child Protection Register to see if they are previously know to social services and, if so, why.

In all cases, make detailed notes of any injuries, including a diagram where possible, outlining the site, size, shape and colour of lesions.

Bruising

- accidental bruises: front of the legs, knees, hands, extensor surface of the arms, forehead and bony prominences
- unusual accidental bruising: ears, neck, lower back or buttocks.

It is not possible accurately to determine the age of bruises, and you must consider alternative possible explanations, such as Henoch–Schönlein purpura, thrombocytopenia, coagulation disorder or meningococcal infection.

Fractures and internal injury

In children and infants, fractures require a significant amount of force and, when accidental, are most often seen in those over the age of 5 years. Spiral fracture of a long bone, especially when there is an inappropriate history or mechanism of injury, is very suspicious of physical abuse. Any fracture in an infant should raise the suspicion of potentially serious internal injury (abdomen, brain) and appropriate investigations should be undertaken. If you have any concerns about the mechanism of injury you should discuss the case with a senior colleague.

Burns and scalds

Burns and scalds are common in children; however, certain aspects of the injury or the history may alert you to a possible non-accidental nature. Again, the history may be inappropriate to the developmental stage of the child, inconsistent with the injury or change when recounted to different people. The following are features which may be associated with inflicted burns:

- circular burns, which are deep and suggestive of contact with cigarettes
- burns to both upper and/or lower limbs, often roughly symmetrical in nature
- burns which have a distinct shape or pattern, suggestive of contact with an object
- burns caused by being immersed in hot water, which may be in a glove or stocking pattern and may have no splash marks (if the child was held still).

Most burns or scalds are likely to be due to a brief lapse in normally protective and caring parents or carers. The significance of these injuries potentially constituting abuse is if they or other similar injuries occur repeatedly, or you suspect may have been caused deliberately.

Emotional abuse

Emotional abuse is very difficult to detect, especially if it is in isolation from other forms of abuse. Those at risk may be from a family with a history of alcohol or drug abuse, mental or other ill health. The history can be extremely variable and can range from the withdrawn, quiet, non-demanding infant, through to the bad-tempered, violent child. Growth may be affected with failure to gain weight sufficiently or short stature relative to parental heights.

Neglect

Various forms of neglect exist. It may involve failing to meet the child's needs to an appropriate standard in areas such as clothing, cleanliness and nutrition. There may be an obvious lack of supervision, allowing the child to place themselves at risk. It may be seen in younger children who are not offered appropriate stimulation or an educational environment. The child may not be presented to health services when necessary. As noted with emotional abuse, it can be difficult to substantiate in isolation, but frequently occurs alongside other types of abuse. Suspicious signs might include poor weight gain or short stature, inappropriate clothing for the prevailing weather, developmental delay or delayed presentation of an unwell child.

If you suspect a child may be suffering from either emotional abuse and/or neglect, but are unsure, contact the local child protection representative. You may also be able to gain more information from other members of the healthcare team, such as health visitor or general practitioner.

Sexual abuse

Children or young people who are being, or have been, sexually abused may present in many different ways, to a number of agencies. They are often threatened by the abuser, so may not make a clear disclosure or may deny that it is occurring. The following are suggestive of, but not diagnostic of, sexual abuse: vaginal irritation, redness or bleeding; rectal bleeding; anogenital warts; inappropriate sexualized behaviour. More obvious indicators include infection with a sexually transmitted disease.

While it may be appropriate to examine the genitalia of children for certain conditions such as urinary tract infection, abdominal pain or reported injury to the perineum, it is essential to be accompanied and to gain specific permission for that element of the examination. If you suspect sexual abuse, it is best to leave the examination of the genitalia to a senior and experienced clinician. In the initial examination(s) of a child with suspected sexual abuse, it is inappropriate to examine a child internally or to use instruments such as a speculum. This should always be deferred to those with specialist training.

MENTAL HEALTH ACT

To whom the Act applies

The legislation covering mental health varies across the UK, especially since the introduction of the Mental Health Act (Scotland) 2003. However, the definition of what constitutes a mental disorder is largely the same, e.g. a mental disorder is any mental illness, personality disorder or learning disability, however caused or manifest.

Note that a person cannot be judged to be mentally disordered or subject to detention under a Mental Health Act by reason of any of the following:

- sexual orientation
- sexual deviancy
- transsexualism

- transvestism
- dependence on, or use of, alcohol or drugs
- behaviour that causes, or is likely to cause, harassment, alarm or distress to any other person, or acting as no other prudent person would act.

Current legislation also emphasizes the need for any action to be in the best interest of the patient and achieved with the minimum possible restriction. Likewise, principles of respect for diversity, non-discrimination and patient involvement in their management apply.

Detention

Different sections of the Mental Health Acts relate to different situations, a summary of which is given below. Comprehensive coverage of the detail in relation to these can be found on the relative Department of Health websites. Comments regarding the sections for England and Wales are listed followed by those for the corresponding section in Scotland.

Removal to a place of safety

- Section 136: for police to arrest and detain an individual who is at risk to themselves or others for up to 72 h
- Scotland: Section 300; similar but for 24 h.

Short-term detention

- Section 2: admission of a patient with a mental disorder, for assessment; applies for up to 28 days and requires formal application, by a doctor, close relative or social worker on the basis of two medical recommendations, one of whom should be an approved doctor in accordance with Section 12 of the Act, e.g. a psychiatrist, and one of whom should know the patient, e.g. a GP.
- Scotland: Short-term Detention Certificate (Section 44); requires examination by an approved medical practitioner (psychiatrist) and approval by Mental Health Officer (specially trained social worker); lasts 28 days.

Emergency detention

- Section 4: permits admission and detention of patients outside of hospital; only one medical recommendation is necessary; applies for up to 72 h after which conversion to Section 2 or 3 is necessary with a second recommendation
- Section 5(2): detention, by the doctor in charge of the ward, of a voluntary patient already in hospital, where they have a mental disorder and are at risk of causing harm to themselves or other by leaving; lasts 72 h
- Scotland: Emergency Detention Certificate (Section 36); any medical practitioner in consultation with the Mental Health Officer; lasts 72 h (from the time of admission if not already admitted) and can be extended by an Extension Certificate while a compulsory treatment order is prepared.

Compulsory detention

- Section 3: admission for treatment of an established mental disorder; applies for up to 6 months and also requires two medical recommendations, as per Section 2; use of this section must only be considered where hospital treatment is appropriate and likely to yield benefit and it is necessary for the health of others that the patient is detained
- Scotland: Compulsory Treatment Order (Section 64); requires approval by a Tribunal after a report by the Mental Health Officer; follows recommendation by two practitioners, one of whom should be the patient's GP and the other an approved medical practitioner (psychiatrist); lasts 6 months, although it must be reviewed formally 2 months before it is due to expire; an extension lasts 6 months, after which review is annually

and by a Tribunal every 2 years; an Interim Compulsory Treatment Order, lasting 28 days, can be granted to allow due consideration by the Tribunal; a Restriction Order (Section 59 of Criminal Procedure Act 1995) can be added to a compulsory order, making it without limit of time.

Nurse powers

- Section 5(4): for psychiatric nurses to detain patients, currently in hospital voluntarily, for up to 6 h pending examination
- Scotland: Section 299; similar but allows only for 2 h, with 1 h extension for the examination itself.

DRIVING

Legislation

The key legislation that can restrict driving in the UK because of medical conditions is contained in the Road Traffic Act 1988. Detailed and current guidance on what is covered by the current regulations can be found in the 'medical rules' section of the DVLA website.

Two types of licence exist and the potential for a condition to affect an individual's right to hold a licence is different for both in some circumstances. Group 1 licences relate to motor cars and motorcycles. Group 2 licences are granted for drivers of large lorries and buses. As well as different groups of licence, the Act describes different levels of disability:

- prescribed: a disability with a legal bar to the holding of a licence, e.g. epilepsy
- relevant: a disability likely to make the driver dangerous, which therefore requires the removal of a licence, e.g. visual field defect
- prospective: a disability which, by being unpredictable or progressive, may cause a prescribed or relevant disability in time; licence holding may continue, but is subject to the attainment of certain conditions, which are kept under interval medical review, e.g. diabetics on insulin.

Your responsibilities

If a patient has a condition that affects their right to hold a licence, you must advise them that they have a legal duty to notify the DVLA. If they are not capable of understanding this advice, for example due to dementia, you must notify the DVLA yourself.

If the patient understands the advice, but is not willing to accept it, you can advise them to seek a second opinion, but not to drive until that opinion has been given. If a patient continues to drive, despite being told not to drive, you should make every effort to persuade them to stop. Where this continues to be unsuccessful, you should advise the patient that you will notify the Medical Advisor at the DVLA, in confidence, and advise the patient, in writing, when this is done.

Common conditions

Table 13.1 contains a list of common conditions and their impact on driving with a group 1 licence (some reference to group 2 is included in the cardiac section). Not all conditions listed require notification to the DVLA. Those that do are indicated by '[N]' (notifiable).

The list is not exhaustive. In particular, the additional effect of a diagnosis on group 2 holders is worth checking on the official DVLA website. Moreover, any condition impairing any aspect of a patient's visual, mental or physical capacity to drive, to whatever extent and for even a brief duration, should prompt consideration of their fitness to drive.

Table 13.1 Common conditions affecting driving status

Neurological	
First single fit (repeat fits = single if within 24 h of initial one)[N], or fit after drugs or alcohol[N], or fits related to neurosurgical conditions[N]	1 year off driving. Restored if symptom free after medical review
Simple faint	No reporting necessary
Unexplained collapse, no markers of fit and normal ECG[N]	4 weeks off
Unexplained collapse, abnormal ECG or injury at wheel or more than one episode in 6/12 or structural heart disease[N]	4 weeks off; and can resume if cause identified *and* treated. Otherwise 6 months off
Unexplained collapse but possible fit, e.g. tongue biting; amnesia >5 min, post-ictal, injury, headache post attack, incontinence[N]	1 year off
Sudden dizziness, e.g. Ménière's[N]	Stop until controlled
Stroke/TIA	4 weeks off; resume without notifying DVLA if no residual deficit. Otherwise notify[N]
Multiple TIAs[N]	Off until 3 months elapsed since last attack
Serious head injury, e.g. compound depressed fracture[N]	6–12 months off
Intracranial haemorrhage (subdural/extradural, intracerebral)[N]	6–12 months off
Subarachnoid haemorrhage[N]	Depends on whether cause identified and level of deficit remaining
Cardiac[a] *Group 2 will usually require further assessment before re-starting*	
Angina: notification not required group 1, required group 2	Cease if symptoms at wheel and re-start when under control, group 1; group 2[a,N]
Angioplasty: notification not required group 1, required group 2	Off 1 week, group 1; 6 weeks, group 2[a,N]
CABG: notification not required group 1, required group 2	Off 4 weeks, group 1; 3 months, group 2[a,N]
MI: notification not required group 1, required group 2	Off 4 weeks, group 1; 6 weeks, group 2[a,N]
Non-ST: MI notification not required group 1, required group 2	Stop until 1/52 post-successful angioplasty, group 1; group 2, 6 weeks after angioplasty[a]
Aortic aneurysm[N]	DVLA to be notified for aneurysms >6 cm, group 1; banned if >5.5 cm, group 2
Arrhythmia: no notification required group 1 unless distracting/disabling symptoms; notify group 2[N]	Driving to cease if condition is or is likely to be incapacitating. Can restart if condition identified and controlled for 4 weeks. (Group 2 more stringent guidance)
Hypertension: no notification, group 1; notify, group 2[N]	Driving fine, group 1, unless problems with side-effects of treatment; group 2, stop if resting SBP >180 and/or DBP >100 mmHg
Pacemaker[N]	Off 1 week, group 1; 6 weeks, group 2[a]

(Continued)

Table 13.1 Common conditions affecting driving status—cont'd

Diabetic	
On insulin[N]	No restriction as long as recognizes hypoglycaemia and can meet visual standards, but licence length may be capped and require interval review
On tablets; possible[N]	As above. Notification depends on whether laser treatment to eye needed or circulation or neuropathy problems in legs
On diet only	No notification required; drive if well
Frequent hypoglycaemia[N]	Cease until controlled. Re-start following GP/consultant report
Impaired symptoms of hypoglycaemia[N]	Stop until evidence obtained that normal awareness has returned
Psychiatric	
Drug use (alcohol, drugs of abuse)[N]	Persistent = off until 6 months (cannabis, amphetamines, ecstasy, hallucinogens, alcohol misuse) –12 months (opiates, methadone, benzodiazepines, methamphetamines, cocaine, alcohol dependency) abstinence achieved. Specialist report may be required
Suicidal intent (persistent)[N]	Cease until controlled and pending medical enquiry
Psychosis/hypomania/schizophrenia[N]	Cease until compliant and well 3/12 and pending specialist medical report
Dementia	Not specified, depends on level of capacity. If has poor short-term memory, lack of insight and judgement, or disorientation, should not drive and should notify[N]
Visual	
The legal level of acuity required of all drivers is that they can read, in good light, from a distance of 20 m (using glasses if necessary) a registration mark fixed to a motor vehicle containing letters 79 mm high and 50 mm wide. Registration for sight impairment is normally thought to be incompatible with holding a licence	
Diplopia[N]	Cease on diagnosis. Re-start when controlled
Visual field defect[N]	Depends on extent and likelihood of progression
Monocular vision (complete loss in one eye, including light perception)[N]	Cease until clinical report advises patient has adapted to condition with remaining eye. Re-starting assumes other eye normal
Respiratory	
Sleep disorders, including obstructive sleep apnoea[N]	Cease until clinical advice received confirming satisfactory control
Cough syncope[N]	Cease until control confirmed by medical advice
Chronic renal failure[N]	Driving usually not restricted, unless dizzy or cognitively impaired

[a]Scotland: separate mechanism for enhanced surveillance.

[N]Notifiable.

NOTIFIABLE DISEASES

The legal requirement to notify certain infectious diseases was introduced in the UK in 1889. The principal aims of this legislation were to control potential outbreaks and reduce the then significantly high mortality associated with infectious disease. A secondary benefit of notification has been the wealth of epidemiological data generated from returns. These allow accurate local and national statistics to be compiled regarding a variety of illnesses.

The list of notifiable diseases has increased over the years and now stands at over 30 (Table 13.2). The lists in England and Wales are similar to those in Scotland, but not identical.

When and how to notify

The prime purpose of notification is to rapidly detect potential outbreaks, and diseases should therefore be notified on clinical suspicion. If a diagnosis subsequently proves to be incorrect the record can be amended or cancelled. The notification should be made to the local Proper Officer of the Local Authority, in England and Wales; often a Consultant in Communicable Disease Control (CCDC), or, in Scotland, to the Consultant in Public Health Medicine (CPHM) at the Health Board.

Written notification, using specific forms, may be adequate in many cases. However, an additional telephone call is required for suspected outbreaks or other situations where urgent action is required, e.g. cases of meningococcal and *E. coli* 0157 infection. A fee is payable for each case notified.

Statutory powers for health protection

The aim, in all cases, is to offer the patient effective treatment and to protect the public in a spirit of collaboration. Occasionally, this collaborative approach fails. Certain legal powers, including removal to hospital, can be invoked by medical staff over patients with a notifiable disease who pose a significant risk to the community, e.g. a patient with multi-drug-resistant pulmonary tuberculosis who is not complying with treatment. However, such measures are rarely needed in clinical practice and are extremely difficult to implement.

Non-statutory reporting and surveillance

New infectious diseases are emerging, while many of the traditional notifiable diseases are now very rare. Furthermore, drug resistance in common organisms is becoming an increasing public health threat. Therefore, the statutory notification system is no longer adequate, by itself, for disease surveillance.

Additional surveillance of non-notifiable pathogens, such as *C. difficile* and MRSA, is undertaken between laboratories, infection control teams and public health services. This practice has become increasingly important over recent years. Indeed, the entire framework for notification and public health legislation is currently under review and may change significantly in the near future.

HIV TESTING

The acquired immune deficiency syndrome (AIDS) results from infection with human immunodeficiency virus (HIV-1) and is defined by the development of specific opportunistic infections or malignancies. Although AIDS remains the leading cause of death in Africa, HIV infection has a good prognosis in patients with better access to highly active antiretroviral therapy (HAART). The ethics of HIV testing have changed to reflect this new reality.

Table 13.2 Notifiable diseases in England and Wales, and in Scotland

Disease	England/Wales	Scotland
Acute encephalitis	X	
Acute poliomyelitis	X	X
Anthrax	X	X
Chickenpox	X	X
Cholera	X	X
Diphtheria	X	X
Dysentery	X	X
Erysipelas		X
Food poisoning	X	X
Legionellosis		X
Leptospirosis	X	X
Lyme disease		X
Malaria	X	X
Measles	X	X
Membranous croup		X
Meningitis – meningococcal	X	X
Meningitis – all other forms	X	
Meningococcal septicaemia (without meningitis)	X	X
Mumps	X	X
Ophthalmia neonatorum	X	
Paratyphoid fever	X	X
Plague	X	X
Puerperal fever		X
Rabies	X	X
Relapsing fever	X	X
Rubella	X	X
Scarlet fever	X	X
Smallpox	X	X
Tetanus	X	X
Toxoplasmosis		X
Tuberculosis[a]	X	X
Typhoid fever	X	X
Typhus fever	X	X
Viral haemorrhagic fever	X	X
Viral hepatitis – all forms	X	X
Whooping cough	X	X
Yellow fever	X	X

[a] Scotland: separate mechanism for enhanced surveillance.

The test

Failure to offer a test for a treatable disease such as HIV should not be considered ethically acceptable and there is currently a strong drive to 'normalize' the process of testing and enhance uptake. The main reasons for offering an HIV test are:

- routine part of clinical care, e.g. blood, semen and organ donation (mandatory), during pregnancy, GUM clinic or patients being considered for dialysis
- asymptomatic individuals with risk factors, e.g. sexual risk factors, IV drug users
- symptomatic individuals with a condition potentially related to HIV (see p. 246)
- as requested by insurance companies, employers, or for visa applications.

Consent

Informed verbal consent must always be obtained prior to testing for HIV, except in a few very exceptional circumstances, e.g. testing a child where consent from a parent may be distorted because they are the cause of the child's infection.

Pre-test discussion

A diagnosis of HIV can have serious social and financial implications, in addition to the obvious medical consequences for the patient. Therefore, before seeking consent for an HIV test, you should perform a risk assessment of the likelihood of a positive test and discuss the following issues with your patient:

- the benefits of testing, e.g. early diagnosis, effective treatment available
- the 'window-period' concept; see below
- the implications of a positive and negative result, e.g. as mentioned above and below
- confidentiality
- consent
- how and when the result will be given.

Patients identified as being at high risk or those with particular concerns can be offered more in-depth discussion. Aim to dispel any myths, such as the ongoing belief that a negative HIV test will prejudice life insurance; it will not.

Results

Most HIV test results will be negative and the patient can be reassured. Nevertheless, life-style modification aimed at avoiding future risk should be advised. If the test was undertaken within the 3-month 'window-period' from the episode of risk-related activity, a follow-up test should be arranged since false negatives can occur.

A positive test result will be very upsetting for the patient and skills in breaking bad news will be helpful (see 'Communication with patients and families', p. 386). Seek specialist advice ahead of the discussion, as there may be specific questions that you are unable to answer. In general, be reassuring and positive about the prognosis. Partner notification and contact tracing is important, but should be performed by somebody who is trained and experienced in this area.

COMPUTERS AND DATA PROTECTION

Computer use

The computers that you use at work are part of the NHS network and are crucial to the functioning of the hospital. In many cases, hospitals utilize firewalls and other restrictions to protect their systems from viruses or server overload. NHS networks may have a limited bandwidth and computer terminals with relatively low functionality.

Local policies will apply to your use of such systems and you should not expect a similar internet connection to that which you have outside work. You should not download material from the internet or install non-approved software (e.g. screen savers, games, etc.) that take up unnecessary space or interfere with other functions of the computers needed for ward work.

You are expected to use NHS computers for work activity and in accordance with what would be expected of a professional doctor. You should not expect any privacy in regard to e-mails or documents you create on hospital systems and should be aware of the standard practice to monitor website visits and downloads performed by hospital staff.

You should note that the Computer Misuse Act 1990 permits prosecution in regard to unauthorized access to computer systems and deliberate transfer of viruses and other malicious code.

Data protection

The Caldicott Report 1997 and the Data Protection Act 1998 cover the handling of sensitive patient data. You have a responsibility to ensure that all data about patients is kept confidential, whether in your head, on paper or on a computer. Case-files should not be removed from the hospital or left unsecured in non-clinical areas. Lists you make of patient details should also be kept safe.

Electronic communication about patients should not contain identifiable information. Logbooks or portfolios should not contain patient data other than case numbers. In addition, you should note that you cannot store any information about a patient in a computer database or file without their consent and that any stored information can only be used for the purposes outlined at the time of consent.

Looking after yourself 14

OCCUPATIONAL HEALTH DEPARTMENT AND PERSONAL HEALTH

The contact that doctors have with patients on a daily basis increases the risk of both contracting and spreading infection. Therefore, it is a personal and professional responsibility to wash your hands, use alcohol disinfectant hand gel (see 'HAI', p. 441) and wear appropriate protection when performing practical procedures, as described in the relevant chapter.

An awareness of your own health is also essential. You should be able to recognize when your capacity to work is limited by physical, mental or emotional difficulties and be prepared to take appropriate action.

Occupational health

Occupational Health (OH) departments help to ensure that NHS staff are physically and mentally able to undertake the work required of them. However, they are not a substitute for a GP and you should ensure you are registered with a local practice. The main contacts you can expect to have with OH are:

- when you are required to demonstrate that your immunity to hepatitis B infection is satisfactory: every time you move into a new health board
- for assessment and advice in the event of illness or injury that has occurred as a direct consequence of your employment, e.g. infectious diarrhoea, needlestick injury
- for assessment and advice regarding a prolonged illness or a condition that may be adversely affected by work, e.g. back or joint injury; stress or depression
- for vaccination against organisms other than hepatitis B, e.g. influenza.

Hepatitis B status

You need to be immunized against hepatitis B infection and have a booster every 5 years. You will need to provide proof of such immunity before you can work. Therefore, you should keep and present a copy of your vaccination certificate when required.

Exposure to blood-borne viruses

Where you are exposed to blood or blood-contaminated body fluids, take the following immediate action:

- mucocutaneous exposure: where skin, nose, eyes or mouth are affected, rinse with copious amounts of water (or a saline drip into eyes and nose)
- needle-stick injury: squeeze around the wound to induce bleeding, but avoid pressing on it directly; then wash with soap, but without scrubbing.

Further action

This will be dictated by the risk posed by the patient. Therefore, they should be questioned (not by you) regarding risk factors for blood-borne virus (BBV) infection, e.g. intravenous drug use, body piercing and tattoos (especially if performed overseas), high-risk sexual contact and previous transfusions. The incident should be documented in the patient's case-notes in addition to their consent, if given, for BBV testing. A clinical incident report form should be completed. Thereafter, you should contact OH (or A&E out of hours), who will coordinate the following as appropriate:

- sampling of your own blood for viral testing
- antiretrovirals, a hepatitis booster or hepatitis immunoglobulin depending on the perceived risk based on the patient's history
- a review a few days later with the results of the patient's blood tests to determine if a high risk exposure has taken place; if so, you may be advised to give further blood for testing in a few months, not to donate blood, to practise safe sex and to avoid undertaking surgical procedures.

A stressful job

Stress is a normal part of our everyday lives. Our physiological responses are inbuilt and have evolved to help us survive situations involving actual or potential physical danger. However, the same physiological response may be triggered by psychological stress.

In small amounts, stress can be helpful, making us more efficient or helping us rise to a challenge, e.g. dealing with a cardiac arrest. However, more persistent stress levels are rarely helpful and usually occur when we feel unable to cope with what is required of us. This perception varies from individual to individual and from day to day. It is influenced by external and personal factors and the coping strategies we have learned. The individuality of stress means it can happen in any branch of medicine. Furthermore, a change of career path may not reduce your stress levels if you have not learned how to recognize stress and modify it.

A situation at work is more likely to cause stress when it happens in the context of other personal problems, fatigue or hunger. In addition, a desire to please everyone and a need for perfection can magnify problems out of all perspective. Stress is cumulative: a small stress on top of others can be all it takes for your performance at work to be affected, for you to feel overwhelmed or become ill.

Recognizing the signs of stress

Stress affects different people in different ways:

Physical

- cardiorespiratory: increased heart rate, fast and shallow breathing
- gastrointestinal: nausea and vomiting, heartburn, diarrhoea, changes in appetite
- general: headaches, back pain, blurred vision, cold or sweaty hands and feet, dry mouth, increased number of minor illnesses, change in libido or sleeping patterns, fatigue.

Psychological and behavioural

- inability to concentrate, forgetfulness or restlessness
- increased errors or clumsiness, e.g. ordering a test for the wrong patient, a 'near-miss' in the car
- increased emotional lability, irritability, irrational thinking, loss of perspective
- increased compulsive behaviour, e.g. cleaning, smoking
- negative thoughts or defensiveness.

Coping during times of stress

- recognize that you are stressed
- recognize that you have a choice: control it or allow it to control you
- fix a time in your mind when you will pay special attention to yourself and any stresses; then focus on the current tasks, one at a time
- take extra care to be polite, considerate and pleasant
- take special care when undertaking complicated tasks, e.g. ask for assistance with a procedure; drive slowly
- accept help and delegate where appropriate
- if possible, take a few minutes alone to pause, breathe and reflect on what has gone well recently, or on something that you particularly enjoy
- get as much sleep as you can and try to fit in some exercise, even walking
- do not skip breakfast
- eat regularly but avoid heavy meals
- avoid large amounts of coffee, alcohol or chocolate.

Stress debrief

When we are stressed is it easy to forget what it is like to be 'normal'. You can address this with simple measures, e.g. observe and take pleasure in 'small' things (less traffic on the road to work, a lovely view, thanks from a patient); keep in touch with your friends; sleep lots and exercise. Specific stress reduction techniques fill many books, the following are only a few suggestions:

It helps to share feelings of frustration, fear or anxiety with others. They may well feel the same. Try to share humour or find something positive from situations. Beware the general 'whingeing' session. Being overly negative can exhaust your energy further. Also, do not expect such sessions to deal with your problems properly: everyone has enough of their own.

If you are stressed, take time out. Stop and reflect on why you were stressed and what part of that was your reaction to something, rather than just what happened. Writing down individual reasons for stress can be helpful. Consider why each is stressful and ask yourself which of them is really reasonable for you to be stressed about. Identify those that you can do something about and those that you need help with. Plan when and how you can take any action.

Support

Use the BMA and other telephone counselling services. If you persistently feel you are not coping, sit down with your supervisor and talk about it.

AGGRESSION AND VIOLENCE

Prevention

Environmental factors can contribute to aggressive behaviour, particularly temperature, noise, lighting and space. Consider your own safety when meeting with patients and relatives:

- avoid seeing patients and families alone; where this is necessary make sure that someone else is aware of the meeting

- choose a seating position that places you rather than the patient nearest to the door
- know how to summon help and exit the room.

Aim to reduce any aggression through your behaviour in all aspects of the consultation:

- consider what effect a condition or situation may be having on a patient
- explain all your intentions and actions to the patient in advance
- communicate well (with an interpreter where necessary)
- adopt a position that is on the same eye level as a patient, e.g. both sitting
- adopt a calm and self-controlled manner; focusing on controlling your breathing may help
- adopt calm and non-threatening non-verbal behaviour: avoid sudden movements
- do not compromise a patient's personal space without permission.

Early suspicion

Aggressive or violent behaviour is more likely in those affected by:

- alcohol and drugs
- physical pain, trauma or traumatic stress
- fear, anxiety or psychosis
- not being heard, sense of neglect or inattention
- disorientation or confusion
- sleep disturbance and fatigue
- provocation by staff, patients or others
- boredom or frustration
- an aggressive coping mechanism, restrictive expression or a previous history of aggressive behaviour
- physical illness, e.g. epilepsy.

Warning signs

Warnings that behaviour may become violent include:

- increased restlessness or pacing
- increased muscle tone, or clenching of fists
- increased volume or speed of speech or refusal to communicate
- erratic movements, gestures or movement towards you
- facial expressions of tension or frustration
- verbal threats or expressions of feelings of anger or upset
- lack of concentration or unclear thought processes
- delusions or hallucinations.

Restraint

The decision to use chemical or physical restraint should only be taken as a last resort by an experienced health professional trained in aggression management. Take advice from senior nursing staff or medical colleagues and do not get involved in physical restraint until you have been properly trained. Never take part in a restraint procedure if you are pregnant.

It is beyond the scope of this text to detail the various breakaway and restraint manoeuvres possible. However, where physical restraint is being used, note that there must be at least one member of staff of the same sex as the patient and at no time should pressure be applied to the patient's neck, chest or back. The patient's airway should be protected at all times, especially if the patient is placed (for what should only be a very short time) on the floor.

A debriefing following such an incident is very important. You should participate in this if you have been involved.

DIFFICULT COLLEAGUES AND COLLEAGUES IN DIFFICULTY

Problems with colleagues may arise when:

- they are not working well within the team
- you have concerns about their clinical care
- they have physical or mental dependence or illness
- the problem is you.

A problem within the team

The non-coping colleague

Acute medical care is busy and challenging and, while some people thrive, others find it very stressful. Individuals who prefer to tackle problems one at a time or who cannot rest until everything is done often struggle and can also find it difficult to ask others for help.

The working life of every doctor involves stressful and difficult situations, for which some feel more personally responsible than others, especially when a patient dies. Some people find it difficult to talk about how they are coping or feeling, and misplaced guilt or a fear of appearing weak can lead to significant emotional distress.

When a colleague is clearly not coping there is often a temptation to give them less to do. Rather than helping, this may simply cut them off from the group and exacerbate the problem. It also places more work unfairly on the other members the team. Group support, and the sharing of difficult experiences among colleagues, can help doctors 'in difficulty' cope with their stress and appreciate that they are not alone. However, persisting concerns should be discussed with your colleague's educational supervisor; see below.

The lazy or disorganized colleague

Some people do only what is asked of them and nothing more. They may not see anything wrong with sitting in the coffee room when their work is done, rather than helping a colleague who is having a particularly busy day. Of course, lazy colleagues simply find themselves without help when they need it, but as overall effectiveness directly influences patient care, lazy doctors need to appreciate the value of better team work. Speak to them directly about this.

A different problem, which may have a similar effect on patient care, is the colleague who cannot organize their work. If you are naturally organized, it is easy to feel frustrated and to suspect that your colleague is simply not trying hard enough. However, stupid people do not get into medical school and doctors have different strengths and ways of working. Share examples of how you run your ward; introduce them to short-cuts and tools; if necessary remind them they are doing the journal club. Persisting concerns should be discussed with your colleague's educational or clinical supervisor; see below.

The bully

This can be an extension of the 'lazy' doctor, e.g. a colleague who pressurizes you to swap into their bad shift on the rota, but refuses to swap into a similar shift in return. Most clinical teams will not tolerate such behaviour and should attempt, as a group, to approach the individual and make it clear that it is unacceptable. However, bullying behaviour can have serious consequences later in a doctor's career and it may be in their interests to involve their supervisor early.

A problem with clinical competence

During your career you are certain to come across colleagues who you would not want to look after a member of your own family, perhaps due to a lack of clinical knowledge or judgement, persistent carelessness or a rude and uncaring attitude. In cases where patients are at risk, you have a responsibility as part of your own 'duties of a doctor' (see 'GMC', p. 463) to advise your colleague's supervising consultant or their educational supervisor of your concerns; see below.

A problem with dependence or illness

Anything that interferes with a doctor's capacity to provide effective and safe patient care becomes a shared responsibility as soon as you are aware of it. Medical graduates are as susceptible to mental illness or dependence on alcohol or drugs as the rest of the population. This natural tendency may be exacerbated by the stress associated with work. If you have suspicions that a colleague is suffering from psychological illness or drug dependence you should discuss your concerns as soon as possible with their supervisor; see below.

In addition, what may have seemed reasonable behaviour as a student, e.g. a night out drinking after a hard week, is not acceptable where the student has become a doctor with responsibilities for patient care the next day. If your colleague is smelling of alcohol or is unfit for work, they should be sent home. Consider also whether their supervisor should be informed; see below.

Likewise, it is not being a 'good doctor' to turn up for work suffering from a gastrointestinal infection or loaded up with cough medicines. It is hard enough for the team to stay fit without everyone sharing their infections and 'I had a cold' is not a satisfactory excuse, in court or in front of the GMC, for clinical errors. Where your colleague is ill, they should be sent home until fit.

A problem with you

When you are having problems with a colleague, consider the reasons for this. You may simply have a different way of working from them or have very different personalities. Alternatively, your own behaviour may be the problem.

It is important to try to maintain a functioning working relationship with those with whom you work regularly. Sit down with them to discuss how you both feel. Try to discuss the problem in terms of how their behaviour or attitude is making you feel, even if they did not intend that. Do not just list a series of things they are doing or not doing to your liking. Do not use the words 'always' or 'never' in reference to them. Explore how they think you could work better together.

Speaking to a supervisor

When you have a concern about a colleague it is important that you speak to their supervisor as soon as is practical. However, presenting a general 'feeling' is not helpful or appropriate. Ideally, you should be able to substantiate your concerns with dates, times and patient cases or names of staff involved. In the case of a serious concern, it may be wise to follow this with a written note to the supervisor, summarizing your meeting and its discussion. Keep a copy of this, in case you are involved in any more formal proceedings later.

COMPLAINTS HANDLING

Prevention of a formal complaint

Good complaints handling is largely about the prevention, or defusing, of an informal complaint. Many complaints are initiated by a relative rather than the patient themselves. Over half of those that reach an independent review panel involve the death of a patient. The handling of a family before and after a death is very important. Likewise, the sensitive and supportive communication of bad news, in an appropriate environment, is vital (see 'The 'bad news' discussion', p. 387).

In the case of elderly or terminally ill patients, there may be little that can be done to reverse the underlying processes. However, good palliative care and consideration of issues such as nutrition, cleanliness, analgesia, privacy and assistance in discharge planning or home care are important, especially to families.

The majority of complaints that prove difficult to resolve informally relate to one of the following:

Poor communication

- lack of information: try to keep patients and families aware of what will affect them ahead of it happening and make sure you know all the facts before you speak with them
- different information given to family members: establish who the patient's next of kin is and communicate with other family members through that person; ensure that the patient gives consent to their next of kin being told information and that this person will share crucial information, such as a diagnosis of cancer, with other key family members
- an apparent 'cover up' of something that should not have happened: if a family member claims something happened that you were not aware of, do not deny it; explain you were not aware of it, offer to investigate it and meet with them again
- insensitive communication of bad news or an apparent lack of respect of family wishes as to how the news is told; for more details on appropriate communication, see 'The 'bad news' discussion', p. 387
- lack of courtesy: if the clinic is running late or there has been a long wait in A&E, apologize for keeping them waiting.

Poor record-keeping

Poor record-keeping in itself does not normally lead to complaints, but can lead to difficulty resolving a complaint because of a lack of sufficient evidence to refute it. In particular, conversations in person or on the phone with patients or their families should be recorded in the notes.

The record should note the name of the person(s) involved, their relationship with the patient, the date, time and venue and the substance of the communication. With regard to conversations with family members, note should also be made of the advance permission granted by the patient, assuming they are competent to do so.

Missed or late diagnosis

There is an increasing public expectation that doctors can diagnose and treat all illness quickly. Where a patient is in hospital for more than a few days with an illness that is not straightforward or is slow to resolve, you should expect that families will ask for information. It is worth anticipating this and offering to meet ahead of their request.

Poor initial complaints handling

Many people find complaining stressful. By the time they do raise a problem they may have been concerned about it for a while and its importance to them may have grown out of all proportion. Also, the stress they feel in raising the complaint with you can make them appear angry or tense. You need to allow for this.

It is important to respond promptly to any request to discuss a concern and to listen sympathetically and dispassionately. Where possible, relatives should be referred to the most senior doctor involved for any detailed discussion about the case. Be prepared to offer an apology for any obvious errors, e.g. keeping them waiting or inaccurate information. However, you should not apologize for something you do not think happened or happened as they describe it. You could instead express that you are sorry that 'they have been upset by X' or 'that they have that impression'. In addition, if the concern involves another member of staff, you should not be drawn into a discussion regarding this. You can note your appreciation of the relatives' concern and give a commitment to pass this information to a senior colleague.

Dealing with a formal complaint

Normally, you will receive notice of a formal complaint from the hospital complaints department. If you receive a formal complaint directly, you should not respond to it yourself, but pass it immediately to the complaints department. You may simply be asked to prepare a written statement. Be aware that this may be shared with the patient/family. It should be factual, non-judgemental and comment only on what you were personally involved with.

You should also be prepared to meet with the patient or family, although it is advisable to do this with the consultant. Before any statement or meeting:

- read the letter and consider what the complainant wishes and what should be done: are they looking for information or an apology; should things have been handled differently; what lessons can be learned?
- obtain the notes: make sure you know everything that happened and its sequence; make your own notes if necessary
- speak to any other staff who were involved with the case
- discuss with the consultant what happened and what you might need to say.

Developing a career

15

CHOOSING A CAREER

Many people spend more time deciding where to go on holiday than choosing their career. As you are probably going to have to work for the next 30 years or so, it is worth making sure that you embark on a career that is going to satisfy you. However, choosing your career can seem like a daunting decision. Breaking it down into stages using the REDI model - Review, Explore, Decide and Implement - provides a structured way of working through the process and updating and reviewing as your career and life develop.

Review

Review is concerned with assessing where you are now. An easy way to begin is to start a 'career reference' file. This can be in any form that suits your way of thinking and recording information, for example a mind map, a list, a grid. If you have an e-portfolio, you can incorporate details from it.

Educational background

Think about what you did, what you enjoyed, why you enjoyed it and, conversely, what you did not enjoy and why. What were you good at and what you did you find more difficult? Why was this?

Previous work experience

List the tasks and activities that you have been involved in. What tasks and activities did you most enjoy and why? Include all your work experience, paid or unpaid, even if it does not initially seem relevant to medicine. What did you not like doing? If you chose the experience, why did you choose it? What skills have you developed? How did you get on with people that you were working with? Are there any additional skills or experience that you might need? Do not just use your own assessments: record feedback that you have been given by others.

Your achievements

Examples can be drawn from any area of your life. What made them an achievement for you?

Your interests

What do you spend your time doing outside medicine? Have you been involved in the same activities for a long time or do you prefer to change your interests regularly? Are you involved in team activities? Do you enjoy competitive hobbies? Is there any aspect of your interests that you would like to be part of a job? What skills have you developed?

Your strengths and weaknesses

It is important to know your strengths so that when you are researching different specialties you can identify those which would make best use of them. However, it is equally important to be aware of your weaknesses and to identify areas that you may wish to develop. Which qualities and attributes would you like to use in a job? Ask other people what they think you are good at.

What sort of person you are

Some jobs and ways of working suit certain personalities better than others. Consider the following questions and rate your answers on a scale of 1 to 10. Use your answers alongside information that you gather from other sources to refine your thinking about potential careers.

- Have you enjoyed working in teams?
- Do you like to plan ahead?
- Do you prefer to wait until a deadline is approaching before you are motivated into action?
- Do you like a lot of variety?
- Would you describe yourself as competitive?
- Do you prefer to work independently?
- Do you enjoy working in areas that demand great attention to detail or do you prefer to be able to take a broader view?
- What role do you typically take in a group?
- Do you like to influence people?
- Do you enjoy working with concepts and theories or prefer more practical activities?

Explore

This stage of the process focuses on visualizing where you would like to be, finding out what opportunities exist and researching more about those that appeal.

Where do you want to be?

Take 10 min to visualize what sort of life you would like to have in 10 years' time. Think about the sorts of tasks and activities you would be doing, what knowledge and skills you would be using, where you might be, what sort of lifestyle you might have.

Generating ideas

If you are struggling to generate ideas or want to widen your horizons, go back to the Review section and select something that interests you or a skill that you would like to use in a job. Draw a spider diagram with this word at the centre and add ideas of jobs that contain that element as a key feature to the diagram, so that they radiate from the centre. Doing this with a colleague will produce more ideas as they will have had different experiences. A key point when looking at the results is to keep an open mind about the ideas generated. Do not be put off by preconceived ideas of a specialty. With any ideas that you have, find out which other specialties involve those aspects that most appeal.

How to find out more

Read specialty information, case studies, and person specifications. Get in touch with specialty contacts that your deanery may have and apply for a taster. Bear in mind, when you speak to someone about their job, that what they like about it might be different from what you might like. Useful resources include the BMJ and NHS careers websites and the career sections of deanery websites, e.g. the London deanery.

What else do you need to know?

Explore how the specialties that you are considering are changing. How are they going to develop over the next 10 years? What technological changes or changes in service development might affect the careers that you are thinking of? Find out the competition ratios for the different specialties.

Decide

Compromise

No job is ever 100% what you want it to be. The key is to select jobs that minimize the components that you do not like so much and maximize those that you do. Address any compromises that might involve your personal life.

Constraints

Think about the constraints that you feel are inhibiting your choice and decision-making. Is there anything that you can do to overcome them? For example, if you own a flat but need to move, you could consider renting it out.

Decision-making aids

Now is the time to synthesize your research and conclusions. You could use a simple list of pros and cons, or a SWOT (Strengths, Weaknesses, Opportunities, Threats) analysis. Try to identify five or so specialties that might fit what you have in mind. Talking your ideas over with a tutor or careers adviser, who can offer an objective perspective, is particularly useful at this stage.

Implement

People who have made well thought out decisions can still fail at the implementation stage, by leaving insufficient time to research the job market and prepare for applications and interviews. It is up to you to find out when and how to apply. Read through the next section on 'Applications, CV and interviews' for tips on how to make the best of what you have to offer.

APPLICATIONS, CV AND INTERVIEWS

As the saying goes, 'fail to prepare and prepare to fail'. Few people devote enough time to this stage of the job-seeking process with the consequence that even good candidates can be unsuccessful. Refer back to your career reference file (see 'Choosing a career', above), review your experience and choices and consider which aspects of your background are best suited to provide evidence of the skills and motivation required.

Application form

The challenge is to distil what you have to offer into succinct, interesting answers. Re-read the person specification and note ideas of evidence you might present within the application form headings. Do not forget your non-clinical experience for aspects that might make you stand out as a candidate. When completing your application form:

- use the CAR technique; it is a good way of structuring your answers: describe the Context, the Action that you took and the Result
- remember that the information you give is all the selector knows about you and saving important information to tell them about in an interview is likely to mean that you will not get an interview
- read the question: if you are only asked for one example, offering three is wasting space that could be used for expanding the one piece of evidence that will count; equally check that you have answered all parts of a question
- check that all the vital pieces of information or evidence are there: once you have submitted your application you will not be allowed to make additions and amendments
- do not repeat or paraphrase the question: you are just wasting valuable space.

Curriculum vitae

Decide what messages you want to convey and what headings you are going to use. It is usual to include the following topics:

- education and qualifications
- awards and prizes
- work experience, include all clinical and relevant non-clinical jobs; use the CAR technique to structure your description of each post; include what you have learned from any experiences or activities listed, as this is as important as what you have done
- clinical skills, e.g. central line insertion
- research experience
- publications, presentations or posters at conferences
- interests: avoid topics that are likely to polarize opinion, e.g. religion, politics and sporting allegiances; try to make your activities outside work sound different or interesting, e.g. rather than, you 'like to eat out', say you have an interest in Asian cooking and cuisine; include activities that demonstrate attractive qualities, e.g. energy, commitment, depth, an interest in mixing with people of different cultures, leadership qualities
- professional memberships
- referees: two are usually sufficient
- personal details: including your GMC registration status.

Select evidence from your career reference file and allocate space within your CV according to the relevance of the information. Two or three pages should be enough for the whole CV. Consult examples on your deanery or careers website.

Top tips

- have a clear, easy to read layout with plenty of white space that breaks up the text
- avoid font sizes of less than 11 pt and stick to one font type throughout
- use headings that stand out and help the reader to skip through and pick out whether you meet the essential criteria
- avoid underlining your headings or using lots of block capitals as they both make text more difficult to read
- do not start every sentence with 'I'
- do not use exclamation marks when describing experiences
- avoid unexplained gaps in your background
- only include anything you can talk about in detail at interview
- get someone else to proofread it before you send it.

Interviews

This is where the selectors find out if you are as you appear on your application. Consult your career reference file and the copy of your application. Consider points that you can use to substantiate the claims made on your application and, if possible, expand on these. It is important to anticipate those areas that you will be asked about:

- motivation for, and knowledge of, the specialty: why do you want this job; what are the aspects of this specialty that most appeal to you?
- clinical skills, personal skills and qualities: bear in mind that all the candidates coming to the interview will have been short-listed because they meet the essential criteria and you will have to provide evidence that you meet them; consider also what you can describe that shows extra commitment or ability
- interests: what makes you different and worth knowing; what shows your energy, perseverance, pursuit of excellence or leadership qualities?
- probity and issues relevant to the career and employer: what do you know of the NHS and important NHS-related bodies and structures?
- your career to date: why were there any gaps; why did you choose the posts you did; how will any research or overseas experience enhance your work now?

You will usually be interviewed by more than one person and may have two or three short interviews. Consider how you come across. It is important to sound enthusiastic and genuinely interested. You should appear professional and capable. Remember that there may also be lay people interviewing you as well as clinicians: any answers that you give should be understandable to all involved.

Before the interview

- do not wait until you have been informed that you have an interview to start preparing because the timescales can be short
- think about your answers to each of the sections above
- practise beforehand: ask friends or family to go through some questions with you
- prepare a couple of questions that you would like to ask.

On the day

- wear something smart and restrained, but ideally something you have worn before and are comfortable in
- avoid excessive perfume or aftershave
- turn up on time: if you are delayed, ring and explain
- do not offer to shake hands unless the interview panel do this
- think briefly before you reply to questions and project your voice adequately
- speak to the whole panel when you answer, not just the questioner
- avoid fiddling, counting on fingers, playing with your tie or hair
- remember that you only have a few minutes to impress the interviewers with your qualities as a doctor and a person as compared to the next candidate.

APPRAISAL AND ASSESSMENT

All doctors in training now follow curricula set within a competency-based framework. Final certification of completion of both general and specialist training can only be given by the PMETB (see p. 464) following satisfactory attainment of the relevant competencies. Individual assessments inform this decision, some of which are discussed in this chapter.

Appraisal

Appraisal is the process through which assessments of a doctor by others can be shared constructively, with each individual doctor, compared with their own self-assessment and used to shape their personal development plan. Such plans identify targets that the individual agrees are relevant for them to pursue, within a specified period of time, in regard to various aspects of their professional and personal learning or skills.

When

Each trainee should have a designated Educational Supervisor with whom time can be set aside for an appraisal discussion. This should take place at the beginning and end of each post and, where possible, also at a mid-point. It is important to set enough time aside for the discussion (usually 1 hour, without bleeps) and to ensure all paperwork for the meeting is prepared well ahead.

What

Appraisal is an opportunity to appreciate what is expected during the post you are in, how well you are doing while you are in it and what you might need to improve. However, appraisal itself is *not* an assessment or something that can be passed or failed. It is a formative, not summative, process. It is also an opportunity to gain advice on the relevant pursuit of specific areas that interest you and to see if support is available for you to undertake these. It is a time to focus on your career objectives, not to complain about your colleagues or accommodation, etc.

How

From the outset of each post, it is important to become familiar with your curriculum and its assessment process; to ensure your portfolio is up-to-date; and to book appraisal meetings with your supervisor sufficiently well in advance. As outlined in most educational contracts, it is the opportunity and responsibility of each trainee to pursue their career according to the curriculum that applies to their specialty. The process is designed to be 'trainee' rather than 'supervisor' driven.

Ahead of each meeting, you should complete any specified self-assessment documentation or portfolio pages and collect any relevant curriculum-defined assessments. You should also spend some time considering any issues you are concerned about and any questions you want to ask.

During the appraisal, your supervisor will use your documentation and discussion to explore your views on your development, often working to a framework based on each of the areas outlined in the GMC's 'Good Doctor' publication. A combined supervisor and trainee documentation of the meeting is then completed and the items within your next personal development plan agreed.

Assessment

There is a variety of assessment tools available and their use varies from specialty to specialty. The common tools are described below.

Mini-clinical evaluation exercise (Mini-CEX)

These are brief, 15 min, snapshots of doctor–patient interaction with, ideally, a different (medical) observer for each encounter. Each should represent a different clinical problem. Immediate feedback is given by the observer rating the trainee. Trainers and trainees agree strengths, areas for development and an action plan.

Direct observation of procedural skills (DOPS)

These assess procedural skills over the space of about 20 min. Each DOPS should represent a different procedure. The trainee chooses the timing, procedure and, ideally, a different observer for each.

Case-based discussion (CbD)

These provide systematic assessment and structured feedback of a trainee's case assessment, management and documentation. Two case records are presented from patients the trainee has recently seen and in whose notes they have made an entry. The assessor will select one of these for the case-based discussion session. The trainee can choose the timing, the cases and a medical assessor, but the direct supervising consultant should be one of the observers.

Multi-source feedback (MSF)

Mini-Peer Assessment Tool (Mini-PAT) and Team Assessment Behaviour (TAB) are two MSF tools usually used to collate views from a range of co-workers for 360° assessment. The trainee chooses the specified number of relevant medical or paramedical assessors and the collated, anonymized results are discussed with the supervisor.

End-of-post assessment

Following the series of appraisal meetings, a final end-of-post and/or annual assessment is usually made. There, a decision must be reached (based on the portfolio of assessments undertaken during the post) about whether the doctor has completed this stage of their training satisfactorily and can progress to the next stage. Such meetings are called ARCP (annual review of competence progression) and were previously called RITA.

RESEARCH

A working knowledge of research methodology and the critical appraisal of published evidence are essential skills for all doctors whose clinical practice and patient care are based on the evidence presented before them. You should use every available opportunity to be involved in clinical research. The experience will aid your learning, broaden your experience and enhance your CV.

Research as part of all training posts

Most units are involved in some form of research. Much of this will be clinical rather than laboratory-based and those undertaking it will have to do so in their own time rather than during work. Research is time consuming and to be involved in a study from design to completion is difficult to achieve in a 4- or 6-month post unless planned ahead. This is especially true if the study proposal needs to be submitted to an ethics committee. Even if you have not arranged something in advance, look for opportunities to help with data or sample collection, patient questioning, or study analysis in ongoing research projects. Try to do enough to be included as an author in any papers that result. Better still, you may get the chance to write up previous work done in the department or contribute to the preparation of a case report.

Research training posts

MMC placed a new emphasis on the structure of academic medicine training programmes and the support of trainees interested in pursuing a career in research and academia. These pathways are set out in the Department of Health document 'New academic training pathways for medical and dental graduates'. They define a shift in emphasis towards a more coordinated and progressive training programme and are designed specifically for those trainees who show an interest and aptitude for academia at an early stage.

These changes aim to define more clearly academic medicine as a specialty. They will create entry points into academia, provide formal training and pathways for career progression. In addition, they will help to reduce the pressure on doctors to undertake a higher degree purely to advance a clinical career.

Basic clinical years

Stand-alone 4-month academic attachments have been proposed for doctors who are keen to pursue an interest in a given specialty or gain a taste of research before deciding to pursue a career in academic medicine. In addition, dedicated, 1- and 2-year, integrated academic/clinical programmes are also being developed and are intended for trainees who know that they want to pursue a long-term career in this field.

Academic specialty training posts

Well defined specialty training pathways are available, providing a clear entry point into academic specialist training. These posts are available to all specialties and are comprised of two phases.

Phase 1

Academic Clinical Fellowship (ACF): a 3-year post (4 years maximum for GP academic trainees) with concurrent clinical and academic training. The first year is dedicated to clinical experience with increasing research sessions thereafter, designed to facilitate achievement of a higher degree (MD or PhD).

Phase 2

Clinical lectureship: a 4-year post running concurrently with clinical training; available to those who have satisfactorily completed clinical and academic training during an ACF and attained an MD/PhD, or those in possession of a National Training Number or other eligibility for specialty training. They provide an opportunity for postdoctoral research with broadly equivalent time in clinical and academic environments.

Other research posts

Entry to specialist training and consultant-level posts is likely to remain competitive, so trainees may still require the advantage and broader experience that a higher degree brings. Although the academic posts described above are the favoured means of achieving this, it is likely that standalone research posts, for periods of 2–3 years, will still be funded by external sources and make the achievement of an MD or PhD possible. However, the accreditation of such a post towards clinical training is less certain. Therefore, before embarking on such a route, you should check with a local training programme director, or the relevant Deanery.

TEACHING AND LIFE-LONG LEARNING

Teaching

All medical careers involve some element of teaching. The responsibility for patient care brings with it a responsibility for sharing what knowledge you have with those working around you. Moreover, teaching a topic enhances your own understanding of it and evidence of teaching activity is an important domain in the short-listing criteria for most posts. In addition, enabling others to learn is a very rewarding privilege.

How to teach well

Doctors are expected to do more teaching as they increase in seniority. However, length of experience itself does not result in good teaching and, however good your natural style, you can be better by taking time to consider how you teach. Much has been written about the art and theory of teaching and learning. The following is a brief introduction to a constantly developing topic.

Learning from your own student experience

Who do you remember; what aspects about their teaching made an impact and for what reason? Teachers must know their subject well, but the learner must also become interested in order to absorb what is being taught. Enthusiastic teachers, who are passionate about their subject and inspire or entertain their audience, can make what is taught seem much more memorable and worthwhile.

Preparing ahead

Consider who you are teaching: their previous and common knowledge; their expectations of the session; the size of the group. Also, what are the objectives of the session, for you and for those you are teaching? These might include the delivery of key points or the attainment of procedural competence or increased personal confidence. To plan how to achieve these, identify as many of these as possible, and write an outline, breaking each into their components:

- what the order of the lesson should be
- what you want students to prepare ahead
- how and where the teaching should be delivered
- what resources you will need
- what can be interactive
- how you will summarize and conclude the session
- what post-lesson learning or practice would be involved
- how you and they will evaluate the lesson.

In addition, where it is part of a whole course, unnecessary duplication should be avoided and overall curriculum objectives considered.

Engaging your audience

- providing preparatory work may make the group feel more involved
- make the lesson objectives clear (if possible allow the group to shape them)
- make the content relevant to the group concerned, e.g. their specialty, training needs, age group and interests
- try to vary your use of teaching formats and media in the session; e.g. lecture, small-group work, role-play, visual or auditory illustration
- use discussion, questions and answers during the lesson to draw out key points
- ensure all members are involved: specifically encourage those that are more reticent to contribute, instead of those who are always speaking
- encourage reflection on what has been covered and outline any further steps learners can take.

Clinical skills teaching

The following structure has been shown to enhance skills-based learning, usually within a laboratory setting:

- the teacher demonstrates the skill
- the teacher demonstrates the skill while talking through each step
- the teacher demonstrates the skill while the learner talks through each step
- the learner performs the skill themselves while talking through each step.

Life-long learning

Most doctors started medicine with an interest in medical science and/or practice, a questioning mind and a search for knowledge. 'Life-long learning' aims to preserve this, despite the hassles of routine clinical work. It is an attitude rather than a concept: a self-discipline of reflection to identify a learning need; action to acquire learning, application of the new learning and further reflection. Although such learning is self-directed, appraisal can help the life-long learner focus on their needs.

It may seem an unaffordable luxury to apply a life-long learning cycle, but medics work in a science-based discipline practising evidence-based medicine. The science and evidence changes from year to year and our career path may also involve new areas of sub-specialist practice. The GMC requires us to keep our 'professional knowledge and skills up-to-date' and our own job satisfaction will be greater where we are masters of the area we practise.

In addition, each day brings new challenges and sometimes adverse events for us or our immediate colleagues. In any other aspect of life, we would learn from negative experiences. We should ensure that our future patients benefit from a similar approach to clinical events. Therefore, active learning in a medical career does not stop with graduation, a post-graduate exam or a consultant appointment, but is a constant and integral part of our patient care, self-development and personal satisfaction.

MAKING AND GIVING PRESENTATIONS

Giving a good presentation is an art form. Good presentation skills are important for all doctors, not just academics. Formal presentations can be intimidating experiences, but they also help doctors learn to speak with confidence and authority in more routine clinical environments, for example during arrests or in meetings with relatives or colleagues.

Presentations come in a variety of guises. Some are impromptu and little preparation is possible, for example the presentation of a new admission on the post-receiving ward round or a case at a radiology meeting. Others are scheduled well in advance and more preparation can be made, e.g. the critical analysis of a paper in a journal club or a research presentation at a scientific meeting. In the latter, you will be expected to have an understanding of audio-visual aids and presentation software, such as Microsoft® PowerPoint®. However, giving a good presentation is much more than producing a set of pretty slides. A career enhancing presentation must be properly structured, rehearsed and delivered. This section summarizes the principles required to achieve this.

Know your audience and tailor your approach

If you are asked to present a new admission on the ward round you should be aiming to go beyond delivering the entire contents of your notes. Instead, you could focus on the presenting complaint, relevant points from the history and examination, a problem list and your intended initial investigations and management. Adopting a tailored approach is just as applicable in preparing for a formal presentation; consider:

- who your audience will be
- what they will already know about the topic
- how formal they will expect you to be, e.g. do not use jokes unless you know that this approach is acceptable.

Know your subject

This seems obvious, but there are countless doctors, many now very senior, who can recall the pain of public embarrassment when they gave a journal club presentation without properly reading the paper beforehand, never mind looking up its references and other relevant articles or books on the topic. Preparation is the key, but concentrating on the detail of one source should not be at the expense of acquiring an overall understanding of the key points.

Organizing your presentation

There is no point in preparing 50 slides for a 10 min talk. Equally, if you are to speak for 10 min, rushing through in 5 min shows you have prepared poorly and leaves a dangerously big gap for questions. If you are using visual aids, allow about 2 min for every slide; remember to rehearse and time your delivery at least a few days ahead.

It is crucial to decide what the key message(s) are. This should allow you to structure your presentation into a beginning, middle and end. It is best to draft your outline on paper before you start and then to consider if any points would be better illustrated using an image or diagram rather than a complicated section of text.

Presentation structure

- title: brief and to the point
- objectives of talk: the headings of each section of the talk, like a 'contents list'; often this part is best put together after the rest are done
- background and scene setting: previous work done on the area of research; key facts that put the topic into context; an attention-grabbing picture or headline; aims of any study/audit you have done; project planning
- what was actually done or should be done: method of study; statistical analysis; how to make the diagnosis of X; how to treat X; case examples
- the results and key messages of your whole talk: best kept to 5 or 6 points; aim to have the key points on one slide if possible; make sure they answer the objectives set at the start of the talk.

Once you have this outline, try to add in as many as possible of the subheadings you want to include under each heading. Then check if you think any headings should be moved, deleted or new ones added. Next, build in your initial thoughts on slides and timings. Consider, as you do this, the points regarding delivery below.

Preparing your presentation

When preparing your presentation, do not assume that the venue will have your PC's version of PowerPoint®. Animation features or special fonts may not work with the version at the venue. Consider the following general points:

Colours and fonts

- choose a simple and effective colour scheme
- make sure diagram colours can be appreciated by anyone who is colour blind
- use dark blue or white backgrounds if possible
- do not have patterns behind text
- avoid garish or indistinct colours and fancy bullets
- avoid using upper case for the points on the slide
- avoid more than two font types on one slide.

Layout

- make a maximum of five points on any one slide
- limit each point to one line: about six words
- change the layout of a slide occasionally, e.g. change your usual side-adjusted text to centred text in a new font
- do not include anything you have to apologize for, e.g. a table that is too small to read
- do not have everything you are going to say on the slide and read it verbatim.

Animation

- at first it is best to avoid animation
- if you use it, use it sparingly and avoid silly forms, e.g. 'light speed' entrance
- switch off any sounds attached to your animations
- check how each slide actually runs with your animations.

Flow

- a blank slide at the beginning and end can be useful
- have something that indicates that you have reached the end of each slide to stop you going on to the next slide by mistake, e.g. a full stop at the end of last point
- try to speak to the first point of your next slide, e.g. 'this is shown by the graph on the next slide'.

Illustrations

- avoid using clip art and do not use images from the internet that may be copyright
- do not use a picture joke that takes a long time to grasp or has small writing.

What to take on the day

- multiple copies of your talk, e.g. e-mail it to the meeting coordinator, have it on a memory stick, have a paper copy you can speak from
- consider making handouts of the main points of your talk, to distribute at the end.

Rising to the challenge of speaking to an audience

In addition to mastering the use of visual aids, speaking to an audience requires two sorts of skills:

- oratory: use of the voice, emphasis, pauses, timing
- self-control: staying calm and composed.

Oratory

The travel of sound and its perception by the human brain are influenced by pitch and speed. A deeper voice at a slower pace will project and be understood better than a higher pitch spoken fast. It is not necessary to shout to present well; however the following skills and factors are important.

Caring for the voice

Avoid alcohol, a lot of caffeine, spicy or very fatty foods within the 24 h before a big presentation as all of these can affect the quality of your voice and lead to catarrh and a dry throat.

Creating interest

Vary your pace and tone a little during your talk: points in a talk that are lighter or humorous can be faster or lighter pitched, those that are more serious can work better if slower or deeper in tone. Identify any special points you want to emphasize and practise doing so. This can be by raising the volume slightly, slowing down or pausing slightly just before you reach them.

Timing

A change of pace and the use of pauses can be used to emphasize particular points, e.g. 'the next slide shows the results we obtained during this study' and then, when you turn to that slide, pause for a few seconds to allow the audience to absorb the table before you comment on the points illustrated. Timing is also crucial for humour but, generally speaking, you are either funny or you are not. If you cannot tell a joke well in the coffee room, do not try to use one in your talk.

Notes

Unless you are already a practised speaker, consider writing out what you will say with each slide, in full. Read these notes over a few times and write down key points from your notes for each slide on a few small cards. With practice, the number of cards will be less and you may not need to write out the 'speech' in full. It is not a good idea to take a full speech to your presentation. Reading from such a full text is very restricting, preventing movement around the podium, eye contact and reducing the impression of confidence in what you are doing.

Self-control

To help you look, and feel, more in control:

- wear something you have worn before and are comfortable in
- keep your hands on the podium or by your side
- shuffle your notes only when you need to turn a page
- do not use a laser pointer if you are very nervous
- make eye contact to engage your audience
- smiling where appropriate can make your voice sound warmer and make you look more confident
- do not put off your preparation hoping the date of the talk will go away: being properly prepared is the most important element in controlling your nerves on the day.

Answering questions

Before the presentation, think of yourself as if you were different members of your audience, particularly those you know often ask questions. What would they ask? Write them down and prepare your answers. If you are presenting a paper or audit study, read about other work in the same area.

When you are faced with something you have not prepared, give yourself time to think about a response with phrases like 'thank you for that question', 'that's an interesting question/thought'. Also, the audience may not have heard the question if the questioner has not used a microphone. It is a good stalling technique, and helpful to the audience, to repeat out loud the question being asked. You may then have had time to think of a response.

As always, listen to the question well and answer it exactly. Never argue with an individual in public. Express that you have a different point of view on the subject and offer to discuss it with them at the end. Keep your answers short and never make them up. If you really do not know the answer, say so.

SECTION 4
Everyday life as a junior doctor

16 Working as part of the system of care

THE GOOD DOCTOR

When considering what makes a good doctor, we need to identify the qualities we would expect from doctors if we ourselves were patients.

Imagine you are the patient and you discover a potentially cancerous lump. How do you choose a doctor? Do you care that they are 'nice' or do you want someone who runs a good and quick service, knows their stuff and delivers good results?

You are now in the clinic room waiting to be seen. You are sitting undressed behind a flimsy curtain. Does it matter if the doctor marches in with a collection of juniors and students unannounced? Do you excuse the roughness of the internal examination on account of their professorial title? Do you leave uncertain of what is happening next, but too intimidated to ask?

Duties of a doctor

The general public often assume that the doctor they are going to see knows how to treat them. This trust in the doctor's clinical capability is closely interwoven with their trust in him or her as a person. Just as some doctors can elicit a placebo effect by a kind touch or word of reassurance, others can hinder the recovery of their patients through poor communication or an insensitive manner.

The importance of the doctor–patient relationship and its contribution to successful medical treatment is acknowledged in the GMC's outline of the 'duties of a doctor'.

- make the care of your patient your first concern
- protect and promote the health of patients and the public
- provide a good standard of practice and care: keep knowledge and skills up-to-date; work within the limits of your competence; work with colleagues in the ways that best serve patients' interests

- treat patients as individuals and respect their dignity: respect a patient's right to confidentiality and treat them politely and considerately
- work in partnership with patients: listen and respond to their concerns and preferences; give them information in a way they can understand; respect their right to reach decisions with you about their treatment and care; support them as they try to improve and maintain their health
- be honest and open and act with integrity: act without delay if you have good reason to believe that you or a colleague may be putting patients at risk; never discriminate unfairly against patients or colleagues; never abuse your patients' trust in you or the public's trust in the profession.

Some of your colleagues might expect 'special treatment' when they or their families become unwell. In this situation, some might suggest that a good doctor treats a sick colleague just as they would any other patient. Perhaps, however, a good doctor should treat all patients as if they were a colleague.

CLINICAL GOVERNANCE

Clinical governance is the structured process through which systems, and the staff working within them, identify lessons to be learned, with the aim of improving care. This is done through evaluation of clinical service structure and outcomes and of the staff delivering them. Substandard care can present in a variety of different ways:

- completely unexpected adverse events, not directly attributable to the clinical systems within which they happened, e.g. the accidental administration of the wrong drug
- patient or staff complaints regarding chronic service suboptimal performance, e.g. incidence of MRSA
- potentially poor staff performance, e.g. unexpectedly high postoperative mortality rates.

The lessons learned could be good examples of clinical care for broader dissemination, areas where systematic modification of clinical practice can be used to improve service delivery and areas where serious incidents or complaints have highlighted a need for new approaches.

Regular clinical audit and recognition of the importance of evidence-based medicine (EBM), e.g. as outlined in clinical guidelines, are central tenants of clinical governance: EBM theoretically ensures uniformity of access to quality care based on scientific research instead of established local practices.

PATIENT SAFETY AND RISK MANAGEMENT

Ensuring patient safety is of paramount importance in clinical practice. As doctors, what we cause to happen intentionally, or in error, impacts directly on the health of individuals and their eventual outcome. Equally, working in the health service can be hazardous to staff and issues related to safety in the workplace are as applicable to medicine as they are to other industries.

The principle

Errors occur either because of individual mistakes or because of failings in the system. Risk management is the process through which NHS staff can analyse errors that have occurred, or were narrowly avoided, and thereby reduce the risk of them happening again.

A structured risk management approach, first developed in the commercial aviation industry, has been integrated into the NHS in recent years. The process may seem laborious and even threatening to busy clinicians, but its purpose is not to apportion blame or identify poor performers. Rather, it is designed to identify systematic failures in working practice and to protect patients.

Definitions

- hazard: something that potentially causes harm or loss
- risk: the possibility that the hazard will cause harm or loss
- critical incident: an event that has caused harm or loss.

Critical incidents

Critical incidents may be 'clinical' and occur in the course of treating a patient such that the patient is directly affected. They may, however, be 'non-clinical' and relate to service personnel or system functionality and not directly affect patients, e.g. a needle-stick injury or computer failure. A near-miss is an event in either category that has the potential to cause a critical incident, but for whatever reason does not.

Steps in the risk management process

- identify the hazard
- determine who may be harmed by the hazard in future and how it might happen
- evaluate the risk related to the hazard, in terms of the likelihood of it causing harm or loss and the seriousness of the consequences if it happened
- determine the actions that are necessary to prevent the hazard from causing harm or loss and those to be taken in the event of it occurring
- formulate a plan that places the above actions within a practical clinical context
- communicate the plan to the staff who may cause or be affected by the hazard
- audit the implementation of the plan and update it if necessary.

Contributing to risk management

Most hospitals use a designated incident reporting form. This may be in paper or electronic form and you have a responsibility to know how to access them, where to send them and how to use them routinely. If possible, attend risk management meetings: they offer a valuable opportunity to learn from your mistakes and those of others.

HEALTHCARE-ASSOCIATED INFECTION

Healthcare-associated infection (HAI) affects an estimated 1 in 10 patients in the NHS every year. Intravenous and urinary catheters, surgical wounds and other breaches to host defences are important risk factors for HAI in these patients. The high incidence of HAI is a major source of concern for patients and their relatives and, as a result, hospital cleanliness and the control of HAI have become major political issues in the UK.

Prevention of HAI

All healthcare workers, with the support and direction of local 'infection control' teams, have a responsibility to ensure that standard (or universal) infection control precautions (SICP) are followed. This includes careful attention to environmental hygiene:

- high standards of hygiene in clinical practice, including handwashing care in the use of medical devices, e.g. urinary catheters, CVP lines and peripheral IV cannulae

- safe use and disposal of sharps
- use of personal protective equipment
- prudent use of antibiotics
- active surveillance and audit of HAI.

Good hand hygiene is exceptionally important and all clinical staff should use effective handwashing techniques. Detailed guidance on SICP is provided in Table 16.1; this advice provides adequate protection for the majority of patients. However, a brief risk assessment should be performed in all patients admitted to hospital, as more comprehensive precautions may be necessary in some, e.g. contact and/or air-borne transmission precautions.

Contact transmission precautions

These should be used in addition to SICP when there is particular concern about transmission of infection by direct or indirect contact. Typical clinical examples include certain gastrointestinal infections, including *C. difficile*, and MRSA.

Table 16.1 Key aspects of standard infection control practice (SICP)

Hospital environmental hygiene	
Hospital cleaning	Hospitals should be clean and acceptable to patients, visitors and staff
Instrument decontamination	Shared clinical equipment must be decontaminated appropriately after each use
Hand hygiene	
Indication	Hands should be decontaminated before and after every direct patient contact
Alcohol hand-rub	Preferable to washing unless hands are visibly soiled
Handwashing with liquid soap and water	Indicated if hands are visibly soiled or potentially grossly contaminated and after several applications of alcohol gel
Personal protective equipment	
Gloves	All invasive procedures, contact with sterile sites, non-intact skin, mucous membranes, and during all activities that carry a risk of exposure to blood, body fluids, secretions and excretions
Plastic aprons	When close contact is anticipated and there is a risk of clothing becoming contaminated
Full-body gowns	Should be worn where there is a risk of splashing of blood, body fluids, secretions or excretions
Facemasks and eye protection	Where there is a risk of blood, body fluids, secretions or excretions splashing into the face
Respiratory protective equipment	Particulate filter masks must be correctly fitted and used for the care of patients with respiratory infections transmitted by air-borne particles
Sharps disposal	
Handling of sharps	Needles should not be recapped or disassembled after use and sharps should be handled as little as possible and not passed directly from hand to hand
Sharps bins	Sharps must be discarded into an appropriate sharps container which must not be overfilled

To reduce environmental contamination, infected patients should be isolated and gloves and aprons should be used by all staff during patient contact.

Air-borne transmission precautions

These are used in addition to SICP for infections that are readily transmitted by air-borne droplets, such as tuberculosis and chickenpox. Patients should be nursed in a side-room and further specific precautions depend on the known or suspected infective agent. Stringent respiratory isolation procedures are required for infections such as multi-drug-resistant tuberculosis (MDRTB), including the use of a negative pressure cubicle and personal respiratory protection for staff.

Management of HAI

It is important to distinguish between simple colonization and clinical infection. This is a frequent clinical dilemma in patients with MRSA, particularly in intensive care or chronic disease settings.

Colonization

Management should include SICP and contact transmission precautions. Where possible, topical rather than systemic therapy should be used since complete eradication of colonizing organisms is often difficult. Any attempt at complete eradication should be directed by infection control teams.

Clinical infection

HAIs, e.g. hospital acquired pneumonia, UTI related to catheterization and wound infections should be anticipated in patients with known risk factors. These include antibiotic use, prolonged hospital stay, chronic lung disease, tracheal intubation or other instrumentation, heavy sedation or a depressed conscious level. Antibiotics should be started promptly and the choice of empirical agent should reflect the increased frequency of drug resistance in HAIs, e.g. MRSA, vancomycin-resistant enterococcus (VRE) and various multi-resistant Gram-negative organisms. Follow your local guidelines and seek senior microbiological advice at an early stage.

C. difficile-associated diarrhoea (CDAD) is an increasing problem in UK hospitals. Prevention should be the primary goal: avoid the unnecessary use of broad-spectrum antibiotics (e.g. third-generation cephalosporins), particularly in the elderly, and pay careful attention to SICP. Follow your local protocols for the diagnosis and treatment of *C. difficile* (see p. 171).

AUDIT

Throughout your career you will be involved in clinical audit: 'a quality improvement process that seeks to improve patient care and outcomes through systematic review of care against explicit criteria and the implementation of change'. Regular audit is a central component of the wider 'clinical governance' framework that underpins good reflective medical practice (see 'Clinical governance', p. 440).

Why and how

Audit improves patient care and your understanding of it. In addition, a clinical audit project is an opportunity to enhance your CV and become more involved in any specialty that interests you. Most units you work in will be continually involved in local and national audit programmes. Take the opportunity to discuss potential audit projects with your supervisors.

In contrast to a piece of research with a defined end-point, audit projects are self-perpetuating. Each single audit is undertaken as part of a continuous 'audit cycle' (see below) driving ongoing improvement in patient care, through analysis, action and further evaluation.

The 'audit department'

Most hospitals in the UK will have a clinical audit team and many will have a clinician designated as the 'clinical audit lead'. These individuals provide access to data collection tools, guidance on local audit policy and may offer you advice and support during data collection and analysis. They also disseminate the results of local audits to management and healthcare teams to ensure that clinical practice improves.

The audit cycle

Stage 1: choosing a topic

Identify a problem or area of particular interest. If the problem spans across specialties or departments consider organizing a joint audit; this makes implementing changes more feasible and avoids uninvolved parties feeling 'blamed'.

Stage 2: identifying an audit standard

Identify a relevant standard of care or baseline data set that can be used for comparison. This could be a clinical guideline, e.g. NICE or SIGN, published clinical research, a previous audit or other standard of care, e.g. a patient's charter.

Stage 3: planning

Pose a specific question, or set of questions, to be addressed by the audit, e.g. are national targets for secondary prevention following acute MI being met? It helps if the question can be measured numerically.

- choose the variables you will use to answer the audit question; they should be valid (the variable is able to measure what it is intended to measure), reliable (consistent), applicable to all relevant cases and simple to collect
- identify what resources are available to you, e.g. access to case-records, clerical support
- check what local approval/permissions are necessary before an audit can be undertaken and that all clinicians affected by the audit are aware that it will be taking place; consider the implications of 'Data protection', see p. 417, and 'Consent', see p. 441
- secure a 'sponsoring' consultant to advise you and support your approval and record access requests
- determine the size of the sample you will need to answer the question posed, e.g. perform a power calculation; statistical power may have to weighed against practical issues and the time available for data collection
- ensure you have enough time in your current post to complete the audit
- consider what you will do with the results: if you hope to present them at a meeting, check the submission deadline for abstracts.

Stage 4: data collection and analysis

This may be time-consuming and it is often useful to seek some guidance from senior colleagues and your local clinical audit department regarding the most efficient method, e.g. if a questionnaire is being used, some audit departments may be willing to advise on its construction. Where possible, consult multiple sources since individual clinical records (e.g. case-notes) are often incomplete. Ensure the data are stored securely and consider how you will analyse the data; with prior consultation your audit department may be willing to help (see also 'Reporting results', p. 446).

Stage 5: reviewing your findings

Once data analysis is complete you should compare your findings with the audit standard. Identify key messages, targets for improvement and potential objectives for further audit. Consider presenting your findings to your unit or hospital department; this will facilitate the next stage in the process.

Stage 6: implementing change

Once the findings of an audit have been disseminated, changes should be made to correct any areas of deficiency. Make an action plan and identify who should do what and when.

Stage 7: closing the audit loop

An audit is not complete until you have 'closed the loop' by re-auditing after implementing any action points identified in the first audit, to evaluate the impact of the actions undertaken.

EVIDENCE-BASED MEDICINE, STATISTICS AND GUIDELINES

The practice of evidence-based medicine links information derived from research to clinical practice. Its application requires an understanding of research methodology and its clinical relevance.

Study type

Different types of study can be used to answer the same clinical question. However, these may have major methodological differences that can affect how you interpret their results:

Case–control studies are retrospective analyses that allow a large number of cases to be identified quickly, potentially achieving the statistical power required to answer clinical questions (see below). However, they are subject to recall bias where errors arise in retrospective data collection.

Cohort studies are prospective, minimizing recall bias; however, they are more difficult to perform because more time is necessary to enrol sufficient patients to achieve statistical power. They are also subject to observer bias as the investigator is aware of the different interventions made in each group.

Randomized controlled trials (RCTs) minimize recall and observational bias but may, like case–control and cohort studies, still be subject to confounding variable bias. This is where the condition being studied may be influenced by factors other than the one manipulated by the investigators. Although a statistical technique called multivariate analysis can be used to adjust for confounding variables, the method itself is subject to error.

Study design

The validity of the question

The question must be relevant to the outcomes that are being measured and must be valid.

- external validity: the degree to which the conclusions in the study hold for other persons in other places at other times
- internal validity: how good the assessment tools used are at measuring the variable of interest, e.g. asking people 'how much do you smoke?' may not be as internally valid as asking them to keep and submit all of their empty cigarette packets.

The study population

The study population should be representative. If not selected appropriately, bias can be introduced, e.g. it would not be appropriate to study a new mode of delivering insulin in patients with diabetes by only recruiting patients attending an adolescent clinic.

Power

The power of a study describes its ability to detect a result that would be reproduced if the entire population were studied. A very large study is required for statistical significance to be achieved when the effect of the intervention is small. Statistical power can be increased by enlarging the sample size, improving the precision of the measurements or changing the size of the effect being measured.

Randomization

This is an essential component of all RCTs. The randomization process must be robust to ensure that the baseline characteristics of the two groups are similar.

Observer bias

Double-blind trials avoid this by ensuring patients and investigators are unaware of the designated study group.

Withdrawal bias

Withdrawal bias occurs when study participants are lost to follow-up or withdraw from the study for whatever reason, e.g. refusal of treatment, death, drug intolerance. Those that remain for analysis at the end of the study may not be representative of the group that was originally included. All subjects should be analysed as part of the group they started in: this is known as an intention-to-treat analysis.

Publication bias and competing interests

Researchers and journals have a tendency towards publishing only positive results, creating bias. Many major journals have insisted that trials that began enrolling patients after July 2005 must register in a public trials registry to be considered for publication.

Reporting results

Some understanding of data analysis and the appropriateness of the tests used is essential to allow you to interpret research studies.

Descriptive statistics

Data types

Before deciding on the most appropriate test to use to answer a clinical question, you must first know what type of data has been collected.

- continuous data are either: interval data (consecutive numbers measured on a graded scale, e.g. BP); ordinal data (ranked lists of data, e.g. quartiles of BP)
- categorical data express the results of experiments or interventions that can have only one of two outcomes, e.g. BP target achieved or BP target not achieved.

Distribution

Large biological data sets commonly have a 'normal' or Gaussian distribution due to the random effect of sampling variability. The results of many statistical tests can only be extrapolated to larger populations if the studied population is also normally distributed. However, this may not be the case with small samples and categorical or ordinal values. Normal distribution should therefore be verified by plotting the frequency of each value on a histogram; normally distributed data will form a bell-shaped curve.

Central tendency and spread

The mean, which is simply the average value, describes the central tendency of normal distributed data. The median is the mid-point of any data set arranged in order and is used for this purpose in non-normally distributed data. The standard deviation and range describe the spread of normally and non-normally distributed data sets, respectively.

Confidence intervals

Confidence intervals (CI) describe how well a sample mean or the effect of an intervention within a sample describes the true mean or true effect in the general population. It is usually given as a 95% CI (calculated by a specific statistical equation). This means that there is a 95% chance that the true mean or effect for a population lies within the resulting range of values.

Statistical tests

Choosing a statistical test that is appropriate to your study format and data is important to the validity of the results achieved. This should be considered before beginning a study. Many universities have departments of medical statistics that are willing to advise on study design and tests before you begin.

Correlation

When looking for relationships between variables, tests of correlation are required:

- Pearson's: used when the distribution of both variables is normal
- Spearman's rho: used when either one or both variables have non-normal distributions.

Regression is a more complicated method that can be used to describe the relationship between variables in detail. Linear regression should be used for continuous variables. Logistic regression is more appropriate for non-continuous data.

Comparing means

Comparative tests are used when looking for differences between variables. A test called the one-way ANOVA is necessary when comparing three or more means. When comparing two variables, the test chosen depends on the type and distribution of the variables (Table 16.2).

Measures of efficacy

The efficacy of a treatment can be defined by various statistical descriptors and it is important to understand what they mean.

Event rate

This is the percentage of patients in each population (e.g. control and active treatment) who experience an event (e.g. death).

Relative risk reduction (RRR)

This is calculated as the difference in event rate between the groups, expressed as a proportion of the event rate in the control group. For example, if the event rates in the placebo and active treatment groups were 25% and 20%, respectively, the RRR in the treatment group would be [(25 – 20)/25] = 0.2, which could also be described as a RRR of 20%.

Absolute risk reduction (ARR)

This is the arithmetic difference between the two event rates. In the example given above the ARR is 5% (i.e. 25 – 20%). In general, the ARR is a more useful value than the RRR, as it takes into account the event rate and, therefore, the clinical

Table 16.2 Comparative statistical tests

Type of variable	Distribution of the variables	Test
Dependent or 'paired', e.g. BP before and after treatment	Both normal Either or both non-normal	Dependent or 'paired' *t* Wilcoxon
Independent or 'unpaired', e.g. BP in two groups of patients	Both normal Either or both non-normal	Independent or 'unpaired' *t* Mann–Whitney

importance of the result. To illustrate this, if the event rate in each group was 10 times less frequent in the above example (2.5% and 2.0%, respectively), the RRR would be identical ((2.5 – 2.0)/2.5) = 0.2) but the ARR would only be 0.5% (i.e. 2.5 – 2.0%), indicating that the result is likely to be less clinically important.

Number needed to treat (NNT)

This is the number of patients who would need to receive the active treatment for one of them to benefit. It is calculated as 1 divided by the ARR (expressed as a fraction). In the original example above, the NNT would be 1/0.05 = 20; in the second example, with less frequent events, the NNT would be 1/0.005 = 200.

Interpreting measures of efficacy in clinical trials

It is important to note that, when there is a low event rate, the relative risk reduction may appear highly significant in statistical terms, but its clinical importance may be low. Therefore the ARR and the NNT are more robust measures of the clinical importance of treatment effects in clinical trials.

Sensitivity and specificity

Results are often described as normal/abnormal or positive/negative. However, there is often an overlap between ranges of values found in patients with and without disease. This results in false-negative or false-positive results, which must be interpreted properly. All diagnostic tests have the following characteristics:

- sensitivity: the ability of the test correctly to identify patients with disease: number of true-positives divided by the total number of people with the disease
- specificity: the ability of the test correctly to identify patients without disease: number of true-negatives divided by all those without the disease
- positive predictive value: the likelihood of having the disease if the test is positive: number of true-positives divided by the number of positive tests
- negative predictive value: the likelihood of not having the disease when the test is negative: number of true-negatives divided by the number of negative tests.

Guidelines

Guidelines should be concise, easily accessible and clinically useful. Most specialist professional bodies produce guidelines on relevant topics as do national organizations such as NICE (National Institute for Health and Clinical Excellence) and SIGN (Scottish Intercollegiate Guidelines Network). These guidelines can be accessed at the relevant websites. The recommendations given reflect the strength of the evidence on which they are based:

- Ia: meta-analysis of randomized controlled trials
- Ib: at least one RCT
- IIa: at least one well-designed controlled study without randomization
- IIb: at least one other type of well-designed quasi-experimental study
- III: well-designed, non-experimental descriptive studies
- IV: expert committee reports or opinions and/or clinical experiences of respected authorities.

DIVERSITY, RELIGION, CULTURE AND DISABILITY

Throughout your undergraduate training you will have met patients and doctors from diverse backgrounds in a wide variety of clinical settings. You may well have come across cases where issues of religion or culture influenced the presentation or management of a condition, from either the patient's or the doctor's perspective. As you become more senior it is important that you reflect on your knowledge, skills, attitudes and behaviour in these areas and consider how they impact on practice.

Diversity

As a doctor, you are expected to respect any differences in culture, religion or preference that might exist among patients and colleagues. In addition, you must ensure, wherever it is practical, that arrangements are made to meet patients' language and communication needs. Most NHS employers have policies in place regarding discrimination in the workplace which you should be familiar with. In general these will involve:

- treating one another with respect
- giving other people their dignity
- respecting each other's right to privacy and confidentiality
- accepting and being sensitive to each other's differences
- being professional in relations with each other
- building constructive working relationships
- working with and supporting each other.

Equal opportunities legislation

Equal opportunities legislation gives these principles a legal framework and is implemented by all UK employers: 'the prevention, elimination or regulation of discrimination between persons on the grounds of sex or marital status, on racial grounds, or on grounds of disability, age, sexual orientation, trade union membership or activity, language or social origin or of other personal attributes, including beliefs or opinions, such as religious beliefs or political opinions'.

Sex Discrimination Act 1975

Prohibits discrimination (direct or indirect) on the grounds of sex or marriage and applies to men and women.

Race Relations Act 1976

Makes both direct and indirect discrimination on the grounds of race, colour, nationality (including citizenship), ethnic or national origin unlawful.

Equal Pay Act 1970

Prohibits different pay for men and women doing the same work, work rated as equivalent, or work of equal value.

Disability Discrimination Act 1995

Deals with discrimination against disabled people, i.e. when someone treats a disabled person less favourably than someone else, with justification related to their disability. Discrimination also occurs if, without justification, a 'reasonable adjustment' for the disability is not made. The Act applies to all those who provide goods, facilities and services to the public.

Trade Unions and Labour Relations (Consolidation) Act 1992

Protects employees from discrimination on the grounds of trade union activities or membership, or of non-trade union membership.

Employment Relations Act 1999

Includes a number of 'family friendly' measures, e.g. legislation to cover the European Parental Leave Directive. The Act provides employees with rights to paternal leave and time off work in family emergencies and also simplified and improved maternity rights.

Asylum and Immigration Act 1996

Makes it a criminal offence for an employer to recruit individuals who do not have permission to work in the UK. Prospective employees should expect to be asked for a birth certificate or passport to establish their eligibility to work in the UK.

Part-time Workers Regulations 2000

Prohibit discrimination against part-time work at all skill levels and responsibility.

Employment Equality (Sexual Orientation) Regulations 2003

Make it unlawful to discriminate either directly or indirectly on the grounds of sexual orientation. It is also unlawful to harass and victimize people at work on the grounds of their sexual orientation.

Employment Equality (Religion or Belief) Regulations 2003

Outlaw direct and indirect discrimination and harassment and victimization on the grounds of religion or belief.

Others

A variety of other acts also relate to discrimination:

- Sex Discrimination (Gender Reassignment) Regulations 1999
- Rehabilitation of Offenders Act 1974
- Human Rights Act 1998.

Religion or culture

Religion may influence behaviour through cultural influences, and it is important to recognize how these can impact on many branches of medicine. Different belief systems may have a major influence on how patients view illness. For example, some religions view illness as a punishment for previous wrongdoing, while others may view it as a challenge to be accepted, as God's will, or even as a route to spiritual enlightenment. An appreciation of these differences may help your understanding of patients' attitudes to illness and treatment.

In addition, religions may affect what treatments patients are willing to accept, e.g. blood products such as whole blood, packed red cells, white cells, plasma and platelets are unacceptable to Jehovah's Witnesses. However, non-blood volume expanders or re-infusion of their own blood is often permitted.

Religious and cultural factors may also influence how patients present and report symptoms and doctors should be aware of this, e.g. Hindu or Muslim women may be reluctant to discuss genitourinary or bowel symptoms with a male doctor or if their spouse is present. Considerations like the timing of appointments around periods of fasting should be made and the provision of an acceptable chaperone may be necessary in certain settings.

There are also cultural differences regarding the acceptability of eye contact and touching (even shaking hands), or examination of the body after death. For example, use gloves when touching the bodies of deceased Hindu, Jewish and Muslim patients; avoid touching the bodies of Jewish patients for 20 min after death; note that the Islamic faith prevents women from touching a dead body for 40 days after the delivery of a baby, even if it is a stillborn child.

You should pay particular attention to names. When names are unfamiliar to you, always check what is the person's preferred name and form of address. This applies both to patients and to colleagues. Consider your own religious and cultural beliefs too and whether these aid or hinder your interactions with patients. You may encounter situations where your duty as a doctor is at odds with your religious beliefs or customs. How will you deal with that?

Spirituality can have a major impact on how patients deal with illness, and acknowledging this is a central part of holistic care in many settings. Recognizing the importance of familiar customs and rituals, at a time when patients and relatives face major illness or death, provides some patients with additional valuable support and coping strategies. The hospital chaplains can be a valuable source of support to some patients and guidance to you on how to manage dead and dying patients. As in any other area of medicine, if you find yourself in a difficult situation and you are not sure how best to proceed, remember the general principle of mutual respect for patients and colleagues. Use what resources are available to get knowledge about the facts of the situation and seek advice from relevant senior colleagues.

Disability

Disabled patients

The rights of disabled people have been given considerable priority in recent years. They have been the focus of significant legislation (e.g. the Disability Discrimination Acts of 1995 and 2005 and the Mental Capacity Act 2005) and other measures such as the establishment of the Disability Rights Commission. This is a complex area but, as doctors, some of the issues we should consider when treating disabled people include:

- the preferred method of communication
- barriers that prevent disabled people getting access to healthcare, e.g. physical barriers such stairs, or as a result of prejudice or attitudes
- involvement of carers while recognizing the autonomy of the disabled person
- organizations or equipment that could help disabled people
- those with long-term conditions or impairment are often expert in dealing with their medical problems and can bring valuable expertise to the consultation
- not all health needs are related to the disabled person's disability and new symptoms should be given as much credence as those developing in a non-disabled person.

Disabled doctors

If you are a doctor with a disability, you should speak in confidence to your local occupational health service about local sources of support. The GMC has recently published guidance on disabled doctors and most employers will have policies on the rights of disabled staff. You can expect reasonable adaptations to be made to accommodate your disability under the terms of the Disability Discrimination Act.

PRIMARY AND SECONDARY CARE INTERFACE

The concept of an interface between primary and secondary care implies that the two are distinct. However, in reality, they are both integral parts of a continuum of medical care for patients.

Partnership

For care to be most effective, there needs to be a close partnership between primary and secondary care. Much of this depends on proper and prompt communication. Each party must consider what information the other needs to know, whether it is in written or verbal form. Common interactions of this sort include referrals to hospital from general practice and discharge summaries from the ward (see 'Written communication', p. 389). In addition, it is important that secondary care doctors respect the role of the general practitioner, and vice versa. Although general practitioners may not be familiar with new working practices within a particular specialty, many will have broad or specialist understanding of a range of disciplines. Moreover, the GP is likely to know the patient and their family much better than you do. They will also be the person the patient listens to for advice when they have left the hospital.

Pathways of care

For many chronic conditions and some acute presentations, protocol-based care and shared care have softened previous barriers between primary and secondary areas. Pathways that are available to patients and carers allow them to be more aware of which group of doctors or other staff are responsible for each aspect of care for a condition. In addition, such pathways provide for more structured involvement of non-medical staff. Moreover, they have enabled services with a specialty focus to develop within a primary care environment, either as part of shared specialty care or in accordance with locally agreed policy.

In both acute and primary care, there is a variety of services and multidisciplinary staff who are important in ensuring effective patient care. Indeed, in some situations they can be of more benefit to the patient than their medical care. For different conditions, both types of clinician can find themselves at the centre of clinical care coordination for a patient. However, both also need to be prepared to adopt a more peripheral position in the process which may be better coordinated by another medical, or indeed non-medical, clinician.

EPIDEMIOLOGY, SCREENING AND HEALTH PROMOTION

Epidemiology

Epidemiology is the study of the causes, distribution and control of disease in the population. It can be used to identify populations at greater risk of a disease, e.g. mesothelioma in those exposed to asbestos. Such information also improves public understanding of disease pathogenesis, e.g. the link between hypercholesterolaemia and stroke allows patients to make lifestyle choices. Factors related to disease epidemiology include:

- prevalence: total number of cases as a percentage of the whole population at risk
- incidence: number of new cases in the population at risk over a specific time period
- population characteristics: variation of incidence by sex, age, social class, occupation, housing, lifestyle
- environmental risk: including the relative risk of a disease occurring in an exposed population and the attributable fraction, which is the percentage of the disease that can be attributable to this risk:

$$\text{Relative risk} = \frac{\text{incidence in exposed population}}{\text{incidence in non-exposed population}}$$

$$\text{Attributable fraction} = \frac{\text{incidence in exposed population} - \text{incidence in non-exposed population}}{\text{total population at risk}} \times 100$$

Screening

Screening is used to identify serious illness, to prevent further spread of disease and to target interventions. For screening to be worthwhile, there must an effective treatment for the condition. For it to be widely used it must be cost-effective. Any judgement on cost-effectiveness is influenced by the prevalence of the disease, the cost of the test, its sensitivity and specificity, the availability and effectiveness of the available treatments and the cost of not detecting and treating the condition.

Whenever screening is undertaken, it must be performed within a supportive environment; this is especially so in the case of genetic testing. Patients must be counselled about the implications of the results and specific informed consent may be necessary. Screening programmes are used in a variety of settings:

- genetic disease, e.g. Huntington's disease, familial cancer syndromes
- pre-natal detection of conditions, e.g. Down's syndrome, neural tube defects
- post-natally, e.g. phenylketonuria, cystic fibrosis

- child development, e.g. childhood hearing and eye tests
- infection, e.g. TB
- cancer, e.g. cervical, breast
- complications of disease, e.g. diabetic retinopathy.

Health promotion

Many diseases can be prevented or modified by health promotion strategies. Most of this activity is based within the community and coordinated by general practice, community paediatric and public health departments. Health promotion programmes in secondary care include:

Vaccination

Hepatitis B vaccination is essential for all health professionals; see p. 418. Vaccinations against typhoid and other infectious diseases are also commonly provided in travel clinics. There are also general vaccination programmes targeted at specific population groups, e.g. childhood illness, anti-tuberculosis, influenza and anti-HPV.

Smoking

Smoking cessation is a key management goal in a variety of chronic diseases. For example, it is the only simple or pharmacological intervention that has been proven to prolong survival in patients with COPD. However, smoking is highly addictive and both chemical and behavioural components must be addressed if the patient is to be successful in quitting. There is some evidence that medical advice given during an acute illness may be better received by smokers than that given during times of better health. During a hospital admission, it is therefore important to emphasize the potential benefits to be gained:

- 50% reduction in the risk of heart attack after 1 year
- 50% reduction in the risk of lung cancer after 10 years
- 25% reduction in risk of miscarriage and stillbirth
- reduction in risk of smoking-related impotence and infertility.

Useful tips for smokers who are planning to quit include:

- identify reasons why they want to quit, e.g. health benefits, financial savings, positive effects on others, for example their children
- fix a date for stopping
- tell others their plans; they can give support
- identify times that they normally look for a cigarette and plan ahead how they will manage cravings
- consider pharmacological aids; see below.

Pharmacological therapy

Pharmacological treatment should only be offered to smokers who have committed to a stop date and may not be necessary in those who smoke <5 cigarettes/day.

Nicotine replacement therapy (NRT)

NRT is available in the form of chewing gum, tablets, lozenges, patches, a nasal spray and an inhalator. Patches are available in a variety of strengths and can last for up to 24 h. These patches are particularly useful for smokers who experience strong morning cravings; others can manage with 16 h patches, which are removed at night. The nasal spray is usually only recommended for very heavy smokers.

NRT should be avoided in patients with significant cardiovascular disease and used with caution in hepatic or renal impairment, pregnancy and breast-feeding mothers. Blood sugars must be monitored in diabetics. Dose and dose duration depends on cigarette consumption and the chosen format of NRT (see the BNF for detailed guidance).

Other drugs

- Bupropion hydrochloride (Zyban®): originally used as an antidepressant; the mechanism of its effect as a smoking cessation adjunct is unclear. It is contraindicated in patients with eating disorders or at risk of seizures, including epilepsy, alcohol abuse and drugs that lower seizure threshold, e.g. systemic corticosteroids, theophylline, antidepressants. Bupropion should be commenced 1–2 weeks before the patient's proposed stop date and used for a period of 7–9 weeks in total
- Varenicline (Champix®): selective nicotine receptor partial agonist; avoid in patients with a history of depression or renal impairment, pregnancy or breast-feeding.

Cravings

Patients should plan ahead for coping strategies for any cravings they experience. Potentially useful measures include sipping water, chewing gum, using a stress-ball, going for a walk, brushing teeth, reaching for a packet of cigarettes that is securely sealed with layers of tape.

Alcohol and drugs

Alcohol and drug abuse is common. Therefore, it is important to consider whether they may contribute to some of your patients' problems. Specific, but sensitive, questioning should be undertaken, ideally away from other family members. Features that suggest alcohol dependence or its development include: organizing a lifestyle around drinking, effects on work or other commitments related to previous drinking, being unable to remember a night drinking, injury related to drinking, alcohol withdrawal symptoms, drinking in the morning, a compulsion to keep drinking, difficulty stopping drinking.

Excess anxiety, sweating, mydriasis, abdominal upset or cramps, tachyarrhythmias, premature myocardial ischaemia, hallucinations, seizures, confusion, ataxia, mood swings, rhinorrhoea and peri-oral sores can suggest drug or solvent abuse or withdrawal.

Patients suspected of drug or alcohol abuse should be offered referral to community addiction teams. Where medical effects (e.g. on heart, liver or brain) appear related to such abuse, the patient should be made aware of the risks of continued exposure, the potential benefits of altering their lifestyle and the support that is available, both through NHS organizations and independent bodies such as Alcoholics Anonymous.

Diet

Both obesity and anorexia pose risks to health (see 'Nutrition', p. 183). Obesity is more common, but often develops over many years with multiple contributing factors. An acute illness, e.g. angina, TIA, or the need for an operation for which there is now greater risk can prompt patients to see that a sustained change in lifestyle is needed. It is important to use these opportunities to discuss, in a supportive context, the contribution of the patient's weight to their illness and what reduction in risk could be achieved by weight loss. Dietetic input can also be offered.

In a similar fashion, patients who present with hypercholesterolaemia should be offered advice on the benefits of dietary or drug intervention.

Sexual health

Sex workers or their clients, frequent travellers, drug abusers and homosexuals are more prone to sexually transmitted disease (STD). Check for evidence of rashes, urinary symptoms, pelvic pain or discharge. Consider STD in those with scabies or genital warts and offer referral to specialist genitourinary services.

Young adults with previous teenage pregnancy or admissions relating to alcohol or drugs are also at greater risk of ongoing unprotected sexual intercourse. Sensitive questioning should be undertaken and advice offered where appropriate.

REHABILITATION

Orthopaedic rehabilitation

Orthopaedic rehabilitation should commence as soon a possible following injury or surgery. Nutritional needs, pain control, the re-establishment of walking and the activities of daily living are the first priorities. Multidisciplinary collaboration is needed between orthopaedic surgeons, care of the elderly physicians, physiotherapists, occupational therapists, dieticians and nurses.

The identification of patients who require more intensive rehabilitation in Geriatric Orthopaedic Rehabilitation Units (GORU) should be guided by an assessment of premorbid function and mobility, available social support, current relevant clinical conditions and mental state. Those who require further rehabilitation, but are relatively fit and alert, can be discharged with formal home support schemes after discussion with the patient and their family. Patients with greater incapacity, either physical or mental, may require more intensive, inpatient rehabilitation and admission to GORU.

Stroke and care of the elderly rehabilitation

Care of the elderly clinicians coordinate large multidisciplinary teams whose aim is to maximize functional recovery. This includes an improvement in the ability to carry out the activities of daily living and, where possible, facilitating discharge to the patient's own home. The home environment and the level of support available from the family are important considerations when planning this process. A range of disciplines should be involved, including physiotherapy, occupational therapy, social work, speech and language therapy, dietetics, nursing and doctors. Therefore, when you are working in such wards, you will be involved in multidisciplinary meetings to discuss patient progress and further treatment plans. The GP should also be involved in the plans that develop for discharge.

Cardiac rehabilitation

This is recommended following myocardial infarction, coronary revascularization and in patients with stable angina or LVF who have limiting symptoms or have had a new event recently. Such patients should be referred for assessment during their first admission for these problems. Cardiac rehabilitation programmes include exercise training (twice a week for 8 weeks), education on diet, smoking and heart disease, and psychological support and intervention.

Pulmonary rehabilitation

This is particularly used for patients with COPD, but can also be of benefit to those with other forms of chronic respiratory disease. It includes a 6–12-week programme of aerobic, often lower limb, exercise, education and psychological and social intervention. The exercise prescription is individualized and based on the patient's performance during progressive exercise testing or shuttle-walk testing. The effect of the programme is assessed using objective measures of quality of life and symptom scores. Despite the potential benefit of pulmonary rehabilitation in other forms of chronic lung disease, competition for places usually limits availability to those with severe or moderately severe COPD, in whom there is the strongest evidence base.

COMPLEMENTARY AND ALTERNATIVE THERAPY

Western medicine prides itself on its scientific evidence base, with each new treatment developed and tested through a process of deductive research. Complementary therapies have, instead, often developed over centuries and their effectiveness tends to be subjectively, rather than objectively, measured. Nevertheless, many patients report considerable benefits especially in pain control, smoking cessation and relaxation.

Given the prevalence of cancer, orthopaedic pain and stress-related illnesses, it is helpful to have an appreciation of the complementary role such therapies can offer patients. However, while some are available within the NHS and, indeed, may be practised by physiotherapists, podiatrists or GPs, the majority of therapies are only available on a private basis.

Therapies

- acupuncture: Chinese in origin; aims to treat disruptions or imbalance of the flow of 'Qi' through the body by the insertion of fine needles at specific points in the body; often used in pain control and smoking cessation
- aromatherapy: natural 'essential' oils are extracted from plants; different oils are said to have different effects on mood, mental activity or have medicinal qualities, e.g. antisepsis; oils must be diluted before application or inhalation and are used in relaxation therapy, especially cancer care
- Ayurveda: Indian with a basis in Hinduism, Ayurveda is a medical system rather than a single treatment; it involves whole patient assessment and diagnosis where dietary regimes and treatments, including massage, are used to treat a range of illnesses including stress
- chiropractic: centrally regulated in the UK, this aims to treat the nervous system as well as improving skeletal mobility by spinal manipulation; used in migraine, repetitive strain, back pain, sciatica
- healing: colour therapy crystals, music and spiritual healing are thought to harness energy or power and create harmony; used in a variety of situations, especially cancer care and stress-related conditions
- herbalism: a multitude of therapies can be bought over the counter, e.g. echinacea for viral infections, feverfew for migraine, St John's wort for depression; side-effects and interactions with prescribed medications may not be appreciated by the user, e.g. warfarin can be affected by gingko biloba, ginseng, ginger and garlic; true herbalism involves consultation and assessment with prescriptions addressing the whole person
- homeopathy: uses very dilute solutions which are based on a principle that what makes a healthy person unwell can be used to treat the same symptoms; although available over the counter, ideally involves a consultation with a practitioner; used for various illnesses including asthma, eczema, arthritis
- hypnotherapy: can induce a trance-like state or deep relaxation through which the practitioner may influence the unconscious mind; used in combination with counselling to treat stress-related illnesses, phobias, habits, e.g. smoking
- kinesiology: aims to restore a natural healing balance; muscle testing is used where the strength or weakness of a muscle (corresponding to body systems) indicates areas for treatment, e.g. with massage
- magnet therapy: thought to stimulate natural healing processes and enable more rapid elimination of toxins; used for joint and muscle injury, back pain, migraine
- osteopathy: centrally regulated in the UK; soft tissue massage and manipulative stretching techniques are used for sports injuries, muscle and joint pain

- reflexology: reflex points on the hands or feet are thought to correspond to every part of the body; massage aims to break down crystalline deposits at nerve endings and is used for stress, migraine, asthma, sinusitis, back and general pain
- Reiki: Japanese, with a basis in Buddhist teaching; 'initiates' act as channels for a natural healing energy thought to be drawn to areas of imbalance in others
- shiatsu: popular in Japan, originally from Chinese Buddhists; uses pressure on acupuncture points to promote the flow of 'life energy', prevent illness or allow natural healing; mostly used for stress-related problems, sinusitis, asthma, headaches, muscle and backache.

Working in the UK 17

THE NEW POST

Every hospital is unique and the first few days may be stressful, especially if you are also trying to settle in a new geographical area and make new friends. This section provides some advice, from people who have been through it, on how to make the start of your new job as stress-free and uncomplicated as possible.

Preparation

Shadowing

Most hospitals run 'shadowing' schemes for incoming pre-registration doctors. These may now also include aspects of what was covered previously during the hospital 'induction programme'. If your hospital does not run such a programme, ask if you can visit the ward informally and speak to the team working there. Introduce yourself to the current junior doctors and nursing staff and ask:

- when are the ward rounds and what are you expected to do?
- is there a phlebotomist, what hours do they work and where should requests be left?
- where can you find needles, venous cannulae and blood culture bottles?
- where are forms kept: drug and fluid prescription sheets, consent forms, death certificates and any forms used to refer to other departments?
- how can ECGs, radiographs and emergency procedures, e.g. endoscopy or theatre, be arranged out of hours?
- what are the pharmacy opening hours; when should discharge prescriptions be completed; how can you contact a pharmacist during and out of hours; where is the hospital drug formulary kept; are there any specific drug nomograms or policies?
- what should be put on any ward notice boards or charts that show patient details, e.g. is any system or colour used to code different types of patient, and who is expected to update the details?
- do any of the consultants have any specific 'do's and don'ts', e.g. specific drugs or tests they prefer to be used?
- when you are on-call, who takes the calls from GPs and, if it is you, is there anyone or any place you are expected to notify about incoming admissions?

- when on-call, are you also expected to be looking after your ward?
- where are rotas kept and how do you know which member of senior staff to contact for help during the day and out of hours and how is this done routinely?
- are there any rules around how or when certain staff are contacted out of hours?
- how do you contact or refer to other departments?
- where can you get something to eat (especially out of hours)?
- when and for how long can you take breaks and are you supposed to tell someone when you go for one?
- where is the library and when/where are any departmental teaching, audit and X-ray meetings held?

Professional organizations

Register with a Medical Defence Organization (e.g. MDU, MPS, MDDUS). The BMA can be useful for advice regarding rotas and working regulations.

Outside work

If you are moving into a new area, sort out your accommodation early and do not rely on hospital accommodation, as many hospitals no longer provide this. Register with a local GP and a dentist. Plan your route to work to avoid being late on your first day and check what transport is available for the end of later shifts.

Rota

Check if your rota is available and if you are scheduled to work out of hours in the first few days. If you are planning any leave, contact the rota coordinator ahead and, ideally before you book it, to see whether this is possible (see 'Leave', p. 461).

First day

Turning up

- be on time: remember that you need to park the car, find the ward, get your belongings organized and may even want a cup of coffee before really starting work
- bring a stethoscope, pens, a note-pad, (money to buy) your lunch, qualification documents, GMC certificate and any professionally related health certificates, e.g. hepatitis status
- wear something appropriate and smart avoiding exposed mid-rifts, excessive jewellery, jeans or tops bearing obvious logos; women should also avoid short skirts, low-cut tops and high heels.

Induction

The 'hospital induction programme' can run over the first couple of days. Some hospitals may already have covered much of this during 'shadowing'.

Check that you have passwords for the relevant hospital systems. Check how your pager works and note any guidance given on using the labs (including blood transfusion), radiology and pharmacy departments. Make yourself aware of the fire procedures.

Someone from your department should introduce you to the staff with whom you will be working, departmental policies and procedures and your educational supervisor. You may be expected to attend Occupational Health for a check-up and/or verification of any vaccination certificates.

On the wards

Take the time to introduce yourself to the nursing staff, pharmacists, physiotherapists. Listen to their advice and be courteous. Your reputation in your hospital matters and news of it quickly spreads from ward to ward. Adopting an 'I'm the doctor and I'm in charge' attitude never helps and will only upset experienced staff, regardless of whether you think you are correct (and you will probably, in fact, be wrong). The more you get a reputation for being pleasant, readily contactable, prompt and helpful in your responses, conscientious, sensible and concerned about your patients, the more other staff will go out of their way to help you with the tasks you have to do.

Colleagues

Get to know your colleagues early: you will all be subject to the same pressures and can be of enormous support to each other. Try to find time to have coffee or lunch breaks together and, if possible, organize an early night out so that everyone can get to know each other.

FINANCE

Money coming in

Payslips and expenses

Your net salary will be paid to you after all necessary deductions have been made from your gross salary by your employer, e.g. tax, pension contributions, NI, student loan repayments, charges for accommodation or telephone. It is your responsibility to check that the calculations are correct. It is worth noting:

- at the start of your employment you may be on an emergency tax code and what you are receiving net may need to be adjusted later
- deaneries and trusts often have time limits within which expenses can be claimed and maximum rates for mileage between two specific points or for accommodation as part of meetings; check the policy, make sure you claim what you can, but do not assume everything you claim will be paid
- if you are part-time, the slip will often show what the WTE (whole time equivalent) salary is for your grade and the average hours you are contracted to do on which your pay is calculated
- if you have been paid too much, it will be discovered sooner or later and taken back; it is better to declare what may be a problem early and negotiate a gradual return.

Other forms

- P60: a summary of your taxable income for each year; you need this for your tax returns
- P45: sent when you cease work with one employer, i.e. move health boards.

Income protection

Early in your career, your income is only protected by the NHS for a few weeks. When you have regular fixed outgoings, e.g. mortgage and car payments, it is important to ensure that these will still be paid in the event of temporary illness. Likewise, if you became seriously ill and are unable to work, the life-time income potential you have studied hard to achieve will be lost. Income protection and critical illness policies are available to protect you in such circumstances. Check that they cover the illnesses you might contract while working, pregnancy-related conditions if you are female and whether you will be covered if you are still fit enough to do any type of work.

Money going out

Budgeting

It seems obvious, but only spending what you can afford is important. A medical salary can seem quite large after life as a student. However, before you decide what car, flat, holidays and gadgets you can afford, make sure you have paid off any high-interest debts, e.g. credit cards and overdrafts; made plans to pay soon any medium-interest debts, e.g. bank loans; and allowed for any other debts like student loans, if not already deducted.

Remember that the out-of-hours banding you receive may fall or vanish as you move from post to post. Fix your most crucial outgoings around your 'basic' salary income. Equally, interest rates may rise or you may need to move region and sell your flat incurring legal and estate agent fees. Make contingency plans for sudden demands on your income: try to fix your regular outgoings such that you can also regularly contribute to a savings plan. Ideally, invest in savings that you can access immediately, as well as those intended to be kept for a longer term.

Tax

If you have any additional income, this must be declared, e.g. statutory fees such as cremation certificates. However, you can claim (with receipts) certain expenses that you incur solely because of your work against your tax deductions, i.e. those expenses for which you would not have any other personal use, e.g. stethoscope, professional subscriptions, books. Having to dress smartly does not count! Although not required every year by the treasury, it is advisable to make an annual tax return on account of the variations in your additional income or expenses in any one year and the impact of this on your tax code. Otherwise one year's code will simply be extended to the next year, and you will end up paying too much or too little, requiring adjustment later.

Insurance

Life insurance is worth considering and is important when you have dependants. Equally, when you are in a long-term relationship or have family, it is important to make a will.

Pension

On no account leave the NHS scheme. By all means consider a top-up pension, especially if you are part-time. It is worth starting pensions and indeed all saving schemes early in your career, but only if you have spare income.

Money management

It takes time to check your outgoings against your budgets and income, and experience to know how to invest or choose a policy. Accountants and financial advisors can help with this. Ideally, pick one with experience of medics. Senior colleagues should be able to recommend good local professionals and some can also be found through union or defence organizations.

LEAVE

Annual leave

Junior doctors are entitled to 5 weeks' annual leave (AL) plus days in lieu of bank holidays. AL taken in complete weeks should consist of seven consecutive days. For AL taken in individual days a calculation is required because junior doctors, due to on-calls, work more than the traditional 5-day week. The method endorsed by the British Medical Association (BMA) is as follows:

- entitlement in days = number of weeks entitled to (5) × number of days per week when there is a contractual commitment to be met
- example: an FY1 working a 1 in 10 rota would therefore be entitled to 26 AL days: 5 weeks × 5.2 days/week (calculated as 5 days (Monday–Friday) + 0.2 days at weekend: 2 days/10 people in rota).

Planning annual leave

It is very unusual to be allowed to take more than 2 weeks at a time. In some hospitals, only 1 week at a time is the norm. Time for leave is also often fixed within a particular rota slot. Therefore, before you start your post, it is essential that you contact the team with whom you will be working, if you have holidays planned in advance. They can then assign you to an appropriate slot on the rota, avoiding complicated swaps later on.

Where allocations are more flexible, remember that Trusts need to plan the allowance of AL such that a limited number of doctors are away from duty at any one time and any clinics or theatre lists trainees might do are cut. After informing you of the conditions under which leave is granted, Trusts can refuse a leave request. In addition, requests often need to be made ≥6 weeks in advance. Check the local policy and whether there is a form to be signed by your consultant and submitted.

Untaken annual leave

Do not expect to be able to take your leave just because you have some left at the end of your post. If other trainees are already away, Trusts can refuse to allow you the time off. Time can be carried forward to another post, but only at the discretion of your new employer and no more than four untaken AL days can be carried forward. If, despite adequate planning, you cannot take your leave before the end of your post, you will be paid for it.

Maternity, paternity and parental leave

Maternity leave provision in the NHS is complicated. Details on the new 'NHS scheme' are available from HR departments or the British Medical Association. In general, doctors who have been with the NHS for 12 months' continuous service before the due date of birth can expect:

- to return to their previous job after childbirth if they wish to do so
- a period of paid maternity leave (8 weeks on full pay, 18 weeks on half pay)
- a further period of unpaid leave (26 weeks) assuming they have spent enough time working in the NHS.

Doctors are required to notify their employer no later than 15 weeks before the due date of birth of their intention to take maternity leave and their intention to return to work for at least 3 months after the end of such leave. In the UK, a MATB1 form is needed from the GP or midwife to confirm the due date of birth. Expectant mothers also have a right to paid leave for antenatal care.

Fathers who have worked continuously for their employer for 26 weeks before the 15th week ahead of the due date of birth are entitled to a maximum of two consecutive weeks' paternity leave at statutory paternity rates of pay (note this is not full pay). This can be taken from a chosen date, later than the first day of the week containing the due date of birth, until 56 days after the actual birth.

Either parent, if they have worked for more than 12 months continuously in the NHS, can take up to 13 weeks' unpaid parental leave in respect of children aged <14 years.

Study leave

Study leave (SL), in contrast to AL, is granted at the discretion of your Trust and Postgraduate Deanery. The Clinical Director of your unit will need to be satisfied of the merits of the proposed leave and that clinical commitments can be met in your absence.

- pre-registration: often no formal study leave allowance, but there is an expectation of release from working hours to attend clinical meetings, grand rounds, teaching sessions, etc.
- specialty trainees: maximum of 30 days per year, but usually inclusive of time for formal, e.g. deanery or postgraduate teaching sessions, ALS and tasters; additional time to sit an exam may be allowed.

Sick leave

Notify your HR department or directorate office as soon as you are unable to work because of illness. For leave of >3 days, you also need to submit a statement (self-certificate) about the illness, within 7 days of beginning leave. After 7 days, a certificate from your GP is required. Pay entitlement during sick leave is as follows:

- year 1: after 4 months' service trainees are allowed 1 month sick leave at full pay; 2 months at half pay
- year 2: 2 months at full pay, 2 months at half pay.

Thereafter, pay entitlement increases incrementally in accordance with length of service.

Special leave

Leave for situations such as to make funeral arrangements, attending the funeral of a close relative or armed forces reserve training is at the discretion of the employing authority. Local policies may apply, but reasonable requests for short periods are usually granted and paid.

IMPORTANT PROFESSIONAL BODIES

The General Medical Council

The General Medical Council (GMC) has the responsibility of regulating doctors to ensure patient and public safety and has a statutory role through controlled entry to the medical register. All doctors are required to register with the GMC. Annual fees are required for this.

Passing your final medical examinations allows you provisional registration with the GMC. Provisional registration allows newly qualified doctors to undertake the general clinical training needed for full registration. A doctor who is provisionally registered is entitled to work only in junior house officer posts in hospitals or institutions that are approved for the purpose of pre-registration house officer (PRHO) or Foundation Year 1 (FY1) service.

If you achieve the required level of competence at the end of your first Foundation Year, you will be eligible for full registration with the GMC, needed for unsupervised medical practice in the NHS or private practice in the UK. Some doctors qualifying from outside the UK may be eligible to apply directly for full registration. The requirements which need to be met by Foundation Doctors applying for full registration are laid out in the GMC publication 'The New Doctor 2007'.

Since 1 January 1997, it has been a legal requirement that, in order to take up a consultant post (other than a locum consultant appointment) in a medical or surgical specialty in the NHS, a doctor must be included in the specialist register. You are eligible to apply to join the specialist register if you have completed specialist training. It is not possible to hold specialist registration without also holding full registration.

Since 1 April 2006, all doctors working in general practice in the health service in the UK, other than doctors in training, such as GP Registrars, are required to be on the GP Register.

Regulation of all doctors in the UK is currently under review and a new framework for medical regulation was proposed in the Government White Paper entitled 'Trust, Assurance and Safety – the Regulation of Health Professionals in the 21st Century'. This introduces the concept of re-licensing (for all practising doctors) and re-certification (for those on the specialist and GP registers).

The generic standards required for remaining on the medical register are laid out in the publication 'Good Medical Practice'. The procedures for investigating and taking action against doctors whose performance or behaviour does not meet those standards is currently under review. The GMC has also published other guidance on professional practice under the collective title 'Duties of a Doctor'. These cover areas of practice such as research, management, consent, ethics and confidentiality.

Postgraduate Medical Education Training Board (PMETB)

The PMETB was established as an independent statutory body, responsible for promoting the development of postgraduate medical education and training for all specialties, including general practice, across the UK. The PMETB assumed its statutory powers on 30 September 2005. It took over the responsibilities of the Specialist Training Authority of the Medical Royal Colleges and the Joint Committee on Postgraduate Training for General Practice.

The PMETB is responsible for establishing and raising standards and quality in postgraduate medical education and training. Specific responsibilities include:

- approval of postgraduate medical education and training programmes and courses
- accreditation of postgraduate education, training institutions and trainers
- quality assurance of the postgraduate medical education and training system
- ensuring that assessments and examinations undertaken as part of training are reliable and fair
- issuing certificates to doctors meeting the standards it sets for successful completion of training
- assessing the equivalence of the qualifications, training and experience of doctors seeking a statement of eligibility to apply for entry to the Specialist or General Practice Registers of the General Medical Council.

Therefore, the PMETB is responsible for ensuring the quality of Foundation and Specialty training programmes. Following the 'Tooke' report in 2007, it has been agreed that the PMETB will cease to function independently of the GMC, but will continue to operate as part of the GMC. The GMC will become the final responsible authority for both undergraduate and postgraduate medical education and training.

The medical Royal Colleges and specialty societies

The medical Royal Colleges and specialty societies have an important role in setting standards for medical practice, frequently through specialist examinations. Each represents a body of specialists in their field, who have first-hand knowledge of the issues affecting the practice of their discipline. They bring an important clinical perspective to decisions on specialty training curricula or assessment. In addition, they can best appreciate the continuing professional development (CPD) needs of fully trained specialists. Hence, they are involved in setting CPD standards and in the monitoring of CPD activity undertaken by clinicians.

College accreditation of any one specialty trainee, against the relevant College curriculum standards, is required before PMETB will issue a certificate of completion of specialty training. Equally, College verification that a specialist is undertaking sufficient and appropriate CPD activity is likely to be required for specialist re-certification.

The British Medical Association

The BMA is the union organization of doctors in the UK which provides a political voice for medical opinion. As a union, it is involved in the negotiation of rights in regard to pay and working conditions. Individual advice and representation, in regard to contract and job plan negotiations, is available to members. Although often thought as being particularly relevant to trainees, the BMA also has sections within it for consultants, staff grades and associate specialists.

Medical indemnity insurers

Indemnity is provided by the NHS, but will only cover you for costs in relation to mistakes you make at work. However, the legal perspective on what is best for your employing authority in such circumstances may be different to personal legal advice you could receive on what is best for you. This and individual representation in court, together with indemnity for any medical action you perform away from work, e.g. a car crash, are available through separate indemnity insurers. These include the Medical Protection Society, the Medical Defence Union and (as Scottish legal representation may be best, given the variations of Scottish Law in Scotland) the Medical and Dental Defence Union of Scotland.

Index

Please note that page references relating to non-textual content such as Figures or Tables are in *italic* print